Lecture Notes in Artificial Intelligence 9413

Subseries of Lecture Notes in Computer Science

More information about this series at http://www.springer.com/series/1244

Grigori Sidorov · Sofía N. Galicia-Haro (Eds.)

Advances in Artificial Intelligence and Soft Computing

14th Mexican International Conference
on Artificial Intelligence, MICAI 2015
Cuernavaca, Morelos, Mexico, October 25–31, 2015
Proceedings, Part I

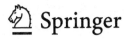 Springer

Editors
Grigori Sidorov
Instituto Politécnico Nacional
Centro de Investigación en Computación
Mexico City
Mexico

Sofía N. Galicia-Haro
Facultad de ciencias
Universidad Autónoma Nacional
México, DF
Mexico

ISSN 0302-9743   ISSN 1611-3349 (electronic)
Lecture Notes in Artificial Intelligence
ISBN 978-3-319-27059-3   ISBN 978-3-319-27060-9 (eBook)
DOI 10.1007/978-3-319-27060-9

Library of Congress Control Number: 2015955365

LNCS Sublibrary: SL7 – Artificial Intelligence

Springer Cham Heidelberg New York Dordrecht London

Printed on acid-free paper

Springer International Publishing AG Switzerland is part of Springer Science+Business Media
(www.springer.com)

Preface

The Mexican International Conference on Artificial Intelligence (MICAI) is a yearly international conference series organized by the Mexican Society of Artificial Intelligence (SMIA) since 2000. MICAI is a major international artificial intelligence forum and the main event in the academic life of the country's growing artificial intelligence community.

MICAI conferences publish high-quality papers in all areas of artificial intelligence and its applications. The proceedings of the previous MICAI events have been published by Springer in its *Lecture Notes in Artificial Intelligence* series, vol. 1793, 2313, 2972, 3789, 4293, 4827, 5317, 5845, 6437, 6438, 7094, 7095, 7629, 7630, 8265, 8266, 8856, and 8857. Since its foundation in 2000, the conference has been growing in popularity and improving in quality.

The proceedings of MICAI 2015 are published in two volumes. The first volume, *Advances in Artificial Intelligence and Soft Computing*, contains 46 papers structured into eight sections:

- Invited Paper
- Natural Language Processing
- Logic and Multi-agent Systems
- Bioinspired Algorithms
- Neural Networks
- Evolutionary Algorithms
- Fuzzy Logic
- Machine Learning and Data Mining

The second volume, *Advances in Artificial Intelligence and Its Applications*, contains 46 papers structured into eight sections:

- Invited Papers
- Natural Language Processing Applications
- Educational Applications
- Biomedical Applications
- Image Processing and Computer Vision
- Search and Optimization
- Forecasting
- Intelligent Applications

This two-volume set will be of interest for researchers in all areas of artificial intelligence, students specializing in related topics, and the general public interested in recent developments in artificial intelligence.

The conference received for evaluation 297 submissions by 667 authors from 34 countries: Argentina, Australia, Brazil, Canada, Chile, China, Colombia, Cuba, Czech Republic, Ecuador, France, Germany, India, Iran, Israel, Italy, Japan, Kazakhstan,

Table 1. Distribution of papers by topics

Track	Submitted	Accepted	Rate
Applications	73	29	40 %
Pattern Recognition	58	15	26 %
Machine Learning	54	18	33 %
Data Mining	46	21	46 %
Natural Language Processing	41	15	37 %
Computer Vision and Image Processing	38	9	24 %
Genetic Algorithms	35	13	37 %
Expert Systems and Knowledge-Based Systems	30	6	20 %
Knowledge Representation and Management	30	12	40 %
Neural Networks	27	10	37 %
Hybrid Intelligent Systems	21	10	48 %
Planning and Scheduling	20	4	20 %
Fuzzy Logic	18	7	39 %
Robotics	18	5	28 %
Bioinformatics and Medical Applications	17	5	29 %
Multi-agent Systems and Distributed AI	14	2	14 %
Ontologies	13	5	38 %
Sentiment Analysis and Opinion Mining	12	2	17 %
Constraint Programming	10	6	60 %
Knowledge Acquisition	9	3	33 %
Intelligent Tutoring Systems	8	5	62 %
Uncertainty and Probabilistic Reasoning	8	4	50 %
Logic Programming	7	5	71 %
Intelligent Interfaces: Multimedia, Virtual Reality	5	2	40 %
Intelligent Organizations	4	–	–
Automated Theorem Proving	3	2	67 %
Spatial and Temporal Reasoning	3	2	67 %
Case-Based Reasoning	2	1	50 %
Model-Based Reasoning	2	2	100 %
Non-monotonic Reasoning	1	–	–
Philosophical and Methodological Issues of AI	1	–	–
Qualitative Reasoning	1	1	100 %

Mexico, Pakistan, Peru, Poland, Portugal, Romania, Russia, Saudi Arabia, Slovakia, Spain, Switzerland, Taiwan, Tunisia, Turkey, UK, and USA; the distribution of papers by topics is shown in Table 1. Of those submissions, 89 papers were selected for publication in these two volumes after a peer-reviewing process carried out by the international Program Committee. The acceptance rate was 29.9 %.

In addition to regular papers, the volumes contain three invited papers by the keynote speakers Alexander Gelbukh (Mexico), Gennady Osipov (Russia), and Zita Vale (Portugal).

The international Program Committee consisted of 172 experts from 27 countries: Australia, Azerbaijan, Belgium, Brazil, Canada, Colombia, Czech Republic, Denmark, Finland, France, Germany, Greece, India, Israel, Italy, Japan, Mexico, New Zealand, Poland, Russia, Singapore, Spain, Sweden, Switzerland, Turkey, UK, and USA.

MICAI 2014 was honored by the presence of renowned experts who gave excellent keynote lectures:

- Alexander Gelbukh, Instituto Politécnico Nacional, Mexico
- Gennady Osipov, Higher School of Economics, Russia
- Paolo Rosso, Universitat Politècnica de València, Spain
- Ruslan Salakhutdinov, University of Toronto, Canada
- Juan M. Torres Moreno, Université d'Avignon et des Pays de Vaucluse, France
- Zita Vale, Politécnico do Porto, Portugal

The technical program of the conference also featured tutorials presented by Roman Barták (Czech Republic), Ildar Batyrshin (Mexico), Alexander Gelbukh (Mexico), Isai Rojas González (Mexico), Luis Enrique Sucar (Mexico), Zita Vale (Portugal), and Ivan Zelinka (Czech Republic), among others. Four workshops were held jointly with the conference: the 8th Workshop on Hybrid Intelligent Systems, HIS 2015; the 8th Workshop on Intelligent Learning Environments, WILE 2015; the Second International Workshop on Recognizing Textual Entailment and Question Answering, RTE-QA 2015; and the First International Workshop on Intelligent Decision Support Systems (DSS) for Industry Application.

The authors of the following papers received the Best Paper Award based on the paper's overall quality, significance, and originality of the reported results:

First place:	"Detecting Social Spammers in Colombia 2014 Presidential Election," by Jhon Adrián Cerón-Guzmán and Elizabeth León (Colombia)
	Prize from Springer: € 400; prize from SMIA: € 400
Second place:	"Dynamic Systems Identification and Control by Means of Complex-Valued Recurrent Neural Networks," by Ieroham Baruch, Victor Arellano Quintana, and Edmundo Pérez Reynaud (Mexico)
	Prize from Springer: € 300; prize from SMIA: € 300
Third place:	"Inferring Sentiment-Based Priors in Topic Models," by Elena Tutubalina and Sergey Nikolenko (Russia)
	Prize from Springer: € 200; prize from SMIA: € 200

The authors of the following paper selected among all papers of which the first author was a full-time student, excluding the papers listed above, received the Best Student Paper Award:

First place:	"Place Recognition-Based Visual Localization Using LBP Feature and SVM," by Yongliang Qiao, Cindy Cappelle, and Yassine Ruichek (France)
	Prize from Springer: € 100; prize from SMIA: € 100

The awards included significant monetary prizes sponsored by Springer and by the Mexican Society of Artificial Intelligent (SMIA).

We want to thank everyone involved in the organization of this conference. In the first place, the authors of the papers published in this book: it is their research work that gives value to the book and to the work of the organizers. We thank the track chairs for their hard work, the Program Committee members, and the additional reviewers for their great effort spent on reviewing the submissions.

We would like to thank the Polytechnic University of Morelos (Upemor) for hosting the workshops and tutorials of MICAI 2015; in particular, we thank Dr. Mireya Gally Jordá, the rector of the university, and Dr. Yadira Toledo, the academic secretary, for their support and generosity. We also thank the Tecnológico de Monterrey Campus Cuernavaca for the hospitality and for opening its doors to the participants of MICAI 2015; we would especially like to thank Dr. Mónica Larre, the director of professional studies, for her support. We thank the INAH Delegación Morelos, Secretary of Culture of Morelos, and Secretary of Tourism of Morelos, particularly Mr. Manuel Zepeda Mata, Ministry of Promotion of the Arts, and Mr. Sergio Perea Garza, Director for Tourism, for their support in carrying out the cultural activities of MICAI 2015. We also want to thank the staff of the Electrical Research Institute (IIE) and the National Center for Research and Technology Development (CENIDET) for their support in the organization of this conference.

We gratefully acknowledge the sponsorship received from Springer for monetary prizes handed to the authors of the best papers of the conference. This generous sponsorship demonstrates Springer's strong commitment to the development of science and their sincere interest in the highest quality of the conferences published with them.

We are deeply grateful to the conference staff and to all members of the local committee headed by Gustavo Arroyo Figueroa, Yasmín Hernández, and Noé Alejandro Castro Sánchez. We acknowledge support received from the project CONACYT 240844. The entire submission, reviewing, and selection process, as well as preparation of the proceedings, was supported for free by the EasyChair system (www.easychair. org). Finally, yet importantly, we are very grateful to Springer staff for their patience and help in the preparation of this volume.

October 2015

Grigori Sidorov
Sofía N. Galicia-Haro
Obdulia Pichardo Lagunas
Oscar Herrera Alcántara
Gustavo Arroyo Figueroa

Conference Organization

MICAI 2015 was organized by the Mexican Society of Artificial Intelligence (SMIA, Sociedad Mexicana de Inteligencia Artificial) in collaboration with the Instituto de Investigaciones Eléctricas (IIE), the Centro Nacional de Investigación y Desarrollo Tecnológico (CENIDET), the Universidad Politécnica del Estado de Morelos (Upemor), the Tecnológico de Monterrey Campus Cuernavaca, the Centro de Investigación en Computación del Instituto Politécnico Nacional (CIC-IPN), the Unidad Profesional Interdisciplinaria en Ingeniería y Tecnologías Avanzadas del Instituto Politécnico Nacional (UPIITA-IPN), the Universidad Autónoma de México Azcapotzalco (UAM), and the Universidad Nacional Autónoma de México (UNAM).

The MICAI series website is www.MICAI.org. The website of the Mexican Society of Artificial Intelligence, SMIA, is www.SMIA.org.mx. Contact options and additional information can be found on these websites.

Conference Committee

General Chair

Grigori Sidorov	Instituto Politécnico Nacional, Mexico

Program Chairs

Gustavo Arroyo Figueroa	Instituto de Investigaciones Eléctricas, Mexico
Sofía N. Galicia-Haro	Universidad Autónoma Nacional de México, Mexico
Oscar Herrera Alcántara	Universidad Autónoma Metropolitana Azcapotzalco, Mexico
Obdulia Pichardo Lagunas	Instituto Politécnico Nacional, Mexico
Grigori Sidorov	Instituto Politécnico Nacional, Mexico

Workshop Chairs

Obdulia Pichardo Lagunas	Instituto Politécnico Nacional, Mexico
Noé Alejandro Castro Sánchez	Centro Nacional de Investigación y Desarrollo Tecnológico, Mexico

Tutorials Chair

Félix Castro Espinoza	Universidad Autónoma del Estado de Hidalgo, Mexico

Doctoral Consortium Chairs

Miguel Gonzalez Mendoza	Tecnológico de Monterrey CEM, Mexico
Antonio Marín Hernandez	Universidad Veracruzana, Mexico

Keynote Talks Chair

Sabino Miranda Jiménez	INFOTEC, Mexico

Publication Chair

Miguel Gonzalez Mendoza   Tecnológico de Monterrey CEM, Mexico

Financial Chair

Ildar Batyrshin   Instituto Politécnico Nacional, Mexico

Grant Chairs

Grigori Sidorov   Instituto Politécnico Nacional, Mexico
Miguel Gonzalez Mendoza   Tecnológico de Monterrey CEM, Mexico

Organizing Committee Chairs

Gustavo Arroyo Figueroa   Instituto de Investigaciones Eléctricas, Mexico
Yasmín Hernández   Instituto de Investigaciones Eléctricas, Mexico
Noé Alejandro Castro   CENIDET, Mexico
  Sánchez

Area Chairs

Natural Language Processing

Grigori Sidorov   Instituto Politécnico Nacional, Mexico

Machine Learning and Pattern Recognition

Alexander Gelbukh   Instituto Politécnico Nacional, Mexico

Data Mining

Miguel Gonzalez-Mendoza   Tecnológico de Monterrey CEM, Mexico
Félix Castro Espinoza   Universidad Autónoma del Estado de Hidalgo, Mexico

Intelligent Tutoring Systems

Alexander Gelbukh   Instituto Politécnico Nacional, Mexico

Evolutionary and Nature-Inspired Metaheuristic Algorithms

Oliver Schütze   CINVESTAV, Mexico
Jaime Mora Vargas   Tecnológico de Monterrey CEM, Mexico

Computer Vision and Image Processing

Oscar Herrera Alcántara   Universidad Autónoma Metropolitana Azcapotzalco,
  Mexico

Robotics, Planning and Scheduling

Fernando Martin   Universidad Veracruzana, Mexico
  Montes-Gonzalez

Neural Networks and Hybrid Intelligent Systems

Sergio Ledesma-Orozco   Universidad de Guanajuato, Mexico

Logic, Knowledge-Based Systems, Multi-Agent Systems and Distributed AI

Mauricio Osorio   Jose Raymundo Marcial Romero

Fuzzy Systems and Probabilistic Models in Decision Making

Ildar Batyrshin   Instituto Politécnico Nacional, Mexico

Bioinformatics and Medical Applications

Jesus A. Gonzalez   Instituto Nacional de Astrofísica, Óptica y Electrónica, Mexico
Felipe Orihuela-Espina   Instituto Nacional de Astrofísica, Óptica y Electrónica, Mexico

Program Committee

Juan C. Acosta-Guadarrama   Universidad Autónoma del Estado de México, Mexico
Teresa Alarcón   Universidad de Guadalajara, Mexico
Fernando Aldana   Universidad Veracruzana, Mexico
Jesus Angulo   Ecole des Mines de Paris, France
Marianna Apidianaki   LIMSI-CNRS, France
Alfredo Arias-Montaño   Instituto Politécnico Nacional, Mexico
Jose Arrazola   Universidad Autónoma de Puebla, Mexico
Gustavo Arroyo   Instituto de Investigaciones Eléctricas, Mexico
Victor Ayala-Ramirez   Universidad de Guanajuato, Mexico
Alexandra Balahur   European Commission Joint Research Centre, Italy
Sivaji Bandyopadhyay   Jadavpur University, India
Maria Lucia Barrón-Estrada   Instituto Tecnológico de Culiacán, Mexico
Rafael Batres Prieto   Tecnológico de Monterrey, Mexico
Ildar Batyrshin   Instituto Politécnico Nacional, Mexico
Albert Bifet   University of Waikato, New Zealand
Igor Bolshakov   Russian State University for the Humanities, Russia
Ramon F. Brena   Tecnológico de Monterrey, Mexico
Eduardo Cabal-Yepez   Universidad de Guanajuato, Mexico
Hiram Calvo   Instituto Politécnico Nacional, Mexico
Nicoletta Calzolari   Istituto di Linguistica Computazionale – CNR, Italy
Erik Cambria   Nanyang Technological University, Singapore
César Cárdenas   Tecnológico de Monterrey, Mexico
Michael Carl   Copenhagen Business School, Denmark
Heydy Castillejos   Universidad Autónoma del Estado de Hidalgo, Mexico
Oscar Castillo   Instituto Tecnológico de Tijuana, Mexico
Felix Castro Espinoza   Universidad Autónoma del Estado de Hidalgo, Mexico

Noé Alejandro
  Castro-Sánchez
Centro Nacional de Investigación y Desarrollo
  Tecnológico, Mexico

Hector Ceballos   Tecnólogico de Monterrey, Mexico
Gustavo Cerda-Villafana   Universidad de Guanajuato, Mexico
Niladri Chatterjee   Indian Institute of Technology Delhi, India
Stefania Costantini   Università degli Studi dell'Aquila, Italy
Heriberto Cuayahuitl   Heriot-Watt University, UK
Erik Cuevas   Universidad de Guadalajara, Mexico
Oscar Dalmau   Centro de Investigación en Matemáticas, Mexico
Guillermo De Ita   Universidad Autónoma de Puebla, Mexico
Maria De Marsico   University of Rome La Sapienza, Italy
Asif Ekbal   Indian Institute of Technology Patna, India
Hugo Jair Escalante   Instituto Nacional de Astrofísica, Óptica y Electrónica,
                                    Mexico

Ponciano Jorge
  Escamilla-Ambrosio
Instituto Nacional de Astrofísica, Óptica y Electrónica,
  Mexico

Vlad Estivill-Castro   Griffith University, Australia
Gibran Etcheverry   Universidad de Sonora, Mexico
Denis Filatov   Instituto Politécnico Nacional, Mexico
Juan J. Flores   Universidad Michoacana de San Nicolás de Hidalgo,
                                    Mexico

Andrea Formisano   Università di Perugia, Italy
Anilu Franco-Arcega   Instituto Nacional de Astrofísica, Óptica y Electrónica,
                                    Mexico

Claude Frasson   University of Montreal, Canada
Alfredo Gabaldon   Carnegie Mellon University, USA
Sofia N. Galicia-Haro   Universidad Nacional Autónoma de México, Mexico
Ana Gabriela
  Gallardo-Hernández
Universidad Nacional Autónoma de México, Mexico

Carlos Garcia-Capulin   Instituto Tecnológico Superior de Irapuato, Mexico
Ma. de Guadalupe
  Garcia-Hernandez
Universidad de Guanajuato, Mexico

Raúl Garduño Ramírez   Instituto de Investigaciones Electricas
Alexander Gelbukh   Instituto Politécnico Nacional, Mexico
Onofrio Gigliotta   University of Naples Federico II, Italy
Eduardo Gomez-Ramirez   Universidad La Salle, Mexico
Arturo Gonzalez   Universidad de Guanajuato, Mexico
Miguel Gonzalez-Mendoza   Tecnológico de Monterrey CEM, Mexico
Felix F. Gonzalez-Navarro   Universidad Autónoma de Baja California, Mexico
Efren Gorrostieta   Universidad Autónoma de Querétaro, Mexico
Carlos Arturo
  Gracios-Marin
CERN, Switzerland

Joaquin Gutierrez   Centro de Investigaciones Biológicas del Noroeste
                                    S.C., Mexico

Yasunari Harada   Waseda University, Japan
Rogelio Hasimoto   Centro de Investigación en Matemáticas, Mexico

Antonio Hernandez	Instituto Politécnico Nacional, Mexico
José Alberto Hernández Aguilar	Universidad Autónoma de Estado de Morelos, Mexico
Yasmín Hernández Pérez	Instituto de Investigaciones Eléctricas, Mexico
Oscar Herrera	Universidad Autónoma Metropolitana Azcapotzalco, Mexico
Dieter Hutter	DFKI GmbH, Germany
Pablo H. Ibarguengoytia	Instituto de Investigaciones Eléctricas, Mexico
Oscar G. Ibarra-Manzano	Universidad de Guanajuato, Mexico
Diana Inkpen	University of Ottawa, Canada
Héctor Jiménez Salazar	Universidad Autónoma Metropolitana, Mexico
Laetitia Jourdan	Inria/LIFL/CNRS, France
Pinar Karagoz	Middle East Technical University, Turkey
Ryszard Klempous	Wroclaw University of Technology, Poland
Olga Kolesnikova	Instituto Politécnico Nacional, Mexico
Konstantinos Koutroumbas	National Observatory of Athens, Greece
Vladik Kreinovich	University of Texas at El Paso, USA
Angel Kuri-Morales	Instituto Tecnológico Autónomo de México, Mexico
Mathieu Lafourcade	Le Laboratoire d'Informatique, de Robotique et de Microélectronique de Montpellier (UM2/CNRS), France
Ricardo Landa	CINVESTAV Tamaulipas, Mexico
Dario Landa-Silva	University of Nottingham, UK
Bruno Lara	Universidad Autónoma del Estado de Morelos, Mexico
Monica Larre Bolaños Cacho	Tecnológico de Monterrey Campus Cuernavaca, Mexico
Yulia Ledeneva	Universidad Autónoma del Estado de México, Mexico
Yoel Ledo Mezquita	Universidad de las Américas, Mexico
Eugene Levner	Ashkelon Academic College, Israel
Rocio Lizarraga-Morales	Universidad de Guanajuato, Mexico
Aurelio Lopez	Instituto Nacional de Astrofísica, Óptica y Electrónica, Mexico
Virgilio Lopez-Morales	Universidad Autónoma del Estado de Hidalgo, Mexico
Omar López-Ortega	Universidad Autónoma del Estado de Hidalgo, Mexico
Tanja Magoc	University of Texas at El Paso, USA
J. Raymundo Marcial-Romero	Universidad Autónoma del Estado de México, Mexico
Luis Martí	Pontifícia Universidade Católica do Rio de Janeiro, Brazil
Lourdes Martínez	Tecnológico de Monterrey CEM, Mexico
Francisco Martínez-Álvarez	Universidad Pablo de Olavide, Spain
R. Carolina Medina-Ramirez	Universidad Autónoma Metropolitana Iztapalapa, Mexico
Patricia Melin	Instituto Tecnológico de Tijuana, Mexico
Ivan Vladimir Meza Ruiz	Universidad Nacional Autónoma de México, Mexico
Efrén Mezura-Montes	Universidad Veracruzana, Mexico

Mikhail Mikhailov	University of Tampere, Finland
Sabino Miranda	INFOTEC, Mexico
Raul Monroy	Tecnológico de Monterrey CEM, Mexico
Manuel Montes-y-Gómez	Instituto Nacional de Astrofísica, Óptica y Electrónica, Mexico
Carlos Montoro	Universidad de Guanajuato, Mexico
Jaime Mora-Vargas	Tecnológico de Monterrey CEM, Mexico
Eduardo Morales	Instituto Nacional de Astrofísica, Óptica y Electrónica, Mexico
Guillermo Morales-Luna	CINVESTAV, Mexico
Masaki Murata	Tottori University, Japan
Michele Nappi	Italy
Jesús Emeterio Navarro-Barrientos	Society for the Promotion of Applied Computer Science (GFaI e.V.), Germany
Juan Carlos Nieves	Umeå University, Sweden
Roger Nkambou	Université du Québec À Montréal, Canada
Leszek Nowak	Jagiellonian University, Poland
C. Alberto Ochoa-Zezatti	Universidad Autónoma de Ciudad Juárez, Mexico
Ivan Olmos	Benemérita Universidad Autónoma de Puebla, Mexico
Ekaterina Ovchinnikova	KIT, Karlsruhe and University of Heidelberg, Germany
Partha Pakray	National Institute of Technology Mizoram, India
Ivandre Paraboni	University of Sao Paulo, Brazil
Mario Pavone	University of Catania, Italy
Ted Pedersen	University of Minnesota Duluth, USA
Héctor Pérez-Urbina	Google, USA
Obdulia Pichardo	Instituto Politécnico Nacional, Mexico
David Pinto	Benemérita Universidad Autónoma de Puebla, Mexico
Volodymyr Ponomaryov	Instituto Politécnico Nacional, Mexico
Marta R. Costa-Jussà	Universitat Politècnica de Catalunya, Spain
Risto Fermin Rangel Kuoppa	Universidad Autónoma Metropolitana Azcapotzalco, Mexico
Ivan Salvador Razo-Zapata	Université libre de Bruxelles, Belgium
Orion Reyes	University of Alberta Edmonton AB, Canada
Alberto Reyes Ballesteros	Instituto de Investigaciones Eléctricas, Mexico
Erik Rodner	Friedrich Schiller University of Jena, Germany
Arles Rodriguez	Universidad Nacional de Colombia, Colombia
Alejandro Rosales	Instituto Nacional de Astrofísica, Óptica y Electrónica, Mexico
Paolo Rosso	Universitat Politècnica de València, Spain
Horacio Rostro Gonzalez	Universidad de Guanajuato, Mexico
Jose Ruiz-Pinales	Universidad de Guanajuato, Mexico
Chaman Sabharwal	Missouri University of Science and Technology, USA
Luciano Sanchez	Universidad de Oviedo, Spain
Edgar Sánchez	CINVESTAV Unidad Guadalajara, Mexico
Abraham Sánchez López	Benemérita Universidad Autónoma de Puebla, Mexico
Marino Sánchez Parra	Instituto de Investigaciones Eléctricas, Mexico

Guillermo Sanchez-Diaz	Universidad Autónoma de San Luis Potosí, Mexico
Antonio-José Sánchez-Salmerón	Universitat Politècnica de València, Spain
Jose Santos	University of A Coruña, Spain
Oliver Schuetze	CINVESTAV, Mexico
Friedhelm Schwenker	Ulm University, Germany
Shahnaz Shahbazova	Azerbaijan Technical University, Azerbaijan
Oleksiy Shulika	Universidad de Guanajuato, Mexico
Patrick Siarry	Université de Paris 12, France
Grigori Sidorov	Instituto Politécnico Nacional, Mexico
Bogdan Smolka	Silesian University of Technology, Poland
Jorge Solis	Waseda University, Japan
Thamar Solorio	University of Houston, USA
Juan Humberto Sossa Azuela	Instituto Politécnico Nacional, Mexico
Efstathios Stamatatos	University of the Aegean, Greece
Josef Steinberger	University of West Bohemia, Czech Republic
Johan Suykens	Katholieke Universiteit Leuven, Belgium
Hugo Terashima	Tecnológico de Monterrey, Mexico
Leonardo Trujillo	Instituto Tecnológico de Tijuana, Mexico
Alexander Tulupyev	St. Petersburg Institute for Informatics and Automation of Russian Academy of Sciences, Russia
Fevrier Valdez	Instituto Tecnológico de Tijuana, Mexico
Edgar Vallejo	Tecnológico de Monterrey CEM, Mexico
Manuel Vilares Ferro	University of Vigo, Spain
Aline Villavicencio	Universidade Federal do Rio Grande do Sul, Brazil
Francisco Viveros Jiménez	Instituto Politécnico Nacional, Mexico
Panagiotis Vlamos	Ionian University, Greece
Piotr W. Fuglewicz	TiP Sp. z o. o., Poland
Nicolas Younan	Mississippi State University, USA
Carlos Mario Zapata Jaramillo	Universidad Nacional de Colombia, Colombia
Ramon Zatarain	Instituto Tecnológico de Culiacán, Mexico
Alisa Zhila	Independent Researcher, Russia
Reyer Zwiggelaar	Aberystwyth University, UK

Additional Reviewers

Akiko Aizawa	Brenda L. Flores-Rios
Haneen Algethami	Mercedes García Martínez
Miguel Ángel Álvarez Carmona	Marcos Angel González-Olvera
Leticia Cagnina	Braja Gopal Patra
Francisco De Asís López-Fuentes	Esteban Guerrero
Miguel Angel De La Torre Gomora	Oznur Kirmemis
Oscar H. Estrada	Pramod Kumar Sahoo

Wasakorn Laesanklang
Rodrigo Lankaites Pinheiro
Luis M. Ledesma-Carrillo
Misael Lopez Ramirez
Pascual Martínez-Gómez
Miguel Angel Medina Pérez
Gabriela Ramírez-De-La-Rosa

Claudia A. Rivera
Jorge Rodas
Salvador Ruiz-Correa
Karan Singla
Yasushi Tsubota
Pavel Vorobiev

Organizing Committee

Local Chairs

Gustavo Arroyo Figueroa	Instituto de Investigaciones Eléctricas, Mexico
Yasmín Hernández	Instituto de Investigaciones Eléctricas, Mexico
Noé Alejandro Castro Sánchez	CENIDET, Mexico

Finance Chair

Gustavo Arroyo Figueroa	Instituto de Investigaciones Eléctricas, Mexico

Sponsorships Chair

Yasmín Hernández	Instituto de Investigaciones Eléctricas, Mexico

Logistics Chair

Yasmín Hernández	Instituto de Investigaciones Eléctricas, Mexico

Registration Chair

Yasmín Hernández	Instituto de Investigaciones Eléctricas, Mexico

Design and Print Chair

Luis Arturo Domínguez Brito	Instituto de Investigaciones Eléctricas, Mexico

Promotion Chair

Noé Alejandro Castro Sánchez	CENIDET, Mexico

Website

Sara Edith Pinzon Pineda	Instituto de Investigaciones Eléctricas, Mexico

Members

Yadira Toledo Navarro	Universidad Politécnica del Estado de Morelos, Mexico
Mónica Larre Bolaños Cacho	Tecnológico de Monterrey Campus Cuernavaca, Mexico
Jose Alberto Hernández Aguilar	Universidad Autónoma del Estado de Morelos, Mexico

Contents – Part I

Logic and Multi-agent Systems

Bioinspired Algorithms

Neural Networks

Best Paper Award, Third Place

Evolutionary Algorithms

Fuzzy Logic

Machine Learning and Data Mining

Contents – Part II

Educational Applications

Biomedical Applications

Image Processing and Computer Vision

Best Student Paper Award

Search and Optimization

Forecasting

Intelligent Applications

Invited Paper

Signs-Based vs. Symbolic Models

Gennady S. Osipov[✉]

Federal Research Center "Computer Science and Control" of the Russian
Academy of Sciences, pr. 60-letiya Octyabrya, 9, Moscow, Russia
gos@isa.ru

Abstract. In this paper a sign-based or semiotic formalism is considered. The
concept of sign arose in the framework of semiotics. Neurophysiological and
psychological researches indicate sign-based structures, which are the basic
elements of the world model of a human subject. These elements are formed
during his/her activity and communication. In this formalism it was possible to
formulate and solve the problem of goal-setting, i.e. generating the goal of
behavior.

Keywords: Sign · Image · Significance · Meaning · Relationship on the set of
signs · The synthesis of behavior

1 Introduction

In the area of artificial intelligence there are problems which are difficult to solve in a
symbol-based paradigm. Planning of goal-oriented behavior is one of these problems.
Under certain conditions, it belongs to the class of nondeterministic polynomial time
complete problems. The problem definition includes, in particular, setting the goal of
behavior. At the same time, in cognitive research, goal-oriented behavior also means
generating the goal of behavior. However, in artificial intelligence research, the latter
problem is not even set. Presumably, this is due to limitations related to symbol-based
formalism.

Here we consider a fragment of the formalism that may be called a sign-based or a
semiotic one. It is based on the concept of sign that originated in the semiotics [1, 2]
and that is used, in an informal way, in cognitive psychology [3]. The results of a
number of researches in the field of neurophysiology [4, 5] also indicate the possibility
of existence of sign structures in a world model of the subject of activity. Moreover, in
the paper [6] the transition from the neurophysiological level on the psychological one,
i.e. appearing of consciousness is connected with formation of signs. In [7] neurophysiological mechanisms of some cognitive functions and their relations with formation of a world language model are considered. Paper [8] is devoted to the appearing
of mechanisms of communication on the basis of semiotics approach. In [9] D. Roy
offers a sign model of the world as a basis for an operational component of the robot
manipulator.

In the present paper the concept of sign is defined accurately. Moreover, the family
of relationships and operations on the set of signs are considered. Within the formalism

© Springer International Publishing Switzerland 2015
G. Sidorov and S.N. Galicia-Haro (Eds.): MICAI 2015, Part I, LNAI 9413, pp. 3–11, 2015.
DOI: 10.1007/978-3-319-27060-9_1

it was possible to describe a number of world models and cognitive functions. One of them – the function of goal-setting (generation of a behavior goal) is described in the report as an example.

2 Sign

Let us define a set S that will be referred to as the set of signs. Each element $s \in S$ has the form: $s = <n, p, m, a>$ where $n \in N$, $p \subseteq P$, $m \subseteq M$, $a \subseteq A$. Here N is a set of words of finite length in an alphabet that we will refer to as the set of names; P is a set of closed atomic formulas for first order predicates calculus that we will refer to as a set of properties. M and A are sets of actions each of which, as it is accepted in artificial intelligence research, is represented using a rule. M is referred to as a set of significances and to A as a set of meanings. The overlap of the sets M and A is, generally speaking, non-empty.

Note 1. The terms 'significance' and 'meaning' or, more accurately, 'personal meaning' are taken from psychology. In that sphere they denote the assignment of the item (or phenomenon) to reality and the way of using (applying) the item that is preferred by the actor, respectively [10, 11].

Note 2. It follows from the note 1 that each sign corresponds to an item (phenomenon) in reality. Each item, from the actor's perspective, possesses a name, image, general cultural significance (assignment), and personal meaning (hereafter, the meaning) with regards to the actor.

Let us remember that the rule [12] means an ordered triad of sets: $r = <C, A, D>$ where C is a condition of the rule r, A is a set of the facts added by the rule r, and D is the set of the facts removed by the rule r. Generally, each of those sets is a set of the atomic formulas for first order predicates calculus.

Let us introduce next *linking* operators:

$\Psi_p^m : 2^P \to 2^M$ is the operator of linking images p to significances m: $\Psi_p^m (p^{(i)}) = m^{(i)}$ so that $m^{(i)} = \{r | \mathcal{P}(r) \subseteq \mathcal{P}(p^{(i)})\}$ where $\mathcal{P}(r)$ is a set of different predicate symbols of the condition C or the rule r, $\mathcal{P}(p^{(i)})$ is a set of predicate symbols of image $p^{(i)}$; $p^{(i)} \in 2^P$, $m^{(i)} \in 2^M$, 2^P and 2^M are power sets P and M, respectively.

Second operator: $\Psi_m^a : 2^M \to 2^A$ links significances to meanings:

$\Psi_m^a (m^{(i)}) = a^{(i)}$ so that $a^{(i)} = \{r^* | \mathcal{P}(r) \cap \mathcal{P}(r^*)\} \neq \emptyset$ where $\mathcal{P}(r^*)$ is a set of predicate symbols of the r^*, $m^{(i)} \in 2^M$, $a^{(i)} \in 2^A$, 2^A being power set A.

Third operator $\Psi_a^p : 2^A \to 2^P$ links meaning to images so that $\Psi_a^p (a^{(i)}) = p^{(i+1)}$ where $p^{(i+1)} = \bigcup_j \mathcal{P}(r_j^*)$, $a^{(i)} \in 2^A$, $p^{(i+1)} \in 2^P$, and J is the number of the rule in the set $a^{(i)}$.

Generally, $p^{(i+1)} \neq p^{(i)}$. One can show that for some initial approximation this iterative process converges to some p. We have then $\forall r$ and $\forall r^* \; ||\mathcal{P}(r) \cap \mathcal{P}(r^*)|| \geq 2$. The sufficient condition of convergence is $\mathcal{P}(r) \subseteq \mathcal{P}(r^*)$.

If we introduce an operator $\Psi_m^p = \Psi_a^p \Psi_m^a$, one can see that the pair of operators Ψ_p^m and Ψ_m^p form Galois correspondence. The following proposition holds:

Proposition. The sign is a fixed point of the Galois closure of the operators Ψ_p^m and Ψ_m^p.

3 Relations Over a Set of Signs

3.1 Relations Over a Set of Signs Generated by Their Images

Let $S = \{s_1, s_2, \ldots, s_k\}$ be a set of signs, $p = (\pi_1, \pi_2, \ldots, \pi_g)$ and $q = (\vartheta_1, \vartheta_2, \ldots, \vartheta_h)$ are images of signs s_p and s_q, respectively.

The ordered sets $\tau_p = <i_1, i_2, \ldots, i_g>$ and $\tau_q = <j_1, j_2, \ldots, j_h>$ will be referred to as types of the images of signs s_p and s_q, respectively.

Definition 1. If, for signs s_p and s_q, $\tau_p = \tau_q$ and $\forall i\ \pi_i = \vartheta_i$, $(i \in 1, 2, \ldots, g)$, then $R_1 := R_1 \cup \{(s_p, s_q)\}$.

One can readily see that relation R_1 is the relation of equivalence over the set of images of signs form S. The relations R_2, R_3, and R_4 are the relations of inclusion, similarity, and opposition, respectively.

Definition 2. If, for signs s_p and s_q, $\tau_p \subset \tau_q$ and $\forall i \in \tau_p$, we have $\pi_i = \vartheta_i$, then $R_2 := R_2 \cup \{(s_p, s_q)\}$ is the relation of inclusion.

Definition 3. If, for signs s_p and s_q, $\tau_p \cap \tau_q \neq \varnothing$ and $\forall i \in (\tau_p \cap \tau_q)$, we have $\pi_i = \vartheta_i$, then $R_3 := R_3 \cup \{(s_p, s_q)\}$ is the relation of similarity.

Definition 4. If, for sign s_p and some sign s_q, $\tau_p \cap \tau_q \neq \varnothing$ and $\forall i \in (\tau_p \cap \tau_q)$, we have $\pi_i \neq \vartheta_i$, then $R_4 := R_4 \cup \{(s_p, s_q)\}$ is the relation of opposition.

It is clear that each of the relations defined above is a subset S^2.

The definitions specified above are essentially the procedures for generating new elements of relations over a set of signs. Applied whenever the set of signs is extended by adding a new sign (or the usage of the set of signs begins), the described procedures either create a new relation or enhance some of the relations over symbols with a new element. This means that interaction of images of different signs results in creating an heterogeneous semantic network [13]. It contains four types of relations: equivalence of images, inclusion of images, similarity of images, and opposition of images.

3.2 Relations Over the Set of Signs Generated by Their Significances

Over a set of signs one can define a number of relations generated by their images. Here one of the relations, which in author's opinion is the most important one, is described.

In accordance with the abovementioned, the significance is a set of actions which the actor can perform with the item that is described by using any sign. However, each action corresponds to a set of some roles that are substituted by participants of the action in, approximately, the way described by Fillmore [14]. (This corresponds to the situation in the human language where action is usually represented by using a verb, or a deverbative, or a participle, or gerund that may be characterized using a set of semantic valences).

Therefore, we will associate the significance of each sign with some ordered set that will be referred to as the set of its roles. It is clear that each role may be substituted with a sign. This approach is the basis for creating relations over the set of signs that are generated by the significances of the signs. It would be reasonable to refer to that relation as a script-based one. So, if $I = \{i_1, i_2, \ldots, i_q\}$ is a set of all possible roles, the significance of each sign is a subset of that set. (For simplicity it is assumed that each significance includes one action.). Let now s_p be a sign with the significance $m(s_p) = <i_1, i_2, \ldots, i_k>$ where $i_1, i_2, \ldots, i_k \in I$, and s_q is a sign.

Definition 5. If, for signs s_p and s_q, we have s_q/i_j, (the sign s_q substitutes role i_j), $i_j \in m(s_p)$, then $R_5 := R_5 \cup \{(s_p, s_q)\}$. As it was stated above, it is reasonable to refer this relation as the scenario-based one. It is clear that the relation R_5 enables one to generate complex constructions, i.e. scenarios that are essentially the networks of signs related by the significances and names of those signs.

3.3   Relations Over a Set of Signs Generated by Their Meanings

Over the sets of signs (personal meanings), there is a natural way for generating relations of subsumed and opposition on the basis of their meanings (personal meanings).

It should be reminded that each meaning is associated with a set of actions. As before, here for simplicity we assume that each meaning is associated with one action described by the rule r = <C, A, D>.

Let, as before, $S = \{s_1, s_2, \ldots, s_k\}$ be a set of signs and a1 and a2 be the meanings of signs s_1 and s_2, respectively.

We define the following relations over the set of personal meanings:

1. $\sqsubseteq(a1, a2)$ or $(a1 \sqsubseteq a2)$ (read 'meaning a1 is subsumed by meaning a_2'), if $A(r_1) \subseteq A(r_2)$ or $D(r_1) \subseteq D(r_2)$ where $A(r_1)$, $A(r_2)$, and $D(r_1)$, $D(r_2)$ are sets of the facts added or removed by the rules r_1 and r_2, respectively; then $R_6 := R_6 \cup \{(s_1, s_2)\}$
2. $\perp(a_1, a_2)$ or $a_1 \perp a_2$ (read 'meaning a_1 is opposed to meaning a_2'), if $\forall P(x_1, x_2, \ldots, x_n) \subset \Lambda(r_1) \exists P(x_1, x_2, \ldots, x_n) \in D(r_2)$; then $R_7 := R_7 \cup \{(s_1, s_2)\}$.

4   Operations Over a Set of Signs

Let us consider as an example the operation of *generalization*.

The operation of generalization Θ is defined over the set of pairs of signs that belong to the relation R_3; applying the operation Θ yields a new image that includes all *common* features of the initial images. Namely, if π is a set of images, $p_1, p_2 \in \pi, p_1 = (x_1, x_2, \ldots, x_g)$ and $p_2 = (y_1, y_2, \ldots, y_h)$, then $\Theta : \pi \times \pi \to \pi$ so that for each $p_1, p_2 \in \pi$ such that $(p_1, p_2) \in R_3 \Theta (p_1, p_2) = p_3$, where $p_3 = (z_1, z_2, \ldots, z_l)$ so that for $\forall i \exists j$, k such that $z_i = x_j = y_k$.

The image generated as a result of generalization may be used as a basis for creating a new sign. A description of the corresponding procedure is contained in item 1. One can show that R_3 is a lower semi-lattice with respect to operation Θ.

Operation of closure over significances of $\Pi(s_1, i_j, s_2)$. If s_1 is a sign with a significance $m(s_1)$ and $i_j \in m(s_1)$ is a role of that significance, the operation creates a new sign s_1^* where role i_j is substituted with the sign s_2 (s_2/i_j). In this case, the meanings and significances of the initial signs are combined.

Operation of agglutination $\nabla(s_1, s_2) = s_3$. If s_1, s_2 are signs and a_1 and a_2 are their meanings, the operation of agglutination creates a new sign s_3 with meaning a_3 where $A(r_3) = A(r_1) \cup A(r_2)$ or $D(r_3) = D(r_1) \cup D(r_2)$. It is clear that in both cases $C(r_3) = C(r_1) \cap (r_2)$ where $C(r_3)$ are the set of conditions of the rules r_3, r_1, and r_2 and A and D are the sets of the facts that are added and removed by the rules r_1 and r_2, respectively.

5 Applications to Cognitive Psychology and Synthesis of Behavior

5.1 Actor's Model of the World

It was shown above that, over the set of signs, three main types of the structure are formed so that they are generated by the families of relations on images, significances, and meanings. In accordance with [13], it is reasonable to refer to each of them as an heterogeneous semantic network.

Therefore, we have a semantic network H_P over a set of images, semantic network H_A over a set of personal meanings, and semantic network H_M over a set of the significances of the signs.

We will refer to the triad of objects $H = <H_P, H_A, H_M>$ as a *semiotic* network.

As it follows from the above, the transitions between the networks H_P, H_A, H_M are implemented using the procedures Ψ_m^a, Ψ_a^p, and Ψ_p^m described earlier.

The level of the names of signs may inherit any of the semiotic networks described above. Owing to such inheritance, one can speak about creation of a semantic network on the level of signs (and not on the level of their components alone).

Note that in psychology, there is a concept of the *Model of the World* of the actor. Three types of the Model of the Worlds may be distinguished: the rational one, the common life, and the mythological one [15].

We have seen that, over the network H_P, one can define the operations of generalization (and classification) over features. This set of operations characterizes the rational Model of the World. Based on these considerations and a number of psychological experiments (the description of which is beyond the topic of this report), one may assume that this network is over the set of images (and its inheritance of the level of the names of signs) that underlies the rational Model of the World. The importance of the term 'underlies' is to be stressed. All types of the World Models use networks over images, meanings, and scripts. However, there is some 'controlling' network that is used for defining a goal, searching for adequate actions, calling up scripts, and changing personal meanings. For example, in the rational Model of the World, in the network over images, first, a goal is set. Then, on the network over significances, appropriate roles are looked for in a script as a condition for performing actions to attain the goal. Next, the meanings of the objects are taken into account. They may perform motivations or obstacles or means for attaining the goals. Degenerated World Models in which two networks instead of three are used, are known as well.

The characteristic feature of the common-life Model of the World consists in following some stereotypes or scenarios of behavior. Thus, inheritance to the level of the names of signs in the network results in forming a *common-life* Model of the World. It should be noted here that the network of significances is only a leading one: for example, the bureaucrats' Model of the World is based on two networks, scripts and personal meanings. Therefore, if a new object matter of need appears (for example, allocation of resources for science and culture), a script is found in which the meaning of the goal transforms from an ambivalent one into the meaning of obstacle. Since this process does not involve images, the corresponding Model of the World may be considered as a degenerate one. Generally, in the common-life Model of the World, the selected script (on the network of significances) is extended using the images of those objects (also including partners). In the best possible way (in accordance with the assessment on the network of meanings), they may perform the roles prescribed by the script. For example, the head of a project selects performers for a new team to ensure 'good' execution of the new type of work or a groom and bride choose guests to the wedding ceremony in accordance with their understanding of what is a 'good' wedding.

In the mythological Model of the World, each role has an invariable meaning and an image associated to it, i.e. in this case the network over meanings is the leading one. In other words, inheritance of the network H_A to the level of names of signs results in forming a *mythological* Model of the World.

It should be added here that it is the actors' Models of the World are the environments in which different cognitive functions are implemented such as introspection, reflection, and goal setting. We describe below one of the most important functions, the goal setting function as an example.

5.2   The Problem of Goal Setting

We apply the formalism developed above to the problem of goal setting – defining a new goal for behavior.

Goal setting is a complicated process that also involves, in addition to finding a goal, determination of the conditions and specific way for attaining that goal. As it was told above, the character of the goal setting process is determined by the type of the actors' Model of the World. In case of a common-life Model of the World, the leading component is *significance*, i.e. the actor bases on the structure of subject matter and roles and uses already existing signs to select a suitable situation that will be the goal-setting one.

To denote operations of transitions over the networks of significances, images, and personal meanings, we introduce an operator Tr. We denote the left composition of the operator Ψ_x^y where $x, y \in \{m, a, p\}$ with the operator of transition over the network as

$\underline{\Psi}^y_x$: $\underline{\Psi}^y_x = \Psi^y_x \circ Tr(x)$ where $Tr(x) = x'$, $x \in A$, $x \in P$ or $x \in M$ and $x' \in A$, $x' \in P$ or $x' \in M$. The right composition of operator Ψ^y_x where $x \in \{m, a, p\}$, $y \in \{m, a, p\}$ with the operator of transition over network y is denoted as $\bar{\Psi}^y_x$: $\bar{\Psi}^y_x = Tr(y) \circ \Psi^y_x$ where Tr $(y) = y'$, $y \in A$, $y \in P$ or $y \in M$ and $y' \in A$, $y' \in P$ or $y' \in M$. For example, the left composition of operator Ψ^m_p with the operator of transition over the network of images may be presented as $\underline{\Psi}^m_p = \Psi^m_p \circ Tr(p)$.

The process of goal setting is performed as part of an activity when the motive of the activity is recognized; i.e. the sign of the object matter of need is included in the actor's Model of the World. Then the significance (m) of this sign (in the common-life Model of the World) is the motive of the activity. The motive is satisfied if there exists a sign such that the application of the right composition of operator Ψ^p_a with the transition operator ($Tr(p) \circ \Psi^p_a$) to the personal meaning of that sign yields the image of the sign of the object matter of need.

The sign will be referred to as the goal sign when the application to it of the right composition of operator Ψ^p_a with the transition operator yields the image of the sign of the object matter of need. Thus, the goal setting process consists of building a sequence that ends with the sign from which motive may be attained, i.e. the need is satisfied.

In accordance with the aforementioned, the significance of the sign will be represented as a set of pairs 'action – role of the item in that action' and image (p) of that sign as a set of features, i.e. pairs 'attribute – attribute significance'. Personal meaning (a) will be represented as a rule that corresponds to the action of the actor with the item; the condition and effects of the action of the rule are specified as a set of properties.

Next, denote s^* a sign if the significance m^* is motive.

In the algorithm described below, we use both synthetic and semantic considerations without emphasizing this circumstance.

Step 1: transition $m^* \rightarrow a_1$ (operator $\underline{\Psi}^a_m$ is applied). Significance m_1 is searched for over a subset of significances (in the script with generating sign s^*) such that its sign s_1 possesses personal meaning a_1 such that the action in the set of added parameters p_{add} that it interprets contains the set of attributes p^* of sign s^*:

$$\underline{\Psi}^a_m : m^* \rightarrow a_1 \text{ where } a_1 \text{ is such that } p^* \subseteq p_{add}(a_1).$$

If the sign s_1 does not coincide with the sign s^*, the identified goal sign with its personal meaning is a goal and the algorithm ends its operation otherwise we go to step 2.

Step 2: transition $a_1 \rightarrow \bar{p}_2$ (operator $\bar{\Psi}^p_a$ is applied). The set of attributes p_2 of sign s_2 is searched for on the subset of images which has the maximum power. It is a subset of the set of attributes of condition p_{cond} of the rule that interprets the personal meaning a_1 of the sign s_1 found at step 1. The combination of the attributes of the image p_2 of the sign s_2 with any attribute (one or more) from the set $p_{cond} \backslash p_2$ will be referred to as the extended image $\bar{p}_2$:

$\bar{\Psi}^p_a : a_1 \rightarrow \bar{p}_2$ where $\bar{p}_2$ is such that $p_2 \subseteq \bar{p}_2$ и $\bar{p}_2 \subseteq p_{cond}$.

Step 3: transition $\bar{p}_2 \rightarrow m_3$ (operator $\bar{\Psi}^m_p$ is applied). Significance m_3 is selected among the significances of the sign s_3 the image of which coincides with the set of attributes $\bar{p}_2 \backslash p_2$ such that:

(1) The script $M_{est}(s_3)$ generated by the sign s_3 coincides with a script generated by the sign s_2 found at step 2 up to signs s_2 and s_3 (without taking them into account);

(2) The personal meaning a_3 that corresponds to the significance m_3 is interpreted by the action such that the set of the attributes of its effect contains the set of the attributes of the image p_3 of the sign s_3 itself.

$\bar{\Psi}_p^m : \bar{p}_2 \rightarrow m_3$ where m_3 is a significance in the set M_{scen} of the scenario $M_{est}(s_3)$ and $\exists M_{est}(s_2)$ such that $M_{est}(s_2) = M_{est}(s_3)$ without consideration for signs s_2 and s_3.

Step 4: transition $m_2 \rightarrow a_2$ (operator Ψ_m^a is applied). The personal meaning a_2 is found that corresponds to the significance m_2 of the sign s_2. The algorithm operation ends.

Running the algorithm yields a sign not identical to the sign of the object matter of need the personal meaning of which is interpreted by the action that results in satisfying the need. Thus, sign s_2 with personal meaning a_2 becomes the goal.

6 Conclusion

In this paper, the basis of a new formalism that correlates with the available neuro-physiological and psychological data on the structure and function of the actor's Model of the World, is considered. The proposed formalism enables describing a number of cognitive functions, such as introspection, reflection, goal setting, and some others, and enhancing the extent of understanding cognitive processes. A description of a cognitive function, the goal setting function, is provided. Further development of the formalism is related to handling multi-agent and robotic systems, in which Models of the World may be generated in automatic (or semiautomatic) way as a result of communication, interaction of visual and audio systems. On this basis it becomes possible to distribute tasks and coordinate goals in cognitive robots coalitions. Implementation of such functions will enable one to boost the extent of autonomy of such systems and their coalitions.

Acknowledgments. This work was supported by the Russian Foundation for Basic Research (project no. 15-07-06214_a).

References

1. Peirce, C.S.: Issues of Pragmaticism. In: The Monist, vol. XV, no. 4, pp. 481–499. The Open Court Publishing Co., Chicago, IL, October 1905
2. Frege, G.: On sense and reference. In: Geach, P.T., Black, M. (eds.) Philosophical Writings of Gottlieb Frege. Blackwell (1892/1952) (Original work published in 1892)
3. Leontyev, A.N.: The Development of Mind. Erythros Press and Media, Kettering (2009)
4. Edelman, G., Mountcastle, V.: The Mindful Brain. Cortical Organization and the Group-Selective Theory of Higher Brain Function. The MIT Press, Cambridge (1978)

5. Desmedt, J., Tomberg, C.: Neurophysiology of preconscious and conscious mechanisms of the human brain. Abstr. Xth Intern. Congr. Electromyography Clin. Neurophysiol. Kyoto, Japan. Electroenceph. Clin. Neurophysiol. **97**(4), S4 (1995)
6. Ivanitsky, A.M.: Information synthesis in key parts of the cerebral cortex as the basis of subjective experience. Neurosci. Behav. Physiol. **27**(4), 414–426 (1997)
7. Friederici, A.D., Singer, W.: Grounding language processing on basic neurophysiological principles. Trends Cogn. Sci. **19**(6), 329–338. http://doi.org/10.1016/j.tics.2015.03.012 (2015)
8. Loula, A., Queiroz, J.: Synthetic semiotics : on modelling and simulating the emergence of sign processes. In: AISB/IACAP World Congress 2012: Computational Philosophy, Part of Alan Turing Year 2012, p. 102129. Birmingham (2012)
9. Roy, D.: Semiotic schemas: a framework for grounding language in action and perception. Artif. Intell. **167**(1–2), 170–205 (2005). http://doi.org/10.1016/j.artint.2005.04.007
10. Nilson, N.J.: Principles of Artificial Intelligence. Tioga Publishing, CA (1980)
11. Osipov, G.S.: Formulation of subject domain models: Part 1. Heterogeneous semantic nets. J. Comput. Syst. Sci. Int. 1–11 (1992) (Scripta Technica Inc., New York)
12. Osipov, G., Panov, A., Chudova, N.: Semiotic foundations of consciousness functions. In: Proceedings of the First Conference of the International Association for Cognitive Semiotics (IACS 2014), p. 211. Lund University, Lund, 25–27 September 2014
13. Osipov, G.S., Panov, A.I., Chudova, N.V.: Behavior control as a function of consciousness. I. World model and goal setting. J. Comput. Syst. Sci. Int. **53**(4), 517–529 (2014)
14. Fillmore, C.J.: The case for case. In: Bach, E., Harms, R. (eds.) Universals in Linguistic Theory, pp. 1–88. Holt, Rinehart, and Winston, New York (1968)
15. Chudova, N.V.: Conceptual description of world view for the task of consciousness-based behavior simulation. J. Artif. Intell. Decis. Making Russ. Acad. Sci., Iskusstvennyi intellect i prinyatie reshenii **2**, 51–62 (2012). (In Russian)

Natural Language Processing

SynFinder: A System for Domain-Based Detection of Synonyms Using WordNet and the Web of Data

Matteo Lombardi and Alessandro Marani[✉]

School of Information and Communication Technology, Griffith University,
170 Kessels Road, Nathan, QLD 4111, Australia
{matteo.lombardi,alessandro.marani}@griffithuni.edu.au

Abstract. The detection of synonyms is a challenge that has attracted many contributions for the possible applications in many areas, including Semantic Web and Information Retrieval. An open challenge is to identify synonyms of a term that are appropriate for a specific domain, not just all the synonyms. Moreover, the execution time is critical when handling big data. Therefore, it is needed an algorithm which can perform accurately and fast in detecting domain-appropriate synonyms on-the-fly. This contribution presents SynFinder which uses WordNet and the web of data. Given a term and a domain in input, WordNet is used for the retrieval of all the synonyms of the term. Then, synonyms which do not appear in web pages related to the domain are eliminated. Our experimentation shows a very good accuracy and computation performance of SynFinder, reporting a mean precision of 0.94 and an average execution time lower than 1 s.

Keywords: Synonyms · Semantic Web · Synonyms extraction · Domain-based synonyms detection

1 Introduction

The extraction of synonyms is a current and popular topic in literature for the many possible applications in different areas of Semantic Web (SW), from query expansion to ontology matching [17,20]. In SW, the identification of lexical relationship of terms is a critical task because different words can have the same or similar meaning.

A first approach for the retrieval of synonyms is the usage of traditional dictionaries such as WordNet [10] and Wiktionary[1] among others. WordNet is a well-established English lexical database that provides meaning and synonyms of a term in different contexts. The structure of WordNet is mainly based on the synonym relationship among words. These synonyms are grouped into sets

---

[1] http://www.wiktionary.org accessed on 27-06-2015.

© Springer International Publishing Switzerland 2015
G. Sidorov and S.N. Galicia-Haro (Eds.): MICAI 2015, Part I, LNAI 9413, pp. 15–28, 2015.
DOI: 10.1007/978-3-319-27060-9_2

called Synsets formed by words that (i) have the same meaning, and (ii) are interchangeable in different contexts. Presently, WordNet contains more than 110,000 Synsets.

Wiktionary is a free-content multilingual dictionary that, similarly to Wikipedia, allows users to modify translations, definitions, synonyms and other information available in it. It currently offers 4,039,912 entries with English definitions from over 1550 languages[2]. However, as reported in the next section, most of the dictionary-based works for the retrieval of synonyms use WordNet.

Another possible source of synonyms is the web. On one side we have Google Translate that may represent a valid tool for synonyms retrieval using data from the web. Unfortunately, at the time of this study, the APIs of Google Translate[3] offers a service for translation purposes only, with no possibility to retrieve synonyms of terms using such service. On the other side, a part of the research community utilizes web pages for the extraction of synonyms via patterns [20,21]. This approach promises the identification of synonyms as they are actually used on the web, but it cannot be used for real-time synonyms extraction, due to the time that is required to parse the web. Another important consideration is that those contributions do not focus on domain-based detection of synonyms.

Therefore, an interesting challenge is the development of a technique that uses both dictionaries and the web for a proper retrieval of synonyms of a term in a short time. In fact, dictionaries can offer the reliability of a correct set of synonyms, and the web can be used to refine the synonyms according to a domain, current trend of usage and other criteria. In particular, the identification of synonyms of a term appropriate for a specific domain is helpful for the construction of domain ontologies, query expansion process, and any other application of Information Retrieval (IR) and SW techniques where it is worth to have a reduced set of synonyms according to a domain.

In this paper it is proposed a new approach for synonyms detection that is (i) focused on a domain, (ii) performed in a short time to be suitable for real-time applications, and (iii) based on reliable sources of lexical relationships. To achieve those criteria, in this study it is addressed an hybrid solution based on IR methods that uses both a dictionary and the web of data. From a dictionary, for example WordNet, a set of synonyms of a term in different contexts is retrieved, with the assurance of correctness of the retrieved set. Then, such set is reduced to only those synonyms that appear in web pages related to the specific domain. This approach aims to produce quickly a set of synonyms that are appropriate for the domain of interest, instead of all the possible synonyms reported by the dictionary. In this way, the proposed approach may be used by any IR or SW system that is domain based, without a significant impact on the performance of the system in terms of execution time.

---

[2] https://en.wiktionary.org/wiki/Wiktionary:Main_Page accessed on 27-06-2015.

[3] https://cloud.google.com/translate/v2/using_rest accessed on 29-06-2015.

2 Background and Related Works

The problem of detection of synonyms, especially domain-based extraction of synonyms, finds multiple applications in IR and SW as discussed along this section. In order to have a more clear picture of such applications, Table 1 reports an overview of some significant studies where techniques for the extraction of synonyms have been proposed or applied. It is particularly reported the purpose for which synonyms have been useful and what source of lexical relationships is used. Most of the analysed contributions detect synonyms from ready-to-use dictionaries and the most popular is WordNet (refer to Table 1). Other studies try to define patterns for conducting the extraction of new synonyms from the web. These solutions are expected to produce more recent sets of synonyms than current dictionaries like WordNet. However, that process requires time and it is not applicable for real-time synonyms detection applications, which is the focus of this paper.

Table 1. An overview of some contributions which use techniques for synonyms detection.

Paper (Year)	Purpose	Lexical relationship source
[6] (2008)	Ontology matching	WordNet
[19] (2010)	Relationships among concepts	WordNet
[5] (2011)	Ontology matching	Wiktionary
[12] (2011)	Domain ontologies creation	WordNet
[13] (2012)	Extraction of key concepts from ontologies	WordNet
[9] (2013)	Creation of a reverse dictionary	WordNet
[15] (2013)	Query expansion	WordNet and Linked Data
[1] (2013)	Sentiment analysis	WordNet
[11] (2013)	Textual entailment recognition	WordNet
[2] (2014)	Most frequent sense of a word	WordNet
[21] (2014)	Synonyms extraction	Corpus-driven
[3] (2014)	Query generation and expansion	Query logs
[16] (2015)	Sentence similarity	WordNet
[7] (2015)	Query expansion	WordNet
[20] (2015)	Query generation and expansion	Query logs
[4] (2015)	Synonyms extraction	Web

The English language, as other languages, has many terms that have the same or similar meaning. For this reason, the refining of the set of synonyms for a domain is a critical task for the improvement of the retrieval phase of IR systems and ontology management in SW.

For example, a user query has to be well expanded in order to effectively retrieve all the items that meet the query. Many techniques have been proposed for query expansion based on users' characteristics, web navigation history and background knowledge among others [3, 7, 8, 18, 20], some of them using synonyms of terms [3, 7, 20]. In fact, once the domain of interest of the user has been deducted, the issue is to identify key terms for the query expansion process, including synonyms. Also the construction process of domain ontologies can benefit of a real-time domain-based synonyms detection [12].

As Table 1 shows, the most current popular techniques for synonyms detection are based on: query logs, web and dictionaries. The query logs of users are mostly used when it is conducted a query expansion or generation. For such task, the query logs allow to have a set of alternative words that have been used by users in the past to formulate queries about a topic. Instead, the web is mainly involved for studies that aim to improve current dictionaries with the most recent usage of terms and their synonyms. Finally, the most widespread source of lexical relationships of words are the dictionaries, especially WordNet. They are mostly used because they offer reliable relationships in a very short time. WordNet also provides APIs which make an integration in IR and SW systems easy. More interesting, such dictionary has been involved in several studies about ontologies, from domain ontologies creation to extraction of key concepts from ontologies [6, 12, 13].

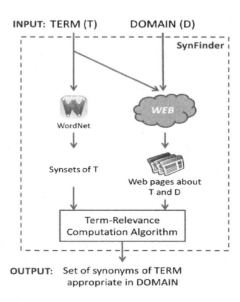

Fig. 1. The structure of SynFinder.

However, to the best of our knowledge, no studies about domain-based detection of synonyms have been proposed. Therefore, in this study it is suggested a novel approach for domain-appropriate synonyms detection which promises a highly reliable synonyms identification in a short time. As current studies use WordNet and other dictionaries to get synonyms quickly but correctly, those criteria have been the guidelines for the design and development of the system proposed in this contribution, called SynFinder. It combines the reliability of WordNet with the web for the computation of synonyms relevance in a domain. The main goal is to perform such task with high accuracy but low execution or computation time. In this way, the research community can benefit of such system for getting domain-appropriate synonyms in a time that is only a bit longer than just using a present dictionary.

3   Structure of the System

This section reports the main characteristics of SynFinder and discusses a specific configuration of its settings for an effective domain-based deduction of relevant synonyms.

Figure 1 shows the structure of SynFinder, where it is possible to identify the most important parts of the system: *Input Data, Dictionary, Web Dataset, Term-Relevance computation algorithm* and *Output Data*. These parts of SynFinder are described in the following paragraphs.

Input data. The data in input to SynFinder are two strings: the term (T), and the domain of interest (D).

Dictionary. SynFinder uses a dictionary to get all the synonyms of T in different contexts. For this phase, SynFinder can use any dictionary that offers APIs, like WordNet does.

Web Dataset. SynFinder queries the web through current search engines. In this regard, search engines are used as access points to the huge amount of data in the Internet. In addition, search engines provide a structure and an order to the information retrieved from the web, allowing to select only the top-N results that are closer to a query instead of millions of web pages, without losing valuable information. Having less data to analyze, the speed of the synonym detection process can be significantly improved. To query the search engine, T and D are concatenated and given in input to the search engine for retrieving a set of web pages about the term T in domain D. Again, any search engine can be used to perform this task, and it is even possible to combine the results from different search engines in order to consider different sources of information, as shown in Fig. 2.

Term-Relevance computation algorithm. The computation of domain-appropriate synonyms is mainly performed by the *Term-Relevance computation algorithm*, designed and implemented during this study. Currently, this algorithm considers only title and snippet of the documents in input, because title and snippet report short descriptive information about the content of web pages that is close to the query. It is expected that title and snippet contain the term T and/or its appropriate synonyms in domain D. Most of the current popular search engines structure the results presenting, among other information, the title of the page, and the snippet composed using parts of the page where some of the keywords in the query, and/or their synonyms, appear. A first analysis of the problem could lead to compute the relevance of a synonym in a set of web pages using the well-known TF-IDF score. Such score is very popular in IR and it is useful to evaluate the relevance of a term in a set of text-based documents [14]. However, for the purpose of this study it is useful to calculate, for each candidate synonym of T, how many documents contain the synonym in the title or the snippet compared to the number of total retrieved documents; in essence, the document frequency of a synonym. Hence, the score used in this algorithm consists only of the Document Frequency df, calculated for each synonym s as follow:

$$df(s) = \frac{\mid PostingsList[s] \mid}{\mid Docs \mid} \qquad (1)$$

where $Docs$ is the set of documents, and $PostingsList$ is a dictionary of terms that records the list of documents where the term appears. Such postings list is built prior to the computation of the document frequency of terms considering only the title and snippet of the web pages in $Docs$. An important characteristic of the document frequency is that $df(s) \in [0,1]$. Using Formula 1 and the documents retrieved from the web, the algorithm computes the domain-relevance of all the synonyms of T coming from the dictionary (WordNet in the case of SynFinder).

Output Data. After the computation of the relevance of each candidate synonym, only the synonyms with relevance higher than 0 are grouped to form the output of SynFinder. As result, the output of SynFinder is a dictionary of domain-relevant synonyms of term T reporting the document frequency of each synonym.

3.1   Parameters of SynFinder

The architecture of SynFinder is formed by different modules, as presented in Fig. 1 and discussed at the beginning of this section. Those modules can work at different settings, so it is possible to choose some parameters for running SynFinder. The most relevant parameters of the proposed system are:

- **Dictionary**: it is a reliable database of lexical relationship of terms. In this study WordNet has been chosen among others due to the established popularity and the offered APIs for a fast retrieval of set of synonyms.
- **Web Dataset**: it is the access point to the web and it has the critical task to retrieve web pages that are related to the term and domain given in input to SynFinder. For this aim, after few tests of SynFinder with different *Web datasets*, we have observed that YAHOO! and Google perform nearly the same, but YAHOO! is surprisingly faster. Hence, YAHOO! has been selected for the implementation of SynFinder using the BOSS Search APIs[4].

---

[4] https://developer.yahoo.com/boss/search/.

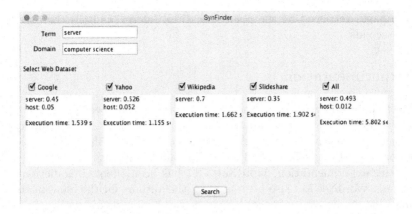

Fig. 2. The *Comparative GUI* of SynFinder.

- **Number of results**: A search engine may retrieve millions of web pages for a query, thus, for a low execution time of SynFinder, only the top 20 web pages are considered. Before to establish such number, the system has been tested with few terms considering the top 10, 20 and 30 web pages of the query results. The top 10 pages are not enough, instead with 20 and 30 top pages SynFinder produces the same set of synonyms, only the document-frequency values are different. Therefore, the configuration with top 20 has been preferred mostly for keeping low the execution time.
- **Features of the results**: Most of current search engines structure the results offering, among other features, title and snippet. These two features are sufficiently good for expressing the content of a web page that is related to a query. So, title and snippet have been selected as the features to be considered by the *Term-Relevance computation algorithm* of SynFinder.
- **Score**: it is used by the *Term-Relevance computation algorithm* to calculate the relevance of the synonyms for the input domain. An appropriate score proposed in this study for this task is the *document frequency* presented earlier in Formula 1.

The configuration of SynFinder presented here is the one used for the experimentation, so more details are reported in Sect. 4.

Every parameter is very important for the execution of SynFinder, but the *Web Dataset* is the most important. Indeed, it determines the quality and significance of the set of web pages that are in input to the *Term-Relevance computation algorithm*. For this reason, SynFinder is presently provided with a *comparative GUI*, showed in Fig. 2, for the comparison of the results that SynFinder produces with different *Web Datasets* (the other parameters are in common).

In particular, the developed GUI offers the possibility to specify the term, domain and web sources. The resulting synonyms are presented in the text areas below the name of the selected search engines. In each text area is also reported (i) the document frequency of the synonyms (in the range *[0,1]*) according to the web pages retrieved by the respective *Web dataset*, and (ii) the execution time in seconds.

4 Experimentation

The performance evaluation of the proposed system has been conducted with an experiment to test the accuracy and computation time of SynFinder. The experiment has been run on an iMac machine with 2.66 Ghz Intel Core 2duo processor, 4 gigabyte of RAM and OS X Yosemite V.10.10.3.

For this experimentation, WordNet V3.1 has been adopted as dictionary of the system. WordNet has also been used by the authors for the identification of possible different domains of a word, looking at the contexts of meaning proposed by such dictionary for a term. Before running the experiment, we have used the *comparative GUI* presented in Sect. 3.1 for the execution of SynFinder with few terms just for selecting the search engine for this experiment. As result, YAHOO! and Google produced nearly the same results but YAHOO! resulted faster, thus YAHOO! has been selected as search engine for the exploration of the web. In addition, the best results were achieved considering the first 20 web pages retrieved by the search engines. Hence, for this experimentation the following system's parameters have been used:

– Search engine: YAHOO!
– Number of web pages analysed: 20
– Score for term relevance: Document Frequency
– Dictionary: WordNet V3.1

4.1 Methodology

The objective of this experimentation is to report the accuracy and computation performance of SynFinder. Both performance evaluations of the system have been conducted with a test set of domain-related synonyms of terms manually defined by the authors themselves. Each element of the test set is a triple made by term, domain and the set of synonyms as retrieved from the dictionary. In addition, each synonym has a flag that says if it is appropriate or not for the domain as decided by the authors. The appropriateness of a synonym has been decided considering the *sense* of the set of synonyms as retrieved from WordNet. For example, the term 'array' has synonyms 'raiment' and 'regalia' for the *sense* 'especially fine or decorative clothing'. Moreover, from a *sense* it is possible to deduct the domain, in that case 'clothing'. Hence, the synonyms 'raiment' and 'regalia' are appropriate for the term 'array' in domain 'clothing'. With such approach, 32 triples have been produced and used as test set for this experimentation, a small sample is reported in Table 2. For the evaluation of the accuracy performance of the system, it has been adopted the cosine similarity, precision and recall which are common accuracy measures of IR systems [14]. For each entry of the test set, such measures have been calculated for comparing the set of

Table 2. A sample of the test set reporting the term, domain and a list of synonyms as retrieved by WordNet with their domain-relevance flag (0 non-relevant, 1 relevant).

Term	Domain	Set of synonyms
server	computer science	server:1;waiter:0;host:1
server	hospitality	server:1;waiter:1;host:0
array	social science	array:1;raiment:0;regalia:0;range:0;lay out:0;set out:0;align:1
array	clothing	array:1;raiment:1;regalia:1;range:0;lay out:0;set out:0;align:0
tumor	medicine	tumor:1;tumour:1;neoplasm:1
term	architecture	term:1;condition:0;full term:0;terminus:1;terminal figure:1
term	law	term:1;condition:1;full term:0;terminus:0;terminal figure:0

relevant synonyms produced by SynFinder against the correct ones as stated in the test set. In this experimentation all the synonyms with document frequency greater than 0 have been assigned the value 1. The reason is that if a synonym occurs even once in a very small piece of information of the web (only title and snippet of 20 web pages), then the synonym is likely appropriate for the domain. The cosine similarity has been used to compute the similarity between the vector of relevant synonyms of the test set and the relevance values produced by the system. In practice, the similarity is calculated between two vectors with only zeros and ones. The formula of the cosine similarity between vector A and B is the following:

$$CosineSimilarity(A, B) = \frac{A \cdot B}{\|A\| \|B\|} = \frac{\sum_{i=1}^{n} A_i * B_i}{\sqrt{\sum_{i=1}^{n} (A_i)^2} * \sqrt{\sum_{i=1}^{n} (B_i)^2}} \qquad (2)$$

Precision and recall are here useful for further insights of the quality of the results produced by SynFinder. Precision shows the actual relevance of the set of synonyms suggested by the system, recall depicts the capability of the system in retrieving all the relevant synonyms, defined as follow:

$$Precision = \frac{\#true\ positives}{\#true\ positives + \#false\ positives} \qquad (3)$$

$$Recall = \frac{\#true\ positives}{\#true\ positives + \#false\ negatives} \qquad (4)$$

Where *true positives* are the synonyms correctly labelled as relevant, *false positives* are those synonyms wrongly labelled as relevant by the system and *false negatives* are relevant synonyms considered non-relevant by SynFinder.

Moreover, for the evaluation of the computation performance, the execution time of each call to the system has been recorded. During the execution of each triple it has been registered the time when the system received the input (T_s) and the time when the output was given back (T_e). The difference between the T_e and T_s is the *completion time* for the detection of domain-appropriate synonyms.

4.2   Results

In this subsection we report the accuracy and computation performance of Syn-Finder recorded during the experimentation. Table 3 shows the minimum, maximum and average values of precision, recall and cosine similarity measures registered during the experimentation. Overall, the system performed well having an average precision of 0.94 and average recall of 0.64. Such high precision means that most of the synonyms retrieved by SynFinder are actually relevant for the domain, and, as expected, a high precision causes a low recall. However, a value of 0.64 for recall says that more than 60 % of relevant synonyms are detected by the system, which is not a low recall at all. In addition, the experimentation was run considering only title and snippet of the first 20 results presented by YAHOO!. So, more results can be considered and the web page can be fully analysed in order to increase the recall, but it may lead to a lower precision as well as an increase of execution time. For the application of the synonyms detection problem in IR and SW areas, we believe that the precision is more important than the recall, otherwise the proposed system does not make any significant difference than using only WordNet. We also highlight that some terms are not so popular on the web, thus a low recall may just reflect a disuse of some synonyms in current English. For example, for the term *word* in the domain *social science* we registered a precision of 1 but a recall of 0.25 because SynFinder has retrieved only the term itself, leaving out three other relevant synonyms. One of these is *give-and-take* retrieved by WordNet V3.1 as a synonym of *word* when people exchange different views on a topic. However, that exact syntactic structure may result not common on the web language. Also *discussion* is a valid synonym left out by SynFinder, but it might be present in the body of a web page returned by the search engine, thus a full analysis of web pages instead of only title and snippet may detect it. Anyway, a recall value lower than 0.5 occurs only for 7 out of 32 records. Therefore, a mean value of recall equal to 0.64 is not a big issue and it is better to keep it as it is than lowering the precision of the system.

Table 3. Minimum, maximum and average value recorded for precision, recall and cosine similarity.

	Minimum	Maximum	Average
Precision	0.6	1.0	0.94
Recall	0.25	1.0	0.64
Cosine Similarity	0.5	1.0	0.75

About precision, the lowest recorded value of precision is 0.6 for the term *instrument* in *law* and the term *tone* in *art*; only for those two cases we recorded that value of precision.

With more details about the accuracy performance of SynFinder, Figs. 3 and 4 show the accuracy performance of the system recorded for each element

Table 4. Percentage of cases where precision, recall and cosine similarity have been recorded equal or greater than the respective average values.

	Precision	Recall	Cosine Similarity
Test cases with measure equal or greater than average	84 %	38 %	38 %

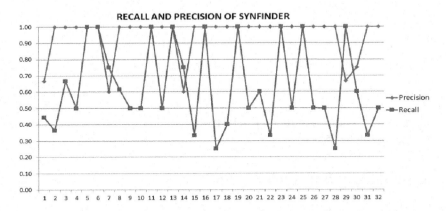

Fig. 3. Accuracy performance of SynFinder in terms of precision and recall.

of the test set. In addition, Table 4 reports another interesting finding about the percentage of entries of the test set for which it has been recorded a value of precision, recall and cosine similarity equal or greater than the respective mean values. Very interesting, for more than 80 % of terms SynFinder detected domain-relevant synonyms with a precision of at least 0.94. From a perspective of computation performance, SynFinder performs well according to the statistics of execution time recorded in this experimentation and reported in Table 5. A very encouraging result is that the longest recorded execution time is less than 2 s, with a very positive average execution time of 0.71 s, very close to the minimum time recorded (0.57 s).

Table 5. Recorded minimum, maximum and average execution time in seconds.

	Minimum	Maximum	Average
Execution time (seconds)	0.57	1.96	0.71

Therefore, at the end of this experimentation we have a very positive analysis of SynFinder performance, showing that it performs very well in terms of both accuracy and execution time, promising a novel valid approach for domain-based detection of synonyms.

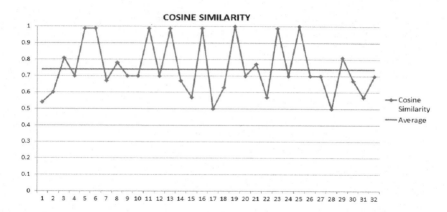

Fig. 4. The cosine similarity between the relevant synonyms as established by Syn-Finder and the actual relevant ones, together with the average value recorded among the 32 cases of the test set.

5   Conclusions and Future Work

At the end of this study, it has been described the SynFinder system and proved its significant effectiveness as a tool for the detection of domain-appropriate synonyms. The combination of a very reliable and popular dictionary, like Word-Net is, with the web has been successful for the proposal of a new and valid approach for the discovery of synonyms of terms suitable for a domain. The experimentation conducted in this study confirms it, with very positive results about both the accuracy and computation performance of SynFinder. Other possible configurations of the system can be evaluated to see whether or not SynFinder significantly benefits of the analysis of entire web pages instead of title and snippet only as proposed in this study. However, the configuration here proposed and analysed performs very well, with a mean precision measure of 0.94 and average execution time lower than 1 s. Therefore, the proposed SynFinder is ready to be integrated or used for systems in SW and IR that would benefit of such a tool.

In this regard, SynFinder should be available online via REST APIs in order to be automatically used by the research community. So, the next step is the deployment of SynFinder as web service for domain-based synonyms retrieval guaranteeing high accuracy of the results and low response time, as reported by the experimentation. Currently, to the best of our knowledge, no other online system offers a domain-based synonyms detection through APIs, neither Google Translate that has APIs for translation purposes only.

In conclusion, SynFinder represents a novel contribution in the field of SW for improving and speeding up the detection of domain-relevant synonyms using WordNet and the web of data.

References

1. Batool, R., Khattak, A.M., Maqbool, J., Lee, S.: Precise tweet classification and sentiment analysis. In: IEEE/ACIS 12th International Conference on Computer and Information Science (ICIS), pp. 461–466. IEEE (2013)
2. Calvo, H., Gelbukh, A.: Finding the most frequent sense of a word by the length of its definition. In: Gelbukh, A., Espinoza, F.C., Galicia-Haro, S.N. (eds.) MICAI 2014, Part I. LNCS, vol. 8856, pp. 1–8. Springer, Heidelberg (2014)
3. Cheng, T., Chakrabarti, K., Chaudhuri, S., Xin, D.: Robust discovery of entity synonyms using query logs, 3 June 2014. US Patent 8,745,019
4. Hu, F., Shao, Z., Ruan, T.: Self-supervised synonym extraction from the web. J. Inf. Sci. Eng. **31**, 1133–1148 (2015)
5. Lin, F., Krizhanovsky, A.: Multilingual ontology matching based on wiktionary data accessible via sparql endpoint (2011). arXiv preprint arXiv:1109.0732
6. Lin, F., Sandkuhl, K.: A survey of exploiting wordnet in ontology matching. In: Bramer, M. (ed.) Artificial Intelligence in Theory and Practice II, pp. 341–350. Springer, US (2008)
7. Lu, M., Sun, X., Wang, S., Lo, D., Duan, Y.: Query expansion via wordnet for effective code search. In: IEEE 22nd International Conference on Software Analysis, Evolution and Reengineering (SANER), pp. 545–549. IEEE (2015)
8. Makvana, K., Shah, P.: A novel approach to personalize web search through user profiling and query reformulation. In: International Conference on Data Mining and Intelligent Computing (ICDMIC), pp. 1–10. IEEE (2014)
9. Méndez, O., Calvo, H., Moreno-Armendáriz, M.A.: A reverse dictionary based on semantic analysis using wordnet. In: Castro, F., Gelbukh, A., González, M. (eds.) MICAI 2013, Part I. LNCS, vol. 8265, pp. 275–285. Springer, Heidelberg (2013)
10. Miller, G.A.: Wordnet: a lexical database for english. Commun. ACM **38**(11), 39–41 (1995)
11. Pakray, P., Neogi, S., Bandyopadhyay, S., Gelbukh, A.: Recognizing textual entailment in non-english text via automatic translation into english. In: Batyrshin, I., Mendoza, M.G. (eds.) MICAI 2012, Part II. LNCS, vol. 7630, pp. 26–35. Springer, Heidelberg (2013)
12. Pariente Juarez, S., Esquivel, H.E., Rebollar, A.M., Suárez-Figueroa, M.C.: CreaDO–A methodology to create domain ontologies using parameter-based ontology merging techniques. In: 10th Mexican International Conference on Artificial Intelligence (MICAI), pp. 23–28. IEEE (2011)
13. Rospocher, M., Tonelli, S., Serafini, L., Pianta, E.: Key-concept extraction for ontology engineering. In: ten Teije, A., Völker, J., Handschuh, S., Stuckenschmidt, H., d'Acquin, M., Nikolov, A., Aussenac-Gilles, N., Hernandez, N. (eds.) EKAW 2012. LNCS, vol. 7603, pp. 413–416. Springer, Heidelberg (2012)
14. Shani, G., Gunawardana, A.: Evaluating recommendation systems. In: Ricci, F., Rokach, L., Shapira, B., Kantor, P.B. (eds.) Recommender Systems Handbook, pp. 257–297. Springer, US (2011)
15. Shekarpour, S., Hoffner, K., Lehmann, J., Auer, S.: Keyword query expansion on linked data using linguistic and semantic features. In: IEEE Seventh International Conference on Semantic Computing (ICSC), pp. 191–197. IEEE (2013)
16. Shin, Y., Ahn, Y., Kim, H., Lee, S.-G.: Exploiting synonymy to measure semantic similarity of sentences. In: Proceedings of the 9th International Conference on Ubiquitous Information Management and Communication, p. 40. ACM (2015)

17. Shvaiko, P., Euzenat, J.: Ontology matching: state of the art and future challenges. IEEE Trans. Knowl. Data Eng. **25**(1), 158–176 (2013)
18. Sieg, A., Mobasher, B., Burke, R.: Web search personalization with ontological user profiles. In: Proceedings of the Sixteenth ACM conference on Information and Knowledge Management, pp. 525–534. ACM (2007)
19. Sorrentino, S., Bergamaschi, S., Gawinecki, M., Po, L.: Schema label normalization for improving schema matching. Data Knowl. Eng. **69**(12), 1254–1273 (2010)
20. Tannebaum, W., Rauber, A.: *PatNet*: a lexical database for the patent domain. In: Hanbury, A., Kazai, G., Rauber, A., Fuhr, N. (eds.) ECIR 2015. LNCS, vol. 9022, pp. 550–555. Springer, Heidelberg (2015)
21. Yıldız, T., Yıldırım, S., Diri, B.: An integrated approach to automatic synonym detection in Turkish corpus. In: Przepiórkowski, A., Ogrodniczuk, M. (eds.) Advances in Natural Language Processing. LNCS, vol. 8686, pp. 116–127. Springer, Switzerland (2014)

Ro-PAAS – A Resource Linked to the UAIC-Ro-Dep-Treebank

Cenel-Augusto Perez[1], Cătălina Mărănduc[1,2(✉)], and Radu Simionescu[1]

[1] Faculty of Computer Science, Al. I. Cuza University, Iaşi, Romania
{augusto.perez, catalina.maranduc, radu.simionescu}@info.uaic.com
[2] Academic Institute of Linguistics
Iorgu Iordan – Al. Rosetti, Bucharest, Romania

Abstract. Ro-PAAS is a resource which contains the Romanian verbs and their specific argument and adjunct structures. This resource is linked to our dependency Treebank; we have extracted these structures to the trees and each structure has a list of examples. In this paper, we intend to describe the resource and the modalities in which it can be used in other projects. First, we intend to extract rules for building a hybrid, rule and statistic based parser to quickly increase the dimensions of our Treebank. In the second step, the syntactic structures are in relation with the meaning of the predicates; the structures can be used in programs which need a sense disambiguation. In the third step, we intend to start a comparative study on syntactic structures in the old Romanian language pointing out its differences from the contemporary Romanian, and building some tools rule based for processing old Romanian Language.

Keywords: Pattern of relations · Hybrid parser · Predicate argument · Predicate adjunct · Syntactic structures · Universal dependencies

1 Introduction

This paper describes a new resource for Romanian, created following the example of other languages. Both the linguists and the computer scientists conclude that predicate structure is an important element of the generation and the organization of natural language sentences.

This set of frames for each (category of) verb is manually written in .xml format and content mandatory, facultative and forbidden dependencies followed by examples extracted from UAIC-RoTb, sentences with morphosyntactic annotation in form of trees. Ro-PAAS is linked to another resource which we will increase, the UAIC Romanian Treebank (UAIC-RoTb). We are extracting predicate structures from it and from the Electronic Thesaurus Dictionary of Romanian [3] and we intend to create models of arguments and adjuncts of the most important verbs. The purpose is to create such structures for the majority of Romanian verbs, to establish a categorization of Romanian verbs and an electronic dictionary of Romanian predicate structures. Finally, all the predicates of UAIC-RoTb were linked with one of the structures in Ro-PAAS;

© Springer International Publishing Switzerland 2015
G. Sidorov and S.N. Galicia-Haro (Eds.): MICAI 2015, Part I, LNAI 9413, pp. 29–46, 2015.
DOI: 10.1007/978-3-319-27060-9_3

programs and frameworks will be created in order to establish these links in an automatic way, and we will supervise these operations.

The idea of this project is born from the need to develop the UAIC-RoTb [14, 18]. This important resource for Romanian had only 3 600 sentences a year ago. Now, we supervise the last hundreds for attending 10 000 sentences, but it is still insufficient for the training of a statistical parser. Our parser, based on a variant of the Malt parser created for Romanian by Hall et al. [6], only reaches an accuracy about 70 % for the head precision and slightly lower for the label precision, because our corpus has an average of 20 words per sentence and complicated syntactic structures; we aim to convey the natural language complexity and the specific of Romanian.

We decided to include both mandatory and optional dependencies in our patterns, because there are verbs with mandatory local, temporal, quantitative modifiers and the difference between "mandatory" and "facultative" cannot be made. The dependencies belonging to the first category are called arguments, while the dependencies belonging to the second category are called adjuncts; for this reason, we named our resource first PAS, and then PAAS, after introducing the adjuncts into the predicate structure of dependencies.

In our NLP group, there were created resources such as Romanian Frame-Net [24] and Romanian Verb-Net [2], by importing and translating English resources. Such enterprise has the advantage of a parallel corpus, easy to align. It is easy to establish correspondences between Romanian and English structures. But translating important structures of English, we obtain peripheral unused structures in Romanian; we cannot restore the complexity of Romanian structures and the specific of our language, which was the purpose of our research, might slip through our fingers. We opted not to translate the PDEV (Pattern Dictionary of English Verbs) model [17], but to introduce structures of Romanian [16] in this format.

2 Extending the Sense of the Term "Predicate"

2.1 Categories of Words Which Can Be Logical Predicates

The natural language is a means of communication between humans. The content of communication can be analyzed as a string of logic judgments. Each judgment is composed of a theme and a predicate. The theme is the grammatical subject, the information known, and the predicate is the information added, the new information communicated. We can assign to this judgment a truth value, 1 for true or 0 for false, and then we can compose the more complicated structures by adding a lot of judgments.

So, the predicate is the element through which we communicate, the center around which the new information is organized and which guides the selection of certain linguistic elements to complete its information. The syntactic parser which we intend to optimize has a tendency to select wrongly these centers of communication, the root and the other judgments coordinated with the root, the syntactic tree top, and, consequently, the structure of the tree is disorganized and cannot be recovered.

The conclusion is that we must integrate in this program a dictionary of the syntactic particularities [25] of Romanian predicates and we must study these particularities in the quotations in as many examples of Romanian as possible. Therefore, the head of the sub-trees is not ever a main verb: it can be an infinitive, gerundive, participle verb or even an adjective, adverb, interjection or a function word (for the dependency systems of annotations which accept these words as heads). We intend to consider all these words as predicates and to study the types of mandatory or facultative dependencies which they accept.

In the example in Fig. 1, there are no relations between the direct object "caprele" *(the goats)* and the local "dreapta" *(to the right)*, so we need a new verbal center and we translate the structure of arguments to the verb "pune" at the conjunction "iară" by means of coordination:

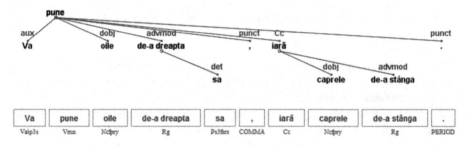

Fig. 1. Example of a conjunction as head for a sub tree. (He will put the sheep to his right and the goats to the left.)

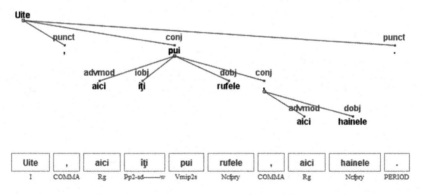

Fig. 2. Example of an interjection as head for a sub tree. (Look, here you put the laundry, the clothes here.)

In Fig. 2, the local optional determiner "here" is in relation with a single direct object in each of his two occurrences, so we must translate by coordination the information of the verb "put" through a comma, in the second case. The comma is the substitute for the repetition of the verb.

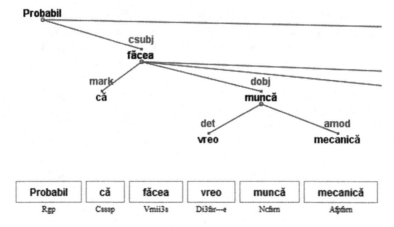

Fig. 3. Example of an adverb as head for a sub tree. (Probably she had some mechanical job.)

In Fig. 3, the adverb "probably" is an abbreviation of the predicate "to be probable" with the copula "to be" and the predicative "probable", and this pattern has a subjective clause as mandatory dependency.

In the last example (Fig. 4), a complicated syntactic structure is subordinated to the participle "cleft", annotated as adjective by some POS-taggers. The participle has passive meaning and it requires a mandatory agent complement, although in some sentences it may be elliptical.

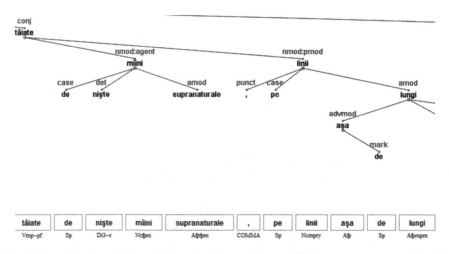

Fig. 4. Example of a verbal participle as head for a sub tree. (Cleft by some supernatural hands, on such long lines.)

We intend to carefully inventory and describe these categories of patterns in our Ro-PAAS. The examples above are extracted from the UAIC-RoDepTb.

2.2   The Dependency Status of Function Words

There are still many countries that build dependency grammar based corpora, because this convention of annotation is economical and flexible; but syntactic phenomena are viewed differently by the authors of different corpora. Therefore all follow the four axioms of dependency grammars, each dependency system of conventions is adjusted to the language of the corpus, or it can illustrate different views on the relevance ranking of linguistic information, annotated or not.

For example, the status of function words can vary significantly from one dependency system of annotation to another. Tesnière [23] took many function words to be the head of the content word. The Word Grammar [8] positions most of the function words as heads over the related content words. Since the Dependency Grammar does not accept the existence of transformations between a deep structure and a surface one, we cannot situate the function words at the surface structure. Some computational models like the Stanford Dependencies emphasize the word content and, therefore, subordinate function words to content words, and the UD (Universal Dependencies) system of annotation adopts this model.

We intend to affiliate our Treebank to the UD group, which aims to unify the different dependency systems of the twenty countries affiliated for being compatible. The compatibility of systems is profitable for making comparisons between data from different languages and for popularizing our research results.

Before deciding its affiliation to UD[1], UAIC-RoTb was built considering the relational words as heads for the linguistic elements which they insert in the text. In this way, the trees have a greater number of levels of subordination, which is a disadvantage for the economy of the description. Another disadvantage is losing the annotation of the syntactic function that relative pronouns, adjectives and adverbs have in the subordinate sentence that they introduce because they are considered their head.

However, the method has some advantages that cannot be neglected. The relational words are less numerous in all languages. If we intend to build a hybrid, statistical and rule-based parser, it is very simple to formulate a limited number of rules for the interpretation of a limited number of words, especially the subordinate conjunctions and the other relational words with a subordinate role.

For each syntactic parser, an important issue is the root node detection, and the correct parsing of the sentences which are coordinated with it, representing the higher levels of the dependency tree. We can prescribe rules relating to each of the words that have a subordinate role, which cannot insert fully meaningful sentences, and, consequently, cannot be coordinated with the top of the tree.

In order to join the consensus of the 20 UD participant countries, which do not accept to consider the relational words as head, we trained our parser with an obsolete

---

[1] http://universaldependencies.github.io/docs/.

form of our corpus in which relational words were annotated as subordinate at the head of the sentence they insert for a first set of 1 200 sentences, automatically annotated and previously supervised by experts, we may notice a decrease in the root node and independent clauses detection accuracy.

The score of root detection was 36.8 %. Of course, this result is due to an insufficient training on a small corpus, and this score will increase, but the root detection is really more difficult if the relational words are not considered important. In fact, they govern/guide the relationship. Examples:

El nu ştie *ce* face, *ce* drege."He does not know *what* he builds, *what* he restores."

$$(1)$$

In the sentence (1), the parser annotated "ce" *(what)* as a subordinate element of "face" *(does)*, "drege" *(restore)*; the predicates "ştie" *(know)*, "face", "drege" become in this way at the same level of importance, and, consequently, "drege" is automatically annotated as the root; and "ştie" becomes subordinated to "face", in the reverse order to the real one.

Era odată într-o oaste trei cătane *care* erau bătute.
"There was once in an army three soldiers *who* were beaten".

$$(2)$$

In the sentence (2)[2], the parser annotated "care" *(who)* as subordinated of "erau" *(were)* and "erau" is annotated as root. Therefore, we intend to formulate rules to prohibit the location in the root position of a predicate with a subordinate conjunction.

3 Related Works

Large-scale lexical semantic resources, such as Word-Net, have been developed and put to use for approximate semantic modeling in many applications. The Ro-WN was obtained by mapping Princeton Word-Net synsets on Romanian [1] and then, the English VerbNet, created following the Beth Levin's classification of verbs [12] was imported into Romanian and linked by the Ro-WN [2].

The PropBank project develops lexical semantic resources that focus on the modeling of predicate-argument structure. The importance of the task is confirmed by the emergence of international competitions concerned with the recognition of semantic roles (for the English language), based on PropBank predicate-argument structures (Shared Tasks of CONLL 2005–2009).

Since 2010, a greater number of countries have developed resources describing the PAS (Predicate Argument Structures) for their language. There are papers which describe corpora of PAS for Italian [10], German [20], and Japanese [4, 26]. Other papers present various types of automatic parsing tools based on PAS, using decision

---

[2] In folk language uses, there is no concord between subject and predicate, sometimes, in existential sentences; here, we have rendered this in English by 'There was', instead of 'There were'.

lists [4], or discriminative classifiers for deterministic dependency parsing [6]. Many papers describe another task: the automatic procedure for obtaining the PAS from corpora. The PAS are extracted using graphical models [13], or semantic space models [15]. Other papers show the connection between the syntactic annotation and the semantic one, based on syntax [10]. Of course there is a strong relationship between automatically parsing syntactic arguments and parsing semantic roles [19, 22].

We were particularly interested in the article describing the Italian resource [11], called T-PAS (Typed Predicate Argument Structures), obtained, just as in our case, by a large corpus of quotations using a lexicographic procedure called CPA (Corpus Pattern Analysis) [7, 10] and human annotators experts. They have developed techniques for evaluating the annotators' agreement. The arguments of their corpus also contain a specification for the expected semantic type. Example:

$$[\text{Human}]] \; guida \; [[\text{Vehicle}]]. \; (\text{Human } drive \; \text{Vehicle}) \qquad (3)$$

A very important model for our approach is the PDEV (The Pattern Dictionary of English Verbs).[3] This dictionary has 1 276 completely analyzed verbs, 433 verbs in progress and 3 687 not yet started verbs; the dictionary intends to treat 5 602 English verbs. The format of this dictionary contains a variable number of patterns formed by a semantic structure of core determiners (with the statistic of its frequency); it has no syntactic information, an implicature (or presupposition extract by the meaning and an example):

We can easily complete the syntactic information so we can use this pattern from the model for our resource. One must notice that in Fig. 5 there is a code of colors: the black Aldine is the color of labels, the black Italic is for the examples, the orange means semantic categories of nouns, the green means verbs and the violet is the color for some grammatical categories.

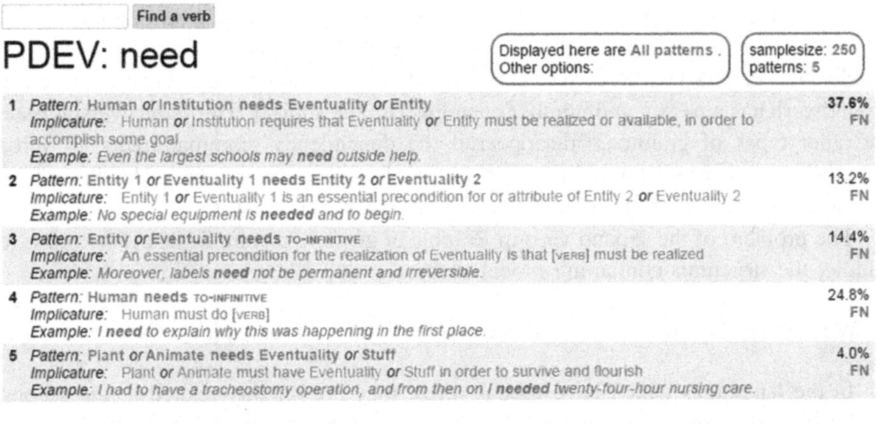

Fig. 5. The patterns of the verb "need" in the PDEV dictionary (Color figure online).

---

[3] http://pdev.org.uk/#browse?q=need;f=A;v=.

We quit citing the large number of papers which describe applications of this type of resources: for the automatic translations, for information extracting, resuming, question answering, etc.

4 Description of Ro-PAAS

4.1 The Verb "a putea" (Can)

We commenced to build the format or our Ro-PAAS by studying the verb "can". It is at the top of the list with the most frequent verbs in Romanian [9]. We think that, if we establish the format of our resource beginning with the most complicated verb, we will not omit a category that will prove necessary for the other verbs. This verb is not part of the 40 verbs whose syntactic structure hasbeen described [16]. We began by the extraction and the annotation of 114 quotations from eDTLR without omitting any sense glossed in this dictionary. We introduced them in our Treebank. There are in it a lot of sentences which contain this verb, but we created a table in xlsx format containing only the quotations extracted from eDTLR. These structures have maximum 3 arguments and 3 adjuncts.

A specific syntactic feature noticeable for the general appearance of a text in Romanian is the modality of binding the second verb. In English and in French the second verb is main infinitive directly related or related with a preposition: Example:

$$Il \; cesse \; de \; parler. \; / \; He \; ceases \; to \; speak. \; / \; El \; \text{încetează} \; s\breve{a} \; vorbeasc\breve{a}. \qquad (4)$$

The structure with the second infinitive verb is related to the main one with a preposition "Noi încetăm de a vorbi" is possible in Romanian but less frequent and obsolete. The Romanian second verb is subjunctive and has a person and number inflexion:

$$Nous \; cessons \; de \; parler \; / \; We \; cease \; to \; speak \; / \; Noi \; \text{încetăm} \; s\breve{a} \; vorbim. \qquad (5)$$

So in Romanian we have two clauses in terms of classical grammar because the second verb has a person and number concord with the subject. This controversial issue for other types of grammars disappear if the dependency grammar treats all verbs identically. A gerund, an infinitive, a participle can have the dependencies of an indicative, so they form gerundival, infinitival, participial clauses.

The problem of the second verb in Romanian gets more complicated if we place in parallel the structures containing modal verbs:

$$We \; must \; eat \; / \; Il \; faut \; manger \; / \; Trebuie \; s\breve{a} \; m\hat{a}nc\breve{a}m. \; / \; Trebuie \; plec^* \; (incorrect) \qquad (6)$$

In the languages which have modal verbs, they are directly related to the second main verb infinitive. In Romanian there is a single verb, "a putea" (can) which accepts this syntactic behavior, as well as the usual one in Romanian, the second verb being main subjunctive:

$$\text{Putem scrie / Putem să scriem / We can write.} \qquad (7)$$

There are a number of syntactic phenomena conducive to the conclusion that in Romanian "a putea" is the only verb that becomes in a process of transition to the status of modal verb. We can even formulate the hypothesis that in Romanian "a putea" is a verb halfway between ordinary syntactic behavior and a modal verb. We try to demonstrate this hypothesis. The structures in which "can" is followed by a main infinitive are synonymous and commutable with those where it is followed by a main subjunctive.

$$\text{Poate scrie / Poate să scrie / He can write.} \qquad (8)$$

We performed a preliminary statistical study using only the 110 examples containing this already studied verb. In this small corpus of quotations we have three categories of structures. In 33 % of these sentences, the verb "a putea" has a syntactic behavior similar to that of all the verbs in Romanian; it is determined by a second subjunctive verb. In 25 % of occurrences, the verb is not followed by a second verb; it is placed at the end of the sentence. In this case, the structure is elliptical, but we can reconstruct the missing verb following the meaning of the sentence. More frequently, it is expressed by the head of the verb "a putea". Example:

Scapă cine poate / escape / whoever can. this means: escape / whoever can escape.

$$(9)$$

In these cases, the expected verb after "a putea" as the second verb can be both a main infinitive without a conjunction or a main subjunctive. Example:

The text: *Ar vrea să fugă dacă ar putea* / (He) would like to run if he could can be continued either with *dacă ar putea (să fugă)*, or with *dacă ar putea (fugi)*. (He) would run if he could (run)

$$(10)$$

In these situations, "a putea" cannot be classified as a modal auxiliary or as an ordinary verb. In 43 % of the sentences analyzed the verb is already a modal auxiliary followed by a directly related main infinitive verb. Its syntactic structure has many specific features. There are a lot of dependencies of the modal "a putea" that are advanced in the text, i.e. these dependencies are located next to the verb "a putea" and appear to be subordinated to it, but in fact they are the dependencies of the subordinate verb. That is sometimes visible in their agreement.

Problema țărănească nu se poate rezolva "the /rural/problemnot/refl.pass./can solve"

$$(11)$$

The issue of the subject advanced in the head of the nominal subject clause has already been studied (Pană Dindelegan 2013 [5]). But in our sentences there are direct

(10) or indirect objects (11) advanced, too. The negation and the reflexive pronoun are amalgamated, they appear once affecting both the modal "a putea" and the directly related second verb. Examples (Fig. 6):

$$\text{Cartea se poate citi The book / can be read} \tag{12}$$

$$\text{(scrisoarea) pe care a putut-o adresa (the letter) that could / it / address} \tag{13}$$

$$\text{(El) nu-mi putea da o cameră (He) not/me/can/give a room} \tag{14}$$

There are in (10) a reflexive with passive meaning, expressing the voice of secondary verb "citi" (read) and a nsubjpass "cartea" *(the book);* it is also dependent on the secondary verb. In these cases, "a putea" should be annotated as an auxiliary for circumventing the problem of the head of common and advanced dependencies. The trees containing advanced structures have a complicated architecture difficult to automatically parse.

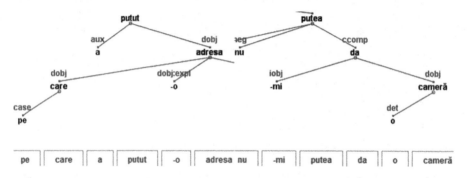

Fig. 6. Structures containing the verb "can" with advanced dobj and with advanced iobj.

As a result of these findings, we decided to change the annotation convention in our Treebank, in the case of the verb "can", considering it as auxiliary when the next verb is directly linked. The trees in the examples above will look as follows (Fig. 7):

So, we modified the table containing the structures of the 110 sentences, drawing two tables, one for the structures with "can" as Modal Auxiliary and another with "can" subordinated/by a clause or without subordination.

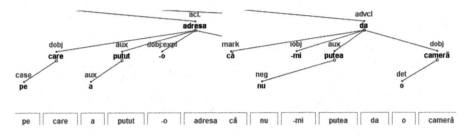

Fig. 7. The structures of Fig. 5 with "can" annotated as auxiliary.

4.2 The Content of .xml Tags

We are obliged to take into consideration, in our format (see the Appendix), the phenomenon of advanced dependencies and the ellipsis of mandatory dependencies. Natural language permits contextual ellipses for all the mandatory dependencies.

The pattern begins with a number of meanings which must be correlated by the numeric code of meaning(s) in eDTLR; any meaning in eDTLR can consequently be expressed by several patterns. The label "form" contains the lemma of the analyzed verb. The label "semantic_pattern" contains a short definition of meaning in this pattern and the label "head" can take the value "irrelevant" for some patterns; but it is nec-essary for those whose occurrence is conditioned by their regent, generally the auxiliary verbs.

The tag "pattern" includes two other tags, "dependencies" and "example"; we include between them a commentary called implicature. The tag "dependencies" includes other four tags. It begins with "restrictions", containing the categories which cannot be found among the dependencies of this pattern. These interdictions strongly influence the structure of the whole pattern. The values of each label may be more, numbered and separated by slash.

The second sub tag of "dependencies" is "advanced_arguments"; it contains the dependencies of the verb subordinated to the verb "can", if they are advanced and are apparently the mandatory dependencies of "can". Beginning with this tag, each syn-tactic dependency tag is followed by its semantic interpretation. If there are many advanced arguments, they are numbered: "type_1", "type_2", "type_3" … and each type is followed by its semantic interpretation, also into the tag "advanced _argu-ments". For the syntactic dependencies we employ the syntactic label of the UD project, which will be ours beginning this autumn; for the semantic interpretation we employ part of the "SEMANTIC TYPES" (the most abstract ones) of PDEV. By adding new verbs, we also form an increasing list of semantic labels employed into Ro-PAAS.

The third tag in the "dependencies" one is "advanced_adjuncts"; it includes advanced facultative dependencies of the subordinate verb, if they are advanced, and are apparently the facultative dependencies of "can". There are some cases in our little corpus of analyzed examples. This tag can also have more types and each of them is followed by a semantic interpretation, i.e. the semantic categories expected to be selected by this kind of syntactic positions. If there aren't any advanced arguments or adjuncts, we complete the tag with "none" and respectively, its semantic interpretation ⁓will be "none" too.

The fourth tag into the "dependencies" tag is "arguments" and contains the mandatory dependencies of "can". The mandatory dependencies of "can" start with type_0 because there are cases in which "can" is part of a multi word expression and this "mwe" (multi word expression) dependency is of primary importance for the selection of others. The argument type_1 is the subject, but its place may be taken by the reflexive pronoun with impersonal value. The argument type_2 is the second verb. The argument type_3 is the direct object or the indirect object and we will employ the type_4 if the two objects are present. An argument is not present in this section if it appears in the tag "restrictions". Otherwise, it takes the value "remnant" which, in the UD system, means "ellipse". Each type is followed by the semantic value which may be taken, i.e. it is expected to be selected.

For example, in Appendix 1, in the pattern id "4", we have two types for the "advanced_arguments", the type_1 = "nsubj" followed by semantic = "Abstract_Entity", and the type_2 = "csubj", followed by semantic = "Action". In the pattern id "6", in the tag "arguments" there are 2 types: the type_1 = "nsubj" to which there correspond two possible values: semantic = "Human/Animate" and the type_2 = "remnant" semantic = "Action", the value "1:Human/Animate" corresponds to "1. nsubj", and the value "2:Action" corresponds to "2.remnant".

The last tag subordinate to the "dependencies" one is "adjuncts", and it contains the facultative dependencies of "can", including the relational words and the formants for the negative, the mode and the time of the verb, the voice, and so on, (because in dependency grammar conventions we must subordinate also these elements, and they are not mandatory). Such dependencies can appear in the first tag subordinated to "dependencies", i.e. "restrictions", and then it cannot be found in the tag "adjuncts". This section can also have more types. We begin the list with the circumstantial dependencies and we finish with the words-tool. Each "adjunct" type is followed by its semantic interpretation, i.e. the semantic values of circumstantial dependencies and the value "Formants" of word-tools.

The "# implicature" is also inspired by PDEV. This pragmatic term, called presupposition in other studies, means things accepted by the participants of the communication and whose non-acceptance makes the communication impossible. We include here the gloss of the lexicographic definition in the most abbreviated and logical formula possible. It is not double information as the semantic_pattern, because the first is destined to be read by the computer and the # implicature is a comment destined for the human user.

Finally, the pattern includes an example, a sentence from the Treebank, annotated in the form of a tree and preceded by the name of the sub-corpus in the Treebank (the name of the xml document) and the id of the sentence in this xml document. The dependency tree for the example in the Appendix looks as follows (Fig. 8):

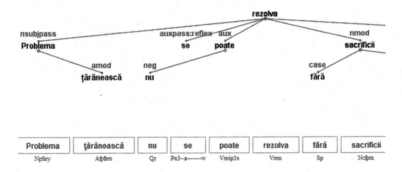

Problema	țărănească	nu	se	poate	rezolva	fără	sacrificii
Npfsry	Afpfsrn	Qz	Px3--s------w	Vmip3s	Vmn	Sp	Ncfpm

Fig. 8. The tree for the example in the Appendix (the peasant problem cannot be solved without sacrifices.)

5 A Tool for Searching Patterns in the UAIC-RoTb: GGS (Graphical Grammar Studio)

Graphical Grammar Studio is a tool oriented towards syntactical analysis, developed in Java [21]. We can first remark that unlike Constituent Grammars, which include grammatical categories as nodes in the trees and whose relationships are based on the inclusion of the words in syntactic groups, dependency grammars are more flexible and they are similar to the automaton with finite states. The automaton with finite state is defined by four elements: A = (S, T, S_0, F). There is a set of transitions (T) among the states (S). There are a finite number of states and a finite number of transition rules between them. There needs to be an initial state (S_0) and a final state (F). A dependency grammar can be defined also by four elements: G = (T, L, R, S_0), namely, T = a finite set of terminal symbols, i.e. words; L = a finite set of relationship types, i.e. grammatical categories, R = a root node, S_0 = a final state (a punctuation element).

A **GGS** grammar is basically a finite state machine which is organized into **GGS** graphs of nodes/states. The GGS matching process takes as input such a grammar and a sequence of tokens and tries to find a path in the grammar from its starting node to its ending node. The nodes of the path must consume input tokens for the path to be considered. For a token to be consumed by a node, it must meet the conditions specified by the node. One can easily search the input text for sequences of tokens which have particular?? certain attributes.

Each **GGS** graph is identified by a name and contains an entry and an exit node. Each **GGS** grammar contains the "Main" graph. The entry and exit nodes of the Main graph are the starting and the final nodes used in the matching process, respectively. A GGS graph node can be one of four types: 1. Empty Node; 2 Token Matching Node; 3 Jump Node; 4 Comment node.

When the matching process reaches the final node, a variable number of input tokens are consumed. These represent the matched sequence. This sequence starts with the first token from the given input. In practice, we need to find multiple matches, some of which start in the middle of a sequence of tokens (a sentence for instance). GGS achieves this by applying the GGS matching process described multiple times, each

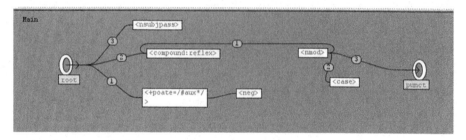

Fig. 9. The GGS graph for the pattern of the example in the Appendix (the peasant problem cannot be solved without sacrifices.)

time incrementing the starting offset by 1 (or by the length of the last match if it is the case). There are many features contained in the GGS, for example annotating matches, changing priorities between paths. Advanced features include look ahead and look behind assertions, running JavaScript code and using variables.

A graph in the GGS system is identical with an automaton with finite states, it has a beginning state and a final one; it can be used as a tool to search for linear sequences, preferably from left to right. The tree structure is not a linear sequence: it has a beginning state, but can have a lot of final states. Those must be conceived as imbricate structures, as parentheses in the principal judgment, and the final state is the final period related to the root, the head of the principal judgment (Fig. 9).

The tool must find the words which have the POS-tag starting with V, memorize their lemma and their id (containing the id of the sentence in the Treebank followed by the id of the word in this sentence); then it must find all the deprel (dependencies) with the identical head at this id. The postag = "V.*" appears 11 319 times in our Treebank. At present, the UAIC-RoDepTb has 7 800 sentences and we continue to validate other automatically annotated ones. We must draw a table with this data, in xlxs, having this head (Table 1):

Subsequently, we apply an alphabetical sort at the first column of this table, grouping in this way all the examples containing the same verb and we obtain the list of dependencies for each verb in the examples annotated in the Treebank. We can also do a statistic of the percent of verbal structures which the GGS had extracted from the Treebank, by rapport to the total number of verbs.

Table 1. The head of the list with the verbs in our Treebank and their dependencies

Lemma	Postag	Form	Id	Head24051	Head24051	Head24051	Head24051	Head24051
Putea	V.*	Poate	24051	Deprel	Deprel	Deprel	Deprel	Deprel

6   Conclusion and Future Works

6.1   Increasing the Size and the Quality of Romanian Resources

Our language has been classified in many reports as having an insufficient degree of computerization. To reduce the lagging, Romanian computer scientists built some resources by translating big English corpora and by importing their accurate annotations [2, 24]. We can learn, in this manner, how to build corpora, but these resources are not representative for our language. Linguists must help the computer scientist to build corpora more representative for our language and correctly annotated, in order to put Romanian in the circle of languages accessible for others.

The automated annotation is the solution, because we don't have big human and financial resources for the manual one. As we do not have large corpora to train the learning machines, we need to create rule based or hybrid tools, i.e. rule and statistical based tools. The linguists aim to formulate these rules in a manner more accessible for the computers. They can translate the important linguistic approach into the computer's language.

So, we have to build modern resources. The resource type structures of arguments and adjuncts for verbs have been recently developed for many languages. This resource (Ro-PAAS) will be used to build a hybrid parser functioning in the top-down direction of annotation and to introduce in the parser rules for the selections at the top of the tree. We intend to transform the Treebank in accordance with the Universal Dependencies conventions of annotation, also keeping the actual Treebank in the form of a semantic annotated one. The semantic annotation which we intend to develop is the superior level after the syntactic one and prepares the information for the discourse level. The treebank must illustrate all the styles of the Romanian language. It is organized in more .xml documents, each of them having about 1 000 sentences illustrating a particular style, journalistic, legal, fiction, social media, etc.

6.2   The Old Romanian Language

Foreign computer scientists talk about Romanian language as of a new language, because they have known it for some time and have no data about its old aspect. There are a lot of Romanian linguists, too, who have no access to the old language. Twenty years ago specialists in structural and transformational grammar considered, that their theories should not be applied to the old language. But in current linguistic theory, too, there is a tendency to apply modern explanatory methods to old languages. These modern theory of grammar specialists, who do not have very much knowledge about the old language, require automatic language processing for old Romanian to extract information by advanced searches.

These instruments can be created only by computer scientists in collaboration with linguists who have sufficient knowledge of the old language. As far as we are concerned, we are ready to begin this laborious activity:

"Biruit-au gândul să mă apuc de această trudă" /The thought overcame me to take up this hard work. (Miron Costin, old Moldavian historian, 1686–1691)

We will provide at the basis of a model for old Romanian the corpus of the eDTLR bibliography, which contains a lot of old texts in new critical editions with indices of words. This old language vocabulary f must contain all the inflected forms of words, which we can find in the corpus by means of a concordancer program. But we need to construct on this basic tools the actual ones for contemporary Romanian; we are aware that their accurate function is very important. The order of priority for us is to increase first the adequacy percentage of automatic morphological and syntactic annotation of texts in contemporary language, then to begin their training with ancient language sentences.

Appendix: The 4-th Pattern of Verb "a putea" in RoPAAS

```
<pattern id="4" form="PUTEA" type="aux" semantic_pattern="Possibility" head="VERB_main_infinitive">
<dependencies>
            <restrictions type="mark"/>
            < advanced _arguments type_1="nsubj" semantic="Abstract_Entity"
                                    type_2="csubj"semantic="Action"/>
            < advanced _adjuncts type="auxpass:reflex" semantic="Passive"/>
            <arguments type="none" semantic="none"/>
            <adjuncts type_1="neg" semantic="Formant" type_2="aux" semantic="Formant"/>
</dependencies>
            # implicature: (Cineva ori nimeni nu) e capabil să modifice starea subiectului pasiv. (One or none) is able
            to modify the state of the passive subject.
<example id="1" corpus="quotations_verbs_1_UD" sentence_id="64"> (The peasant problem can not be solved
without sacrifices.)
            <word id="1" form="Problema" lemma="problemă" postag="Npfsry" head="6" chunk=""
            deprel="nsubjpass"/>
            <word id="2" form="ţărănească" lemma="ţărănesc" postag="Afpfsrn" head="1" chunk=""
            deprel="amod"/>
            <word id="3" form="nu" lemma="nu" postag="Qz" head="5" chunk="" deprel="neg"/>
            <word id="4" form="se" lemma="sine" postag="Px3--a--------w" head="6" chunk=""
            deprel="auxpass:reflex"/>
            <word id="5" form="poate" lemma="putea" postag="Vmip3s" head="6" chunk="" deprel="aux"/>
            <word id="6" form="rezolva" lemma="rezolva" postag="Vmn" head="0" chunk=""/>
            <word id="7" form="fără" lemma="fără" postag="Sp" head="8" chunk="" deprel="case"/>
            <word id="8" form="sacrificii" lemma="sacrificiu" postag="Ncfprn" head="6" chunk=""
            deprel="nmod"/>
            <word id="9" form="." lemma="." postag="PERIOD" head="6" chunk="" deprel="punct"/>
</example>
</pattern>
```

References

1. Cristea, D., Mihăilă, C., Forăscu, C., Trandabăţ, D., Husarciuc, M., Haja, G., Postolache, O.: Mapping Princeton WordNet synsets onto Romanian WordNet synsets. Rom. J. Inf. Sci. Technol. **7**, 125–145 (2004). (Special Issue on BalkaNet)
2. Curteanu, N., Moruz, M., Trandabat, D., Bolea, C., Dornescu, I.: The structure and parsing of Romanian verbal group and predicate. In: Proceedings of the 4th European Conference on Intelligent Systems and Technologies, ECIT (2006)

3. eDTLR (Romanian Thesaurus Dictionary). http://85.122.23.96/
4. Fujita, S., Nagata, M.: A Japanese predicate argument structure analysis using decision lists. In: Proceedings of EMNLP, pp. 523–532 (2008)
5. Pană Dindelegan, G. (ed.): The Grammar of Romanian. Oxford University Press (2013). http://ukcatalogue.oup.com/product/9780199644926.do
6. Hall, J., Nivre, J., Nilsson, J.: Discriminative classifiers for deterministic dependency parsing. In: Proceedings of the 21st International Conference on Computational Linguistics and 44th Annual Meeting of the Association for Computational Linguistics, pp. 316–323 (2006)
7. Hanks, P.: Corpus pattern analysis. In: Williams, G., Vessier, S. (eds.) Proceedings of the XI EURALEX International Congress, pp. 87–98. Francepp, Lorient (2004)
8. Hudson, R.: Language Networks. The New Word Grammar. Oxford University Press, Oxford (2007)
9. Ion, R., Irimia, E., Ştefănescu, D., Tufiş, D.: ROMBAC: the Romanian balanced annotated corpus. In: Proceedings LREC 2012, Istanbul, Turkey (2012)
10. Jezek, E.: Acquiring typed predicate-argument structures from corpora. In: Bunt, H. (ed.) Proceedings of the Eighth Joint ISO - ACL SIGSEM Workshop on Interoperable Semantic Annotation ISA-8, pp. 28–33. Università di Pisa – CNR, Pisa (2012)
11. Jezek, E., Magnini, B., Feltracco, A., Bianchini, A., Popescu, O.: Structures for linguistic analysis and semantic processing. In: Proceedings of LREC, pp. 890–895 (2014)
12. Levin, B.: English Verb Class and Alternations: A Preliminary Investigation. University of Chicago Press, Chicago (1993)
13. Lippincott, T., Séaghdha, D.O., Korhonen, A.: Learning syntactic verb frames using graphical models. In: Proceedings of the 50th Annual Meeting of the Association for Computational Linguistics, pp. 420–429 (2012)
14. Mărănduc, C., Perez, A.-C.: A Romanian dependency treebank. In: Communication at the Conference CICLing 2015, Cairo, Egypt (2015)
15. Pado, S., Lapata, M.: Dependency-based construction of semantic space models. Comput. Linguist. **33**(2), 161–199 (2007)
16. Pană Dindelegan, G.: Transformational Syntax of Verbal Group in Romanian. Academy Press, Bucureşti (1974)
17. PDEV (Pattern Dictionary of English Verbs). http://pdev.org.uk/#browse?q=need;f=A;v=
18. Perez, A.-C.: Linguistical resources for natural language processing. Ph.D. thesis, "Al. I. Cuza" University, Iaşi (2014)
19. Punyakanok, V., Roth, D., Yih, W.-T.: The importance of syntactic parsing and inference in semantic role labeling. Comput. Linguist. **34**(2), 257–287 (2008)
20. Schulte im Walde, S., Brew, C.: Inducing German semantic verb classes from purely syntactic subcategorisation information. In: Proceedings of the 40th Annual Meeting of the Association for Computational Linguistics, Philadelphia, USA (2002)
21. Simionescu, R.: Graphical grammar studio as a constraint grammar solution for part of speech tagging. In: The Conference on Linguistic Resources and Instruments for Romanian Language Processing (2011)
22. Surdeanu, M., Johansson, R., Meyers, A., Marquez, L., Nivre, J.: The CoNLL-2008 shared task on joint parsing of syntactic and semantic dependencies. In: Proceedings of the 12th Conference on Computational Natural Language Learning (2008)
23. Tesnière, L.: Elements of structural syntax, Editions Klincksieck; Éléments de syntaxe structurale, Paris, Klincksieck, deuxième édition (1959, 1966)
24. Trandabăţ, D.: Natural language processing using semantic frames. Ph.D. thesis, "Al. I. Cuza" University, Iaşi (2010)

25. Xianchao, W., Katsuhito, S., Duh, K., Tsukada, H., Nagata, M.: Extracting preordering rules from predicate-argument structures. In: Proceedings of 5th International Joint Conference on Natural Language Processing, Chiang Mai, Thailand, pp. 29–37 (2011)
26. Yuta, H., Komachi, M., Matsumoto, Y.: Japanese predicate argument structure analysis exploiting argument position and type. In: Proceedings of IJCNLP, pp. 201–209 (2011)

Word-Order Analysis Based Upon Treebank Data

Vladislav Kuboň[(✉)] and Markéta Lopatková[(✉)]

Faculty of Mathematics and Physics, Institute of Formal and Applied Linguistics,
Charles University in Prague, Prague, Czech Republic
{vk,lopatkova}@ufal.mff.cuni.cz

Abstract. The paper describes an experiment consisting in the attempt to quantify word-order properties of three Indo-European languages (Czech, English and Farsi). The investigation is driven by the endeavor to find an objective way how to compare natural languages from the point of view of the degree of their word-order freedom. Unlike similar studies which concentrate either on purely linguistic or purely statistical approach, our experiment tries to combine both – the observations are verified against large samples of sentences from available treebanks, and, at the same time, we exploit the ability of our tools to analyze selected important phenomena (as, e.g., the differences of the word order of a main and a subordinate clause) more deeply.

The quantitative results of our research are collected from the syntactically annotated treebanks available for all three languages. Thanks to the HamleDT project, it is possible to search all treebanks in a uniform way by means of a universal query tool PML-TQ. This is also a secondary goal of this paper – to demonstrate the research potential provided by language resources which are to a certain extent unified.

1 Introduction

The traditional linguistics, see esp. [13], devoted considerable effort to studying various language characteristics which enabled them to classify natural languages according to their properties from various points of view. The results of these investigations have led to a generally accepted system of language types (as, e.g., the classification into four basic language types, namely isolated, agglutinative, inflectional and polysynthetic languages [12,14]).

The language phenomena enabling linguists to classify languages are numerous. Probably the most comprehensible list of features can be found in the World Atlas of Language Structures (WALS) [2], which contains 151 chapters, each describing one language phenomenon and its distribution in the languages of the world. This clearly shows that the classification of languages cannot be based upon a single phenomenon (for example the number of cases or genders or the obligatory presence of a subject in a sentence etc.), they must be characterized by a mixture of typical features.

© Springer International Publishing Switzerland 2015
G. Sidorov and S.N. Galicia-Haro (Eds.): MICAI 2015, Part I, LNAI 9413, pp. 47–58, 2015.
DOI: 10.1007/978-3-319-27060-9_4

In this paper we present an investigation of one particular phenomenon, word order of natural languages which we believe is very important for theoretical research as well as for practical applications. The freedom of word order to a great extent determines how difficult it is to parse a particular natural language (a language with more fixed word order is typically easier to parse than a language containing, e.g., non-projective constructions). Its importance is also indicated by the fact that it constitutes one of the 11 major areas of WALS.

When concentrating on word order, we study the prevalent order of the verb and its main complements. Indo-European languages are thus characterized as SVO (SVO reflecting the order Subject-Verb-Object) languages. English and other languages with a fixed word order typically follow this order of words in declarative sentences; although Czech, Russian and other Slavic languages have a high degree of word order freedom, they still stick to the same order of word in a typical (unmarked) sentence. As for the VSO-type languages, their representatives can be found among semitic (Arabic, classical Hebrew) or Celtic languages, while (some) Amazonian languages belong to the OSV type. These characteristics, which are traditionally mentioned in classical textbooks of general linguistics [15], have been specified on the basis of excerptions and careful examination by many linguists.

Although all these investigation have been based upon a systematic observation of linguistic material, modern computational linguistics has brought into play much larger resources providing huge volumes of language material (which can be studied by means of automatic tools), and thus it may bring a deeper linguistic insight into the language typology. Thanks to a wide range of linguistic data resources for tens of languages available nowadays, we can easily confirm (or enhance by quantitative clues) the conclusions of traditional linguists. This paper represents a step in this direction.

2   Setup of the Experiment

The analysis of syntactic properties of natural languages constitutes one of our long term goals. The phenomenon of word order has been in a center of our investigations for a long time. Our previous research concentrated both on studying individual properties of languages with higher degree of word-order freedom – as, e.g., non-projective constructions (long-distance dependencies) [4] – as well as on the endeavor to find some general measures enabling more precise characterization of individual natural languages with regard to the degree of their word-order freedom [5]. Unlike similar experiments, as e.g. [3], we try to concentrate on a deeper analysis and characterization of identified patterns.

The experiment presented in this paper continues in the same direction. It is driven by the endeavor to find an objective way how to compare natural languages from the point of view of the degree of their word-order freedom. While the previous experiments concentrated on more formal approach, this one builds upon a thorough analysis of available data resources.

When investigating syntactic properties of natural languages, it is very often the case that the discussion focuses on individual phenomena, their properties and their influence on the order of words. In this paper we concentrate upon the analysis of quantitative properties of the word order phenomenon. In order to capture the quantitative characteristic of a particular natural language, we exploit a representative sample of its syntactically annotated data and calculate the distribution of individual types of word order for the three main syntactic components – subject, predicate and object. The statistics is calculated separately for main and subordinated clauses.

2.1 HamleDT and Available Treebanks

The tools and resources we are exploiting in this paper can be found in a repository for linguistic data and resources LINDAT/CLARIN.[1] This repository enables experiments with syntactically annotated corpora, so called treebanks, for several tens of languages. Wherever it is possible due to license agreements, the corpora are transformed into a common format, which enables a user – after a very short period of getting acquainted with each particular treebank – a comfortable search and analysis of the data from a particular language. The HamleDT project[2] (HArmonized Multi-LanguagE Dependency Treebank) [16] has already managed to transform 42 treebanks from all over the world into a common format.

The HamleDT family of treebanks is based on the dependency framework and technology developed for the Prague Dependency Treebank (PDT),[3] i.e., large syntactically annotated corpus for the Czech language [1]. Here we focus on the so-called analytical layer, i.e., the layer describing surface sentence structure (relevant for studying word order properties). The English corpus included in HamleDT is the well known Penn Treebank[4] [7], which was automatically transformed from the original phrase-structure trees into the dependency annotation. The third corpus used in our experiments is the Persian Dependency Treebank (PerDT),[5] the collection of sentences with syntactic and morphological annotations useful for natural language processing of the Farsi language.

Figure 1 shows a sample dependency tree for an English sentence in the HamleDT format and Table 1 summarizes the basic characteristics of all corpora used in our experiment.

2.2 PML-TQ Tree Query

For searching the data, we exploit the PML-TQ search tool,[6] which has been primarily designed for processing the PDT data. PML-TQ is a query language

---

[1] https://lindat.mff.cuni.cz/.
[2] http://ufal.mff.cuni.cz/hamledt.
[3] http://ufal.mff.cuni.cz/pdt3.0.
[4] https://www.cis.upenn.edu/~treebank.
[5] http://dadegan.ir/en/perdt.
[6] https://lindat.mff.cuni.cz/services/pmltq/#!/treebanks.

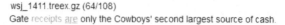

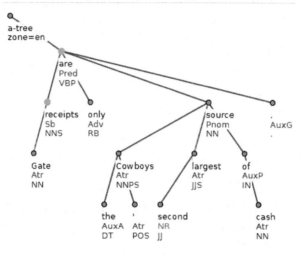

Fig. 1. Sample English dependency tree in the HamleDT format

Table 1. An overview of three treebanks under scrutiny

Corpus	# Predicates	Type	Language	Genre
PDT	79,283	manual	Czech	news
Penn Treebank	51,048	manual	English	economy
PerDT	12.280	automatic	Farsi	news

and search engine designed for querying annotated linguistic data [9]; it allows users to formulate complex queries on richly annotated linguistic data.

Having the treebanks in the common data format, the PML-TQ framework makes it possible to analyse the data in a uniform way   the following sample query in Fig. 2 gives us subtrees with an intransitive predicative verb (in a main clause), i.e. a `Pred` node with a `Sb` node and no `Obj` nodes among its dependent nodes, where `Sb` follows the `Pred`; the filter on the last line (`>> for  $n0.lemma give $1, count()`) outputs a table listing verb lemmas with this marked word order position and number of their occurrences in the corpus.

3   Analysis of Data

Let us now look at the syntactic typology of natural languages under investigation. We are taking into account especially the mutual position of subject, predicate and direct object. After a thorough investigation of the ways how indirect objects are annotated in all three corpora, we have decided to limit ourselves (at least in this stage of our research) to basic structures and to extract and

```
a-node
$n0 := [ afun = "Pred",
    child a-node
    $n1 := [ afun = "Sb",
            $n1.ord > $n0.ord],
    0x child a-node
    [ afun = "Obj"]];
>> for $n0.lemma
        give $1, count()
```

Fig. 2. Sample PML-TQ query and its visualization

analyze only sentences without too complicated or mutually interlocked phenomena. Namely we focus on sentences with the following properties:

– sentences may contain coordinated predicates (but subjects or objects common to coordinated verbs are not taken into account, due to a specific annotation of coordinated structures in the HamleDT scheme);
– we analyze only non-prepositional subjects and objects.

We are analyzing separately two types of clauses in our experiment: (i) main clauses expressing the main proposition, and (ii) subordinated clauses, i.e. clauses expressing predications embedded into the main proposition. While the former type can be easily identified in the data (main predicative verbs are labeled with the **Pred** function in the HamleDT treebanks), the latter type is more tricky: a dependency framework does not explicitly determine clauses [6] thus we approximate subordinated clauses as subtrees rooted in a finite verb (i.e., not infinitive or nominalized form of a verb) with other than **Pred** function. This approach allows us to gain deeper insight into the word order properties of the studied languages, as is documented in the following sections.

3.1 Czech

The highest quality syntactically annotated Czech data can be found in the Prague Dependency Treebank [1];[7] in fact, it is the only corpus we work with that has been manually annotated and thoroughly tested for the annotation consistency. The texts of PDT belong mostly to the journalism genre, it consists of newspaper texts and (in a limited scale) of texts from popularizing scientific journal.

The following Table 2 summarizes the number of sentences with intransitive verbs as well as those with an omitted subject in main clauses in PDT, with respect to the word order positions of **Sb**, verbal **Pred** and **Obj** – we can see that

---

[7] https://lindat.mff.cuni.cz/services/pmltq/pdt30/.

the marked word order (verb preceding its subject or object preceding the verb) is quite common in Czech.

Table 3 displays the distribution of individual combinations of a subject, predicate and a single object. It is not surprising that the unmarked – intuitively "most natural" – word order type, SVO, accounts for only slightly more than half of cases. The relatively high degree of word order freedom is thus supported also quantitatively.

Table 2. Czech sentences with intransitive verbs and sentences with an omitted subject in a main clause

Word order	Number	%
SV	16,032	56.40
VS	12,395	43.60
Total	28,427	100.00
VO	8,616	75.56
OV	2,787	24.44
Total	11,403	100.00

Table 3. Czech sentences with a transitive verb in a main clause

Word order	Number	%
SVO	10,237	51.72
SOV	1,476	7.46
VSO	1,792	9.05
VOS	1,945	9.83
OVS	3,840	19.40
OSV	505	2.55
Total	19,795	100.00

Let us now turn our attention to an investigation whether the word order of subordinated clauses substantially differs from the results collected for main clauses.

As we can see, the distribution is only slightly different. The first interesting result concerns the clauses having a transitive verb on a second position, Table 5. These clauses tend to follow the unmarked word order more often than main clauses; however, the number of clauses with a subject in front (SVO) is higher by an almost equal difference as the number of clauses with the object in front (OVS) is lower. Similar correlation can be found for subordinated clauses either with an omitted subject or without object, Table 4.

The second observation concerns the subordinated clauses starting with a verb – their number is lower compared to the main clauses with the same property, regardless whether the verb is followed by a subject or an object. This drop is compensated by the increase of the cases when the verb is positioned further towards the end of the clause. Actually, the predicate positioned at the end of a main clause beginning with object is quite rare in Czech (only 2.55 % cases) and thus the increase to 7.82 % in Table 5 actually means that this special case of word order is 3 times more frequent in subordinated clauses. This is an interesting result which is not mentioned in Czech grammars.

3.2   English

The statistics concerning the distribution of word-order types for English have been calculated on the Wall Street Journal section of the Penn Treebank [7]

Table 4. Czech subordinated clauses with intransitive verbs and subordinated clauses with an omitted subject

Word order	Number	%
SV	8,625	64.66
VS	4,715	35.34
Total	13,340	100.00
VO	6,080	72.05
OV	2,358	27.95
Total	8,438	100.00

Table 5. Czech subordinated clauses with a transitive verb

Word order	Number	%
SVO	6,266	58.82
SOV	1,179	11.07
VSO	548	5.14
VOS	553	5.19
OVS	1,273	11.95
OSV	833	7.82
Total	381	100.00

whose syntactic structure has been transformed into dependency trees in the HamleDT project.[8] As was mentioned above, the transformation on the surface syntactic layer was fully automatic.

The statistics of different types of word order have been collected in the same manner as in the previous subsection. We have also applied identical filters as for Czech sentences from PDT. Table 6 contains data for sentences with intransitive verbs and sentences with an omitted subject: the total number inadequately increases to 826 subject-less main clauses due to two reasons: first, coordinated subjects are not properly identified because of the specific annotation scheme for coordination in HamleDT; second, for analytical verb forms subject is rendered as dependent on auxiliary verbs, not as a complementation of lexical verb.

Table 6. English sentences with intransitive verbs and sentences with an omitted subject in a main clause

Word order	Number	%
SV	7,633	96.18
VS	303	3.82
Total	7,936	100.00
VO	815	98.67
OV	11	1.33
Total	826	100.00

Table 7. English sentences with a transitive verb in a main clause

Word order	Number	%
SVO	7,749	84.13
SOV	1	0.01
VSO	27	0.29
VOS	3	0.03
OVS	627	6.81
OSV	804	8.73
Total	9,211	100.00

As we can see, the strict word order of English sentences manifests itself in a vast majority of sentences having the prototypical word order of the subject being followed by a predicate. The examples of the opposite word order include sentences containing direct speech with the following pattern *"It's just a matter of time before the tide turns,"* **says** one *Midwestern* **lobbyist**.

---

[8] https://lindat.mff.cuni.cz/services/pmltq/hamledt_en/.

Out of the 303 sentences with the reversed word order, as many as 94 contained the predicate *to say*, 88 *to be*, 38 *to do*, 12 *will*, 11 *to come* and 10 *to have*. Out of all other verbs involved in these constructions, only 7 were represented more than once. A deeper analysis reveals that there are four typical phenomena that cause the marked word order in these cases (in accordance with English grammar books):

- **quotative inversion** (see above);
- **stylistic inversion**, as e.g. ***Not only can they block Wellington*** *from raising money in Japan, ... but they might be able to ... , too.*;
- **locative inversion**, as e.g. ***Here are price trends*** *on the world 's major stock markets, ...*;
- **question**, as e.g. ***And why should holders expect*** *to realize that presumed "worth"?*.

The results for sentences containing transitive verbs, Table 7, also confirm the fact that the SVO order is the prevailing order in standard sentences. The remaining types of word order represent only 15.87 % sentences in the corpus. Some of those cases, especially those with a very low number of occurrences, namely SOV nad VOS, actually represent annotation errors (esp. auxiliary verbs which have been quite often incorrectly annotated as Objects). The queries also revealed an interesting fact concerning the OVS and OSV types of sentences. Again, a vast majority of verbs appearing in these main clauses can be classified as verbs of communication (verba dicendi) – with 566 and 658 appearances of the verb *to say* within OVS and OSV patterns, respectively.

Let us now look at the results collected for English subordinated clauses (Tables 8 and 9). As we can see, for the clauses not containing either a subject[9] or an object, the distribution even more strictly follows the prevailing pattern of main clauses. In these cases, the marked word order VS is again characteristic for (i) verbs of communication, as in *As a result,* **says Mr. Geiger,** *lawyers think twice before appealing a judge 's ruling ...*, and also for (ii) verbs of moving, as e.g. *At 2:43 p.m. EDT,* **came the sickening news:** *....*

The same is actually true also for transitive verbs, where the number of marked subordinated clauses starting with an object substantially decreases in favor of the prototypical word order (SVO). However, in these cases, verbs appearing in marked word order patterns are diverse and cannot be easily characterised with respect to their semantic classes.

3.3 Farsi

We have extracted 12,280 Farsi sentences with the same requirements as for Czech and English.[10] The sentences contain a verbal predicate, no coordination

---

[9] The number of subject-less subordinated clauses is inadequately high due to the same reasons as for main clauses: annotation scheme for coordination and analytical verb forms.

[10] https://lindat.mff.cuni.cz/services/pmltq/hamledt_fa/.

Table 8. English subordinated clauses with intransitive verbs and subordinated clauses with an omitted subject

Word order	Number	%
SV	5,785	98.07
VS	114	1.93
Total	5,899	100.00
VO	3,544	99.49
OV	18	0.51
Total	3,562	100.00

Table 9. English subordinated clauses with a transitive verb

Word order	Number	%
SVO	5,118	96.38
SOV	1	0.02
VSO	1	0.02
VOS	0	0.00
OVS	4	0.08
OSV	186	3.50
Total	5,310	100.00

of dependent words and only non-prepositional objects and subjects. Table 10 contains data for main clauses with intransitive verbs, showing a total dominance of the SV word order; more interesting are the results for main clauses not containing a subject: the position of the object seems to be relatively equally distributed with a slight preference to an object located to the right of the predicate. Quite surprising ale also the results presented in Table 11, namely the low number of sentences containing both a subject and an object. They account only for about 10 % of the entire corpus.

Table 10. Farsi sentences with intransitive verbs and sentences with an omitted subject in a main clause

Word order	Number	%
SV	5,975	99.70
VS	18	0.30
Total	5,993	100.00
VO	947	56.81
OV	720	43.19
Total	1,667	100.00

Table 11. Farsi sentences with a sentences with a transitive verb in a main clause

Word order	Number	%
SVO	447	35.70
SOV	795	63.50
VSO	1	0.08
VOS	0	0.00
OVS	2	0.16
OSV	7	0.56
Total	1,252	100.00

The whole picture looks slightly different if we look at the word order in subordinated clauses. Our query searching for embedded predication with verbal predicate has found 21,649 clauses. A vast majority of them (19,868 clauses) did contain neither subject nor object. Those containing only a subject and a predicate actually confirmed the results for main clauses, i.e., a dominance of the SV word order, Table 12 (top). In case of clauses without a subject, the slight majority has turned into the other direction with almost two thirds of clauses having the OV word order, Table 12 (bottom). Also the subordinated clauses having both object and subject (though rather rare) show similar distribution as in the main clauses, Table 13.

Table 12. Farsi subordinated clauses with intransitive verbs and subordinated clauses with an omitted subject

Word order	Number	%
SV	2,252	99.73
VS	6	0.10
Total	2,258	100.00
VO	443	37.77
OV	730	62.23
Total	1,173	100.00

Table 13. Farsi subordinated clauses with a transitive verb

Word order	Number	%
SVO	101	26.51
SOV	262	68.77
VSO	0	0.00
VOS	0	0.00
OVS	1	0.26
OSV	17	4.46
Total	381	100.00

3.4 Comparison of Results

Let us summarize the statistics presented in the previous section for the main and subordinated clauses separately. The results are displayed in the charts in Fig. 3 for all three languages.

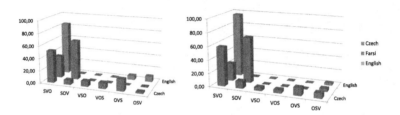

Fig. 3. Comparison of results – main clauses (left) and subordinated clauses (right)

3.5 Application of Results

The analysis of properties of the three languages described in this paper is definitely not a purely theoretical endeavor, it also has numerous practical consequences. One example of such consequence may be the creation of a test suite for a particular language. Unlike ordinary evaluation sets, which are in most cases randomly chosen data set aside from the training set, the test suites aim at more sophisticated selection of sentences or phenomena which should mirror their distribution in a given language. The guidelines for creating natural language test suites were mentioned for example in [8]. The method of corpus data analysis sketched in this paper may provide an important numerical input for particular language phenomena.

Another area where our method may be practically useful is the area of cross-lingual (or delexicalized) parsing where a parser trained on (one or more) syntactically annotated treebank(s) using non-lexical features is applied on a "similar" language with minimal available resources [17]. The notion of language similarity is crucial here: while it is often understood in terms of language relatedness (closely related languages are usually more or less similar) recent experiments show that even languages which are not related may bring useful information, see e.g. [11]. It is quite clear that in order to develop a similarity measure which would allow to determine the degree and the type of similarity, it is impossible to take into account all 151 phenomena of the WALS. One way is to focus on purely statistically-based approaches, like in [10]. Our experiment represents another, more linguistically-based approach to searching for a representative set of characteristics of natural languages.

4   Conclusions

The experiment described in this paper confirmed our initial hypothesis that a quantitative analysis of important linguistic phenomena based upon large scale syntactically annotated resources may bring interesting theoretical and practical conclusions. The ability to exploit a common annotation format of treebanks for queries analyzing individual linguistic phenomena across multiple languages brings observations which cannot be based upon a simple introspective analysis. Some examples of such observations are presented in this paper – the differences between the word order of subordinated clauses in Czech and Farsi compared to the word order of main clauses cannot be discovered solely on the basis of manual analysis of data: a slight shift in the frequency of constructions which are otherwise absolutely syntactically correct can be discovered only on the basis of quantitative data measured on a representative sample of a language.

The investigations described in this paper also represent a first step towards practical applications. In the future, we might be able to discover linguistic phenomena which are decisive for measuring the similarity of natural languages.

The future research will concentrate on two main directions. One is pretty obvious – to apply the queries used in this paper to a larger number of languages. The second one should investigate the possibility to create more detailed queries in PML-TQ enabling even deeper analysis of individual language phenomena.

Acknowledgments. This work has been using language resources developed, stored and distributed by the LINDAT/CLARIN project of the Ministry of Education of the Czech Republic (project LM2010013).

References

1. Bejček, E., Hajičová, E., Hajič, J., Jínová, P., Kettnerová, V., Kolářová, V., Mikulová, M., Mírovský, J., Nedoluzhko, A., Panevová, J., Poláková, L., Ševčíková, M., Štěpánek, J., Zikánová, Š.: Prague Dependency Treebank 3.0 (2013)
2. Dryer, M.S., Haspelmath, M.: The World Atlas of Language Structures Online. Harcourt, Brace and company, Leipzig (2005–2013). http://wals.info, Accessed on 28 June 2015

3. Futrell, R., Mahowald, K., Gibson, E.: Quantifying Word order freedom in dependency corpora. In: Proceedings of the International Conference on Dependency Linguistics (Depling 2015), Uppsala University, Uppsala, Sweden (2015)
4. Holan, T., Kuboň, V., Oliva, K., Plátek, M.: On complexity of word order. Les grammaires de dépendance - Traitement automatique des langues (TAL) **41**(1), 273–300 (2000)
5. Kuboň, V., Lopatková, M., Plátek, M.: On formalization of word order properties. In: Gelbukh, A. (ed.) CICLing 2012, Part I. LNCS, vol. 7181, pp. 130–141. Springer, Heidelberg (2012)
6. Lopatková, M., Homola, P., Klyueva, N.: Annotation of sentence structure: capturing the relationship between clauses in Czech sentences. Lang. Res. Eval. **46**(1), 25–36 (2012)
7. Marcus, M.P., Marcinkiewicz, M.A., Santorini, B.: Building a large annotated corpus of English: the penn treebank. Comput. Linguist. **19**, 313–330 (1993)
8. Oepen, S., Netter, K., Klein, J.: TSNLP - Test suites for natural language processing. CSLI Lecture Notes (1998)
9. Pajas, P., Štěpánek, J.: System for querying syntactically annotated corpora. In: Proceedings of the ACL-IJCNLP 2009 Software Demonstrations, pp. 33–36. Association for Computational Linguistics, Suntec, Singapore, August 2009
10. Rosa, R., Žabokrtský, Z.: KL_{cpos^3} - a Language Similarity Measure for Delexicalized Parser Transfer (2015)
11. Rosa, R., Žabokrtský, Z.: MSTParser Model interpolation for multi-source delexicalized transfer. In: Proceedings of the 14th International Conference on Parsing Technologies, pp. 71–75. Association for Computational Linguistics, Stroudsburg (2015)
12. Sapir, E.: Language: An Introduction to the Study of Speech. Harcourt Brace and Company, New York (1921). http://www.gutenberg.org/files/12629/12629-h/12629-h.htm
13. Saussure, F.: Course in General Linguistics. Open Court, La Salle (1983). (prepared by C. Bally and A. Sechehaye, translated by R. Harris)
14. Skalička, V.: Vývoj jazyka. Soubor statí. Státní pedagogické nakladatelství, Praha (1960)
15. Čermák, F.: Jazyk a jazykověda. Pražská imaginace, Ptraha (1994)
16. Zeman, D., Dušek, O., Mareček, D., Popel, M., Ramasamy, L., Štěpánek, J., Žabokrtský, Z., Hajič, J.: HamleDT: harmonized multi-language dependency treebank. Lang. Res. Eval. **48**(4), 601–637 (2014)
17. Zeman, D., Resnik, P.: Cross-language parser adaptation between related languages. In: IJCNLP 2008 Workshop on NLP for Less Privileged Languages, pp. 35–42. Asian Federation of Natural Language Processing, Hyderabad (2008)

Low-Level Features for Paraphrase Identification

Ekaterina Pronoza[✉] and Elena Yagunova

Saint-Petersburg State University, 7/9 Universitetskaya Nab.,
Saint-Petersburg, Russia
{katpronoza,iagounova.elena}@gmail.com

Abstract. This paper deals with the task of sentential paraphrase identification. We work with Russian but our approach can be applied to any other language with rich morphology and free word order. As part of our ParaPhraser.ru project, we construct a paraphrase corpus and then experiment with supervised methods of paraphrase identification. In this paper we focus on the low-level string, lexical and semantic features which unlike complex deep ones do not cause information noise and can serve as a solid basis for the development of an effective paraphrase identification system. Results of the experiments show that the features introduced in this paper improve the paraphrase identification model based solely on the standard low-level features or the optimized matrix metric used for corpus construction.

Keywords: Paraphrase identification · Low-level feature · Lexical feature · Semantic feature · Matrix similarity metric

1 Introduction

This paper deals with the task of sentential paraphrase identification which is challenging but helpful in many natural language processing (NLP) applications like plagiarism detection, question answering, authorship detection, information retrieval, text summarization, etc. Examples illustrating the use of paraphrase identification in such applications can be found in [6, 7, 15, 17, 25].

We work with Russian but our approach can be applied to any other language with rich morphology and free word order[1]. As part of our ParaPhraser.ru project, we construct a paraphrase corpus, and, having obtained labeled data, we experiment with supervised methods of paraphrase identification. Our corpus is collected from news headlines using an unsupervised metric and includes 3 types of paraphrases: precise paraphrases, loose paraphrases and non-paraphrases. It is annotated via crowdsourcing. This corpus is not a general-purpose one – we intend it to serve as a paraphrase resource for information extraction and text summarization tasks. The description of the corpus and its construction are given in the paper in press [21].

---

[1] In fact, our approach is not restricted to languages with these characteristics (e.g., it can be applied for English as well) but the features we propose in this paper take serious advantage of them, and therefore we recommend using our method for morphologically rich languages with free word order.

© Springer International Publishing Switzerland 2015
G. Sidorov and S.N. Galicia-Haro (Eds.): MICAI 2015, Part I, LNAI 9413, pp. 59–71, 2015.
DOI: 10.1007/978-3-319-27060-9_5

In this paper we experiment with one of the paraphrase identification approaches, namely, the one which uses string, lexical and semantic similarity features, leaving other methods (e.g., vector representations of words) for future work. We focus on simple "single" features (represented by numbers, not vectors), because they have good linguistics interpretation and do not cause information noise. They serve as a solid basis for the development of a paraphrase identification method and can be used in NLP applications. We call such features low-level. Although it might be terminologically incorrect, it is important for us to distinguish these "single" features from vector-based ones, and that is why we call them low-level.

Our aim is to propose an effective paraphrase identification method based on low-level features, and our strategy is as follows. We choose the unsupervised semantic similarity metric used for constructing the corpus as our first baseline and a set of typically used low-level features (calculating the overlap between the sentences) as our second baseline. We introduce another set of features most of which are based on the differences between the sentences, and extend the baselines with these features. It is shown that the model benefits from adding the newly introduced lexical, semantic and part-of-speech-based features.

Today, in sentential paraphrase identification, more and more approaches tend to employ either deep syntactic or vector-based features, while less attention is paid to the low-level ones. We believe that low-level features should not be neglected to such an extent because, despite their obvious simplicity, they can serve as a source of intuition for the key to the paraphrase identification problem. In this paper we focus on the low-level features based on the differences between the sentences (unlike other low-level approaches, based on the overlap between the sentences) which, we believe, lead us to the solution for the paraphrase classification problem.

2   Related Work

The approaches developed in sentential paraphrase identification usually either fall into one of the following groups or use a combination of the respective methods:

1. Low-level features: string overlap, lexical and simple semantic similarity metrics (according to the terminology specified in this paper).
2. Features based on the deep syntactic/semantic structure of the sentences.
3. Distributional models based on vector representations of words and phrases.

In Table 1 we present a brief overview of the low-level features typically used in paraphrase identification. The way these features are calculated usually varies in different papers (most common versions are presented in Table 1 for each feature).

Apart from the string and lexical features (Table 1), there is also a wide range of semantic similarity metrics based on WordNet [20], and most of them exploit hypernymy relations. The description of such metrics can be found, for example, in [13].

The second method is used by Das and Smith [9], Rus et al. [23], Socher et al. [28], etc. and often implies the use of dependency pairs as features (i.e., dependency relations overlap calculated as precision and recall, edit distances between syntactic parse trees, etc.). Sidorov et al. [27] propose to calculate the similarity between texts as the

Table 1. String and lexical features commonly used in paraphrase identification

Feature	Description	References
Sentence length difference (SLD)	The length difference in words or characters	[14,29]
Edit distance (word- or character-based)	The number of operations to transform one sentence into another	[5, 22, 30]
Word/n-gram/character n-gram overlap	The number of overlapping words/n-grams/character n-grams between the sentences	[1, 5, 12, 14, 16, 29]
BLEU precision	Weighted average of n-gram matches between the sentences	[1, 14, 22, 29, 30]
Longest Common Subsequence (LCS)	Length of the longest common sequence of words/characters shared by the sentences	[1, 8, 16, 22, 30]
Skip-grams	The number of overlapping non-contiguous n-grams (of a given length and with a given skip window)	[8, 16, 22]
Cardinal numbers	The number of matching cardinal numbers	[8, 16]
Proper names	The number of matching proper names	[8, 16]

similarity between their respective syntactic n-grams using tree edit distance. However, as such methods use the output of a syntactic parser, they propagate errors made by the parser. The third approach is based on the hypothesis that semantically close words occur in similar contexts. It is represented by count-based models (e.g., the ones based on Latent Semantic Analysis (LSA)) and predictive models like the ones implemented in Word2vec [18, 19]. According to a recent research [2], predictive models outperform count-based ones on a wide range of semantics tasks (semantic relatedness, synonym detection, concept categorization, etc.). The third method, based on vector representations of words, may also cause information noise, while the first method, employing so-called low-level features, does not have this drawback.

The best state-of-the-art result in paraphrase identification known to us (F1 = 85.96 %) is achieved by Ji and Eisenstein [14]. They use a combination of all the approaches described above and evaluate their method against Microsoft Research Paraphrase Corpus (MRPC) [11]. In paraphrase identification community it has become a standard practice to evaluate models against MRPC. It consists of 5801 English sentence pairs labeled as paraphrases and non-paraphrases. This corpus is collected from news clusters and is intended to be a general-purpose one. Introduced more than a decade ago, it has received a lot of criticism since then. Nevertheless it is used as a golden standard by the overwhelming majority of researchers in paraphrase community. Our approach is different: we do not solve an abstract paraphrase identification task – on the contrary, we build a corpus for specific NLP applications and aim to introduce a method which could be used in information extraction and text summarization.

We start with low-level string-based, lexical and semantic features to form a solid basis for our paraphrase identification model and further plan to expand the model by more complex features. Our string-based and lexical features include the ones typically used in paraphrase identification as well as the newly introduced ones. As for semantic features, mostly based on WordNet, there are no analogous resources (of sufficient size) for Russian known to us except for Yet Another RussNet (YARN) [4]. The latter, although lacking hypernymy relations, includes several thousands of synsets, and is a useful synonymy resource for our task. We should also bear in mind morphological issues: they might be of no importance for English, but for Russian the situation is the opposite. There exist a large number of form-based word families, consisting of the words with the same root and various affixes. The words within a family are usually semantically similar. That is why we employ the Russian word formation dictionary by Tihonov [31] while classifying paraphrase sentences.

Thus, starting with a number of simple but accurate low-level features, we are further going to expand them to develop an efficient paraphrase identification method which could be useful in different NLP tasks.

3 Data

Our paraphrase corpus consists of Russian sentence pairs collected from news headlines. Several Russian media sources are parsed every day in real time, their headlines are compared using an unsupervised metric and candidate pairs are included in the corpus. They are further evaluated via crowdsourcing and labeled as precise, loose or non-paraphrases. The corpus is constantly increasing in size. At the moment there are 5503 sentence pairs (1315 precise, 2346 loose and 1842 non-paraphrases).

4 Paraphrase Identification

4.1 Baselines

Our aim is to propose an effective paraphrase identification method based on low-level features. Our strategy is to start with the metric used to construct the corpus (baseline-1) and to expand it with new lexical and semantic features based on the differences between the two sentences. Our baseline-2 consists of the "standard" low-level features. We compare our two baselines and their combination with the full feature set (baseline-1 + baseline-2 + new features). All our features are simple and not noisy; we call them low-level because each of them is represented by a single number.

Our baseline-2 features are the ones typically used in paraphrase identification. They are calculated as described in Table 2, with some amendments. First of all, we divide the values of Cardinal numbers and Proper names[2] by the total number of words in the two sentences. In the SLD feature sentence length is calculated in words. We have 3 variants of BLEU feature, with 1- to 2-grams, 1- to 3-grams and 1- to 4-grams, and 2 variants of skip-grams (with and without preserving word order; skip window = 5). We calculate LCS on the word level and Levenshtein distance on the word and character levels. When calculating word overlap we only take into account notional words. We have two variants of this feature: with the number of notional overlapping

---

[2] We follow a simplified approach and consider any notional title cased word a Proper name.

words divided by (1) the total number of words and (2) the total number of notional words in the sentences. We calculate lemma overlap analogously. And finally, as n-gram overlap is already taken into account as part of the BLEU feature, we only calculate character n-gram overlap. It is incorporated into the Character BLEU feature, with 3- to 5-grams.

The unsupervised metric for corpus construction extends the one proposed by Fernando and Stevenson in 2008 [13]:

$$sim(\vec{a}, \vec{b}) = \frac{\vec{a}W\vec{b}}{|\vec{a}||\vec{b}|},$$

(1)

where W is a similarity matrix and $\vec{a}$ and $\vec{b}$ – word vectors of the two sentences. Each element w_{ij} of the matrix W represents semantic similarity between the words a_i and b_j. Diagonal elements are obviously equal to 1. Other elements are > 0 for similar and equal to 0 for different words. To capture semantic similarity, Fernando and Stevenson use a metric based on the "*is-a*" hierarchy from WordNet [13].

In fact, there exists a generalization of the metric (1) proposed by Sidorov et al. in 2014 [26]. They introduce several versions of soft cosine similarity, and the first version of this similarity measure ("soft_similarity$_1$") is calculated exactly as described in (1). Their soft_similarity$_1$ metric generalizes (1) in the sense that the elements of W can be calculated using any similarity measure (e.g., Sidorov et al. use Levenshtein distance while Fernando and Stevenson employ Word Net relations).

In our research semantic similarity metric is mainly based on the synonymy relation, but also captures string similarity. Unlike [13] and [26], in our approach the elements of W are calculated according to the list of rules. They are described in our paper about the construction of the paraphrase corpus [21]. A detailed description of the improved version of these rules is given in the next section of this paper.

In the baseline version of the similarity metric (baseline-1) we use a Russian synonymy dictionary (about 6 thousand articles). Each article in the dictionary can be treated as a synset, and for each pair of words we calculate the number of times they occur together in the same synset (intuition tells us that the similarity of words correlates with the portion of synsets they occur together in). To compute similarity between the synonyms, we use normalized pointwise Mutual Information (npmi) [3], Dice coefficient [10] and Jaccard index.

Normalized pointwise Mutual Information is calculated as follows:

$$npmi(x, y) = \frac{pmi(x, y)}{- \log_2[p(x, y)]}, pmi(x, y) = \log_2(\frac{p(x, y)}{p(x)p(y)}),$$

(2)

where $p(x)$ denotes relative frequency of x, etc. In our case $p(x)$ and $p(y)$ refer to the relative frequencies of words in the dictionary (in terms of synsets) and $p(x, y)$ to the portion of synsets where the words occur together. Npmi takes values from -1 to 1, but as we need them to be positive, we scale them by subtracting the minimal value and dividing the result by the maximal value. Following the same denotation (with the only difference that frequencies are absolute), we calculate Dice coefficient and Jaccard index:

$$Dice = \frac{2p(x,y)}{p(x)+p(y)} \tag{3}$$

$$Jaccard(x,y) = \frac{p(x,y)}{p(x)+p(y)-p(x,y)} \tag{4}$$

4.2 Extended Features

Advanced Matrix Similarity Metric. In this section we describe the improvements over our two baselines (which are the main results of this part of our research on paraphrase identification, following the work started in [21]).

First of all, we improve the matrix similarity metric (baseline-1) which was used for paraphrase corpus construction. The details of the procedure of its computation (for two words) are described in [21]. We take into account not only synonymy relations, but also substrings, prefixes and title cases. This metric can be further improved by several actions. First of all, we employ YARN [4] – an open WordNet-like thesaurus for Russian, which is about 8 times larger than the synonymy dictionary we initially used. Secondly, we use the Russian word formation dictionary by Tihonov [31] which contains about 3 thousand word families. Each word family includes several words with the same base form, or root, and different affixes.

Synonyms similarity score is calculated using Npmi, Dice and Jaccard coefficients. During our preliminary experiments with this extended metric Dice outperformed Npmi and Jaccard, and therefore was included in the final version of the metric. Finally, we tune the coefficients, and the overall metric calculation procedure is as follows:

- if the two words are identical and title cased, they are assigned 1.1 score (this is a slight bias towards the overlapping of named entities in the sentences);
- if they are just identical, they are assigned 1;
- if the words are synonyms, they are assigned their Dice score multiplied by 0.8;
- if the words belong to the same word formation family, they are assigned 0.8;
- if one of the words is a substring of the other and they are both at least 6 characters long, they are assigned the score equal to the length of the smaller word divided by the length of the larger word, and the score is multiplied by 0.7;
- if the two words have common prefix of at least 3 characters and both words are at least 6 characters long, they are assigned the score equal to the prefix length divided by the length of the lesser word and multiplied by 0.6;
- otherwise, the two words are considered absolutely different and are assigned 0.

Table 2. Comparison of baseline and extended matrix similarity metrics

	Initial similarity metric	Extended similarity metric
Average weighted F1, %	51.79	58.41

We evaluate baseline and modified metrics against our corpus in the 3-classes paraphrase classification task. We split the corpus into training, development and test sets (40 % /30 % /30 %), train Linear Support Vector Machine with default parameters[3] on the training set and evaluate the metrics against the development set.

According to the results presented in Table 2, the extended matrix similarity metric outperforms the initial one. It confirms the idea that the information about word formation families can improve our semantic metric (in the initial metric common prefix and substring scores serve as a rough replacement for the word family overlap).

String-based, Lexical and Semantic Features. Our task is to introduce a basis for the effective paraphrase identification method using low-level string, lexical and semantic features. We suppose that one of the main factors indicating the similarity of the sentences on the low level is the characteristics of the words the sentences differ in. If we examine the sentences and remove the overlapping words, is anything left in the sentences, and what is left?

All the extended low-level features used in our experiments (except for the word2vec-based ones) are obtained the following way: we lemmatize the two sentences and construct the intersection and the symmetric difference of the two sets of lemmas. The lemmas in the symmetric difference (we also call it periphery) are of interest to us as this is what the two sentences differ in.

Although we do not consider distributional features at this stage of the research, we still decided to employ word2vec-based model but as a semantic metric rather than a vector of features. We use it in 3 different ways: (1) first of all, we calculate cosine difference between sentence vectors (*word2vec* feature); (2) we also try a scheme when cosine similarity is calculated between the sentences with the intersecting words pruned (*word2vec_diff* feature); (3) and finally, we use word2vec's similarity between two words as a coefficient in the matrix similarity metric (*word2vec_matrix* feature). In the 1st and 2nd approaches only notional words and particles are considered: it is well known that a negative particle can change the meaning of the whole sentence.

To illustrate our features, we provide an example:

1 *В Красноярске обрушившаяся стена придавила автомобиль: двое погибших.*
   /In Krasnoyarsk a collapsed wall crushed an automobile: two dead. /
2 *При обрушении опорной стены в Красноярске погибли два человека.*
   /Two people died during the collapse of an abutment wall in Krasnoyarsk. /

---

[3] In this section we only show that the modified metric improves over our baseline: we do not solve the task of selecting the optimal classifier, and we simply choose SVM because it is well-known and widely used in NLP. Further in Sect. 5 we present the results obtained in the experiments with other classifiers.

Let us calculate each feature for the two given sentences (see Table 3).

Table 3. Example of features calculation

Feature	Value	Description
POS-based		
adj_periph	2	the number[a] of adjectives at the periphery
advb_periph	0	the number of adverbs at the periphery
noun_periph	3	the number of nouns at the periphery
verb_periph	1	the number of verbs at the periphery
Synonymy-, substring-, word family-based & lexical		
notion_periph	0.57	the number of the notional words at the periphery
substr	0.56	the sum of substring scores of the words from the two peripheries
substr_periph	0.35	the number of words at the periphery after the words with common prefixes are removed
notion_substr_periph	0.35	the number of notional words at the periphery after the words with common prefixes are removed
family	20	the number of pairs of words from the same families at the periphery
family_periph	0.53	the number of the words at the periphery after words from the same families are removed
notion_family_periph	0.53	the number of notional words at the periphery after words from the same families are removed
syn_periph	0.41	the number of the words at the periphery after synonyms are removed
notion_syn_periph	0.41	the number of notional words at the periphery after synonyms are removed
syn_periph_nest	0.18	the number of the words at the periphery after distant synonyms are removed
rest_periph	0	the number of the words at the periphery after synonyms, words with common substrings and overlapping word families are removed
notion_rest_periph	0	the number of notional words at the periphery after synonyms, words with common substrings and overlapping word families are removed
Asymmetry metric		
asym	0	if one of the sentences can be obtained by adding some words to the other sentences, it equals the number of such words (otherwise, 0).
Matrix similarity metric		
dice	0,57	improved matrix similarity metric initially introduced by Fernando and Stevenson
Word2vec-based		
word2vec	0,65	cosine similarity between two sentences represented by average vectors of their word vectors

(Continued)

Table 3. (*Continued*)

Feature	Value	Description
word2vec_diff	0,43	cosine similarity between two sentences represented by average vectors of their peripheral word vectors
word2vec_matrix	1,35	matrix similarity vectors with cosine similarity between word vectors instead of synonymy, substring and other scores

[a]All the features in this table which are calculated as the number of particular words are further divided by the total amount of words in the sentences.

Thus, we introduce 5 types of features, 3 of which are based on the differences between the sentences on the surface lexical, POS- and semantic levels. The other 2 groups of features consist of the simple representation of metrics based on predictive distributional models and an improved version of a semantic matrix similarity metric which performed quite well at constructing our paraphrase corpus.

5   Evaluation

In this section we describe the results of the experiments with our baselines and extended feature sets consisting of typical and the newly introduced low-level features.

To calculate feature values which involve lemmatization and POS-tagging, we use TreeTagger [24]. Word2vec model is trained on the news corpora from 4 different sources. The total news corpus consists of about 4.3 million sentences, 65.8 million tokens and contains news articles from 2012 and 2013 (which are not included in our paraphrase corpus). The context window size is 7 words (i.e., $(-7, +7)$), frequency threshold equals 4, and the dimensionality of feature vectors is set to 300.

All our experiments, including classifiers training, feature selection and parameters tuning, are conducted using scikit-learn.[4]

One of the recent directions for the improvement of standard classifiers involves ensembles of classifiers and we decided to adopt such an approach. We initially experimented with AdaBoost, Random Forests and Gradient Tree Boosting (GTB). The latter performed best, and we adopted it for our experiments.[5]

When constructing a feature set, we omit sentence pairs consisting of the same words in different order as they usually fall into the precise paraphrases class. We scale features, then split our dataset (5503 sentence pairs) into 2 parts: training set (70 %) and test set (30 %). To tune the GTB parameters, we perform grid search using scikit-learn. It is done via 5-fold cross-validation on the training set, and the classifier is tested against weighted F1. Then we evaluate two baseline models (based on the matrix

---

[4] http://scikit-learn.org .

[5] In this paper we do not attempt to select the optimal classifier – we leave the elaborate choice of it for future work.

similarity metric vs. on the commonly used shallow features), their combination, and the full feature set (matrix similarity metric + "standard" shallow features + the features we introduced in this paper) and compare the results (see Table 4).

Table 4. Results with baseline-1, baseline-2 and extended features[b]

Class	Precision, %	Recall, %	Average F1, %
Baseline-1 (1 feature)			
−1	88.48	55.36	68.11
0	52.28	74.78	61.54
1	52.89	42.86	47.35
average	64.92	60.22	60.31
Baseline-2 (14 features)			
−1	86.56	58.88	70.08
0	53.64	*81.90*	64.83
1	59.23	33.99	43.19
average	66.38	62.16	61.31
Baseline-1 + Baseline-2 (15 features)			
−1	83.70	59.58	69.61
0	53.69	78.78	63.86
1	60.78	38.18	46.90
average	65.79	62.16	61.67
Baseline-1 + Baseline-2 + New Features (40 features)			
−1	83.15	65.91	73.53
0	55.71	78.19	65.06
1	63.49	39.41	48.63
average	**67.09**	**64.40**	**63.94**

[b] Precise, loose and non-paraphrases are denoted by 1, 0 and −1 respectively.

It can be seen that the full feature set outperforms both baselines and their combination. It confirms that the paraphrase identification model can benefit from taking into account information about POS tags, word families (such metrics are generally useful for morphologically rich language) and distant synonyms.

As for the two baselines, their scores are similar, with baseline-2 (14 shallow metrics) being slightly better than baseline-1 (one optimized semantic similarity metric), and their combination does not improve over each particular baseline. It can also be noted that baseline-2 yields the best recall on loose paraphrases. Indeed, such features are intended to capture string and lexical overlap between the sentences but are probably not accurate enough and thus are better at detecting roughly similar sentences.

Our paraphrase identification task is a 3-classes classification problem, and it is therefore difficult to compare the introduced approach with other methods which are

Table 5. Binary classification task: results

Class	Precision, %	Recall, %	Average F1, %
0	84.07	63.09	72.09
1	82.82	93.70	87.92
average	**83.25**	**83.14**	**82.46**

usually aimed at solving a binary classification problem. Most approaches also work with English (and the models are evaluated against MRPC) which, compared to Russian, has poor morphology and rather strict word order. However, we still decided to make a rough comparison by uniting precise and loose paraphrases into one class and thus reducing our task to the binary classification problem. We again evaluated our extended model and obtained the following results (see Table 5).

With precise and loose paraphrases united into one class, our corpus has become severely unbalanced (3661 paraphrases and 1842 non-paraphrases) but still the results are comparable (if there could be any comparison at all) with the state-of-the-art results obtained on MRPC.

6 Conclusion and Future Work

In this paper we present an approach to paraphrase identification. Aiming at introducing an effective paraphrase identification method, we start with low-level features which, we believe, form a solid foundation for such a task. Our terminology is a bit different from the common one: our low-level features are the simple features represented by a single number. They include not only shallow string and lexical metrics, but also semantic similarity metrics based on various language resources. Such simple features do not cause information noise, like more complex ones.

Thus, our method is based on string, part-of-speech, lexical and semantic features most of which, to the best of our knowledge, were not previously used in the paraphrase identification task. The results of the experiments show that the "standard" model (the one with commonly used low-level features) benefits from adding these new features.

The proposed metrics are applied to the paraphrase classification task with 3 classes of paraphrases in Russian, but they can also be used for any morphologically rich language with free word order. In the nearest future we plan (1) to conduct a thorough misclassification analysis to improve our current method and (2) to develop a more fine-grained approach to paraphrase identification by introducing feature vectors based on vector space models and syntactic relations, e.g., via syntactic n-grams.

Acknowledgments. The authors acknowledge Saint-Petersburg State University for the research grant 30.38.305.2014.

References

1. Amaral, A.: Paraphrase identification and applications in finding answers in FAQ databases. https://fenix.tecnico.ulisboa.pt/downloadFile/395145918749/resumo.pdf
2. Baroni, M., Dinu, G., Kruszewski, G.: Don't count, predict! a systematic comparison of context-counting vs. context-predicting semantic vectors. In: Proceedings of the 52nd Annual Meeting of the Association for Computational Linguistics, pp. 238–247 (2014)
3. Bouma, G.: Normalized (Pointwise) mutual information in collocation extraction. In: Proceedings of the Biennial GSCL Conference (2009)
4. Braslavski, P., Ustalov, D., Mukhin, M.: A Spinning wheel for YARN: user interface for a crowdsourced thesaurus. In: Proceedings of the Demonstrations at the 14th Conference of the European Chapter of the Association for Computational Linguistics, pp. 101–104. Gothenburg, Sweden (2014)
5. Brockett, C., Dolan, B.: Support vector machines for paraphrase identification and corpus construction. In Proceedings of the 3rd International Workshop on Paraphrasing, pp. 1–8 (2005)
6. Burrows, S., Potthast, M., Stein, B.: Paraphrase acquisition via crowdsourcing and machine learning. ACM Trans. Intell. Syst. Technol. **4**(3), 43 (2013)
7. Callison-Burch, C.: Paraphrasing and Translation. Institute for Communicating and Collaborative Systems. School of Informatics, University of Edinburgh, Edinburgh (2007)
8. Chitra, A., Kumar, S.: Paraphrase identification using machine learning techniques. In: Proceedings of the 12th International Conference on Networking, VLSI and Signal Processing, pp. 245–249 (2010)
9. Das, D., Smith, N.A.: Paraphrase identification as probabilistic quasi-synchronous recognition. In: Proceedings of the Joint Conference of the 47th Annual Meeting of the Association for Computational Linguistics and of the 4th International Joint Conference on Natural Language Processing of the Asian Federation of Natural Language Processing (2009)
9. Dice, Lee R.: Measures of the amount of ecologic association between species. Ecology **26**(3), 297–302 (1945)
11. Dolan, W. B., Quirk, C., Brockett, C.: Unsupervised construction of large paraphrase corpora: exploiting massively parallel news sources. In: Proceedings of the 20th International Conference on Computational Linguistics, Geneva, Switzerland (2004)
12. Eyecioglu, A., Keller, B.: ASOBEK: Twitter paraphrase identification with simple overlap features and SVMs. In: Proceedings of the 9th International Workshop on Semantic Evaluation (SemEval 2015), pp. 64–69 (2015)
13. Fernando, S., Stevenson, M.: A semantic similarity approach to paraphrase detection. In: 11th Annual Research Colloqium on Computational Linguistics UK (CLUK 2008) (2008)
14. Ji, Y., Eisenstein, J.: Discriminative improvements to distributional sentence similarity. In: Proceedings of the Conference on Empirical Methods in Natural Language Processing (EMNLP) (2013)
15. Knight, K., Marcu, D.: Summarization beyond sentence extraction: a probabilistic approach to sentence compression. Artif. Intell. **139**(1), 91–107 (2002)
16. Kozareva, Z., Montoyo, A.: Paraphrase identification on the basis of supervised machine learning techniques. In: Salakoski, T., Ginter, F., Pyysalo, S., Pahikkala, T. (eds.) FinTAL 2006. LNCS (LNAI), vol. 4139, pp. 524–533. Springer, Heidelberg (2006)

17. McClendon, J.L., Mack, N.A., Hodges, L.F.: The use of paraphrase identification in the retrieval of appropriate responses for script based conversational agents. In: Proceedings of the Twenty-Seventh International Florida Artificial Intelligence Research Society Conference (2014)
18. Mikolov, T., Chen, K., Corrado, G., Dean, J.: Efficient estimation of word representations in vector space (2013). http://arxiv.org/abs/1301.3781/
19. Mikolov, T., Sutskever, I., Chen, K., Corrado, G.S., Dean, J.: Distributed representations of words and phrases and their compositionality. In: Advances in Neural Information Processing Systems, pp. 3111–3119 (2013)
20. Miller, G., Fellbaum, C.: Wordnet: An electronic lexical database. MIT Press, Cambridge (1998)
21. Pronoza, E., Yagunova, E., Pronoza, A.: Construction of a Russian paraphrase corpus: unsupervised paraphrase extraction. In: Proceedings of the 9th Summer School in Information Retrieval and Young Scientist Conference (2015). (in press)
22. Rajkumar, A., Chitra, A.: Paraphrase recognition using neural network classification. Int. J. Comput. Appl. 1(29), 42–47 (2010). ISSN: (0975 - 8887)
23. Rus, V., McCarthy, Ph. M., Lintean, M.C.: Paraphrase identification with lexico-syntactic graph subsumption. In: Proceedings of the Twenty-First International FLAIRS Conference, pp. 201–206 (2008)
24. Schmid, H.: Improvements in part-of-speech tagging with an application to German. In: Proceedings of the ACL SIGDAT-Workshop. Dublin, Ireland (1995)
25. Sidorov, G.: Non-linear construction of n-grams in computational linguistics: syntactic, filtered, and generalized n-grams, p. 166 (2013)
26. Sidorov, G., Gelbukh, A., Gómez-Adorno, H., Pinto, D.: Soft similarity and soft cosine measure: similarity of features in vector space model. Computación y Sistemas 18(3), 491–504 (2014)
27. Sidorov, G., Gómez-Adorno, H., Markov, I., Pinto, D., Loya, N.: Computing text similarity using tree edit distance. In: NAFIPS 2015 (accepted paper) (2015)
28. Socher, R., Huang, E.H., Pennington, J., Ng, A.Y., Manning, C.D.: Dynamic pooling and unfolding recursive autoencoders for paraphrase detection. In: Proceedings of the Conference on Neural Information Processing Systems (2011)
29. Wan, S., Dras, M., Dale, R., Paris, C.: Using dependency-based features to take the "Para-farce" out of paraphrase. In: Proceedings of the Australasian Language Technology Workshop, pp. 131–138 (2006)
30. Zhang, Y., Patrick, J.: Paraphrase identification by text canonicalization. In: Proceedings of the Australasian Language Technology Workshop, pp. 160–166 (2005)
31. Tihonov, A.N.: Slovoobrazovatelnij Slovar' Russkogo Yazika v Dvuh Tomah: Ok 145000 Slov. Moscow, Russkiy Yazik, vol. 1, 854 p., vol. 2, 885 p. (1985)

Multilingual Unsupervised Dependency Parsing with Unsupervised POS Tags

David Mareček[(✉)]

Faculty of Mathematics and Physics,
Institute of Formal and Applied Linguistics, Charles University in Prague,
Malostranské náměstí 25, 118 00 Prague, Czech Republic
marecek@ufal.mff.cuni.cz
http://ufal.mff.cuni.cz/david-marecek

Abstract. In this paper, we present experiments with unsupervised dependency parser without using any part-of-speech tags learned from manually annotated data. We use only unsupervised word-classes and therefore propose fully unsupervised approach of sentence structure induction from a raw text. We show that the results are not much worse than the results with supervised part-of-speech tags.

Keywords: Grammar induction · Unsupervised parsing · Word classes · Gibbs sampling

1 Introduction

In recent years, unsupervised methods for building structure of natural language sentences (sometimes called grammar induction), became very popular. Their advantage is that there is no need of manually annotated corpora (treebanks), which is very time consuming, and there are still many languages which has no, or very little such resources.

The unsupervised methods of course does not reach the same results as the supervised methods. However, it is not fair to compare the results comparing the output structures with the manually annotated treebanks, because the outputs of the unsupervised parsers can be linguistically plausible as well, even though the structure is completely different. Better comparison should be done in an extrinsic way in practical application, for example in machine translation.

Many of the ongoing unsupervised natural language parsers uses supervised part-of-speech annotation. Part-of-speech is a category of word assigned to each word in the corpus, e.g. noun, verb, adjective, adverb, preposition, conjunction, etc. This means that the sentences, on which the parser operates, must be pre-processed by manual annotation of part-of-speech tags, or by a supervised tagger, which is trained on another corpus, where the part-of-speech tags are annotated manually. An example of a sentence with manually assigned part-of-speech tags and dependency structure is shown in Fig. 1.

© Springer International Publishing Switzerland 2015
G. Sidorov and S.N. Galicia-Haro (Eds.): MICAI 2015, Part I, LNAI 9413, pp. 72–82, 2015.
DOI: 10.1007/978-3-319-27060-9_6

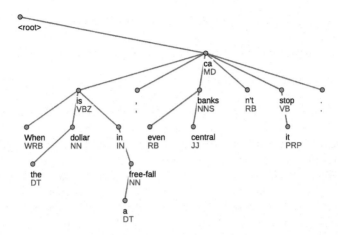

Fig. 1. Example of English dependency structure with manually annotated (gold) part-of-speech tags of the sentence *"When the dollar is in a free-fall, even central banks can't stop it."*

In this work, we do not use any part-of-speech annotation. We use only unsupervised word-classes, which are learned on big, raw (not annotated) language corpus. We show that the unsupervised parser using word classes performs only a bit worse than the one with supervised part-of-speech tags. However, its advantage is the complete independence on any annotated data for particular language.

2   Related Work

We can divide the area of unsupervised parsing research into several groups according to the extent of the degree of supervision.

In the first group, there are so-called delexicalised parsers. Such parsers are in fact supervised, but trained on another language for which a well annotated treebank exists (for example English Penn Treebank [9]). The condition is to use the same part-of-speech (POS) tagset both in the source and in the target language. The parser is then trained on the part-of-speech tags only, since the word forms are of course completely different [13]. The problem of different part-of-speech tagsets is often solved by mapping the original part-of-speech tags to a common (universal) part-of-speech tags. Nowadays the Google Universal part-of-speech tagset [14] become very popular and the part-of-speech mapping exists for many languages. Usage of the delexicalised parsers is therefore very easy.

In the second group, the parsers are also trained on another resource rich language, but they use a projection of dependency structures from the source language to the target language, instead of the common tagset. The procedure is following:

1. Parse the source language (e.g. English) of the parallel treebank using a supervised parser trained on a manually annotated treebank.

2. Project the tree structures of the source language into the target language using the word-alignment links between the words.
3. Train the supervised parser on the target-language projected trees.

See for example [4] for more details.

The third group contains the real unsupervised approaches, in which the grammar is induced from monolingual corpus without annotated structure. Many of these approaches however use the supervised part-of-speech tags. The state-of-the-art dependency parsers are described in [10,20]. Some of the parsers can be called "minimally supervised", because of using some external knowledge of how the individual part-of-speech tags behaves in the structure, for example, they say that the tags beginning by letter "V" represent verbs and therefore have higher probability to be in the root of the trees and govern other words (e.g. [15]). Another work only distinguish nouns by a condition that the most frequent tag in a given part-of-speech tagset is a tag for nouns [11].

The fully unsupervised parsing methods that uses only the raw input texts is for example the work [16]. The most interesting work so far is [17], where the word classes are used, however, only experiments on English are proposed there. In this work, we experiment with word classes as well, but we use different parser and test it over 25 languages, so that we could prove that the method is language universal.

3   Unsupervised Dependency Parser

In our experiments, we use the unsupervised parser described in [10]. This parser is based on Dependency Model with Valence, introduced by Klein and Manning [7] and then improved by Headden et al. [6] and Spitkovsky et al. [18,19]. The Dependency Model with Valence is a generative model using the following two types of probabilities:

– $P_{choose}(w_d|w_g, dir)$ is the probability of the dependent word w_d given the governing word w_g and the direction dir, which represents the *left* or *right* attachment. This generates the words (or the labels of nodes) in the dependency tree.
– $P_{stop}(\cdot|w_g, dir, adj)$, is the probability that a word w_g has another child in the direction dir. This generates the edges in the tree. "STOP" means that no more dependency edge from w_g is going to be generated in direction dir.

The parser uses Gibbs sampling method [5] for the inference of the dependency structures. The authors of the parser also show that it is also beneficial to estimate the P_{stop} probabilities for individual part-of-speech tags (or word classes) using so called reducibility principle [12]. These probabilities are estimated using a big raw not-annotated corpus. For more details, see the work [10][1]

---

[1] The software of the unsupervised parser described in [10] can be downloaded at http://ufal.mff.cuni.cz/udp.

Table 1. Properties of language resources used in our experiments. We used the testing parts of the treebanks only, both for inference and for testing.

Language	Treebank (testing part)		Wikipedia corpus	
	Sentences	Tokens	Sentences	Tokens
bg	398	5,934	926,063	17,879,640
bn	150	812	235,033	3,441,539
ca	1,724	53,015	926,175	26,067,761
cs	286	4,724	1,030,283	19,224,276
da	322	5,852	745,402	15,192,361
de	2,000	32,033	2,751,042	54,184,340
el	197	4,804	891,320	19,966,198
en	1,334	33,368	3,197,902	81,816,887
es	1,655	50,368	1,800,273	51,636,619
et	131	956	705,789	11,000,150
eu	1,121	14,284	767,766	13,347,995
fa	329	6,694	731,625	15,874,092
fi	430	5,425	1,146,736	17,055,452
hi	543	12,616	844,271	17,627,209
hu	390	7,344	1,389,060	24,937,181
it	249	5,096	1,285,478	37,672,036
la	316	4,789	176,421	3,223,187
nl	386	5,585	1,276,722	25,868,666
pt	288	5,867	1,155,717	30,589,567
ro	266	2,640	906,591	21,908,266
ru	402	3,458	1,613,637	32,628,923
sl	402	6,390	668,451	13,103,212
sv	389	5,656	935,304	18,300,709
te	150	597	507,778	7,492,388
tr	300	4,513	1,005,336	15,524,518

4   Data

For testing the dependency parser, we use data from HamleDT collection of treebanks [21]. This collection consists of 29 dependency treebanks, all of them are separated into training part and testing part. We took the testing part to do the inference and evaluation of the dependency trees.[2]

To estimate the p_{stop} probabilities, we use the large collections of Wikipedia articles provided by [8] containing between 10 and 80 million words for each language.

---

[2] We can do the inference and evaluation on the same data, since the correct annotation (labels and dependencies) is not used in the inference (unsupervised training).

The Wikipedia articles must be first preprocessed – tokenized and encoded in the same way as the particular treebank. For many languages, this is not a problem, since they use Latin alphabet and the segmentation into tokens can be simply done by segmentation on whitespaces and separation of the punctuation marks. However, a couple of problems have arisen:

- In the Arabic treebank, the tokenization is a part of morphological analysis, which cannot be used here, since we do not allow any supervised methods trained on any annotated data. The Arabic treebank is therefore not included into our experiments. Similar problem has arisen for Chinese. We did not find any automatic tokenizer which would tokenize the Wikipedia articles in the same way as it is in the treebank. So we excluded Chinese from the experiments as well.
- Tamil treebank has the texts transliterated into Latin, while the Wikipedia articles are not.
- The ancient Greek has very poor resources on Wikipedia and the treebank has also very unintelligible structure, so we excluded it as well.

Because of the aforementioned problems, we perform our experiments on 25 languages only. Their sizes are listed in Table 1.

5   Word Clustering

Instead of using part-of-speech tags for categorizing the words, we use the unsupervised word-clustering tool developed by Alex Clark [3].[3] The clustering is based on distributional and morphological information. It treats words not only as atoms, it goes deeper to the level of letters and takes into account also the similarity of prefixes or suffixes of words. Such morphological information can mainly improve the performance on rare words.

We do the inference of word clusters using both the corpora we have. For each language, the testing part of the treebank is joined with the articles from Wikipedia and such input is passed to the Clark's part-of-speech induction clustering tool. We run it several times for different number of clusters.

6   Experiments and Results

Each experiment comprises the following steps:

1. We tokenize the Wikipedia data in the same way as it is done in the treebank.
2. We concatenate the Wikipedia and the testing data and run the Clark's POS induction tool to make clusters. We perform the experiments for 25, 50, 100, and 200 clusters. From now, each word is categorized to one cluster.
3. We run the script *get_stop_priors.pl* (see [10] for detailed description) on the Wikipedia data with assigned word clusters, and extract the stop-probability estimates for individual clusters and direction. The stop-probability says, how likely a word belonging to a particular cluster has a left or a right dependent.

---

[3] The Clark's tool for unsupervised POS induction can be downloaded at http://www.cs.rhul.ac.uk/home/alexc/pos2.tar.gz.

4. We run the unsupervised parser [10] on the testing data and the inferred word-classes. We use the stop-probability estimates for the dependency tree inference.
5. We compare the resulting dependency structures with the original manually annotated treebank. We measure the accuracy: how many tokens have the correct parent (the parent is the same as in the original treebank).

In Table 2, there are the results for all the 25 languages (treebanks) and four different number of clusters used for unsupervised part-of-speech induction.

Table 2. Parsing accuracy against the manually annotated data for different number of word classes. The best results for each the languages are in bold. The average accuracy over all the languages is computed in the last row.

Punct. classes	Without punctuation				With punctuation			
	25	50	100	200	25	50	100	200
bg	**48.2**	47.9	42.8	34.6	31.4	36.5	26.8	26.3
bn	25.6	30.2	23.4	29.3	18.5	18.6	22.5	**42.1**
ca	**49.8**	49.2	48.4	46.9	43.3	45.1	44.0	45.5
cs	33.6	**38.0**	34.8	32.3	32.1	35.7	29.8	33.3
da	**49.0**	40.8	40.7	41.6	33.4	29.8	25.9	28.2
de	43.6	41.2	**47.6**	38.6	33.9	33.8	34.5	27.7
el	36.8	39.7	**45.1**	36.3	29.3	29.7	33.3	28.9
en	41.6	47.9	**50.5**	47.8	33.1	34.6	38.0	37.9
es	55.6	**60.1**	58.2	56.8	46.9	49.4	45.9	47.2
et	45.1	52.9	**55.9**	52.5	18.6	37.9	21.7	25.0
eu	26.7	28.7	**29.8**	26.0	13.1	26.5	18.4	12.4
fa	23.6	**28.3**	21.9	21.0	20.0	19.6	19.6	19.6
fi	36.4	**39.6**	38.0	31.9	32.8	34.9	25.5	23.6
hi	14.6	13.1	12.8	**25.7**	8.1	7.3	10.5	23.7
hu	**46.2**	24.1	23.4	26.1	33.6	33.8	19.0	16.7
it	40.4	**41.4**	34.6	30.8	30.9	27.2	23.2	23.1
la	22.1	24.1	20.7	17.8	20.1	**22.4**	18.3	16.9
nl	31.0	34.4	27.3	32.1	**47.5**	28.8	27.7	19.9
pt	**40.2**	31.4	30.0	23.5	26.6	20.8	19.0	16.4
ro	47.0	**51.0**	43.8	39.5	48.9	47.6	48.8	39.7
ru	49.4	**50.8**	48.2	47.4	49.3	49.9	49.5	48.3
sl	24.5	18.3	21.2	**28.2**	14.6	19.7	19.0	23.4
sv	54.8	54.9	49.2	46.4	49.5	38.3	37.1	32.8
te	29.2	29.8	32.0	37.1	33.5	26.8	26.1	**45.3**
tr	27.0	**55.0**	54.5	51.5	32.7	26.3	24.4	21.4
avg	37.7	**38.8**	37.4	36.1	31.3	31.2	28.3	29.0

The columns "with punctuation" use the treebanks in their original form. The results in the columns "without punctuation" are on the same texts, but with removed punctuation marks (full stops, commas, hyphens, colons, semicolons, quotations, etc.). The evaluation was also done on the treebank with removed punctuation marks. If a punctuation node was not a leaf in the dependency structure, all its dependents were attached to its parent, so that they did not remain unattached.

Table 3. Comparison of the best results (without punctuation) with parsing baselines and unsupervised parsing with gold part-of-speech tags.

	Left chain baseline	Right chain baseline	Unsup. POS 50 classes	Unsup. POS best classes	Gold POS
bg	18.8	32.5	47.9	*48.2*	**54.9**
bn	**52.0**	5.3	30.2	*30.2*	23.6
ca	23.8	25.9	49.2	*49.8*	**67.0**
cs	26.9	25.2	38.0	*38.0*	**52.4**
da	11.6	**41.9**	40.8	*49.0*	41.6
de	22.4	18.0	41.2	*47.6*	**52.4**
el	33.6	16.9	**39.7**	*45.1*	26.3
en	23.7	25.4	47.9	*50.5*	**55.4**
es	23.6	25.7	60.1	*60.1*	**61.1**
et	28.8	15.5	**52.9**	*55.9*	28.7
eu	24.6	**35.7**	28.7	*29.8*	35.5
fa	17.5	37.6	28.3	*28.3*	**49.0**
fi	34.3	13.9	**39.6**	*39.6*	33.3
hi	21.5	27.8	13.1	*25.7*	**39.4**
hu	**35.9**	6.2	24.1	*46.2*	34.0
it	24.0	**42.8**	41.4	*41.4*	39.4
la	18.6	18.4	24.1	*24.1*	**24.6**
nl	24.7	31.2	34.4	*34.4*	**47.5**
pt	22.9	27.0	31.4	*40.2*	**69.6**
ro	18.0	46.4	**51.0**	*51.0*	45.1
ru	23.3	35.5	**50.8**	*50.8*	40.0
sl	26.8	19.5	18.3	*28.2*	**35.7**
sv	24.8	24.3	**54.9**	*54.9*	54.5
te	**65.5**	2.5	29.8	*37.1*	10.8
tr	**65.5**	1.6	55.0	*55.8*	56.9
avg	27.8	24.4	38.9	*42.5*	**43.8**

We can see, that grammar induction of sentences including punctuation has worse results. It is often caused by the full stop, which is almost in all the sentences and can be easily treated as the root of the sentence, which is not correct with respect to the manual annotations. It is hard to say which number of clusters is ideal for unsupervised grammar induction. There are many languages, for which the number of clusters does not affect the accuracy much. For example Catalan and Russian have both the parsing accuracy on the level about 49 % for all sizes of classes. On the other hand, Turkish have only 27 % accuracy on 25 classes, but more then 51 % accuracy for 50, 100, and 200 classes. Hungarian and Portuguese achieved, however, the best results just on the 25 classes and the results on 50, 100, and 200 are much worse.

Table 3 shows the left-chain and the right-chain baselines and compare them with the unsupervised parsing results. In the left-chain, each word is attached to the following word and the last word is attached to the technical root. In the right-chain, each word is attached to the previous one.

Our best results from Table 2 (inference without punctuation and 50 word classes) are compared to the baselines. We also compare it to the unsupervised parsing with gold part-of-speech tags [10]. The fifth column (in italic) shows the best result over the number of classes for particular language. This is a possibly achievable score, if we were able to automatically infer the best number of classes for each language.

On average, the unsupervised parsing with unsupervised part-of-speech tags has a bit lower accuracy than with gold part-of-speech tags. However, there

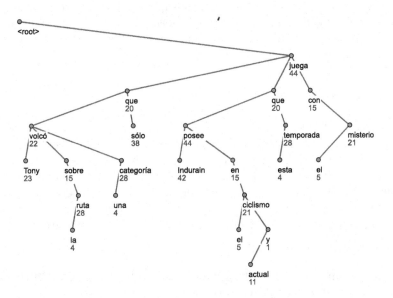

Fig. 2. Example Spanish sentence *"Tony volcó sobre la ruta una categoría que sólo Indurain posee en el ciclismo actual y que esta temporada juega con el misterio"*, parsed and tagged using 50 word-classes. Punctuation marks were removed.

are languages, on which the unsupervised tags perform much better: Greek, Estonian, Finnish, Italian, Romanian, Russian. Very good results and similar to the results with gold part-of-speech tags were achieved on e.g. Spanish (60.1 %), Swedish (54.9 %), and Turkish (55.0 %).

For curiosity, we have computed the correlation coefficient between the parsing results with unsupervised POS tags and the results with gold POS tags. The highest correlation (0.45) was for the best setting, i.e. for 50 classes and without punctuation. The lowest correlation (0.04) was for 200 classes and including punctuation.

There are languages, on which the accuracy of the parser is very low, for example Hindi (13.1 %), Slovenian (18.3 %), Latin (24.1 %), or Telugu (29.8 %). One reason could be lower amount of Wikipedia texts, from which the important stop-probability estimates are computed [10].

Some of the languages have higher baseline score than any of the parser results. It is hard to beat it for the strongly left-branching languages as Bengali, Telugu, or Turkish (Table 3).

7   Conclusions

We described an experiment with fully unsupervised dependency parsing using unsupervised word classes instead of supervised (or gold) part-of-speech tags. We tested it on 25 different languages (treebanks) and four different number of classes (25, 50, 100, and 200). When compared to the manually annotated dependency structures, the results of fully unsupervised parser are slightly worse then when we use gold part-of-speech tags, however, there are some languages, for which the unsupervisedly inferred word classes perform better that the gold, manually designed part-of-speech tags.

8   Future Work

In future, we would like to try also different part-of-speech induction tools, for example the Brown's clusters [2] or the clusters inferred by the Pitman-Yor process [1]. It would be also beneficial to automatically detect the best number of classes. Such mechanism would bring the results to the ones in the fifth column of Table 3. We would also like to bring the unsupervised dependency parsing to the practical applications, for example to the machine translation systems. Measuring the performance extrinsically is more fair than comparing it to the manual annotations.

Acknowledgments. This research has been supported by the grant no. GPP406/14/06548P of the Grant Agency of the Czech Republic.

References

1. Blunsom, P., Cohn, T.: A hierarchical Pitman-Yor process hmm for unsupervised part of speech induction. In: Proceedings of the 49th Annual Meeting of the Association for Computational Linguistics: Human Language Technologies, HLT 2011, vol. 1, pp. 865–874. Association for Computational Linguistics, Stroudsburg (2011). http://dl.acm.org/citation.cfm?id=2002472.2002582
2. Brown, P.F., deSouza, P.V., Mercer, R.L., Pietra, V.J.D., Lai, J.C.: Class-based n-gram models of natural language. Comput. Linguist. **18**(4), 467–479 (1992). http://dl.acm.org/citation.cfm?id=176313.176316
3. Clark, A.: Combining distributional and morphological information for part of speech induction. In: Proceedings of 10th EACL, pp. 59–66 (2003)
4. Ganchev, K., Gillenwater, J., Taskar, B.: Dependency grammar induction via bitext projection constraints. In: Proceedings of the Joint Conference of the 47th Annual Meeting of the ACL and the 4th International Joint Conference on Natural Language Processing of the AFNLP, ACL 2009, vol. 1, pp. 369–377. Association for Computational Linguistics, Stroudsburg (2009). http://dl.acm.org/citation.cfm?id=1687878.1687931
5. Gilks, W.R., Richardson, S., Spiegelhalter, D.J.: Markov Chain Monte Carlo in Practice. Interdisciplinary Statistics. Chapman & Hall, London (1996)
6. Headden III, W.P., Johnson, M., McClosky, D.: Improving unsupervised dependency parsing with richer contexts and smoothing. In: Proceedings of Human Language Technologies: The 2009 Annual Conference of the North American Chapter of the Association for Computational Linguistics, NAACL 2009, pp. 101–109. Association for Computational Linguistics, Stroudsburg (2009)
7. Klein, D., Manning, C.D.: Corpus-based induction of syntactic structure: models of dependency and constituency. In: Proceedings of the 42nd Annual Meeting on Association for Computational Linguistics, ACL 2004. Association for Computational Linguistics, Stroudsburg (2004)
8. Majliš, M., Žabokrtský, Z.: Language richness of the web. In: Proceedings of the Eight International Conference on Language Resources and Evaluation (LREC 2012). European Language Resources Association (ELRA), Istanbul, Turkey, May 2012
9. Marcus, M.P., Santorini, B., Marcinkiewicz, M.A.: Building a large annotated corpus of English: the penn treebank. Comput. Linguist. **19**(2), 313–330 (1994)
10. Mareček, D., Straka, M.: Stop-probability estimates computed on a large corpus improve unsupervised dependency parsing. In: Proceedings of the 51st Annual Meeting of the Association for Computational Linguistics, vol. 1 (Long Papers), pp. 281–290. Association for Computational Linguistics, Sofia, Bulgaria, August 2013
11. Mareček, D., Žabokrtský, Z.: Gibbs sampling with treeness constraint in unsupervised dependency parsing. In: Proceedings of RANLP Workshop on Robust Unsupervised and Semisupervised Methods in Natural Language Processing, pp. 1–8. Hissar, Bulgaria (2011)
12. Mareček, D., Žabokrtský, Z.: Exploiting reducibility in unsupervised dependency parsing. In: Proceedings of the 2012 Joint Conference on Empirical Methods in Natural Language Processing and Computational Natural Language Learning, EMNLP-CoNLL 2012, pp. 297–307. Association for Computational Linguistics, Stroudsburg (2012)

13. McDonald, R., Petrov, S., Hall, K.: Multi-source transfer of delexicalized dependency parsers. In: Proceedings of the Conference on Empirical Methods in Natural Language Processing, EMNLP 2011, pp. 62–72. Association for Computational Linguistics, Stroudsburg, July 2011. http://dl.acm.org/citation.cfm?id=2145432.2145440

14. Petrov, S., Das, D., McDonald, R.: A universal part-of-speech tagset. In: Chair, N.C.C., Choukri, K., Declerck, T., Doan, M.U., Maegaard, B., Mariani, J., Moreno, A., Odijk, J., Piperidis, S. (eds.) Proceedings of the Eight International Conference on Language Resources and Evaluation (LREC 2012). European Language Resources Association (ELRA), Istanbul, Turkey, May 2012

15. Rasooli, M.S., Faili, H.: Fast unsupervised dependency parsing with arc-standard transitions. In: Proceedings of the Joint Workshop on Unsupervised and Semi-Supervised Learning in NLP, ROBUS-UNSUP 2012, pp. 1–9. Association for Computational Linguistics, Stroudsburg (2012)

16. Seginer, Y.: Fast unsupervised incremental parsing. In: Proceedings of the 45th Annual Meeting of the Association of Computational Linguistics, pp. 384–391. Association for Computational Linguistics, Prague, Czech Republic (2007)

17. Spitkovsky, V.I., Alshawi, H., Chang, A.X., Jurafsky, D.: Unsupervised dependency parsing without gold part-of-speech tags. In: Proceedings of the 2011 Conference on Empirical Methods in Natural Language Processing (EMNLP 2011) (2011)

18. Spitkovsky, V.I., Alshawi, H., Jurafsky, D.: Punctuation: making a point in unsupervised dependency parsing. In: Proceedings of the Fifteenth Conference on Computational Natural Language Learning (CoNLL-2011) (2011)

19. Spitkovsky, V.I., Alshawi, H., Jurafsky, D.: Three dependency-and-boundary models for grammar induction. In: Proceedings of the 2012 Conference on Empirical Methods in Natural Language Processing and Computational Natural Language Learning (EMNLP-CoNLL 2012) (2012)

20. Spitkovsky, V.I., Alshawi, H., Jurafsky, D.: Breaking out of local optima with count transforms and model recombination: a study in grammar induction. In: Proceedings of the 2013 Conference on Empirical Methods in Natural Language Processing, pp. 1983–1995. Association for Computational Linguistics, Seattle, October 2013

21. Zeman, D., Mareček, D., Popel, M., Ramasamy, L., Štěpánek, J., Žabokrtský, Z., Hajič, J.: HamleDT: to parse or not to parse? In: Proceedings of the Eight International Conference on Language Resources and Evaluation (LREC 2012). European Language Resources Association (ELRA), Istanbul, Turkey (2012)

Term Dependence Statistical Measures for Information Retrieval Tasks

Francis C. Fernández-Reyes, Jorge Hermosillo Valadez[⊠],
and Yasel Garcés Suárez

Universidad Autónoma del Estado de Morelos, 62209 Cuernavaca, Mexico
{fcaridad,jhermosillo,ygarces}@uaem.mx

Abstract. In the information retrieval (IR) research community, it is commonly accepted that independence assumptions in probabilistic IR models are inaccurate. The need for modeling term dependencies has been stressed in the literature. However, little or nothing has been said on the statistical nature of these dependencies. We investigate statistical measures of term-to-query and document term-to-term pairs dependence, using several test collections. We show that document entropy is highly correlated to dependence, but that high ratios of linearly uncorrelated pairs, do not necessarily mean independent pairs. A robust IR model should then consider both dependence and independence phenomena.

Keywords: Information retrieval · Probability Relevance Framework · Statistical independence tests · Term correlations

1 Introduction

Information Retrieval (IR) is the research field responsible of the study and development of models that handle information collections (image, text, speech) in order to retrieve only the relevant documents for a user need [14].

In our work, we focus on probabilistic IR models, based on the probability of relevance given a document and a query. Illustrative examples are Binary Independence Retrieval (BIR) [13], Poisson [7] and BM25 [5,11] models. All of them share the assumptions of the Probability Relevance Framework (PRF) [11], which consists in assuming essentially term conditional independence.

It has been widely accepted that these independence assumptions are inaccurate. Indeed, the probability of using one term inside a paragraph may be affected by the appearance of other terms in the same context. A term dependency is any relationship between two or more terms. Examples of term dependencies include noun phrases, verb phrases, ordered and unordered windows, spans of text, or any sequence of n-grams [4].

Theoretical and experimental work on term dependency modeling has a long history [10,15]. Term dependencies have been modeled under different approaches, usually finding a compromise between suitable weighting (e.g. [6,9,16]) or better dependency modeling (e.g. [1,8,15]). In order to improve

© Springer International Publishing Switzerland 2015
G. Sidorov and S.N. Galicia-Haro (Eds.): MICAI 2015, Part I, LNAI 9413, pp. 83–94, 2015.
DOI: 10.1007/978-3-319-27060-9_7

effectiveness in ranked document retrieval, several term dependency retrieval models have been proposed in the literature, most of them over query terms [1,2,18].

While several works propose, as an open research problem, dependence modeling, no previous work demonstrates, in a statistical way, that dependence is a main issue for relevant document retrieval [12]. This is the main motivation of our work.

In this paper, we statistically investigate term-to-query and term-to-term independence in relevant and non-relevant documents. The questions we address are: To what extent is term-to-query dependence significant in relevant and non-relevant documents? What is the nature of this correlation and how is it related to relevance? How are term-to-term contextual co-occurrences correlated? A word on this last question is worth to mention. Context has proved to be useful in ranked retrieval [4]. By context we mean a sentence. Two words co-occurring within a sentence would not have the same semantic implication as if they co-occurred in a wider context (e.g. the start and the end of the document). This considerations could have serious implications on document relevance. Thus, we believe our work constitutes a further step towards a better understanding of dependency modeling issues in IR.

The structure of the paper is in order. Section 2 is devoted to define the problem and statistical independence tests techniques we need to use to accomplish our objectives. Section 3 describes the document collections used and the design of our independence tests. It also shows the main results obtained. Finally, Sect. 4 provides some conclusions and directions for future work.

2   Dependence Analysis

Current probabilistic models share the assumptions of independence of terms within a same document (Bag-Of-Words - BOW - assumption)[1] and conditional independence between the document and the query terms. Our main interest is to investigate these hypotheses as well as the nature of the dependence phenomena.

2.1   Problem Statement

Let: $D = \{d_1, d_2, ..., d_m\}$ be the documents set and $Q = \{q_1, q_2, ..., q_n\}$ be the queries set. Let consider $X_{d_i}, i = \overline{1, m}$ and $X_{q_j}, j = \overline{1, n}$ discrete random variables that represent each of the documents and queries respectively. The set of values that could take these variables are the vocabulary terms or words appearing in the document or the query they represent:

$$X_{d_i} = \{t_1^{d_i}, t_2^{d_i}, ..., t_p^{d_i}\} \tag{1}$$

---

[1] This independence assumption is not a marginal one, since the probability of a term, given the knowledge of relevance and the query, is not obtained from the summation over the marginal terms of the joint distribution (see [11] for details). It is unclear however, whether the assumption refers to a pairwise- or a mutually- independence hypothesis.

$$X_{q_j} = \{t_1^{q_j}, t_2^{q_j}, ..., t_q^{q_j}\} \tag{2}$$

where p and q represent the length of the document d_i and query q_j, respectively and $t_k^{d_i}, k = \overline{1, p}$ and $t_k^{q_j}, k = \overline{1, q}$ are the terms of the documents and the queries respectively.

Our aim is to answer the following questions:

1. What degree of dependency exists between pairs (X_{d_i}, X_{q_j}) in relevant and non-relevant documents? This would partially support the PRF hypothesis on conditional dependence of terms given the query.
2. What is the nature of (X_{d_i}, X_{q_j}) pairs correlations? We search for additional insight on those dependencies. Also, we look for possible correlations between the test collection features and relevance.
3. How are the terms of each document in a collection contextually correlated? We investigate on the statistical nature of term-to-term dependencies.

In answering questions 1 and 2, we will perform a test of independence together with a measurement of correlation. The first test assesses whether paired observations on two variables, expressed in a contingency table, are independent from each other. The second test resorts to measures of data association. For document term-to-term dependency (question 3) we propose a mutually-independence test as will be explained in Sect. 3.

Below we proceed firstly to explain some of the existing independence tests and select the most appropriate for the problem at hand. Then we explain the interest of using measures of association or correlation for our purposes.

2.2   Independence Tests

Two events are independent when no event influences the other. That is, knowing that one event has already occurred does not influence the probability that the other event will occur. There are different statistical independence tests for demonstrating that two or more random variables do not have correlations [17]. Statistical independence tests could be classified into parametric tests and non-parametric ones [17].

As we do not adjust the distribution of our data, we use a non-parametric statistical independence test and measures of association in order to demonstrate that, in fact, dependence exists between a query and a document.

Non-parametric Independence Tests. Non-parametric tests focus on order or ranking. There are several tests, we will show a few of them below and describe them shortly.

The Binomial Effect Size Display (BESD) is a method for summarizing the results of a study inside the pattern of a 2×2 contingency table. The cells in a BESD table will vary as a function of the value of the correlation coefficient, but they represent data as percent of the sample size. The method also assumes that subjects of study are broken down into two groups (which represent the two levels of the independent variable). Each row of the 2×2 contingency table represent each of the groups. The columns of the contingency table will represent the two levels of the dependent variable on which a subject can be categorized [17].

The Kolmogorov-Smirnov test compares the distributions of two unmatched groups. This test works by comparing the cumulative frequency distributions of the two groups. It is based on the principle that if there is a significant difference at any point along the two cumulative frequency distributions, it can be concluded there is a high likelihood that the samples are derived from different populations [17].

The Mann-Whitney U test is used with ordinal (rank-order) data. If the result of the Mann-Whitney U test is significant, it indicates there is a significant difference between the two sample medians, and as a result of the latter, it can be concluded there is a high likelihood that the samples represent populations with different median values. For Mann-Whitney U test, one of the following is true regardless of the rank-order data that are evaluated: (a) The data are in a rank-order format; or (b) The data have been transformed into a rank-order format from an interval ratio format [17].

The Chi-square test of independence is employed when a single sample is categorized on two dimensions (or variables). It is assumed that the sample is randomly selected from the population it represents. One of the variables comprises r categories (where $r \geq 2$) which are represented by the r rows of the contingency table, while the second variable comprises c categories (where $c \geq 2$) which are represented by the c columns of the contingency table. The chi-square test of independence evaluates the general hypothesis that the two variables are independent from each other. Another way of stating that two variables are independent of one another is to say that there is a zero correlation between them. A zero correlation indicates there is no way to predict in which category an observation will fall in one of the variables, if it is known which category the observation fell in the second variable [17].

We select Chi-square test because: (a) The experiment involves a single sample which is categorized on two dimensions, with each dimension comprising two mutually exclusive categories; and (b) The data comprises frequencies for each of the $r \times c$ cells in the contingency table.

2.3 Measures of Association or Correlation

Measures of association or correlation are descriptive statistical procedures which describe the relationship between two or more variables. We aim at testing which kind of dependence exists, most of the correlations measures try to find a linear dependence between two random variables.

Several measures of association exist: Pearson Product Moment, Spearman Correlation Coefficient, Kendall's Tau, Kendall's Coefficient of Concordance and

Goodman and Kruskal's Gamma. All but Pearson and Spearman assume normal distributions. Hence in order to develop our experiments we use the Pearson Product Moment and the Spearman Correlation Coefficient.

The Pearson Product Moment is calculated as follows [3]:

$$\rho_{X,Y} = \frac{cov(X,Y)}{\sigma_X \sigma_Y} \tag{3}$$

where X and Y are the two random variables for which the association measure is desired, $cov(X,Y)$ is the covariance between X and Y and σ_X, σ_Y stand for the standard deviation of each variable X and Y respectively. In our case, X, Y are X_{q_j}, X_{d_i} respectively.

The Spearman Correlation Coefficient is calculated as [19]:

$$\rho = 1 - \frac{6 \sum D^2}{N(N^2 - 1)} \tag{4}$$

Where D is the difference between the corresponding statistical $x-y$. N is the number of couples. The Spearman coefficient interpretation is the same as the Pearson correlation coefficient. Ranges from -1 to $+1$, indicate negative or positive associations respectively, zero, means no correlation but not independence.

Results are presented in the following section.

3   Experimental Design and Results

3.1   Test Collection Description

A test collection contains a set of documents, a set of information needs or queries, and relevance judgments. There are several test collections in order to evaluate information retrieval models. Small test collections are held by Glasgow repository[2].

We proceeded to make a characterization of the test collections used as Table 1 shows. The main features obtained were: number of documents, number of queries, subject, number of indexed terms, number of unique terms, entropy (η) based on vocabulary variability and average document length.

From Table 1 we observe that, even though the collections are of a specific domain, they have a high entropy in the vocabulary; which means that the words employed are very different form one document to another, letting us to conjecture that independence would predominate. Moreover, taking into account the ratio between the indexed and unique terms we can divide the test collections into two groups: LISA, NPL, TIME, Medline and ADI which have more than a half of unique terms and Cranfield, CACM and CISI which do not. Therefore, we hypothesize that either dependence must be more significant in the second group or the entropy is correlated somehow.

Below we proceed to design the independence test to demonstrate dependence between a document and a query and between terms inside a document.

---

[2] http://ir.dcs.gla.ac.uk/resources/test_collections/.

Table 1. Test collection characterization: *Docs.* refers to number of documents in the collection, *Qrs.* refers to number of queries in the collection, $\eta(C)$ refers to entropy value for the collection and *A.D.L* refers to average document length of the collection.

Collection	Docs.	Qrs	Subject	Indexed Terms	Unique Terms	$\eta(C)$	A.D.L
LISA	6 004	35	Library Science	44 448	31 225	0.680	46.95
NPL	11 429	64	Elec. Engineering	35 078	23 922	0.670	22.09
TIME	423	83	General articles	35 839	24 508	0.799	293.67
Medline	1 033	30	Biomedicine	13 254	7 167	0.729	83.97
ADI	82	35	Information Science	1 272	897	0.815	38.90
Cranfield	1 400	225	Aeronautics	7671	3 368	0.637	75.38
CACM	3 204	64	Computer Science	10 506	5 168	0.673	33.17
CISI	1 460	112	Information Retrieval	9 958	4 662	0.674	66.95

3.2   Independence Test Design

Query-to-term Dependence Test. In order to show dependence between the documents and the query, we use the two random variables already defined in Sect. 2.1: X_{d_i} and X_{q_j}.

For each combination of document and query, we count the occurrences of terms in the pair (X_{q_j}, X_{d_i}) then we construct a 2×2 contingency table by counting the terms appearing, and not, in the document and in the query submitted to processing (see Table 2).

Table 2. Contingency Table for document-to-query independence test

	X_{d_i}	$\neg X_{d_i}$
X_{q_j}	$|X_{q_j} \cap X_{d_i}|$	$|X_{q_j} \cap \neg X_{d_i}|$
$\neg X_{q_j}$	$|\neg X_{q_j} \cap X_{d_i}|$	$|\neg X_{q_j} \cap \neg X_{d_i}|$

We observe that we cannot assume that all cells will be greater than zero, because there are documents that do not contain terms of the query. Taking this into account we designed a Chi Square test with $\alpha = 0.05$, i.e. our results are produced with 95 % of confidence, based on the following hypotheses:

H_0: X_{q_j} and X_{d_i} are independent.
H_1: X_{q_j} and X_{d_i} are not independent.

Support for the alternative hypothesis suggests that the variables are related, even though the relationship is not necessarily causal, in the sense that one variable "causes" the other. Hence, if H_1 is validated, we also tried Pearson and Spearman Coefficients to find correlations between query and documents. All the results are shown and discussed in Sect. 3.3.

Term-to-term Dependence Test. In order to test the dependence between the terms in documents we turn to the mutually independent events concept: each event occurs independently of any intersection between the others. One event is the occurrence of a term, then we postulate a question: Does one event, in any way, affect the outcome of the other events? In other words, we are interested in knowing whether any two terms appear together or co-occur in more than one sentence. If the response is affirmative, we may conclude that events are dependent, otherwise, they are independent. This is formalized as follows: $\forall d_i, i = \overline{1, m}$: $\exists t_k, t_j \in d_i, k \neq j : P(t_k, t_j) \neq 0$

Our methodology design is explained next:

1. First we divide the document in sentences and find terms that appear in more than one sentence.
2. For each of the terms in those sentences we retrieve the rest of the terms that appear in more than one sentence. That is, we save the other terms co-occurring in more than one sentence.
3. If this set is empty, we may conclude that term occurrences are independent, otherwise, there exist terms that appear in conjunction in more than one sentence so they are dependent.
4. If an effect of dependence appears, it is enough to conclude that the occurrences of terms in the document are not mutually independent, based on the above concept.

For example, consider the following text passage taken from document 017 of TIMES collection:

> *Last week, as they studied the Nassau Accord between president Kennedy and prime minister Macmillan, europeans saw emerging the first outlines of the nuclear nato that the U.S. wants and will support... back from Nassau, the prime minister beamed that Britain now had a weapon that "will last a generation. The terms are very good."...*

The term *Nassau* co-occur always with *prime minister*, also *prime* co-occur with *minister*, in every case. Then, we can conclude that the terms occurrences in this document are not mutually independent.

3.3   Experimental Results Analysis

Query-to-term Dependence Results. For each test collection we create all combination pairs of queries and documents to populate the contingency Table 2. For each combination, we count how many dependence relationships are observed in relevant and non-relevant judgments. This is shown in Table 3. Tables 4 and 5 show the correlation results obtained from cases when some possible correlation exists due to appearance of terms in both query and documents.

We have special interest in the behavior of relevant documents for each query. Tables 3, 4 and 5 allow us to draw some interesting observations:

Table 3. Chi Square Test. The Table shows the % of document-query pairs in each category with a 95 % of confidence.

Collection	Total of pairs		Independent		Dependent	
	Rel	Not Rel	Rel	Not Rel	Rel	Not Rel
LISA	356	209 784	41.29	47.44	58.71	52.56
NPL	1 467	729 989	89.37	92.93	10.63	7.07
TIME	321	34 788	9.97	58.60	90.03	41.4
Medline	696	30 294	19.83	77.64	80.17	22.36
ADI	170	2 700	17.65	44.11	82.35	55.89
Cranfield	1 604	313 396	12.59	55.82	87.41	44.18
CACM	719	204 337	21.14	75.78	78.86	24.22
CISI	3 114	160 406	16.44	39.08	83.56	60.92

Table 4. Pearson Test. The Table shows the % of document-query pairs in each category with a 95 % confidence of being correlated.

Collection	Pairs with Possible Correlations		Uncorrelated		Correlated	
	Rel	Not Rel	Rel	Not Rel	Rel	Not Rel
LISA	203	108 507	69.95	70.25	30.05	29.75
NPL	132	41 149	87.12	88.7	12.88	11.3
TIME	289	14 376	36.68	81.05	63.32	18.95
Medline	556	6 767	62.41	88.8	37.59	11.2
ADI	140	1 511	65.0	68.7	35.0	31.3
Cranfield	1 604	313 396	40.4	7.48	59.6	92.52
CACM	513	34 923	65.89	82.46	34.11	17.54
CISI	2 603	98 547	63.81	77.7	36.19	22.3

1. Except for the NPL collection, the Chi Square test reveals that the proportion of relevant documents showing dependence is greater than those showing independence. The exception of NPL is striking and might suggest that a term association or synonymy phenomenon is having a strong impact on relevance for this collection.
2. The Pearson and Spearman tests indicate that the linear dependencies do not correspond to the dependence suggested by Chi Squared for relevant document-query pairs. Therefore non-linear correlations could be present and should be taken into account. This seems to be confirmed by both correlation tests.

   In order to investigate possible correlations between the test collection characteristics and our Chi Square results, we plot the relevance against entropy in Fig. 1. We did the same for the unique terms ratio in Fig. 2. Lines indicate the correlation inside each group of data (dependent and independent relevant pairs). Most of the

Table 5. Spearman Test. The Table shows the % of document-query pairs in each category with a 95 % confidence of being correlated.

Collection	Pairs with Possible Correlations		Uncorrelated		Correlated	
	Rel	Not Rel	Rel	No Rel	Rel	No Rel
LISA	203	108 507	64.53	66.68	35.47	33.32
NPL	132	41 149	86.36	86.6	13.64	13.4
TIME	289	14 376	32.53	68.71	67.47	31.29
Medline	556	6 767	59.89	86.09	40.11	13.91
ADI	140	1 511	67.86	73.2	32.14	26.8
Cranfield	1 604	313 396	21.95	1.8	78.05	98.2
CACM	513	34 923	63.55	82.07	36.45	17.93
CISI	2 603	98 547	65.5	77.72	34.5	22.28

pairs are dependent in all cases, except for the NPL collection. Some observations are derived from these graphs:

1. The more the collection distributes the vocabulary in the documents, the less independence and therefore the greater dependence emerges on relevant documents for different queries.
2. The more the collection has unique terms, the greater independence and therefore less dependence appears on relevant documents for different queries; which is consistent with the above observation.

These observations allow us suggesting that the term variability as reflected by entropy is highly correlated to the dependency phenomenon. This is also corroborated by the unique terms analysis and by the term-to-term analysis as we show now.

Term-to-term Dependence Results. Table 6 reflects that in most cases there are terms that co-occur inside the same document each time, and this evidence supports that the event joint independent hypothesis for probability computations

Table 6. Mutually exclusive events test

Collection	Independent	Dependent
LISA	1 819	4 185
NPL	11 429	0
TIME	39	384
Medline	110	923
ADI	17	65
Cranfield	226	1 174
CACM	1 941	1 263
CISI	259	1 201

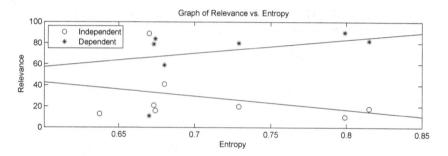

Fig. 1. Correlation for dependent and independent relevance documents for Entropy variable

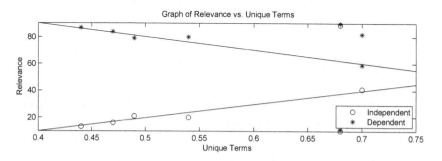

Fig. 2. Correlation for dependent and independent relevance documents for Unique Terms variable

should be reconsidered. NPL and CACM are the only collections that show more independent cases than dependent ones. We believe that this is due to the average size of the documents, and that the smaller this size the less likely is to find co-occurrences. More research should be done in this direction.

4 Conclusions

We investigated dependence between query and documents and between terms inside documents for 8 small collections. Our dependency and correlation tests have proved to be concluding in that there is indeed a dependence issue that should be addressed appropriately.

To the best of our knowledge there is no other study in the literature using statistical tools for proving dependence in IR. We arrived at some interesting conclusions:

1. Relevant documents are correlated with the entropy and the number of unique terms. Collections used had high entropy in the vocabulary; which means that the words employed are very different form one document to another.

2. Term variability as reflected in entropy is highly correlated to the dependency phenomenon. The more the collection distributes the vocabulary in the documents, the greater dependence emerges on relevant documents for different queries. The correlation tests provide information on linear relationships and as such they show higher ratios of linearly uncorrelated pairs. However, this does not necessarily mean independent pairs. A robust IR model should consider both dependence and independence phenomena. More research is needed on this issue.

3. In several collections there are terms that co-occur inside the same document each time, and this evidence supports the widely accepted claim that the event joint independent hypothesis for probability computations should be reconsidered. Accounting for dependency between terms that co-occur in a given context would allow us to identify semantic associations of terms that can be useful for query expansion. We believe this is an interesting research vein to be considered.

Much more remains to be investigated in relation to dependence modeling for IR tasks. Our results are modest but reveal that in order to improve IR systems performance, dependence issues should be addressed beyond proximity heuristics or pair co-occurrence models. Other mathematical tools should be used to produce more effective information retrieval models using statistical techniques accounting for distinct dependence phenomena.

Acknowledgement. This research was partially supported by the Consejo Nacional de Ciencia y Tecnologia (CONACYT) through the scholarship grant No. 296232.

References

1. Bendersky, M., Croft, W.B.: Modeling higher-order term dependencies in information retrieval using query hypergraphs. In: Proceedings of the 35th International ACM SIGIR Conference on Research and Development in Information Retrieval, SIGIR 2012, pp. 941–950. ACM, New York (2012). http://doi.acm.org/10.1145/2348283.2348408

2. Choi, S., Choi, J., Yoo, S., Kim, H., Lee, Y.: Semantic concept-enriched dependence model for medical information retrieval. J. Biomed. Inform. **47**, 18–27 (2014)

3. Galton, F.: Regression towards mediocrity in hereditary stature. J. Anthropol. Inst. G. B. Irel. **15**, 246–263 (1886). http://dx.doi.org/10.2307/2841583

4. Huston, S., Culpepper, J.S., Croft, W.B.: Indexing word sequences for ranked retrieval. ACM Trans. Inf. Syst. (TOIS) **32**(1), 3 (2014)

5. Jones, K.S., Walker, S., Robertson, S.E.: A probabilistic model of information retrieval: development and comparative experiments. Inf. Process. Manage. **36**(6), 779–808 (2000). http://dx.doi.org/10.1016/S0306-4573(00)00015-7

6. Lu, W., Robertson, S., MacFarlane, A.: Field-weighted XML retrieval based on BM25. In: Fuhr, N., Lalmas, M., Malik, S., Kazai, G. (eds.) INEX 2005. LNCS, vol. 3977, pp. 161–171. Springer, Heidelberg (2006)

7. Margulis, E.L.: N-poisson document modelling. In: Proceedings of the 15th Annual International ACM SIGIR Conference on Research and Development in Information Retrieval, SIGIR 1992, pp. 177–189. ACM, New York (1992). http://doi.acm.org/10.1145/133160.133195

8. Metzler, D., Croft, W.B.: A markov random field model for term dependencies. In: Proceedings of the 28th Annual International ACM SIGIR Conference on Research and Development in Information Retrieval, SIGIR 2005, pp. 472–479. ACM, New York (2005). http://doi.acm.org/10.1145/1076034.1076115

9. Mittendorf, E., Mateev, B., Schäuble, P.: Using the co-occurrence of words for retrieval weighting. Inf. Retr. **3**(3), 243–251 (2000). http://dx.doi.org/10.1023/A:1026520926673

10. Rijsbergen, C.V.: A theoretical basis for the use of cooccurrence data in information retrieval. J. Documentation **33**(2), 106–119 (1977). http://dx.doi.org/10.1108/eb026637

11. Robertson, S., Zaragoza, H.: The probabilistic relevance framework: BM25 and beyond. Found. Trends Inf. Retr. **3**(4), 333–389 (2009). http://dx.doi.org/10.1561/1500000019

12. Roelleke, T.: Information Retrieval Models: Foundations & Relationships. Synthesis Lectures on Information Concepts, Retrieval, and Services, Morgan & Claypool Publishers (2013). http://dx.doi.org/10.2200/S00494ED1V01Y201304ICR027

13. Roelleke, T., Wang, J., Robertson, S.: Probabilistic retrieval models and binary independence retrieval bir model. In: Liu, L., Zsu, M.T. (eds.) Encyclopedia of Database Systems, pp. 2156–2160. Springer, US (2009)

14. Saini, B., Singh, V., Kumar, S.: Information retrieval models and searching methodologies: Survey. Information Retrieval **1**(2) (2014)

15. Salton, G., Buckley, C., Yu, C.T.: An evaluation of term dependence models in information retrieval. In: Salton, G., Schneider, H.-J. (eds.) SIGIR 1982. lncs, vol. 146, pp. 151–173. Springer, Heidelberg (1982)

16. Salton, G., Buckley, C.: Term-weighting approaches in automatic text retrieval. Inf. Process. Manage. **24**(5), 513–523 (1988). http://dx.doi.org/10.1016/0306-4573(88)90021-0

17. Sheskin, D.J.: Handbook of Parametric and Nonparametric Statistical Procedures, 4th edn. Chapman & Hall/CRC, New York (2007)

18. Song, R., Yu, L., Wen, J.R., Hon, H.W.: A proximity probabilistic model for information retrieval. Technical report, Citeseer (2011)

19. Spearman, C.: The proof and measurement of association between two things. Am. J. Psychol. **15**, 88–103 (1904)

The Role of *n*-grams in Firstborns Identification

Gabriela Ramírez-de-la-Rosa[1](✉), Verónica Reyes-Meza[2],
Esaú Villatoro-Tello[1], Héctor Jiménez-Salazar[1],
Manuel Montes-y-Gómez[3], and Luis Villaseñor-Pineda[3]

[1] Information Technologies Department,
Universidad Autónoma Metropolitana (UAM) Unidad Cuajimalpa, Mexico, Mexico
{gramirez,evillatoro,hjimenez}@correo.cua.uam.mx
[2] Psychology Department, Universidad Popular Autónoma del Estado de Puebla
(UPAEP), Puebla, Mexico
veronica.reyes@upaep.mx
[3] Language Technologies Laboratory, Computational Sciences Department,
Instituto Nacional de Astrofísica Óptica y Electrónica (INAOE), Puebla, Mexico
{mmontesg,villasen}@ccc.inaoep.mx

Abstract. Psychologists have long theorized about the effects of birth order on intellectual development and verbal abilities. Several studies within the field of psychology have tried to prove such theories, however no concrete evidence has been found yet. Therefore, in this paper we present an empirical analysis on the pertinence of traditional Author Profiling techniques. Thus, we re-formulate the problem of identifying developed language abilities by firstborns as a classification problem. Particularly we measure the importance of *lexical* and *syntactic* features extracted from a set of 129 speech transcriptions, which were gathered from videos of approximately three minutes length each. Obtained results indicate that both bag of words *n*-grams and bag of part-of-speech *n*-grams are able to provide useful information for accurately characterize the language properties employed by firstborns and later-borns. Consequently, our performed experiments helped to validate the presence of distinct language abilities among firstborns and later-borns.

Keywords: Lexical features · Syntactic information · Text classification · Author profiling · Natural language processing

1 Introduction

The study of how birth order influence on several aspects of our lives has been an attractive long-established research topic in the field of psychology. According to some recent publications [1, 2], more than 2 K studies have been performed during the last four decades, aiming at finding why firstborns are normally compared favorably to later-borns. Generally, it is said that birth order plays a key role in the development of a wide variety of acquired abilities, such as cognition and language advantages as well as with the presence of some personality traits.

© Springer International Publishing Switzerland 2015
G. Sidorov and S.N. Galicia-Haro (Eds.): MICAI 2015, Part I, LNAI 9413, pp. 95–106, 2015.
DOI: 10.1007/978-3-319-27060-9_8

As part of his personality theory, Adler [3] suggested that the situation into which a person is born, such the family size, sex of siblings and birth order, plays an important role in our personality development. He was able to identify common characteristics among firstborns, such as their inclination to be more conservative, always follow the rules and submit to authority as well as more motivated to greater achievements than later-borns. However, more recent studies [1,2,4] state that such acquired abilities might be result of several other aspects in addition to the birth order, such as the social context in which a child was raised.

Regarding the birth order, in [1] it is mentioned that firstborns appear to have an early advantage in the development of vocabulary and syntax, but later-borns may have an advantage in the development of conversational skills. In addition, it has been found that later-borns tend to produce a higher number of personal pronouns than firstborns [5]. Nonetheless, most of the collected evidence of a general firstborn advantage in early vocabulary development comes from studies performed in children between 8 and 30 months old [1,5,6]. Consequently, there is no clear evidence with respect to longer term vocabulary differences associated with birth order, *i.e.,* there is no similar studies among teenagers neither among grown-ups.

Traditionally, in order to correlate the acquisition of some (*language*) abilities among firstborns and later-borns, psychologists apply a set of well-defined questionnaires to the subjects that are being analysed [2,3,7]. By means of measuring certain factors such as attitudes and opinions, tastes and interests, studies or work information, personality, etc., it is possible for psychologists draw conclusions regarding the behaviour, abilities or even the personality of firstborns. Although there are some works [5,7–9] that measure some language related factors (*e.g.,* vocabulary length, use of pronouns and some morphological cues, as well as some syntactic aspects), these works rely on the answers provided by the subjects in a predefined questionnaire, which is afterwards manually reviewed by psychologists.

In order to overcome some of the main drawbacks of the current work in the field of psychology, and with the aim of providing concrete evidence regarding the differences (until nowadays just barely proved) of language abilities among firstborns and later-borns, in this paper we present an empirical analysis on the pertinence of classical Author Profiling (AP) techniques for automatically identify firstborns. As known, AP main goal is to obtain as much information as possible from authors by means of analyzing their written text [10]. For instance, in [10,11] authors have shown that it is possible, to some extent, automatically detect *age* and *gender* from authors by just analyzing text documents written by them. More recent works have also proposed AP methods for detecting personality [12] and leadership orientation [13,14]. Therefore, in order to apply AP techniques, we *re*-formulate the problem of identifying language developed abilities by firstborns as a classification problem, *i.e.,* once we compute a set of *lexical* features (word n-grams) and *syntactic* features (POS n-grams), we train a classification model to distinguish firstborns from later-borns. Performed experiments among 129 subjects, between 11 and 16 years old, demonstrate that our proposed methodology is able to accurately characterize the language properties employed by firstborns and later-borns.

In this paper we investigate which of these features are more discriminative in the posed task. Consequently, the research questions we aim to answer are: *(i) Is the firstborns vs. later-borns detection a special case of AP?, (ii) Are there any differences in the use of lexical and syntactic elements between firstborns and later-borns?*

The rest of this document is organized as follows. Section 2 presents some related work concerning to the author profiling task. Section 3 describes some important aspects of the employed data for performing our experiments, as well as some statistics regarding this corpus. Then, Sect. 4 describes our followed methodology, experimental setup and obtained results. Next, Sect. 5 provides a brief discussion over our principal findings. Finally, Sect. 6 depicts our conclusions and some future work directions.

2   Related Work

As we have mentioned before, we face the problem of distinguish language characteristics developed by firstborns and later-borns as an Author Profiling task. In this context, our AP task is approached as a single-labeled classification problem, where the different profiles (*firstborns* vs. *later-borns*) stand for the target classes. It is important to mention that the posed problem is not addressed as a traditional thematic classification task neither as an Authorship Attribution task since we are not interested in the content of the documents nor in the specific writing style of each author. On the contrary, the AP methodology will allow us to model more general sociolinguistic features that apply to groups of authors, revealing how both type of authors use different linguistic features.

Most of the recent work on AP focuses in two particular problems that have gained interest during the last years, *i.e.,* identifying age an gender from writers [10,11]. However, there are more sophisticated problems that have been addressed using similar AP approaches, such as detecting personality traits [12] and leadership identification within social media [14]. At the end, the underlying idea behind AP techniques represent the likelihood of revealing as much as possible information from a given author's text (*e.g.,* age, gender, cultural background, native language, etc.). In general, the AP problem has been approached from different areas, including psychology where the work described in [15] might be considered amongst the most representative. Nevertheless, we will only explain some of the most representative approaches from the Natural Language Processing perspective.

Traditionally, the AP pipeline can be summarized in three steps: *(i)* extracting a specific set of features from the text, *(ii)* building an appropriate representation (*e.g.,* BoW-like) and, *(iii)* building a classification model for the target profiles (classes). It is worth mentioning that second and third steps are usually addressed by means of standard representations (*e.g.,* BoW) and well defined classifiers (*e.g.,* Support Vector Machines, Naïve Bayes, etc.) respectively. Nonetheless, the research community has centered its efforts in the first step, *i.e.,* determining which are the most pertinent set of features that can be extracted from the documents. Accordingly, most of the employed textual features used in AP fall into two general categories: lexical (*e.g.,* content and functional words), and syntactical (*e.g.,* POS tags). One of the first published works in demonstrating the pertinence of such features is [10], where a combination of function words and POS based features achieved approximately 80 % of accuracy for gender prediction in formally written texts from the National British Corpus.

In spite of the good results shown by [10], its proposed method it is not suitable for more dynamic environments, such as AP in social media (*e.g.,* blogs, chats, etc.). As shown by [11,14] social media represent a totally different matter, and traditional AP settings are no longer acceptable. In order to overcome such limitations, in [11] authors propose a representation for documents that capture discriminative and subprofile-specific information of terms. Under this representation, documents are represented in a low-dimensional (and discriminative) space which is non-sparse, allowing to obtain good results in the task of *gender* and *age* detection.

Although we are not proposing a new AP approach, our work differs from many of the previous research in that we want to determine if AP is possible within texts that represent literal transcriptions from spontaneous speech phenomena. Additionally, to the best of our knowledge, the evaluation of the firstborns advantage in the development of language abilities through AP techniques has never been addressed. Therefore, the main contributions of this work are: *(i)* an analysis on the pertinence of using *lexical* and *syntactic* features for the identification of firstborns, and *(ii)* the relevance of employing Natural Language Processing techniques within the field of Psychology, particularly for characterizing sociolinguistic features that apply to firstborns.

3 Data Set

The data set used in this research was gathered as part of a master's thesis on Biological Sciences at the Tlaxcala Biology Center of Conduct in the Autonomous University of Tlaxcala [16]. It is important to mention that all participants in the study were teenagers between 11 and 16 years old. Additionally, all participant subjects do not have any twins, half siblings. Their families are formed by more than one member, and none of the subjects reflected any psychiatric or neurological disorder. As part of the followed methodology for gathering the data, we needed an explicit authorization from the legal tutor of the teenagers in order to be part of this experiment, and upon approval by the ethics committee of the Ministry of Health and the Commission for Bioethics at the UNAM (National Autonomous University of Mexico).

As additional information from the analysed subjects, it is worth mentioning that they all belong to a small town in the state of Tlaxcala, Mexico; which is considered by the Secretary of Social Development of Mexico to be below the national average indicators of poverty and social vulnerability. Particularly, 54.7 % of the total population are moderate poverty and 6.2 % extreme poverty. This is an important indicator, since in the literature there are very few studies (if none) that have evaluated populations with these characteristics.

Even though determining birth order from a teenager might seem like an easy task for a psychologist, in practice it is not. Some factors such as being the child of a second marriage, or being a child that was born after five or more years from its last sibling, might alter the purpose of this type of studies. Therefore, after carefully interviewing all candidate subjects, we preserve the data from only 129 participants, from which 48 were labeled as firstborns and 81 as later-borns. In order to acquire the data we were interested in, *i.e.*, spontaneous speech, all participants were interviewed without previous warning. During the interview, subjects were asked to talk about themselves by a period of three minutes length. All interviews were recorded and manually transcribed. As mentioned before, we used the manual transcriptions as the only input for our performed experiments. It is worth mentioning that all the subjects are native Spanish speakers. Table 1 shows some statistics about the employed data set, such as number of words and vocabulary's size.

Table 1. Statistics describing the employed data set. For each profile it is shown the number of words and vocabulary elements. Between parenthesis appears the standard deviation, whilst between brackets there is the minimum and maximum number of words and vocabulary terms respectively.

Profiles	Subjects	Words (SD) [min, max]	Vocabulary (SD) [min, max]
Firstborns	48	274.2 ($\pm$ *123.9*) [56, 521]	120.5 ($\pm$ *42.4*) [42, 205]
Later-borns	81	235.0 ($\pm$ *114.0*) [52, 474]	109.4 ($\pm$ *42.8*) [30, 205]

4   Followed Methodology

As we have mentioned before, our main goal is finding out if there is a distinct use of language in teenagers, such that allows to categorize firstborns and later-borns. This hypothesis has been around in the psychological field for several years, therefore, our designed experiments are oriented to provide some evidence regarding such theory, *i.e.*, that developed language abilities by firstborns are different from those developed by later-borns. The hypothesis behind these experiments is that by means of employing AP techniques, using *lexical* and *syntactic* representations, we can generate good classification models for identifying firstborns subjects and later-borns, and therefore implicitly determine the pertinence of these attributes.

In the following subsections we first describe the general experimental setup and then, we describe in detail each of our performed experiments. In the first experiment we attempt to answer if lexical information by itself can accurately separate subjects into our two classes (firstborns *vs.* later-borns). In a second set of experiments we aim at determining if the use of some grammatical categories reveals patterns that differentiate firstborns language's use from later-borns language's use.

4.1   Experimental Setup

For all performed experiments we employed a BoW-like form of representation using boolean weighting scheme. We choose this representation because is appropriate when using few and short documents. In our case we have 129 transcriptions, each one with 250 words in average (see Table 1). To serve our purpose of analyzing the role of lexical and syntactic information, we use words and POS tags respectively, as atomic units for the BoW-like representation. For constructing the classification model we employed the Weka [17] implementation of the well-konwn Naïve Bayes algorithm and as a validation strategy a 10-*fold-cross-validation* technique.

The pre-processing done to each transcripts was simple and consisted on converting all the text into its lowercase form. We preserve all the stopwords given that these tokens convey important structural information that can be captured through both lexical and syntactic features.

A special treatment was given to all numbers or references to numbers in the transcriptions. Particularly, for our first experiment (analysis of lexical information) we replace all number references with a single tag in order to limit the vocabulary's growth. For our second experiment (employing syntactic information) we intentionally kept the references to numbers since the grammatical category can be different if they refer to an ordinal or cardinal number.

4.2   Lexical Features

This first experiment aims at considering only *lexical* information and determining if it is useful for identifying firstborns. To accomplish this goal, we employed words as atomic units. As we mentioned before, we used classical author profiling techniques to infer if this set of attributes can be useful in identifying firstborns. Accordingly, we experimented with the traditional bag of words representation, and using words n-grams with $n = 2, ..., 5$. As previous research works has shown, using word n-grams up to $n = 5$ allows the inclusion of contextual information, which might result useful for some AP tasks.

Figure 1 shows the obtained performance by this experiment when using different sizes of word n-grams. Notice that when $n = 1$ represents the traditional bag of words configuration, *i.e.*, using single words as features. We report our experimental results in terms of precision, recall and F-score metrics for the positive class only (*i.e.*, firstborns profile).

As can be observed in Fig. 1, adding a wider context to the documents' representation, *i.e.*, using a big value for n, affects the performance of the classification

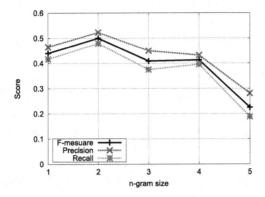

Fig. 1. Obtained performance of the classification model when word *n*-grams ($n = 1$ to $n = 5$) are employed as representation strategy.

Table 2. Results for the firstborns class obtained when IG is applied in order to select the most discriminative lexical features. First row depicts the performance of the best configuration, *i.e.*, word 2-grams. Second row shows obtained results when IG is applied to the best configuration, *i.e.*, word 2-grams+IG.

Features	Vocabulary	Performance metrics		
		Precision	Recall	F-measure
word 2-grams	14,086	0.52	0.48	0.50
word 2-grams+IG	367	1.00	0.88	0.93

process. On the contrary, when small values of *n* are employed ($n = 2$) a better performance is obtained. These results are mainly due to the length of the transcripts, thus it is very unlikely to find large *n*-grams within the texts.

It is worth remembering that our main goals were not directed to obtain a higher classification performance. Instead, by performing this experiment we wanted to validate the existence of some *lexical* features that allow to distinguish how firstborns are able to develop their language abilities in a different manner than later-borns. Accordingly, from the best configuration (*i.e.*, word 2−grams) we compute a new representation considering only the most discriminative features. In order to construct this new representation we employed a widely used attribute selection strategy, namely Information Gain (IG).

Table 2 shows the obtained performance when this reduced form of representation is employed. Even though the most discriminative features were determined through applying IG to the complete data set, obtained results indicate that; on the one hand, there are several *lexical* elements that represent noisy features during the classification process; on the other hand, results support the intuition on the existence of certain *lexical* units (word 2-grams) that help distinguishing how firstborns and later-borns develop their language skills. In other words, there are some combination of words that are specially linked to our different groups of authors.

In a later section (see Sect. 5) we present the list of the top ten more useful word n-grams.

4.3 Syntactic Features

As known, the lexicon contained within a document is usually attached to a particular thematic. Therefore, if we go up one level in the organization of the language production, we encounter the syntactic rules, which convey knowledge such as word's grammatical categories. Accordingly, grammatical categories generalize the use of the language and can enclose different lexical forms under a same category, for instance, the uses of *family, friend, dad, mom*, can be all be labelled as a *noun*.

The main goal of the experiments described in this section was to investigate if using grammatical categories for representing documents it would be possible to discriminate between firstborns and later-borns. Specifically, we used Part-Of-Speech (POS) tags to label each word on the transcripts with its grammatical category. Particularly, we employed the TreeTagger [18] tool with a set of 75 tags for the Spanish language[1].

Similarly to the experiments described in previous section, we build a BoW-like representation using n-grams as main features. For the experiments described here, we employed POS n-grams of different sizes (from $n = 1$ to $n = 10$). Intuitively, larger values of n provide information about the structure (syntax) employed by authors.

Figure 2 shows the obtained performance by the classification model when POS tags are used for representing documents. Contrary to the experiments from previous section, we can notice that for this experiments the context information (*i.e.,* syntactical information) is important, thus the best result was achieved when $n = 5$.

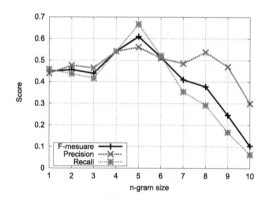

Fig. 2. Obtained performance of the classification model when POS n-grams ($n = 1$ to $n = 10$) are employed as representation strategy.

---

[1] The full set of POS tags and its descriptions can be found at http://www.cis.uni-muenchen.de/~schmid/tools/TreeTagger/data/spanish-tagset.txt.

Table 3. Results for the firstborn class obtained when IG is applied in order to select the most discriminative POS features. First row depicts the performance of the best configuration, *i.e.,* POS 5-grams. Second row shows obtained results when IG is applied to the best configuration, *i.e.,* POS 5-grams+IG.

Features	Vocabulary	Performance metrics		
		Precision	Recall	F-measure
POS 5-gram	25,551	0.56	0.67	0.61
POS 5-gram+IG	464	1.00	0.79	0.88

In the same way we did with the *lexical* features, we applied the IG strategy to preserve the most discriminative POS *n*-grams features. Similarly to the experiments shown in Table 2, Table 3 shows the obtained performance of our classification model after reducing the dimensionality of the POS 5-grams representation. As we have mentioned before, although we were not interested in achieving a higher classification performance, the obtained results help us validating the existence of a particular subset of POS *n*-grams features that are useful describing how firstborns and later-borns compose their sentences, *i.e.,* they have particular syntactic rules when producing spontaneous speech. In Sect. 5 we will discuss about the list of *n*-grams present on the top ten attributes with more discriminative information.

5   Analysis and Discussion

In order to contribute with the understanding of the features that are useful in distinguishing firstborns from later-borns, this section presents an initial analysis on the top ten lexical and syntactic patterns. Table 4 shows the top ten

Table 4. Top ten word 2-grams with more information gain.

Top ten word 2-grams	
Literal *n*-gram	Closest translation
y-la	*(and the)*
papá-y	*(dad and)*
la-música	*(the music)*
va-en	*(goes in)*
porque-por	*(because)*
un-tiempo	*(some time)*
este-me	*(this me)*
que-ya	*(already)*
no-le	*(do not)*
o-lo	*(or it)*

words 2-grams and Table 5 the top most discriminative POS 5-grams. Both tables include some examples with their respective closest translation.

Table 4 shows that the more discriminant words 2-grams are those that function as connectors of utterances. For instance, *y-la* (and the) is a connector that is used as link between clauses. A particular interesting word appearing in the list is *este* that is frequently used as filler. Moreover, the use of *porque por* might indicate hesitation in the speech, since both words in this case can mean *because*).

Regarding the syntactic attributes (see Table 5), our analysis revels the frequent use of personal pronouns. In addition, it is notorious the absence of nouns (NC) in the 5-grams, especially when the average length of a sentence in Spanish is around 5 words. Another interesting aspect to note is that some 5-grams do not have any verbs (*e.g.*, PREP-PPO-NC-CC-PPX, PREP-ART-NC-PREP-

Table 5. Top ten POS 5-grams with more information gain. The POS tag labels in this example are ADV (Adverbs), ART (Articles), CC (Coordinating conjunction), CSUBX (Subordinating conjunction underspecified for subord-type), NC (Common nouns), NEG (Negation), PPO (Possessive pronouns), PREP (Preprosition), PPX (Clitics and personal pronouns), VEinf (Verb *estar*. Finite), VLfin (Lexical verb. Finite) and VLinf (Lexical verb. Infinitive) (See footnote 1).

Top ten POS 5-grams	
Literal *n*-gram	Example (closest translation)
PPX-VLfin-VLinf-ART-NC	me gusta jugar el futbol
	(I like to play the footbal)
CSUBX-NEG-PPX-VLfin-ADV	porque no me gustaba mucho
	(because I did not liked much)
PREP-PPO-NC-CC-PPX	con mis amigos y yo
	(with my friends and I)
ART-NC-CC-PPX-VLfin	una persona y me desquito
	(one person and I take it out)
PPX-VLfin-ADV-VEinf-PREP	me gusta mucho estar en
	(I like a lot to being in)
PPO-NC-CC-PPX-VLfin	su trabajo o me pongo
	(its work or I start)
PREP-ART-NC-PREP-ART	en las calles con los
	(in the streets with the)
VLfin-PREP-VLinf-PREP-ART	voy a hacer en el
	(I'm going to do in the)
VLfin-ADV-VLinf-PREP-PPO	gusta mucho cantar con mis
	(like a lot singing with my)
NC-VLinf-PREP-ART-NC	este platicar con la gente
	(to talk with the people)

ART). We noticed that POS *n*-grams reveal some of the followed rules during the language production of teenagers. Although found patterns, both *lexical* and *syntactic*, represent interesting results, a deeper analysis on these patterns is needed in order to obtain a more complete interpretation of these language phenomena.

6   Conclusions

In this paper we have addressed one of the long-established problems within the psychology field, *i.e.,* determining if there are long term vocabulary and language production differences associated with birth order among teenagers. Accordingly, we faced this problem as an Author Profiling task, where we modeled general sociolinguistic features that apply to our particular group of authors, namely *firstborns* and *later-borns.*

Our performed experiments demonstrate that there is a strong relation between a subset of *lexical* and *syntactic* features and the order of birth. These findings represent an important contribution for both, psychological and computational research fields. On the one hand, we provided empirical evidence on the differences of language use among firstborns and later-borns, and on the other hand, this work represents the first attempt in employing NLP techniques, particularly traditional author profiling techniques, to this concrete problem.

Although good results were achieved, our future work is directed to perform a deeper analysis on found *lexical* and *syntactical* features. A detailed analysis on the meaning of these language production rules will imply an additional research work. In addition, we intend to study if using a higher level of abstraction in the analysis of the language, *i.e.,* a semantical representation, it would help to broaden the differences in the use of the language between these two populations.

Acknowledgement. This work was partially funded by CONACyT under the Thematic Networks program (Language Technologies Thematic Network project no. 260178). Additionally, authors would like to thank to INAOE, UAM Cuajimalpa, UPAEP and SNI-CONACyT for their support.

References

1. Hoff, E.: How social contexts support and shape language development. Dev. Rev. **26**, 55–88 (2006)
2. Healey, M.D., Ellisb, B.J.: Birth order, conscientiousness, and openness to experience tests of the family-niche model of personality using a within-family methodology. Evol. Hum. Behav. **28**, 55–59 (2007)
3. Adler, A.: The practice and Theory of Individual Psychology. Routledge, Trench, Trubner & Co., Ltd., New York (1927)
4. Gustafson, C.: The effects of birth order on personality. Master's thesis, Alfred Adler Graduate School (2010)
5. Oshima-Takane, Y., Goodz, E., Deverensky, J.L.: Birth order effects on early language development: do secondborn children learn from overheard speech? Child Dev. **67**, 621–634 (1996)

6. Zambrana, I.M., Ystrom, E., Pons, F.: Impact of gender, maternal education, and birth order on the dev. of language comprehension: a longitudinal study from 18–36 months of age. J. Dev. Behav. Pediatr **33**, 146–155 (2012)

7. Bornstein, M.H., Leach, D.B., Haynes, O.M.: Vocabulary competence in first and secondborn siblings of the same chronological age. J. Child Lang. **31**(4), 855–873 (2004)

8. Stolt, S., Haataja, L., Lapinleimu, H., Lehtonen, L.: Associations between lexicon and grammar at the end of the second year in finnish children. J. Child Lang. **36**(4), 779–806 (2009)

9. Keller, K., Troesch, L., Grob, A.: First-born siblings show better second language skills than later born siblings. Front. Psychol. **6**, 705 (2015)

10. Koppel, M., Argamon, S., Shimoni, A.R.: Automatically categorizing written texts by author gender. Literary Ling. Comput. **17**(4), 401–412 (2002)

11. López-Monroy, A.P., Montes-y Gómez, M., Escalante, H.J., Villaseñor-Pineda, L.: Using intra-profile information for author profiling. In: Working Notes for CLEF 2014 Conference, vol. 1180, pp. 1116–1120 (2014)

12. Youyou, W., Kosinski, M., Stillwell, D.: Computer-based personality judgments are more accurate than those made by humans. Proc. Nat. Acad. Sci. **112**(4), 1036–1040 (2015)

13. Ramírez-de-la-Rosa, G., Villatoro-Tello, E., Jiménez-Salazar, H., Sánchez-Sánchez, C.: Towards automatic detection of user influence in twitter by means of stylistic and behavioral features. In: Gelbukh, A., Espinoza, F.C., Galicia-Haro, S.N. (eds.) MICAI 2014, Part I. LNCS, vol. 8856, pp. 245–256. Springer, Heidelberg (2014)

14. Cossu, J.-V., Dugué, N., Labatut, V.: Detecting real-world influence through twitter (2015). https://hal.archives-ouvertes.fr/hal-01164453, (hal-01164453)

15. Pennebaker, J.W.: The Secret Life of Pronouns: What Our Words Say About Us. Bloomsbury USA (2011)

16. Cruz-Sanchez, K., Reyes-Meza, V., Martínez-Gómez, M., Hudson, R., Bautista-Ortega, A.: Effects of birth order and number of siblings on personality and stress response. Dev. Psychobiol. **57**, S:10 (2015)

17. Garner, S.R.: Weka: The waikato environment for knowledge analysis. In: Procceding of the New Zealand Computer Science Research Students Conference, pp. 57–64 (1995)

18. Schmid, H.: Probabilistic part-of-speech tagging using decision trees. In: Proceedings of the International Conference on New Methods in Language Processing, Manchester, UK (1994)

Recognition of Paralinguistic Information in Spoken Dialogue Systems for Elderly People

Humberto Pérez-Espinosa$^{(\boxtimes)}$ and Juan Martínez-Miranda

CONACYT Research Fellow – CICESE-UT3, Andador 10 #109,
Ciudad Del Conocimiento, 63173 Tepic, Nayarit, Mexico
{hperez,jmiranda}@cicese.mx
http://idi.cicese.mx/ut3/

Abstract. Different strategies are currently studied and applied with the objective to facilitate the acceptability and effective use of Ambient Assisted Living (AAL) applications. One of these strategies is the development of speech-based interfaces to facilitate the communication between the system and the user. In addition to the improvement of communication, the voice of the elder can be also used to automatically classify some paralinguistic phenomena associated with specific mental states and assess the quality of the interaction between the system and the target user. This paper presents our initial work in the construction of these classifiers using an existent spoken dialogue corpus. We present the performance obtained in our models using spoken dialogues from young and older users. We also discuss the further work to effectively integrate these models into AAL applications.

Keywords: Interactive systems · Speech analysis · Paralinguistic phenomena · Acoustic voice patterns

1 Introduction

The life expectancy has been increased during the past decades in an important number of countries around the world. Although this fact can be considered highly positive, one of the consequences associated to this phenomenon combined with a fertility decline in many countries is the increment of the population aged over 60. According to the United Nations in 1950, just 8 % of the world population was aged 60 years or over; by 2013 that proportion had risen to 12 % and it is expected to reach 21 % (more than 2 billion) in 2050 [1]. This increment brings new challenges in how to improve the quality of life of elderly people, alleviate pressure on formal care services and facilitate the tasks of their informal (family members, close relatives) caregivers. One strategy to address these challenges is the development and use of technologies to assist elder with living in their own home and execute their daily activities in their usual environment. Applications of ambient assisted living (AAL) focused on elderly users have been developed for different purposes including the monitoring of behavioral patterns and management of daily activities at home [2]; the promotion of social interaction [3];

© Springer International Publishing Switzerland 2015
G. Sidorov and S.N. Galicia-Haro (Eds.): MICAI 2015, Part I, LNAI 9413, pp. 107–117, 2015.
DOI: 10.1007/978-3-319-27060-9_9

support mobility [4] or the prevention and management of chronic conditions related with age [5] among some others. Most of these solutions need a continuous and long-term interaction with the users to effectively collect relevant data and to provide useful feedback. The nature of human-computer interaction in this context is a high priority factor to better achieve user acceptance of the technology. Therefore is crucial the design of user interactive interfaces taking into account the sensory, motor, and cognitive changes that are part of the ageing process to achieve the fullest potential of AAL applications. The use of speech and languages technologies is a straightforward interaction modality that could tackle the prevalence of chronic conditions and fine-motor problems in these users.

There is some evidence that elderly consider speech-based interaction less complicated when compared to more traditional forms of interaction, such as using a mouse or a keyboard. The potential of speech to provide a unified way of interacting with different services and different devices was also highly acknowledge by a set of older adults [6]. The development of speech-based interactive systems addressed to the elderly needs to be specifically tuned and configured according to the particular characteristics of their voice to achieve an acceptable performance. In this paper, we present our initial findings on the paralinguistic analysis of speech-based interaction aimed to identify relevant differences in acoustic variation between young and older adults. We argue that the recognition of these differences will contribute to better understand what acoustic characteristics in elder's voice need to be taken into account during the design of a more effective and adaptive speech-based AAL interactive systems. The rest of the paper is organized as follows: in Sect. 2 we put in context our research by presenting some of the related work. Section 3 describes the speech corpora used for experimentation analysis while Sect. 4 details the data analysis process. Then, Sects. 5 and 6 present relevant findings related to the automatic recognition of paralinguistic phenomena and some differences between young and older users respectively. Finally, Sect. 7 discusses some conclusions and further work.

2   Related Work

There have been some research efforts focused on the speech-based interaction of older speakers with computer systems. Some of them have studied mainly the differences between the linguistic aspects of the interaction of young and older adults. For example, the work presented in [7] was intended to answer research questions regarding the differences in the way younger and older users talk to a spoken dialogue system and the effect of system's help prompts. They collected a spoken dialogue corpus obtained from a Wizard-of-Oz (WoZ) scenario. The interactions were transcribed and also annotated with task success and task failure tags. Using a questionnaire, they were able to measure the quality of the spoken interactions with the system. One of the findings in this study was that younger users judged the interaction more positive than older users which also use a different speaking style, closer to human-human communication.

A similar study was carried out by Georgila et al. [8] where they also created a corpus of interactions of older and young users with a WoZ dialogue system. In this case, the corpus was designed and annotated in order to examine the impact of cognitive ageing on users' interactions with this kind of systems. They also find significant differences in the way young and older users interact with the system: older users have a richer vocabulary and use a larger variety of vocal acts. Another work on the topic of older users' interaction with computer systems, is the one by Miller et al. [9]. They wanted to determine which memory and cognitive abilities of older people predict successful interactions with an interactive voice response (IVR) system. They compared the performance of users on cognitive tests and the performance of users on IVR based tasks. An important finding was that adults aged 65 and older experience significant difficulties in interacting with IVR systems. The oldest adults experienced more difficulties and made more mistakes than younger participants. An interesting result was that both working and auditory memory independently predicted the performance of the users. These works present evidence on the differences and particularities between older and young users when interacting with computer systems. The results indicate that young and older people adapt in a different way how they interact with the systems. Furthermore, older users have more difficulties due to changes in cognitive abilities. All the presented works have addressed these differences based mainly on a linguistic analysis of the interactions and on some success measurements of the tasks performed by the users. In the present work, we study the differences in the interaction between young and older users with a spoken dialogue system but based on a paralinguistic analysis of the interactions. Our study does not analyze the words the participants use to interact with the system but the way they speak and the acoustic variations on their voices. We design our experiments based on two research questions:

What paralinguistic events are useful for measuring the success of interactions between computer systems and older users? Can a trained model automatically recognize these paralinguistic events?

Are there significant acoustic differences between these paralinguistic events when expressed by young people than when expressed by older users? How much necessary is to train the models to get a good performance with older users?

3   Data Used for Experimentation

In order to answer the above research questions, we used the JASMIN Speech Corpus collected by Cucchiarini [10]. This corpus was designed to cover a wide range of phonetic, phonological, and discourse phenomena. It contains recordings of children, non-natives and elderly people interacting in Dutch with a spoken dialogue system. The interactions took place in a WoZ scenario to induce the interactions. The corpus was automatically processed to obtain part-of-speech tagging and phonemic transcription. The collected corpus was manually processed to generate orthographic transcription and annotations of speech-based phenomena. The following 12 phenomena were transcribed: hesitations, filled pause, syllable lengthening, self-talk, loud speech, repetition of the system prompt, repetition of the user utterance, accent shift, paraphrasing, restart, hyper-articulation, understanding check. An interesting analysis made on this phenomena annotations was to consider which speaker moods could cause the different phenomena. The authors found three relevant states of mind: (A) Confusion, when speakers start talking to themselves; (B) Uncertainty, when speakers use longer pauses, filled pauses and repetitions in order to gain more time and (C) Frustration, when speakers yell or hyper-articulate. These states of mind were induced by asking unexpected or ambiguous questions, providing insufficient information on what is coming, asking questions with higher cognitive load, and refusing to understand the speaker. The annotations of these phenomena included in the JASMIN corpus are well suited for the purposes of our research. We hypothesize that speech-based phenomena could be used to measure the success of the interactions of elderly people with computer systems, in particular, AAL systems. The presence of these phenomena and their associated states of mind could be used as indicators that e.g. the elder is not having a fluid interaction with the system which can cause unsuccessful completion of the task or session and in the long-term, a poor system's acceptability and effectiveness.

4   Data Analysis

4.1   Segmentation of Interaction Recordings

The first step was to extract the audio segments that encompass the paralinguistic phenomena from the interactions recordings. This was automatically done using the PRAAT software (http://www.praat.org/) and the annotations provided in the JASMIN corpus. Figure 1 shows an example of the annotation of a self-talk segment. The labels shown in tier 3 at the bottom of the figure indicates the start (SLF) and the final (/SLF) of the phenomenon. The text ('k heb niet vers*a) that is shown in tier 2 is the transcription of the users utterances. Tier 1 is the transcription of the system utterances generated by a Text to Speech engine. In the upper panels of the figure, the speech signal is plotted in time and frequency domains. By using these annotations, the samples of phenomena were trimmed out from the complete interaction recordings. For the experiments reported in this work, we used 299 interaction recordings of Dutch speakers, 193 interaction recordings of Flanders speakers and 141 reading recordings of Dutch speakers. As shown in Table 1 we had a total of 7,405 speech segments, where each segment is a single sample of a speech phenomenon.

4.2   Phenomena Selection

We use two criteria to select the speech-based phenomena samples. Fist we classify the phenomena in two types, linguistic and paralinguistic. Linguistic phenomena are related with an interpretation of what the user has said. For example, Rephrasing and Understanding Check are linguistic phenomena, because it

Table 1. Number of segments obtained from interaction recordings

	Recorded sessions	Segments
Interaction NL	299	5,285
Interaction FL	193	1,845
Reading NL	141	275
Total	633	7,405

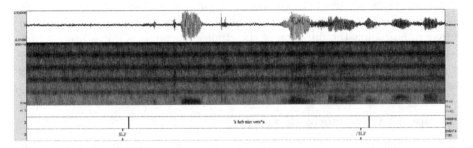

Fig. 1. Example of annotation of the paralinguistic phenomenon Self-Talk (SLF) in the JASMIN Corpus.

Table 2. Average duration of the speech-based phenomena

Speech-based phenomena	Type	Samples	Avg. duration
Rephrasing	Linguistic	254	2.25
Repetition of prompt	Linguistic	415	1.85
Repeat	Linguistic	777	1.73
Incomprehension	Linguistic	221	1.47
Understanding check	Linguistic	349	1.34
Very clear articulation	Para-linguistic	105	1.26
Restart	Para-linguistic	1,758	1.26
Self-talk	Para-linguistic	792	1.19
Stress shift	Para-linguistic	7	1.00
Shouting	Para-linguistic	137	0.66
Syllable lengthening	Para-linguistic	272	0.37
Filler	Para-linguistic	870	0.20

is needed a semantic interpretation of the words used to identify the phenomenon. On the other hand, Shouting and Hyper-articulation are paralinguistic phenomena because it is not important what the user said but only the way it was said. Paralinguistic elements in speech help to contextualize and suggest particular interpretations of verbal communication between people. Paralinguistic information complements the linguistic utterances in verbal communication beyond the content of the message itself. The paralinguistic analysis gives us valuable information about the characteristics and condition of the speaker, for example, clues about the emotional or mental state, user profile, personality traits, or symptoms of depression among some others can be obtained. In the second place, we paid attention in the average duration of the samples of each phenomenon. Our premise is that similar paralinguistic phenomena should have similar durations in order to be compared [11]. As we can see in Table 2 linguistic phenomena are longer than the paralinguistic ones. Furthermore, it is important to take into account the duration of the studied phenomena for future research about real-time automatic segmentation. We have 5 linguistic and 7 paralinguistic phenomena. We selected 6 out of the 7 paralinguistic phenomena discarding Stress shift due to the low number of samples.

4.3 Speech Characterization

We extracted a set of 6,552 acoustic features, mainly prosodic and spectral, using the software OpenSmile [12]. The feature set includes first order functions of low-level descriptors (LLD), such as FFT-Spectrum, Mel-Spectrum, MFCC, Pitch (Fundamental Frequency F0 by ACF), Energy, Spectral, LSP, their deltas and double deltas. Given that speech segments have different lengths, we applied 39 statistical functions to all indices of each sampling window. Some of the applied functions are extremes, regression, moments, percentiles, crossings, peaks, and means. In this way, no matter how many windows are contained in the sample, because the feature vector is composed by statistical functions calculated over all windows, maintaining a fixed number of attributes for each sample. Table 3 shows the number of attributes of each LLD.

5 Automatic Phenomena Recognition

Table 4 shows the results of automatic recognition of paralinguistic phenomena. We used a supervised scheme to create classification models trained on the JASMIN corpus data. We applied the machine-learning algorithm Support Vector Machines, as implemented in WEKA [13], for building a classifier. The model was evaluated by 10 fold cross validation (10-FCV) where 3,934 samples and 255 acoustic attributes were used. As we can see the phenomena with more samples have higher recognition performance. Restart and Filler, the phenomena with more samples 1,758 and 870 also had the highest F-Measure: 84.9 and 77.6 respectively. On the opposite side, Very clear articulation and Shouting which only have 105 and 137 samples also had de lowest F-Measure: 42.0 and 58.4 respectively.

Table 3. Set of acoustic features

LLD	Attribute
Prosodic	
LOG energy	117
Zero crossing rate	117
Probability of voicing	117
F0	234
Spectral	
MFCC	1,521
Mel Spectrum	3,042
Spectral energy in Bands	469
Spectral roll Off point	468
Spectral flux	117
Spectral centroid	117
Spectral max and min	233

Table 4. Recognition performance of unbalanced classes

Phenomenon	Samples	Precision	Recall	F-Measure
Very clear articulation	105	52.1	35.2	42.0
Restart	1,758	82.0	88.1	84.9
Self-Talk	792	71.7	67.0	69.3
Shouting	137	64.6	53.3	58.4
Syllabe lengthening	272	80.4	71.0	75.4
Filler	870	77.2	78.0	77.6

In Table 5 we show the results after balancing the number of samples of each class by applying a resampling algorithm. This method generates synthetic samples for minority classes and randomly chooses samples from majority classes. We obtain 60 % of the sample set. Synthetic samples were created for Very clear articulation and Shouting classes. For the rest of the classes, a subset of the original samples was selected. As expected, F-Measure increased for the classes with synthetic samples and, decreased for the trimmed classes. Interestingly the Self-Talk and Filler phenomenon shown better results though fewer samples were used. This experiment was done using a number of 1,252 samples and 216 acoustic attributes.

6   Differences Between Young and Older Speakers

One of the questions that our experiments aimed to address was to identify relevant differences in the paralinguistic phenomena between young and older

Table 5. Recognition performance after balancing classes

Phenomenon	Samples	Precision	Recall	F-Measure
Very clear articulation	185	79.3	84.9	82.0
Restart	228	78.1	79.8	79.0
Self-Talk	209	78.7	78.0	78.4
Shouting	203	86.8	87.7	87.3
Syllabe lengthening	205	87.1	85.4	86.2
Filler	222	82.7	77.5	80.0

adults. We perform two different experiments using the age of the speakers as the baseline. In the first experiment, we divided the dataset into two subsets: the first one containing the speeches of the individuals aged 75 and older and the second one containing the speeches of adults aged 74 and younger. In the second experiment, we used the speeches of adults aged 65 and older for the first subset and individuals aged 64 and younger for the second subset. The decision to perform two experiments using different ages as the baseline in older adults was based on the evidence that there are acoustic properties that significantly changes as individual ages [14]. The execution of both experiments allows us to compare the performance of the models trained with older and younger voices and to measure the impact of these changes in the automatic recognition of the paralinguistic phenomena.

Table 6 shows the results of both experiments. An interesting finding has been that although the classification performance decreased when the classifiers are trained with the data of young adults and then tested using data from older adults, the obtained performance of the classifiers is still acceptable (above 74 % of precision in both cases). We can argue that although is desirable to get enough set of data with samples of the targeted users for the training of classifiers i.e. elderly people of different ages, it is also possible achieve an acceptable performance training the models with samples of younger adults.

This is important when building speech interfaces in AAL scenarios where there is no available pre-collected data of the target population. For the assessment of successful interactions based on paralinguistic phenomena, initial prototypes can be deployed using speech corpus from public databases and then refine them with collected samples of the target users. Experimentation results show that the datasets containing the voice samples of older users had a better recognition performance. The older than 74 and older than 65 datasets obtained an F-Measure of 81.1 and 80.7 respectively when they were evaluated by 10-FCV. Meanwhile, the younger than 74 and younger than 65 datasets obtained an F-Measure of 76.4 and 77.2 respectively.

Table 6. Recognition performance comparing young and elder speakers

Data set	Validation	Precision	Recall	F-Measure
Older than 74	10-FCV	81.2	81.6	81.1
Younger than 74	10-FCV	76.3	76.9	76.4
Younger than 74	60 % Split	77.2	77.4	77.0
Younger than 74	Older than 74	76.1	76.0	75.6
Older than 65	10-FCV	80.8	81.3	80.7
Younger than 65	10-FCV	77.0	77.6	77.2
Younger than 65	60 % Split	77.1	77.0	76.9
Younger than 65	Older than 65	74.4	73.9	73.6

7   Conclusions

The automatic recognition of paralinguistic phenomena in speech-based user interfaces can be used as an indicator to assess how much successful (and in consequence the level of acceptability) is the interaction between the system and the user. This is particularly important in AAL applications due to the special characteristics of the target users. We described the work performed for the automatic recognition of paralinguistic phenomena using the JASMIN corpus, which include samples of young and older adults. From the obtained results, we can conclude that paralinguistic phenomena are recognizable using automatic methods with an acceptable accuracy rate. The recognition models can be used in interactive systems to infer the states of mind of the users based on the occurrence of these phenomena. Restart, Filler and Syllable Lengthening are the phenomena with the best recognition performance. These three phenomena are good indicators of a hesitation state of mind as they are expressions used when the speaker has doubts about what to do next and when looking for ways of taking time.

Very clear articulation and Shouting are not frequent phenomena during the interaction, but they have good recognition performance when recognition models are trained with balanced classes. These phenomena are good indicators for a frustration state of mind. The phenomenon Self-Talk is a frequent phenomenon related to confusion state of mind but, it has been difficult to recognize, even when classes are balanced. In our experiments, we have found good paralinguistic indicators for two (hesitation and frustration) of the three states of mind induced in the JASMIN corpus. During the experiments, when using sets of data divided by the age of the speakers, we verified that there are not significant acoustic differences between the paralinguistic phenomena when expressed by young and older users. The same acoustic features showed good discrimination properties when used with young and older speakers. Furthermore, the models trained on young speakers showed acceptable recognition performance when tested with older speakers.

Thus, we can conclude that the studied paralinguistic phenomena studied can be automatically recognized when expressed by elderly people, even when the recognition models are trained with samples of younger speakers. Nevertheless, the best recognition performance is obtained when using age-specific recognition models. In order to integrate the developed models for paralinguistic phenomena recognition into interactive systems, it is necessary the development of an automatic speech segmentation method. In the JASMIN corpus, a person performed this segmentation at hand, but it is necessary to implement an automatic mechanism that allows the effective integration of the developed models into AAL applications. The objective of such method will be to capture in separated audio samples the time lapse when the phenomena occur during the conversation.

Another topic to be further explored is the development of a method to evaluate the quality of the interaction between the user and the system based on the occurrence, frequency and appearance order of the paralinguistic phenomena and their associated mental state(s). This evaluation needs to be continuously updated along the interaction and would be used as a complementary input for the background application to determine the next actions to perform during the session with the user. Finally, transfer learning and semi-supervised machine learning techniques will be also explored to evaluate if the current performance of the trained models can be improved.

Acknowledgements. This research work has been carried out in the context of the "Cátedras CONACyT" programme funded by the Mexican National Research Council (CONACyT).

References

1. United Nations. World Population Prospects: The 2012 Revision, Highlights and Advance Tables. Department of Economic and Social Affairs, Population Division (2013). Working Paper No. ESA/P/WP.228
2. Ullberg, J., Loutfi, A., Pecora, F.: A customizable approach for monitoring activities of elderly users in their homes. In: Mazzeo, P.L., Spagnolo, P., Moeslund, T.B. (eds.) AMMDS 2014. LNCS, vol. 8703, pp. 13–25. Springer, Heidelberg (2014)
3. Bisiani, R., et al.: Fostering social interaction of home-bound elderly people: the *easyreach* system. In: Ali, M., Bosse, T., Hindriks, K.V., Hoogendoorn, M., Jonker, C.M., Treur, J. (eds.) IEA/AIE 2013. LNCS, vol. 7906, pp. 33–42. Springer, Heidelberg (2013)
4. Angeletou, A., Garschall, M., Hochleitner, C., Tscheligi, M.: I need to know, i cannot, i don't understand: older users' requirements for a navigation application? In: Assistive Technology: From Research to Practice, vol. 33, pp. 34–39. IOS Press (2013)
5. Tabak, M., Burkow, T., Ciobanu, I., Berteanu, M., Hermens., H.J.: Acceptance and usability of an ambulant activity coach for patients with COPD. In: Proceedings of the IADIS International Conference e-Health 2013, 24–26 July 2013, Prague, Czech Republic, pp. 61–68. IADIS Press (2013). ISBN 978-972-8939-87-8
6. Schlögl, S., Garschall, M., Tscheligi, M.: Designing natural language user interfaces with elderly users. In: Workshop on Designing Speech and Language Interactions, CHI 2014, Toronto (2014)

7. Möller, S., Gödde, F., Wolters, M.: A corpus analysis of spoken smart- home interactions with older users. In: Proceedings of the 6th International Conference on Language Resources and Evaluation, pp. 735–740 (2008)

8. Georgila, K., Wolters, M., Karaiskos, V., Kronenthal, M., Logie, R., Mayo, N., Watson, M.: A fully annotated corpus for studying the effect of cognitive ageing on users' interactions with spoken dialogue systems. In: Proceedings of the 6th International Conference on Language Resources and Evaluation, pp. 938–944 (2008)

9. Miller, D., Gagnon, M., Talbot, V., Messier, C.: Predictors of successful communication with interactive voice response systems in older people. J. Gerontol. Ser. B: Psychol. Sci. Soc. Sci. 68(4), 495–503 (2013)

10. Cucchiarini, C.: The JASMIN speech corpus: recordings of children, non-natives and elderly people. In: Spyns, P., Odijk, J. (eds.) Essential Speech and Language Technology for Dutch, pp. 43–59. Springer, Heidelberg (2013)

11. Batliner, A., Steidl, S., Seppi, D., Schuller, B.: Segmenting into adequate units for automatic recognition of emotion-related episodes: a speech- based approach. Adv. Hum. Comput. Interact. 2010, 15 (2010). doi:10.1155/2010/782802. Article ID 782802

12. Eyben, F., Wöllmer, M., Schuller, B.: Opensmile: the munich versatile and fast open-source audio feature extractor. In: Proceedings of the International Conference on Multimedia, pp. 1459–1462. ACM (2010)

13. Witten, I.H., Frank, E.: Data Mining: Practical Machine Learning Tools and Techniques, 2nd edn. Morgan Kaufmann, San Francisco (2005)

14. Torre, P., Barlow, J.A.: Age-related changes in acoustic characteristics of adult speech. J. Commun. Disord. 42, 324–333 (2009)

Practical Measurements for Quality of Ontology Matching Applying to the OAEI Dataset

Ismail Akbari, Yevgen Biletskiy[✉], and Weichang Du

Faculty of Computer Science, University of New Brunswick, PO Box 4400, C314, 550 Windsor Street, Fredericton, NB E3B 6B9, Canada
{iakbari,biletski,wdu}@unb.ca

Abstract. Nowadays, ontologies are widely used in different research areas. Ontology mapping or ontology matching aims at finding correspondences among different ontologies The Ontology Alignment Evaluation Initiative (OAEI) is an international coordinated initiative that organizes evaluation of the increasing number of ontology matching systems. This campaign consisted of 6 tracks gathering 8 test cases and different evaluation modalities. The present paper describes a work, which defines measurements (factors) to increase the quality of matching results obtained in any ontology matching approach or system. These filtering measures have been applied to the OAEI benchmark dataset and produced promising results.

Keywords: Ontology matching · Quality · OAEI data set · Semantic web

1 Introduction

The current Web is a great success and has significant influences on people's life. The Web almost changed every aspect of today's life. However, it has encountered a new challenge and opportunity: the vast amount of data and documents created in various communities within different contexts. These documents are interpretable by humans, but machine-based interpretation is limited. This volume of data is increasing rapidly every minute; therefore, more and more work is needed to process information gained from the data.

The Semantic Web is supposed to make data located anywhere on the Web, disregarding the language or structure, accessible and understandable to both people and machines. The Semantic Web initiative aims to exploit formal knowledge stored in ontologies at the world scale. Ontology is the core component of the Semantic Web. Ontologies are shared models of a domain that encode a view, which is common to a set of different parties [1]. Web ontologies are usually designed with RDF Schema [2], OWL [3] or other Semantic Web based languages.

Ontology matching is proposed as a possible solution for the knowledge exchange and sharing, by providing a formal mechanism for defining the semantics of data and plays a key role on expanding and utilizing of the Semantic Web based applications [4–6]. In recent years, there have been developed a lot of ontologies in a variety of domains and

© Springer International Publishing Switzerland 2015
G. Sidorov and S.N. Galicia-Haro (Eds.): MICAI 2015, Part I, LNAI 9413, pp. 118–126, 2015.
DOI: 10.1007/978-3-319-27060-9_10

by various people or organizations. Ontologies created in a same domain may even be in different languages, different structures or be different in the level of details.

2   Related Work

The Ontology Alignment Evaluation Initiative (OAEI) dataset has been originally elaborated for the use by ontology matching systems. Ontology mapping or ontology matching aims at finding correspondences among different ontologies. The proposed factors in the current work can be used by ontology matching (OM) algorithms and systems to test and find out their weak and strong aspects. The need for ontology matching is not limited to one particular application. In fact, ontology matching is needed in any application, which uses ontologies. There has been introduced many OM algorithms and methods, which use this data set to evaluate themselves. The UFOme [7] is an ontology mapping framework, which has a library of modules to match two different ontologies. It has four different modules called Lucene ontology matcher (based on the Lucene search engine), string matcher [8], WordNet matcher [9], and structural matcher [7]. The UFOme also uses a prediction module to predict which module(s) it should use to match two given ontologies. The work [10] uses a gradually exploring method to match very big ontologies. It starts from two matched nodes and advances to their neighbours until all concepts are explored, or no new aligned pair is found. The iMatch [11] is a probabilistic scheme, which uses Markov networks to match ontologies. It learns from matched data and also supports semi-automatic matching.

The biomedical sciences are one of the domains, where ontologies are being developed and used to facilitate information exchange and knowledge sharing. The OAEI 2013 data set [12], as well as its previous versions, has a biomedical track, which is called LargeBio test case. This test aims to find alignments between large and semantically rich biomedical ontologies such as FMA, SNOMED-CT, and NCI. The UMLS Metathesaurus has been used as the basis for reference alignments. The 13 systems including AML, HerTUDA, HotMatch and others have participated in this track. The OAEI 2013 also has an anatomy test case. The anatomy real world test case serves for matching the Adult Mouse Anatomy (2744 classes) and a small fragment of the NCI Thesaurus (3304 classes) describing the human anatomy. The Biomedical Ontologies Alignment Technique (BOAT) [13] uses two features to align biomedical ontologies. First feature considers the informativeness of each word in the concept labels, which has significant impact on biomedical ontologies. Another feature selects only concept pairs to compare and find high likelihoods of equivalence, based on the similarity of their annotations.

3   Finding False-Positive Correspondences

One of the major challenges in the current ontology matching algorithms or systems is the quality of the found alignment correspondences. This quality depends on the precision and recall factors, which show how many of the found matches are correct and how many of the existing matches were found, respectively. In this work, we focus on the first case. The presented filtering factors in this work can increase the precision value by filtering out the wrong correspondences found by an ontology matching algorithm. We applied these factors to the results of some of the state of the art algorithms and got promising results. These factors (criteria) are applied as follows:

- Crisscross relation means that if two nodes are matched, then parents of the first node cannot be matched to the children of the second node and, vice versa.
- Node-to-sibling relation means that if two nodes are matched, then first node cannot be matched to the siblings of the second and, vice versa.
- Node-to-parent relation means that if two nodes are matched, then first node cannot be matched to parents of the second and, vice versa.
- Node-to-child relation means that if two nodes are matched, then first node cannot be matched to children of the second and, vice versa.
- Disjoint relation means that if two nodes are matched then first node cannot be matched to the disjoint nodes of the second node and, vice versa.
- Sibling-to-Parent relation means that if two nodes are matched, then siblings of first node cannot be matched to parents of the second node and, vice versa.
- Sibling-to-Child relation means that if two nodes are matched, then siblings of first node cannot be matched to the children of the second one and, vice versa.

To make the above mentioned factors (bulleted list) clearer, the example in Fig. 1 is presented.

The left ontology is the source ontology and the right ontology is the target one, where solid arrow shows IS-A (parent) relation, and dashed arrow shows disjoint relation. Consider that there is a correspondence between node "C" and node "X". Based on criss-cross factor, the node "A" cannot be matched to the node "Z". Node-to-sibling factor indicates that the node "C" cannot be matched to the nodes "W" and "Y" (which are siblings of the node "X"). Factor node-to-parent indicates that the node "C" cannot be matched to the node "V". Based on node-to-child measure, the node "C" should not be matched to the node "Z". Disjoint factor indicates that the node "C" cannot be matched to the node "W". Based on sibling-to-parent relation, the node "B" cannot be matched to node "V". Finally, based on sibling-to-child measure, the node "B" cannot

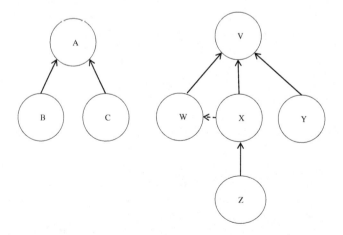

Fig. 1. Source (on left) and target (on right) Ontologies

be matched to the node "Z". The above mentioned factors have been applied to the final results of the algorithms and systems included in the Ontology Alignment Evaluation Initiative (OAEI) [14] campaign. Since disjoint relations in the benchmark test case of OAEI is rare, the factor cannot be applied.

4   Experimental Results

The Ontology Alignment Evaluation Initiative (OAEI) is an internationally coordinated initiative that organizes the evaluation of the increasing number of ontology matching systems [14]. The evaluation organizers provide different kind of ontology matching data sets (tracks). One of these tracks is the benchmark track. This systematic benchmark test set is built around one reference ontology and many variations of it. It consists of 3 categories: simple tests (1xx), systematic tests (2xx) and real life tests (3xx). The first two categories contain respectively 4 and 102 ontologies, which are variations of the reference ontology (ontology #101). The category 3xx consists of 4 real ontologies. The matching systems participating in the benchmark track should compare these 110 ontologies with the reference ontology. The ontologies are described in OWL-DL and serialized in the RDF/XML format. The expected alignments are provided in a standard format expressed in RDF/XML and described in [15].

Table 1 shows the systems that have participated at the benchmark test case and the harmonic mean of precision and recall of their result. Table 2 shows the number of false-positive correspondences, which are dropped correctly by each factor from the final results of these thirteen algorithms participated in the benchmark track of OAEI 2009. The abbreviations used in the first row correspond to crisscross, node-to-sibling, node-to-parent, node-to-child, sibling-to-parent, sibling-to-child, and disjoint relations respectively. The results in Table 2 show that 80 % (284 out of 353) of the dropped matches are dropped correctly.

Where the "+" sign shows the number of false-positive matches (wrong matches which are considered as true) which are dropped correctly by the each factor. The "−" sign shows the number of true-positive matches (correct matches that were considered also as

Table 1. (split in two) Systems that participated at the benchmark test of OAEI [14]

Algorithm	Edna	aflood	AgrMaker	aroma
Precision	0.43	0.98	0.99	0.94
Recall	0.59	0.80	0.62	0.69
Algorithm	kosimap	Lily	MapPSO	RiMOM
Precision	0.91	0.97	0.64	0.93
Recall	0.59	0.88	0.59	0.82

Algorithm	ASMOV	DSSim	GeRoMe
Precision	0.95	0.97	0.91
Recall	0.87	0.66	0.73
Algorithm	SOBOM	TaxoMap	
Precision	0.98	0.86	
Recall	0.44	0.26	

Table 2. Number of false-positive matches found by each factor from the results obtained by participants on the benchmark test case of OAEI

Factor	CC	N2S	N2P	N2C	S2P	S2C	DIS	TOTAL
+	21	70	15	45	63	70	N/A	284
−	0	18	19	12	10	10	N/A	69

Table 3. Number of false-positive matches found by applying the factors on the Edna algorithm from OAEI

Factor	CC	N2S	N2P	N2C	S2P	S2C	DIS	TOTAL
+	13	18	7	6	28	39	N/A	129
−	0	2	0	2	3	0	N/A	7

correct) which were dropped incorrectly. Table 3 illustrates the application of all the factors (except disjoint) on results of the basic algorithm Edna of OAEI, and it shows their effects.

The row with label "+" holds the number of false-positive matches (wrong matches which are considered as true) of the Edna algorithm, which are dropped correctly by the each factor. The row "−" shows the number of true-positive matches (correct matches which were considered also as correct) of the Edna algorithm which are dropped incorrectly by the factors. The appendix shows more details about the number of correctly and incorrectly removed matches using the introduced factors.

Based on the number of correctly removed correspondences (false-positive) and incorrectly removed correspondences from the results of Edna in Table 3, the following Eqs. 2 and 3 are to prove that the precision of Edna algorithm is raised by each filter. To mention that the precision value is calculated using the following formula.

$$precision = \frac{number\ of\ correctly\ found\ alignmnets}{number\ of\ found\ alignmnets} \tag{1}$$

$$f = cf + if \tag{2}$$

where: f is the number of found alignments, cf is the number of correctly found alignments and if is the number of incorrectly found alignments. With respect to the Eq. (1), when the number of found alignments decreases the precision value increases. Based on the Eq. (2) number of found alignments decreases when number of incorrectly found alignments decreases. The new precision value is calculated using the following formula:

$$New\ precision = old\ precision * \frac{\frac{cf_2}{f_2}}{\frac{cf_1}{f_1}} \tag{3}$$

$$cf_2 = cf_1 - ir$$

$$f_2 = f_1 - (cr + ir) \tag{4}$$

where: cf_2 is the new correctly found alignments, f_2 is new found alignments, cf_1 is the old correctly found alignments, f_1 is the old found alignments, ir is incorrectly removed true positive alignments, and cr is correctly removed false positive alignments. Based on Eqs. (3) and (4) the precision value of Edna and other algorithm in Table 1 increases, because the numbers of correctly removed false-positive alignments are more than incorrectly removed true-positive alignments for all the factors that have been introduced. The appendix shows details about the changes on precision and recall values (old and new precision and recalls) of the test cases from OAEI dataset. The appendix also shows details of the number of correctly and incorrectly removed matches using the introduced factors of the test cases that these matches have been removed from. Each table at appendix belongs to one factor.

Disjoint factor has no effect on the algorithms because there is no disjoint relation in the data sets. For space reserving purpose, the details of applying the introduced factors on other algorithms than enda algorithm have not brought in the appendix.

5 Conclusion

Nowadays, ontologies are widely used in different research areas. Ontologies are the backbone of the Semantic Web. Ontology matching is the process of finding correspondences between two or more given ontologies. These correspondences can be between all aspects of ontologies e.g. between named classes and/or properties. A lot of work has been done to match different ontologies, and lots of systems and algorithms have been introduced. However, the matching results of these algorithms may not be quite correct or have low quality (low precision or recall). The proposed work here tries to find incorrect correspondences that have been resulted from ontology matching algorithms, which participated in the Ontology Alignment Evaluation Initiative (OAEI) campaign. The proposed filtering factors find false-positive correspondences and shows a promising result. The introduced factors in the current work can be used by any ontology matching algorithm to raise the quality of their matching results by finding the incorrectly matched entities of ontologies.

Appendix

The appendix shows details of the changes on precision and recall values (old and new precision and recalls) of the test cases from OAEI dataset. The appendix also shows details about the number of correctly and incorrectly removed matches using the introduced factors from test cases that these matches have been removed from. Each following table belongs to one factor (Tables 4, 5, 6, 7, 8 and 9).

Table 4. Effect of Criss-Cross (CC) factor on Edna algorithm

Test case	Old prec.	Old rec.	New prec.	New rec.	Correctly removed	Incorrectly removed
201	0.039	0.041	0.04	0.041	2	0
205	0.336	0.35	0.34	0.34	3	0
209	0.346	0.36	0.35	0.35	3	0
210	0.514	0.54	0.515	0.53	1	0
302	0.306	0.65	0.319	0.65	4	0

Table 5. Effect of Node-to-Sibling (N2S) factor on Edna algorithm

Test case	Old prec.	Old rec.	New prec.	New rec.	Correctly removed	Incorrectly removed
201	0.039	0.041	0.041	0.041	4	0
202	0.019	0.02	0.02	0.02	4	0
205	0.336	0.35	0.329	0.329	2	1
206	0.514	0.536	0.525	0.536	2	0
209	0.346	0.36	0.34	340	2	1
301	0.475	0.786	0.484	0.77	3	0
302	0.306	0.645	0.303	0.625	1	0

Table 6. Effect of Node-to-Parents (N2P) factor on Edna algorithm

Test case	Old prec.	Old rec.	New prec.	New rec.	Correctly removed	Incorrectly removed
205	0.336	0.35	0.34	0.35	1	0
207	0.514	0.536	0.515	0.525	1	0
209	0.346	0.36	0.35	0.36	1	0
210	0.514	0.536	0.51	0.525	0	0
301	0.475	0.786	0.484	0.786	2	0
302	0.306	0.645	0.31	0.645	1	0
304	0.722	0.96	0.73	0.96	1	0

Table 7. Effect of Node-to-Children (N2C) factor on Edna algorithm

Test case	Old prec.	Old rec.	New prec.	New rec.	Correctly removed	Incorrectly removed
205	0.336	0.35	0.333	0.34	1	1
206	0.514	0.536	0.52	0.536	1	0
207	0.514	0.536	0.525	0.536	2	0
209	0.346	0.36	0.343	0.35	1	1
301	0.475	0.786	0.474	0.77	1	0
302	0.306	0.645	0.3	0.625	0	0
304	0.722	0.96	0.72	0.947	0	0

Table 8. Effect of Sibling-to-Parents (S2P) factor on Edna algorithm

Test case	Old prec.	Old rec.	New prec.	New rec.	Correctly removed	Incorrectly removed
201	0.039	0.041	0.04	0.041	1	0
202	0.019	0.02	0.02	0.02	2	0
205	0.336	0.35	0.333	0.329	3	0
206	0.514	0.536	0.51	0.515	1	1
207	0.514	0.536	0.52	0.515	3	1
209	0.346	0.36	0.343	0.34	3	0
210	0.514	0.536	0.515	0.515	2	1
301	0.475	0.786	0.505	0.77	7	0
302	0.306	0.645	0.319	0.625	6	0
304	0.727	0.96	0.721	0.921	1	0

Table 9. Effect of Sibling-to-Children (S2C) factor on Edna algorithm

Test case	Old prec.	Old rec.	New prec.	New rec.	Correctly removed	Incorrectly removed
201	0.039	0.041	0.04	0.041	1	0
202	0.019	0.02	0.02	0.02	2	0
205	0.336	0.35	0.354	0.35	5	0
206	0.514	0.536	0.52	0.525	2	0
207	0.514	0.536	0.536	0.525	5	0
209	0.346	0.36	0.364	0.36	5	0
210	0.514	0.536	0.525	0.525	3	0
301	0.475	0.786	0.461	0.59	8	0
302	0.306	0.645	0.307	0.583	6	0
304	0.722	0.96	0.715	0.894	1	0

References

1. Gruber, T.: Towards principles for the design of ontologies used for knowledge sharing. Int. J. Hum Comput Stud. **43**(5/6), 907–928 (1995)
2. Gómez-Pérez, A., Corcho, O.: Ontology languages for the semantic web. IEEE Intell. Syst. J. **17**(1), 54–60 (2002)
3. Pan, J., Horrocks, I.: RDFS (FA): connecting RDF(S) and OWL DL. IEEE Trans. Knowl. Data Eng. **19**(2), 192–206 (2007)
4. Wang, H., Wang, C.: Ontologies for universal information systems. J. Inf. Sci. **21**, 232–239 (1995)
5. Arch-Int, N., Sophatsathit, P.: A semantic information gathering approach for heterogeneous information sources on WWW. J. Inf. Sci. **29**, 357–374 (2003)
6. Hu, W., Jian, N., Qu, Y., Wang, Y.: GMO: a graph matching for ontologies. In: K-Cap 2005 Workshop on Integrating Ontologies, pp. 41–48 (2005)
7. Pirro, G., Talia, D.: UFOme: an ontology mapping system with strategy prediction capabilities. Data Knowl. Eng. **69**(5), 444–471 (2010)

8. Stoilos, G., Stamou, G., Kollias, S.D.: A string metric for ontology alignment. In: Gil, Y., Motta, E., Benjamins, V., Musen, M.A. (eds.) ISWC 2005. LNCS, vol. 3729, pp. 624–637. Springer, Heidelberg (2005)
9. Miller, G.: WordNet an on-line lexical database. Int. J. Lexicography 3(4), 235–312 (1990)
10. Seddiqui, M.H., Aono, M.: An efficient and scalable algorithm for segmented alignment of ontologies of arbitrary size. Web Semant. Sci. Serv. Agents World Wide Web 7(4), 344–356 (2009). doi:10.1016/j.websem.2009.09.001
11. Albagli, S., Ben-Eliyahu-Zohary, R., Shimony, S.E.: Markov network based ontology matching original research article. J. Comput. Syst. Sci. 78(1), 105–118 (2012)
12. Shvaiko, P., Euzenat, J., Srinivas, K., Mao, M., Jiménez-Ruiz E. (eds.): Proceedings of the 8th International Workshop on Ontology Matching co-located with the 12th International Semantic Web Conference (ISWC 2013), Sydney, Australia. CEUR Workshop Proceedings, vol. 1111. CEUR-WS.org (2013)
13. Wei, W., Chua, K., Kim, J.: BOAT: automatic alignment of biomedical ontologies using term informativeness and candidate selection. J. Biomed. Inf. 45(2), 337–349 (2012)
14. Ferrara, A., Hollink, L., Isaac, A., Joslyn, C., Meilicke, C., Nikolov, A., Pane, J., Shvaiko, P., Spiliopoulos, V., Wang, S.: Results of the ontology alignment evaluation initiative 2009. In: Fourth International Workshop on Ontology Matching, Washington, DC, 1. 16, 33, 74 (2009)
15. Dong, X., Madhavan, J., Halevy, A.Y.: Mining structures for semantics. SIGKDD Explor. 6 (2), 53–60 (2004)

Automatic Phoneme Border Detection to Improve Speech Recognition

Suárez-Guerra Sergio[⊠], Juárez-Murillo Cristian-Remington,
and Oropeza-Rodríguez José Luis

Centro de Investigación en Computación,
Instituto Politécnico Nacional, Mexico City, Mexico
{ssuarez,joropeza}@cic.ipn.mx,
cristianremingtonjm@gmail.com

Abstract. A comparative study of speech recognition performance among systems trained with manually labeled corpora and systems trained with semi-automatically labeled corpora is introduced. An automatic labeling system was designed to generate phoneme labels files for all words within the corpus used to train a system of automatic speech recognition. Speech recognition experiments were performed using the same corpus, first training with manually, and later with automatically generated labels. Results show that the recognition performance is better when the training of selected diccionary, is made with automatic label files than when it is made with manual label files. Not only is the automatic labeling of speech corpora faster than manual labeling, but also it is free from the subjectivity inherent in the manual segmentation performed by specialists. The performance achieved in this work is greater than 96 %.

Keywords: Label detection · ASR applications · Automatic speech segmentation and labeling

1 Introduction

Automatic speech recognition systems require in their front-end to be trained using a dictionary with the words and phonemes that the system will use. For example, a system for the English language requires to be trained with English phonetics, and a dictionary of the words used in the application. The same can be said for all other languages.

Representative patterns of the phonetic content are required for the training of the system; among the most used being the Mel Frequency Cepstral Coefficients (MFCC). It is also important to chose a technique or model to recognize, and one of the most popular is Hidden Markov Models (HMM). The phoneme borders were detected by using forced alignment.

Forced alignment is a well known technique in which speech is aligned, and the borders among phonemes are found based on the phonetic transcription of the utterance and previously trained models that required some amount of hand-made labels to be trained. The evaluation of an automatic labeling and segmentation of a speech corpus is mainly reported by the agreement with respect to the hand-made labeling and segmentation of the very same corpus, i.e., the percentage of correctly placed boundaries

© Springer International Publishing Switzerland 2015
G. Sidorov and S.N. Galicia-Haro (Eds.): MICAI 2015, Part I, LNAI 9413, pp. 127–135, 2015.
DOI: 10.1007/978-3-319-27060-9_11

within a tolerance interval, which is normally 20 ms (Hosom 2000, Toledano 2003). Some applications use HTK modules to obtain automatic phonemes labeles (Poonam Bansal et al. 2014). However, speech recognition has not been widely used to asess the segmentation of a speech corpus quality.

Automatic segmentation can be evaluated directly, comparing it to a reference manual segmentation; or indirectly a recognizer and using the generated recognition percentage.

Various approaches have been proposed to address the problem and in this study were classified into: DTW, connectionist techniques, stochastic evolutionary, diffuse, fractals, wavelets. Most analyzed systems rely on a combination of techniques. But there is a phonetic segmentation that is "correct". The continuous nature of speech prevents the accurate determination of the boundaries between phonemes. Phoneticians, even experts cannot agree on the boundaries of their segments for an arbitrarily small tolerance. The researchers of this issue have chosen to evaluate the quality of a segmentation comparing how similar is the automatic or manual segmentation generated by an expert.

A subjective way of assessing the segmentation quality is to use the corpus segmented speech synthesis where the synthesized speech is judged by a human; best quality segmentation generates speech sounds more naturally than lower quality segmentation.

Speech segmentation has two uses in particular: the first is a critical step in the system continuous speech recognition; the second is the segmentation of a speech corpus. If working for the first case then it is important that segmentation occurs rapidly, but in the second case it is sufficient that the segmentation is faster than manual segmentation, which takes several minutes for each word. Solving the problem of segmentation and labeling is important for the following reasons: In most approaches to speech recognition the signals must be segmented before they can have an appreciation, because this labeling system training recognizer enables the set of words to be used (dictionary). It is assumed that the characteristics of the signal in a given segment are constant (Ziolko et al. 2006), although there are no acoustically uniform phonemes. The segmentation of words and phonemes is one of the key steps in the systems of automatic speech recognition (Fantinato et al. 2008).

In (Fantinato et al. 2008) they implement a system that speaks segmentation based on described fractal, such as the Grieder work and Kinsner, Fantinato et al. They used the fractal dimension, but this time calculated from the discrete wavelet transform (DWT Discrete Wavelet Transform). Symlet wavelets were used, from (Galka and Ziolko 2008) experimentally giving better results. A preprocessing algorithm that forces the dimension is obtained numerically between 1 and 2 because it is not possible to always find a very similar voice to a fractal. The algorithm uses 512 sample windows with 50 % overlap. Finally, the path described by the dimension is analyzed. If there are edges in areas of high energy, then it is interpreted as a transition between phonemes; edges in areas of low energy are interpreted as transitions between words.

In (Ziolko et al. 2006) the derivative of the energy is used in the DWT sub-bands for attempts borders. Meyer wavelet decomposition is used with six levels. Each sub-band the energy is calculated, then the derivative thereof is obtained by using a filter. The algorithm proposes the border points where the energy and its derivative are similar. The algorithm was tested on a corpus of 43 words. The total error was 4.3

(dimensionless). In a word error sample the number of segments was 0.125, and the error in the positions was 2.29.

In (Galka and Ziolko 2008) they also used the DWT. The wavelet used is symlet12. Six-level decomposition is performed for each level and the number of samples is adjusted so that all sub-bands have the same number of samples. Energy is then obtained in each band which is softened by a filter. The sub-bands are sorted from highest to lowest according to their energy content, and this is done for each sample of the sub-bands, called map of importance. Significant changes in the ordering of the sub-bands are called events. Events that are large enough in magnitude are proposed as boundaries between phonemes. Assessments directly and indirectly were made. The best live result was an average error of 8 ms compared to manual borders. The best result in terms of phonemic awareness was 50 %.

In this work, the labeling and segmentation of speech corpus is automatically performed. Such segmentation is asessed by using the agreement with respect to the hand-made labeling and segmentation of those corpora. Are considers that it is not sufficient to compare the automatic segmentation with the manual as there is no guarantee that manual segmentation is correct, so indirect assessments were performed using a speech recognizer; thus, if recognition is high then segmentation can be considered to be of a good quality. Finally, speech recognition is performed training with the same corpus; first with hand-made label files, and later with the automatic ones. The results show that the recognition with systems trained with automatic label files have a higher performance than those trained with hand-made label files. The performance achieved in this work is greater than 96 %.

2 Application Block Diagram

Work steps for application diagram (Fig. 1):

1. *Corpus of words to automatic labeling*

The audio files and its phonetics level-trascription are made in the input. This information is the existent initial words or new words from the same speaker.

2. *MFCCs segments extraction*

Mel Frecuency Cepstral Coefficients are extracted for each 20 ms traslaped segments.

3. *Code Book from the corpus*

Code Book of the corpus of words is obtained.

4. *Sequence Symbols Generation of words*

Using the Code Book and MFFCs segments extraction the sequence symbols of each word is generated.

5. *HMM phonemes of the corpus*

All the phonemes in language of the application work.

6. Use existing HMM or create the new HMM words by phonemes concatenation

It is decided to create new HMM words by phonemes concatenation or use one of the HMM words existent in the application.

7. Re-estimation words HMM

Re-estimation is made from each HMM word using sequence symbols generation for the corresponding word.

8. Automatic Phoneme Border Detection

Using the Viterbi approach of the frame rate symbols sequence the correspondence of symbols secuence for the HMM of word, and the probability of instants ocurrence border phonemes is detected.

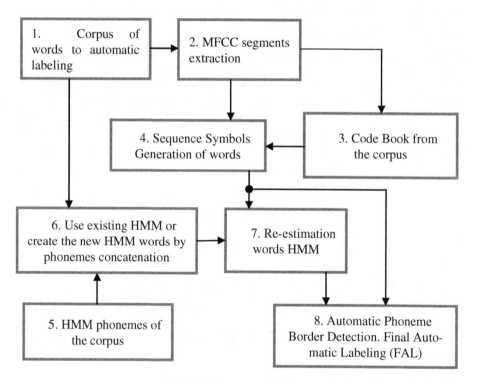

Fig. 1. Diagram applications

3   Automatic Phoneme Border Detection

The methodology followed in this work involves these steps:

- Determine the set of phonemes to be used.
- Build and train a HMM for each phoneme.

- Build and train the HMM model for each word to label.
- Apply the forced alignment algorithm to each speech file to get its automatic label file.

The phonetic alphabet used is Worldbet since it contains symbols equivalent to those from IPA, necessary to transcribe the Spanish language (Hieronymus 1993).

This work focuses on the Spanish spoken in Mexico, where 22 phonemes are used (Pineda et al. 2010). It also took into account 5 allophones, which were the most distinguishable ones. For example, it distinguished between/d/and/ð/because their acoustic features are very different. However, it did not distinguish among the different allophones for/n/since their acoustic features are very similar.

The classes of phonemes and allophones used in this work are (expressed in Worldbet): *a, e, i, o, u, l, r(, r, j, m, n, w, n ~ , tS, dZ, p, t, k, b, d, g, V, D, G, f, s, x, sil, pau*. The closures before a plosive phoneme were labeled as *pau*. Since there is essentially no acoustic difference between a voiceless closure and a pause (Lander 1997), it labeled voiceless closures as *pau*.

The characteristic parameters used are the Mel Frequency Cepstral Coefficients (MFCC). Book Code is generated and the HMMD were trained for each phoneme models with label files manually generated, the HMMD models were subsequently generated for each word of the corpus of words by phonetic concatenation. As can be seen in Fig. 2, each phoneme was modeled with a Bakis type HMM consisting of three observation states (2, 3 and 4) and two dummy or linking states (1 and 5).

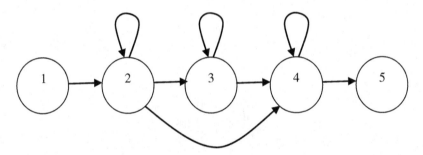

Fig. 2. A HMM states phonemes.

Once a HMM is trained for every phoneme in the corpus, it is necessary to build composite HMM word models which will be used for automatic labeling of each corpus. Such composite models are obtained by concatenating the corresponding necessary phoneme models, taking into account the phonetic transcriptions provided (Becchetti and Ricotti 1999). It is therefore, necessary to have the set of words that compound the dictionary of the application.

The process representation of forced alignment and results is show in Fig. 3.

A result of manual versus automatic labeling for the word 'cero10.wav' is observed in Fig. 4.

The results of the automatic labeling vs the manual shown in Fig. 4, offer a particularity, the addition-correction of the phoneme 'sil' at the beginning of the word

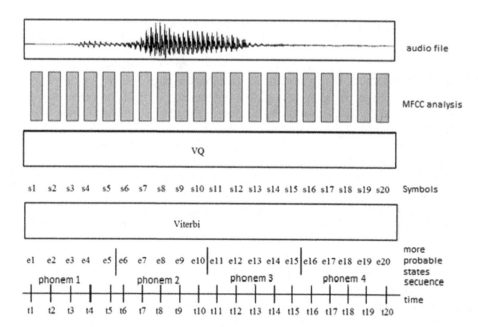

Fig. 3. Forced alignment using Viterbi algorithm

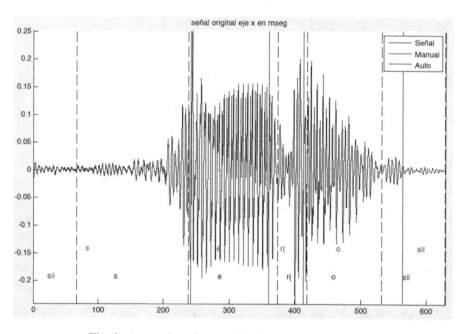

Fig. 4. Automatic and manual labeling of word cero10.wav

'cero10.wav'. This correction possibility of the automatic labeling of the application is an improvement that we have not found in the revised date references.

4 Experiments and Results

Two corpora were used. The first corpus contains spoken digits from 0 to 9; 20 times each digit with 4 speakers (which accounts for 800 files) with a sampling frequency of 11,025 Hz at 16 bits. This corpus is phonetically incomplete. The second corpus contains 150 different types of words, each one repeated 4 times by one speaker (which accounts for 600 files); the sampling frequency is 16,000 Hz at 16 bits. This corpus contains the 22 phonemes spoken in Mexico, plus 5 allophones (Pineda et al. 2010).

In order to assess the recognition performance yielded by systems trained with automatic label files and manual label files, the HTK 3.1 system was used. Both the automatic and manual label files and their corresponding speech files were used by HTK.

The first experiment used the digit corpus with four speakers. As can be seen in Table 1, the corpus itself was divided in two parts: the low and the high. The low part contains the first 10 repetitions of each word, and the high part contains the 10 last repetitions of each word. The automatic labeling system was trained using the low part of the corpus. Once the automatic labeling system was trained, it was used to label the whole corpus. Later, the automatic speech recognition system was also trained using the low part of the corpus; first with manual label files and later with automatic label files. In order to assess the recognition performance, the high part of the corpus was used.

Table 1 shows the recognition performance results comparing systems trained with manual and automatic training label files.

From Table 1 it can be seen that the recognition performance is better when the automatic speech recognition system is trained using automatic label files than when it is trained using manual label files.

In the second experiment all the speakers were mixed, and their files were used at the same time. The automatic labeling system used 25 % of the repetitions of each word to be trained. After that, all the files in the corpus were used to train and evaluate the recognition system. Table 2 shows the results of recognition performance.

The third experiment used the phonetically complete corpus with 150 different types of words, four repetitions of each word. The automatic labeling system was trained with 100 % of the corpus words. The speech recognition system was trained

Table 1. Performance speaker recognition

Speaker 1	Low part	High part	Speaker 2	Low part	High part
Manual label files	100 %	100 %	Manual label files	100 %	92.95 %
Automatic label files	100 %	100 %	Automatic label files	100 %	100 %
Speaker 3	Low part	High part	Speaker 4	Low part	High part
Manual label files	100 %	97.96 %	Manual label files	100 %	97.92 %
Automatic label files	100 %	98.98 %	Automatic label files	100 %	100 %

Table 2. Comparison of recognition performance for systems trained with automatic label files and manual label files for the four speakers mixed.

Concept	Manual label files	Automatic label files
Recognition performance	95.24 %	96.74 %

Table 3. Comparison of recognition performance for systems trained with automatic label files an manual label files for the corpus with 150 different types of words.

Concept	Manual	Automatic
Recognition performance	98.61 %	98.50 %

and tested with all the words in the corpus. As in the last experiment, the difference in recognition performance between the system trained with automatic label files, and the system trained with manual label files is similar, with just a difference of 0.2 %. Table 3 shows the results.

The results shown in Tables 1, 2, and 3 indicate that training automatic speech recognition systems with automatic label files yields superior results compared to those systems trained with manual label files. As automatic labeling implies savings of time, this is a big advantage.

Automatic labeling has a possible use in the fast development of applications in speech recognition.

Manual labeling is the major source of uncertainty and time consumption in the process of building an automatic speech recognition system since it is the most subjective part of the process.

Once HMMs are trained for the phonemes in a corpus and a dictionary for the words is available, it is necessary to train the automatic labeling system with the phonetic transcription of the words that will be used.

An immediate more interesting result is that it can automatically obtain new HMMs of words and their labels when this tool is used with a drastic time savings (Block 6 in the diagram applications).

5   Conclusion

Training automatic speech recognition systems using automatically labeled and segmented speech corpora yields better results than training using manually labeled and segmented corpora. Not only is automatic labeling free from the subjectivity that is always inherent in manual segmentation, but also the necessary time to get the label files is considerably reduced.

Automatic labeling requires minimum interaction from the user. The system requires a list of the words to be recognized and their phonetic transcriptions. The system creates a composite HMM for each word. No specialist is required to phonetically label the words. Given the results of this study it is proposed to create and use an automatic segmentation and labeling system that requires a minimum intervention by the user.

Acknowledgments. We thank National Polytechnic Institute (IPN - Instituto Politécnico Nacional, México), COFAA-IPN, PIFI-IPN SIP-IPN 20141454 and SIP-IPN 20130617; for their academic and financial support.

References

Becchetti, C., Ricotti, L.C.: Speech Recognition. Theory and C ++ Implementation, pp. 305–307. Wiley, New York (1999)

Fantinato, P.C., et al.: A Fractal-based approach for speech segmentation. In: Tenth IEEE International Symposium on Multimedia, ISM 2008, 15–17 December 2008, pp. 551–555 (2008). doi:10.1109/ISM.2008.123

Galka, J., Ziolko, M.: Wavelets in speech segmentation. In: The 14th IEEE Mediterranean Electrotechnical Conference, MELECON 2008, 5–7 May 2008, pp. 876–879 (2008)

Hieronymus, J.L.: ASCII Phonetic Symbols for the World's Languages: Worldbet, pp. 43–44 (1993). http://www.ling.ohio-state.edu/~edwards/WorldBet/worldbet.pdf

Hosom, J.P.: Automatic time alignment of phonemes using acoustic-phonetic information. Oregon Graduate Institute of Science and Technology. Ph.D. thesis, pp. 121–122 (2000)

Lander, T.: The CSLU Labeling Guide. Center of Spoken Language Understanding, Oregon Graduate Institute, pp. 52–56 (1997). http://www.cslu.ogi.edu/corpora/docs/labeling.pdf

Pineda, L.A., et al.: The Corpus DIMEx100: transcription and evaluation. Lang. Resour. Eval. **44**, 347–370 (2009, 2010). doi:10.1007/s10579-009-9109-9

Bansal, P., et al.: Speech synthesis – automatic segmentation. Int. J. Comput. Appl. (0975–8887) **98** (4), (2014)

Toledano, D.T., Gómez, L.A.H., Grande, L.V.: Automatic phonetic segmentation. IEEE Trans. Speech Audio Process. **11**(6), 617–625 (2003). doi:10.1109/TSA.2003.813579

Ziolko, B., Manandhar, S., Wilson, R.C.: Phoneme segmentation of speech. In: 18th International Conference on Pattern Recognition, ICPR 2006, vol. 4, pp. 282–285 (2006). doi:10.1109/ICPR.2006.931

Logic and Multi-agent Systems

Description Logic Programs: A Paraconsistent Relational Model Approach

Badrinath Jayakumar$^{(\boxtimes)}$ and Rajshekhar Sunderraman

Department of Computer Science, Georgia State University, Atlanta, GA, USA
{bjayakumar2,raj}@cs.gsu.edu
http://www.cs.gsu.edu/

Abstract. A description logic program (*dl-program*) consists of a description logic knowledge base (a terminological box and an assertion box) and a set of rules for a logic program. For such description logic programs, instead of providing the fixed-point semantics for *dl-programs* by the immediate consequence operator, we propose an algorithm based on the paraconsistent relational model that mimics the immediate consequence operator of *dl-programs*. We also introduce a dl-paraconsistent relation (*dl-relation*), which is essential for sending information between description logic and logic programs represented in terms of equations containing paraconsistent relations. The first step in our algorithm is to convert rules, which may contain *dl-atoms* that enable the flow of information between description logic and logic programs, into paraconsistent relation equations that contain paraconsistent relational algebraic operators. The second step is to determine iteratively the fixed-point semantics for *dl-programs* using these equations. We will also prove the correctness of both steps of the algorithm.

Keywords: Description logic · Logic programs · Fixed-point semantics · Paraconsistent relational model

1 Introduction

The web ontology language (OWL) [19,30], which is a W3C recommendation, is primarily based on description logic formalism [1], and is a backbone for future information systems. Although description logic is used for modeling the domain of interest, the rule-based systems [42] have many commercial applications [25]. Moreover, both types of formalism (description logic and rule) are based on first-order logic (FOL). This led to the development of the W3C Recommendation rule interchange format (RIF) [7,8].

Many formalisms have been proposed to integrate description logic and rules: SWRL [21–23], DL-Safe rules [31,40,41], DLP [18,48], $\mathcal{AL}$-log [10,11], CARIN [27,28], $\mathcal{DL}{+}log$ [43–47], Horn-$\mathcal{SHIQ}$ [24,26,31], Hybrid MKNF [36–39], *dl-programs* [12–16], disjunctive dl-programs [29], quantified equilibrium logic for hybrid knowledge bases [29], and description graphs [32–35]. We observed that

G. Sidorov and S.N. Galicia-Haro (Eds.): MICAI 2015, Part I, LNAI 9413, pp. 139–157, 2015.
DOI: 10.1007/978-3-319-27060-9_12

no type of formalism employs the paraconsistent relational model [3] to provide the semantics for the integration of rules and description logic.

In this paper, we chose *dl-programs*, which is a loose coupling method (rules may contain queries to description logic) that provides the semantics for the integration of description logic and rules. The integration is achieved through the use of *dl-atoms*, which is a special type of atom that occurs only in the body of the rules. Concretely, the *dl-atom* enables a bi-directional flow of information between description logic and the logic program. The main reason for choosing *dl-programs* in this paper is that the satisfaction of *dl-programs* is an extension of the usual notion of satisfaction of logic programs by Herbrand Interpretation.

Bagai and Sunderraman [3] proposed a data model to represent incomplete and inconsistent information in databases. The paraconsistent logic studied by da Costa [9] and Belnap [6] forms the basis for this data model. Instead of eliminating incomplete and inconsistent information, this model attempts to operate in its presence. The mathematical structures underlying the model, called paraconsistent relations, are a generalization of ordinary relations. Paraconsistent relations represent both positive and negative tuples.

Moreover, using the paraconsistent relation model, Bajai and Sunderraman [3] proposed some elegant methods for determining weak well-founded model [4] and well-founded model [5] for general deductive databases. But, there are not any methods based on the paraconsistent relational model proposed to determine models for *dl-programs*. In this paper, we propose an algorithm to determine the fixed-point semantics of the function free positive *dl-program*. Our idea essentially involves creating a paraconsistent relation for each predicate symbol in the rules and then forming a system of algebraic equations using paraconsistent algebraic operators for all *dl-rules* (ordinary rules containing *dl-atoms*) in *dl-programs*. Then, solve the equations to find the fixed-point semantics of the positive *dl-programs*.

This algebraic approach of finding the fixed-point semantics of a positive *dl-program* has two main advantages: it operates on a set of tuples in contrast to non-algebraic approaches, which operate on a tuple at a time basis; the algebraic expression in the equations can be optimized using various laws of equality, which is very similar to the ordinary relation case where selection and projection are pushed deeper into expressions whenever necessary.

The rest of the paper is organized as follows: in Sect. 2, we briefly introduce the paraconsistent relation model and its algebraic operators; in Sect. 3, we briefly explain *dl-programs*; in Sect. 4, we introduce the *dl-relation*, which is equivalent to *dl-atoms* that are used in *dl-programs*; in Sect. 5, we explain the algorithm that determines the fixed-point semantics of positive *dl-programs* along with its correctness; in Sect. 6, we state the conclusion and future work for this paper.

2   Paraconsistent Relation Model and Its Operators

Paraconsistent relations move forward a step to complete the database. Unlike normal relations where we only retain information believed to be true of a particular predicate, we also retain what is believed to be false of a particular predicate in the paraconsistent relational model. Let a relation scheme Σ be a finite set of attribute names, where for any attribute name $A \in \Sigma$, $dom(A)$ is a non-empty domain of values for A. A tuple on Σ is any map $t \colon \Sigma \to \bigcup_{A \in \Sigma} dom(A)$, such that $t(A) \in dom(A)$ for each $A \in \Sigma$. Let $\tau(\Sigma)$ denote the set of all tuples on Σ. An ordinary relation on scheme Σ is thus any subset of $\tau(\Sigma)$. A paraconsistent relation on a scheme Σ is a pair $<R^+, R^->$ where R^+ and R^- are ordinary relations on Σ. Thus, R^+ represents the set of tuples believed to be true of R, and R^- represents the set of tuples believed to be false.

Algebraic Operators. Two types of algebraic operators are defined here: (i) Set Theoretic Operators, and (ii) Relational Theoretic Operators.

Set Theoretic Operators. Let R and S be two paraconsistent relations on scheme Σ.

Union. The union of R and S, denoted $R \dot\cup S$, is a paraconsistent relation on scheme Σ, given that

$$(R \dot\cup S)^+ = R^+ \cup S^+, (R \dot\cup S)^- = R^- \cap S^-.$$

Complement. The complement of R, denoted $\dot- R$, is a paraconsistent relation on scheme Σ, given that

$$\dot- R^+ = R^-, \dot- R^- = R^+$$

Intersection. The intersection of R and S, denoted $R \dot\cap S$, is a paraconsistent relation on scheme Σ, given that

$$(R \dot\cap S)^+ = R^+ \cap S^+, (R \dot\cap S)^- = R^- \cup S^-$$

Difference. The difference of R and S, denoted $R \dot- S$, is a paraconsistent relation on scheme Σ, given that

$$(R \dot- S)^+ = R^+ \cap S^-, (R \dot- S)^- = R^- \cup S^+$$

Example 1. *Let $\{a, b, c\}$ be a common domain for all attribute names, and let R and S be the following paraconsistent relations on schemes $\{X\}$ and $\{X\}$ respectively:*

$$R^+ = \{\langle a \rangle, \langle b \rangle\}, R^- = \{\langle c \rangle\}$$
$$S^+ = \{\langle c \rangle, \langle b \rangle\}, S^- = \{\langle a \rangle\}$$

$R \dot\cup S$ is

$$(R \dot\cup S)^+ = \{\langle a \rangle, \langle b \rangle, \langle c \rangle\}$$
$$(R \dot\cup S)^- = \{\}$$

$R \dot{\cap} S$ is

$$(R \dot{\cap} S)^+ = \{\langle b \rangle\}$$
$$(R \dot{\cap} S)^- = \{\langle a \rangle, \langle c \rangle\}$$

$\dot{-}R$ is

$$\dot{-}R^+ = \{\langle c \rangle\}$$
$$\dot{-}R^- = \{\langle a \rangle, \langle b \rangle\}$$

$R \dot{-} S$ is

$$(R \dot{-} S)^+ = \{\langle a \rangle\}$$
$$(R \dot{-} S)^- = \{\langle b \rangle, \langle c \rangle\}$$

Relation Theoretic Operators. Let Σ and Δ be relation schemes such that $\Sigma \subseteq \Delta$, and R and S be paraconsistent relations on schemes Σ and Δ.

Join. The join of R and S, denoted $R \dot{\bowtie} S$, is a paraconsistent relation on scheme $\Sigma \cup \Delta$ given that

$$(R \dot{\bowtie} S)^+ = R^+ \bowtie S^+, (R \dot{\bowtie} S)^- = (R^-)^{\Sigma \cup \Delta} \cup (S^-)^{\Sigma \cup \Delta}$$

Projection. The projection of R onto Δ, denoted $\dot{\pi}_\Delta(R)$, is a paraconsistent relation on Δ given that

$$\dot{\pi}_\Delta(R)^+ = \pi_\Delta(R^+)^{\Sigma \cup \Delta}$$

$$\dot{\pi}_\Delta(R)^- = \{t \in \tau(\Delta) \mid t^{\Sigma \cup \Delta} \subseteq (R^-)^{\Sigma \cup \Delta}\}$$

where π_Δ is the usual projection over Δ of ordinary relations.

Selection. Let F be any logic formula involving attribute names in Σ, constant symbols, and any of these symbols $\{==, \neg, \wedge, \vee\}$. Then, the selection of R by F, denoted $\dot{\sigma}_F(R)$, is a paraconsistent relation on scheme Σ, given that

$$\dot{\sigma}_F(R)^+ = \sigma_F(R)^+, \dot{\sigma}_F(R)^- = R^- \cup \sigma_{\neg F}(\tau(\Sigma))$$

where σ_F is a usual selection of tuples satisfying F from ordinary relations.

The following example is taken from Bagai and Sunderraman's paraconsistent relational data model [3].

Example 2. *Strictly speaking, relation schemes are sets of attribute names. However, in this example we treat them as ordered sequence of attribute names so that tuples can be viewed as the usual lists of values. Let $\{a, b, c\}$ be a common domain for all attribute names, and let R and S be the following paraconsistent relations on schemes $\langle X, Y \rangle$ and $\langle Y, Z \rangle$ respectively:*

$R^+ = \{(b, b), (b, c)\}, R^- = \{(a, a), (a, b), (a, c)\}$
$S^+ = \{(a, c), (c, a)\}, S^- = \{(c, b)\}.$

Then, $R \bowtie S$ is the paraconsistent relation on scheme $\langle X, Y, Z \rangle$:

$(R \bowtie S)^+ = \{(b, c, a)\}$
$(R \bowtie S)^- = \{(a, a, a), (a, a, b), (a, a, c), (a, b, a), (a, b, b), (a, b, c), (a, c, a),$
$(a, c, b), (a, c, c), (b, c, b), (c, c, b)\}$

Now, $\dot{\pi}_{\langle X, Z \rangle}(R \bowtie S)$ becomes the paraconsistent relation on scheme $\langle X, Z \rangle$:

$\dot{\pi}_{\langle X, Z \rangle}(R \bowtie S)^+ = \{(b, a)\}$
$\dot{\pi}_{\langle X, Z \rangle}(R \bowtie S)^- = \{(a, a), (a, b), (a, c)\}$

Finally, $\dot{\sigma}_{\neg X = Z}(\dot{\pi}_{\langle X, Z \rangle}(R \bowtie S))$ becomes the paraconsistent relation on scheme $\langle X, Z \rangle$:

$\dot{\sigma}_{\neg X = Z}(\dot{\pi}_{\langle X, Z \rangle}(R \bowtie S))^+ = \{(b, a)\}$
$\dot{\sigma}_{\neg X = Z}(\dot{\pi}_{\langle X, Z \rangle}(R \bowtie S))^- = \{(a, a), (a, b), (a, c)(b, b), (c, c)\}$

In the rest of the paper, relations mean paraconsistent relations.

3   Descripiton Logic Programs

Logic program P, which consists of a set of rules, and description logic L combine to form a description logic program. The rules in logic programs also contain queries to L. In the following, we briefly describe logic programs, description logic, and description logic programs. However, to get an in-depth understanding, we request the readers to read Fitting and Melvin's survey on fixed-point semantics of logic programming [17], $\mathcal{SHOIN}(\mathbf{D})$ [20], and Eiter et al.'s *dl-programs* [12–16].

3.1   Definite Logic Programs (P)

In this subsection, we define the syntax and the fixed-point semantics of logic programs [17].

Syntax. Similar to Eiter et al.'s well-founded semantics of *dl-programs* [12,16], we consider function free first-order vocabulary $\Phi = (\mathcal{P}, \mathcal{C})$, which consists of non-empty finite sets of constants $\mathcal{C}$ and predicate symbols $\mathcal{P}$. In addition to that, let $\mathcal{X}$ be a set of variables. A term is either a variable from $\mathcal{X}$ or a constant from $\mathcal{C}$. An atom is of the form $p(t_1, \ldots, t_n)$ where $p \in \mathcal{P}$ and $t_1, \ldots, t_n$ are terms. In this paper, we consider only POSITIVE logic programs. Therefore, the rules are of the following form:

$$l_0 \leftarrow l_1, \ldots, l_z$$

where $z \geq 1$.

In the above rule, the atom l_0 is the head of the rule and the conjunction of atoms $l_1, \ldots, l_z$ is called the body of the rule. The rule is called a positive rule because it does not have default negated (*not*) atoms. A definite logic program (or logic program) P is a finite set of rules.

In this paper, we do not consider literals in rules. Such restriction is similar to Eiter et al.'s well-founded semantics of *dl-programs* [12,16].

Fixed-Point Semantics. A term, atom, or rule is called ground if it contains no variables. The *Herbrand Universe* of the underlying language is the set of all ground terms. The *Herbrand Base* of the language is the set of all ground atoms; a *Herbrand Interpretation* of the language is any subset of the Herbrand Base. Let I be a Herbrand Interpretation for the logic program P. Let P^* be the ground instances of rules in P. Since P does not have function symbols, P^* is always finite. Then, $T_P(I)$ (immediate consequence operator) is a Herbrand Interpretation, given by

$$T_P(I) = \{l_0 \mid \text{ for some rule } l_0 \leftarrow l_1, \ldots, l_z \text{ in } P^*, \{l_1, \ldots, l_z\} \subseteq I\}$$

It is well known that T_P always possesses a least fixed-point with respect to the partial order of set inclusion. The least fixed-point can be shown to be the minimal model for P. This model is also known to be $T_P \uparrow \omega$, where the ordinal power of T_P is given by:

Definition 1. *For any ordinal* α,

$$T_P \uparrow \alpha = \begin{cases} \emptyset \ if \ \alpha = 0, \\ T_P(T_P \uparrow (\alpha - 1)) \ if \ \alpha \ is \ a \ successor \ ordinal, \\ \bigcup_{\beta < \alpha} (T_P \uparrow \beta) \ if \ \alpha \ is \ a \ limit \ ordinal. \end{cases}$$

The following observation for any logic program is relevant:

Proposition 1. *For any logic program* P, *the upward closure ordinal of* T_P *is finite, i.e. there is a number* $n \geq 0$ *such that* $T_P \uparrow n = T_P \uparrow \omega$.

3.2   Description Logic (L)

In this subsection, we discuss $\mathcal{SHOIN}(\mathbf{D})$, which is the logical underpinning of OWL DL [20].

Syntax. Let E and V be a set of elementary datatypes and data values. A datatype theory $D = (\Delta^D, \cdot^D)$ consists of a datatype (or concrete) domain Δ^D and a mapping $\cdot^D$ that assigns to every elementary datatype a subset of Δ^D and to every elementary data value an element of Δ^D. The mapping $\cdot^D$ is extended to all datatypes by $\{v_1, \ldots\}^{\mathbf{D}} = \{v_1^{\mathbf{D}}, \ldots\}$. Let $\Psi = (A \cup R_A \cup R_D, I \cup V)$ be the vocabulary of the description logic, where A, R_A, R_D, and I are pairwise disjoint sets of atomic concepts, abstract roles, datatype (or concrete) roles and individuals. Table 1 describes the syntax and semantics of $\mathcal{SHOIN}(\mathbf{D})$. In Table 1, $\mathbf{R}_A^-$ is the set of inverses R^- of all $R \in \mathbf{R}_A$. A role is an element of $\mathbf{R}_A \cup \mathbf{R}_D \cup \mathbf{R}_A^-$. Complex concepts are defined inductively from the second part of Table 1. A description knowledge base is a finite set of axioms, where each axiom is one of the axiom from the third part of Table 1.

Semantics. We define the semantics of $\mathcal{SHOIN}(\mathbf{D})$ in terms of first-order interpretation.

Table 1. Syntax and Semantics of $\mathcal{SHOIN}(\mathbf{D})$

Name	Syntax	Semantics
atomic concept	$C \in \mathbf{A}$	$C^{\mathcal{I}} \subseteq \Delta^{\mathcal{I}}$
individual	$a \in \mathbf{I}$	$a^{\mathcal{I}} \in \Delta^{\mathcal{I}}$
abstract role	$R \in \mathbf{R}_A \cup \mathbf{R}_A^-$	$R^{\mathcal{I}} \in \Delta^{\mathcal{I}} \times \Delta^{\mathcal{I}}$
datatype	D	$D^{\mathbf{D}} \subseteq \Delta^{\mathbf{D}}$
concrete or datatype role	$U \in \mathbf{R}_D$	$U^{\mathcal{I}} \in \Delta^{\mathcal{I}} \times \Delta^{\mathbf{D}}$
data values	$v \in \mathbf{V}$	$v^{\mathcal{I}} = v^{\mathbf{D}}$
oneOf	$\{o_1, \ldots, o_n\},\ o_i \in \mathbf{I}$	$\{o_1^{\mathcal{I}}, \ldots, o_n^{\mathcal{I}}\}$
top	$\top$	$\top^{\mathcal{I}} = \Delta^{\mathcal{I}}$
bottom	$\bot$	$\bot^{\mathcal{I}} = \emptyset$
negation	$\neg C$	$\Delta^{\mathcal{I}} \setminus C^{\mathcal{I}}$
conjunction	$C \sqcap E$ where $E \in \mathbf{A}$	$C^{\mathcal{I}} \cap E^{\mathcal{I}}$
disjunction	$C \sqcup E$ where $E \in \mathbf{A}$	$C^{\mathcal{I}} \cup E^{\mathcal{I}}$
exists restriction	$\exists R.C$	$\{x \mid (\exists y)[(x,y) \in R^{\mathcal{I}} \wedge y \in C^{\mathcal{I}}]\}$
value restriction	$\forall R.C$	$\{x \mid (\forall y)[(x,y) \in R^{\mathcal{I}} \rightarrow y \in C^{\mathcal{I}}]\}$
atleast restriction	$\geqslant nR$	$\{x \mid \#\{y \mid (x,y) \in R^{\mathcal{I}}\} \geqslant n\}$
atmost restriction	$\leqslant nR$	$\{x \mid \#\{y \mid (x,y) \in R^{\mathcal{I}}\} \leqslant n\}$
datatype exists restriction	$\exists U.D$	$\{x \mid (\exists y)[(x,y) \in U^{\mathcal{I}} \wedge y \in D^{\mathbf{D}}]\}$
datatype value restriction	$\forall U.D$	$\{x \mid (\forall y)[(x,y) \in U^{\mathcal{I}} \rightarrow y \in D^{\mathbf{D}}]\}$
datatype atleast restriction	$\geqslant nU$	$\{x \mid \#\{y \mid (x,y) \in U^{\mathcal{I}}\} \geqslant n\}$
datatype atmost restriction	$\leqslant nU$	$\{x \mid \#\{y \mid (x,y) \in U^{\mathcal{I}}\} \leqslant n\}$

Axiom	Syntax	Semantics
concept inclusion	$C \sqsubseteq E$	$C^{\mathcal{I}} \subseteq E^{\mathcal{I}}$
role inclusion	$R \sqsubseteq S$ where $R, S \in \mathbf{R}_A$ or $R, S \in \mathbf{R}_D$	$R^{\mathcal{I}} \subseteq S^{\mathcal{I}}$
transitivity	$trans(R)$	$R^{\mathcal{I}} = (R^{\mathcal{I}})^+$
concept membership	$C(a)$	$a^{\mathcal{I}} \in C^{\mathcal{I}}$
role membership	$R(a,b)$ where $b \in \mathbf{I}$ ($U(a,v)$ where v is a data value)	$(a^{\mathcal{I}}, b^{\mathcal{I}}) \in R^{\mathcal{I}}$ $((a^{\mathcal{I}}, v^{\mathbf{D}}) \in U^{\mathcal{I}})$
equality	$a = b(= (a,b))$	$a^{\mathcal{I}} = b^{\mathcal{I}}$
inequality	$a \neq b(\neq (a,b))$	$a^{\mathcal{I}} \neq b^{\mathcal{I}}$

An interpretation $\mathcal{I} = (\Delta^{\mathcal{I}}, \cdot^{\mathcal{I}})$, with respect to a datatype theory $\mathbf{D} = (\Delta^{D}, \cdot^{D})$, consists of a nonempty domain $\Delta^{\mathcal{I}}$ disjoint from Δ^{D}, and $\cdot^{\mathcal{I}}$ is a valuation function defined inductively as shown in the first and second parts of

Table 1. The satisfaction of a DL axiom F in the interpretation $\mathcal{I} = (\Delta^{\mathcal{I}}, \cdot^{\mathcal{I}})$ with respect to a datatype theory $\mathbf{D} = (\Delta^D, \cdot^D)$, denoted $\mathcal{I} \models F$, is given by the third part of Table 1. The interpretation satisfies an axiom F, or the interpretation is a model of F iff $\mathcal{I} \models F$. $\mathcal{I}$ is a model of knowledge base L ($\mathcal{I} \models L$) iff $\mathcal{I} \models F$ for all $F \in L$. L is satisfiable (unsatisfiable) iff L has a model (no model). An axiom $F(\neg F)$ is a logical consequence of L, denoted $L \models F(L \models \neg F)$, iff every model of L satisfies (does not satisfy) F.

3.3   Description Logic Programs (KB)

In this subsection, we review Eiter et al.'s *dl-program* [12–16].

Syntax. The vocabularies of the logic program and description logic in any description logic program are defined in the previous two subsections. An important assumption is that $\mathbf{A} \cup \mathbf{R}_A \cup \mathbf{R}_D$ is disjoint from $\mathcal{P}$ where $\mathcal{P}$ is a set of predicate symbols, while $I_P \subseteq \mathcal{C} \subseteq \mathbf{I} \cup \mathbf{V}$, where I_P is the set of all constant symbols appearing in P. As we said earlier, description logic programs contain *dl-atoms*, which helps to query the description logic knowledge base. A *dl-query* $Q(\mathbf{t})$ is either

1. an inclusion axiom F or its negation $\neg F$ ($\mathbf{t}$ is empty); or
2. a concept $C(t)$ or its negation $\neg C(t)$ ($\mathbf{t}$ is t); or
3. a role $R(t_1, t_2)$ or its negation $\neg R(t_1, t_2)$ where t_1 and t_2 are terms ($\mathbf{t}$ is (t_1, t_2)); or
4. an equality axiom ($= (t_1, t_2)$) or inequality axiom ($\neq (t_1, t_2)$) where t_1 and t_2 are terms ($\mathbf{t}$ is (t_1, t_2)).

A *dl-atom* has the form,

$$DL[S_1 op_1 p_1, \ldots, S_m op_m p_m; Q](\mathbf{t}), m \geqslant 1$$

where each S_i is either a concept or role, $op_i = \{\uplus, \uplus\}$, and $p_1, \ldots, p_m$ are called input predicate symbols. If S_i is a concept, then p_i is a unary predicate symbol; if S_i is a role, then p_i is a binary predicate symbol. $Q(\mathbf{t})$ is called a *dl-query*. $op_i = \uplus$ ($op_i = \uplus$) increases S_i ($\neg S_i$) by the extension of p_i. A rule is called a *dl-rule* if one of the atoms in the rule $\{l_1, \ldots, l_z\}$ is a *dl-atom*. A *dl-program* $KB = (L, P)$ consists of a description logic knowledge base L and a finite set of *dl-rules* P. Since we considered only positive logic program P, KB is referred to positive KB. In this paper, we call positive *dl-programs* (KB) as *dl-programs*.

Fixed-Point Semantics. Let I be a Herbrand Interpretation for the dl-program $KB(KB = (L, P))$. Let P^* be the ground instances of rules in P. Since P does not have function symbols, P^* is always finite. Then, $T_{KB}(I)$ (immediate consequence operator) is a Herbrand Interpretation that is given by:

$$T_{KB}(I) = \{l_0 \mid l_0 \leftarrow l_1, \ldots, l_z \text{ in } P^*, \text{ for all } l_i \text{ where } 1 \leq i \leq z, I \models_L l_i\}$$

An important observation is that l_i is either a ground atom or ground dl-atom. I is a model of l_i under L, denoted $I \models_L l_i$:

– if l_i is a ground atom, then $I \models_L l_i$ iff $l_i \in I$
– if l_i is a ground *dl-atom* $DL[\lambda; Q](\mathbf{c})$, where $\lambda = S_1 op_1 p_1, \ldots, S_m op_m p_m$, then $I \models_L l_i$ iff $L(I; \lambda) \models Q(\mathbf{c})$ where $L(I; \lambda) = L \cup \bigcup_{i=1}^m A_i(I)$ and, for $1 \leqslant i \leqslant m$,

$$A_i(I) = \begin{cases} \{S_i(\mathbf{e}) \mid p_i(\mathbf{e}) \in I\}, & \text{if } op_i = \uplus; \\ \{S_i(\mathbf{e}) \mid p_i(\mathbf{e}) \in I\}, & \text{if } op_i = \between. \end{cases}$$

We say I is a model of a *dl-program* $KB = (L, P)$, denoted $I \models KB$, iff $I \models_L r$ for all $r \in P^*$. We say the KB is satisfiable (unsatisfiable) iff it has some (no) models.

It is easy to show that T_{KB} always possesses a least fixed-point. The least fixed-point is a minimal model for KB ($KB = (L, P)$). This model can also shown to be $T_{KB} \uparrow \omega$, where the ordinal power of T_{KB} is given by:

Definition 2. *For any ordinal α,*

$$T_{KB} \uparrow \alpha = \begin{cases} \emptyset \text{ if } \alpha = 0, \\ T_{KB}(T_{KB} \uparrow (\alpha - 1)) \text{ if } \alpha \text{ is a successor ordinal}, \\ \bigcup_{\beta < \alpha}(T_{KB} \uparrow \beta) \text{ if } \alpha \text{ is a limit ordinal}. \end{cases}$$

Similar to logic programs, the following proposition is true for any *dl-program KB.*

Proposition 2. *For any dl-program KB, the upward closure ordinal of T_{KB} is finite, i.e. there is a number $n \geq 0$ such that $T_{KB} \uparrow n = T_{KB} \uparrow \omega$.*

Proof. The proof is immediate from the fact that the Herbrand Base is finite.   □

The following example is taken from [12, 16], and it is modified to the positive *dl-program.*

Example 3. *Consider $KB = (L, P)$, where $L = \{S \sqsubseteq C\}$ and P is as follows:*
$r(a) \leftarrow DL[S \uplus q; C](a); q(a) \leftarrow p(a); p(a) \leftarrow$

Solution. For $I = \emptyset$, $T_{KB}(I) = \{p(a)\}$. For the second iteration, $I = \{p(a)\}$. Then, $T_{KB}(I) = \{p(a), q(a)\}$. For the third iteration, $T_{KB}(I) = \{p(a), q(a), r(a)\}$. In third iteration, the concept S was extended with a. Now L contains $S(a)$, by *modus ponens*, we say $C(a)$. Hence, the *dl-query* $(C(a))$ is true. Therefore, $r(a)$ is true.

In the following section, we introduce the *dl-relation*, which play a key role in the model construction for *dl-programs*. The main contribution of the paper starts from the following section.

4   Dl-relations

As we already stated in the Introduction section, we will construct a relation for every atom in the rules during model construction. In *dl-programs*, the body of the rules can have *dl-atoms*. It is necessary to have equivalent relations for such *dl-atoms*. It is achieved by redefining *dl-atoms* in terms of paraconsistent relations. To recall, *dl-atoms* are of the form $DL[S_1op_1p_1, \ldots, S_mop_mp_m; Q](\mathbf{t})$, $m \geqslant 1$. Specifically, $p_1, \ldots, p_m$ are input predicate symbols and $Q(\mathbf{t})$ is a *dl-query*. An important observation is that $Q(\mathbf{t})$ performs query entailment and not query answering for a given description logic knowledge base. This is because *dl-atoms* are grounded to determine models [12,16]. As a first step towards modifying *dl-atoms* for our purpose, we will transform constants in $\mathbf{t}$ of dl-queries to variables. By doing so, the *dl-query* performs query answering in the given description logic knowledge base. Next, we create paraconsistent relations for every input predicate symbols. We know that $op_i = \{\uplus, \uplus\}$. In order to denote that $\uplus$ ($\uplus$) adds tuples from relations to concepts or roles, we write $\uplus$ ($\uplus$) as $\dot{\uplus}$ ($\dot{\uplus}$). The update operator $\dot{\uplus}$ takes every tuple from $\dot{\pi}^+_{\{\Sigma\}}(p_i)$, where p_i is a relation, and inserts it in S_i. Similarly, $\dot{\uplus}$ takes every tuple from $\dot{\pi}^+_{\{\Sigma\}}(p_i)$, where p_i is a relation, and inserts it in $\neg S_i$. Hence the *dl-relation* is,

$$DL[S_1o\dot{p}_1\dot{\pi}^+_{\{\Sigma\}}(p_1), \ldots, S_mo\dot{p}_m\dot{\pi}^+_{\{\Sigma\}}(p_m); Q](\mathcal{V}), m \geqslant 1 \tag{1}$$

$p_1, \ldots, p_m$ are relations and $o\dot{p}_i = \{\dot{\uplus}, \dot{\uplus}\}$. $\mathcal{V}$ is the scheme of the *dl-relation* shown in (1). $Q(\mathcal{V})$ is called *dl-query* answering, and $Q(\mathcal{V})$ is a concept assertion or negated concept assertion, a role assertion or negated role assertion, or an equality or inequality axiom. Since $Q(\mathcal{V})$ is a query answering, it returns a set of individuals which is then added as tuples in the positive part of a *dl-relation*.

During model computation, instead of representing the *dl-relation* as shown in (1), we created a new relation for it. For the *dl-relation* shown in (1), the new relation is $R_{DL[S_1o\dot{p}_1\dot{\pi}^+_{\{\Sigma\}}(p_1),\ldots,S_mo\dot{p}_m\dot{\pi}^+_{\{\Sigma\}}(p_m);Q]}(\mathcal{V})$. In a *dl-relation*, we never insert any result of query answering into a *dl-relation* as tuples unless the result is in accordance to the domain values of the *dl-relation*'s scheme. In other words, $I_P \subseteq \mathcal{C} \equiv dom(a) \subseteq \mathbf{I} \cup \mathbf{V}$, where I_P is the set of all constant symbols appearing in P and all $a \in \mathcal{V}$.

In the next section, we will explain two steps for the algorithm to determine the fixed-point semantics of *dl-programs*. In addition to that, we prove that the algorithm is correct and provide an example for it.

5   Fixed-Point Semantics for *Dl-programs*

By using the algebra of the relational model, we present a bottom-up method for constructing models of *dl-programs* that mimics the immediate consequence operator (T_{KB}). The algorithm presented in this paper is based on the construction of well-founded semantics [5] and weak well-founded semantics [4] using the relational model for general deductive database. The model construction involves two steps. The first step is to convert P into a set of relation definitions for the predicate symbols occurring in P. These definitions are of the form

$$p = D_p$$

where p is a predicate symbol of P, and D_p is an algebraic expression involving predicate symbols of P and relation operators. The second step is to evaluate iteratively the expressions in these definitions to construct incrementally the relations associated with the predicate symbols. The first step is called SERI-ALIZE and the second step is called MODEL CONSTRUCTION.

The schemes of the relations are set internally. Hence, the following definition. Let $\Gamma_n = \langle v_1, v_2 \ldots \rangle$ be an infinite sequence of some distinct attribute names. For any $n \geq 1$, let Γ_n be the scheme $\{v_1 \ldots v_n\}$. The following operator renames the scheme of the relation from one to another.

Definition 3. *Let* $\Sigma = \{A_1 \ldots A_n\}$ *be any scheme. Then,*

1. *for any relation R on scheme Γ_n, $R(A_1 \ldots A_n)$ is the relation*

$$\delta_{v_1 \ldots v_n \rightarrow A_1 \ldots A_n}(R)$$

   on scheme Σ, and
2. *for any relation R on scheme Σ, $R(v_1 \ldots v_n)$ is the relation*

$$\delta_{A_1 \ldots A_n \rightarrow v_1 \ldots v_n}(R)$$

   on scheme Γ_n.

Before we get into details of the algorithm, we should replace every *dl-atom* $DL[\lambda; Q](\mathbf{t})$ by a fresh predicate $p_{DL[\lambda;Q]}(\mathbf{t})$ so that it would be easy to create the corresponding *dl-relation*.

Example 4. *Using the same KB from Example 3.*

Solution. $r(a) \leftarrow g_{DL[S \uplus q;C]}(a); q(a) \leftarrow p(a); p(a) \leftarrow$

Here, $g_{DL[S \uplus q;C]}$ is a new predicate symbol.

In the remaining part of this section we describe our method to convert the given *dl-rules* in KB $(KB = (L, P))$ into a set of definitions for the predicate symbol in P.

Algorithm. SERIALIZE
Input. A *dl-rule* (definite rule) $l_0 \leftarrow l_1, \ldots, l_z$. Let l_0 be an atom of the form $p_0(A_{01} \ldots A_{0k_0})$, and each l_i, $1 \leq i \leq z$, be an atom either of the form $p_i(A_{i1} \ldots A_{ik_i})$ or $p_{DL[\lambda;Q]}(\mathbf{t})$[1]. Let V_i be the set of all variables occurring in l_i.
Output. An algebraic expression involving paraconsistent relations.
Method. The expression is constructed by the following steps:

1. For each argument A_{ij} of literal l_i, construct argument B_{ij} and condition C_{ij} as follows:
   (a) If A_{ij} is a constant a, then B_{ij} is any brand new variable and C_{ij} is $B_{ij} = a$.
   (b) If A_{ij} is a variable, such that for each k, $1 \leq k < j$, $A_{ik} \neq A_{ij}$, then B_{ij} is A_{ij} and C_{ij} is true.
   (c) If A_{ij} is a variable, such that for some k, $1 \leq k < j$, $A_{ik} = A_{ij}$, then B_{ij} is a brand new variable and C_{ij} is $A_{ij} = B_{ij}$.
2. Let $\hat{l}_i$ be the atom $p_i(B_{i1} \ldots B_{ik_i})$, and F_i be the conjunction $C_{i1} \wedge \cdots \wedge C_{ik_i}$. Then Q_i is the expression $\dot{\pi}_{V_i} \dot{\sigma}_{F_i}(\hat{l}_i)$.

---

[1] $\lambda = S_1 op_1 p_1, \ldots, S_m op_m p_m$.

As a syntatic optimisation, if all conjuncts of F_i are true (i.e. all arguments of l_i are distinct variables), then both $\dot{\sigma}_{F_i}$ and $\dot{\pi}_{V_i}$ are reduced to identity operations, and are hence dropped from the expression.

If $\hat{l}_i$ is the atom $p_{DL[\lambda;Q]}(\mathbf{t})$, then Q_i is the expression $\dot{\pi}_{V_i}\dot{\sigma}_{F_i}(\hat{l}_i)$ where every input predicate symbol p_i in λ is $\dot{\pi}_{V_{p_i}}(p_i)^+$ in which V_{p_i} refers to a set of variables in p_i.

3. Let E be the natural join ($\bowtie$) of the Q_i's thus obtained, $1 \le i \le z$. The output expression is $(\dot{\sigma}_{F_0}(\dot{\pi}_{V'}(E)))\ [B_{01} \ldots B_{n_{k}n}]$. V' is a set of variables occurring in l_0.

As in step 2, if all conjuncts in F_0 are true, then $\dot{\sigma}_{F_0}$ is dropped from the output expression. However, $\dot{\pi}_{V'}$ is never dropped, as the rule may contain variables not in V'.

From the algebraic expression of the algorithm, we construct a system of equations.

For any *dl-program* $KB = (L, P)$, $EQN(P)$ is a set of all equations of the form $p = D_p$, where p is a predicate symbol, and D_p is the union ($\dot{\cup}$) of all expressions obtained by the algorithm *SERIALIZE* for the rules (*dl-rules*) in P with symbol p in their head. The algebraic expression D_p is also called a *definition* of p.

It is easy to observe that a predicate symbol may have many definitions. We now show that the above method for converting a *dl-program* KB into definitions for its predicate symbols terminates, and that the definitions produced mimics the immediate consequence operator (T_{KB}).

Proposition 3 (Termination). *The procedure of constructing EQN(P) terminates for any dl-program $KB(KB = (L, P))$.*

Proof. The proof is immediate from the fact that P has only a finite number of rules (*dl-rules*) that each rule contains a finite number of atoms (*dl-atoms*) and each atom (*dl-atom*)[2] has a finite number of arguments.   □

The transformation between a relation and an interpretation is necessary for the correctness of the proof.

Definition 4. *Let I be any interpretation and $r(X_1 \ldots X_n)$ be any atom (dl-atom), where the X_i's are distinct variables. Then $I \triangleright r$ is the following relation*
$$r^+ = \langle t \in \tau(\Sigma) \mid r(t(X_1)) \ldots t(X_n)) \in I \rangle$$
$$r^- = \emptyset$$
on scheme $\Sigma = \{X_1, \ldots, X_n\}$. Moreover, for any relation R on scheme Σ, $r\lfloor R \rfloor$ is the following interpretation
$$\langle r(t(X_1) \ldots t(X_n)) \mid t \in R^+ \rangle$$

In the following, we show the correctness of SERIALIZE.

---

[2] *dl-atoms* cannot have more than two arguments.

Proposition 4 (Correctness). *Let $a_1, \ldots, a_n$ be atoms (dl-atoms) occurring in the definition of some equation $p = D_p$ in $EQN(P)$, for any dl program $KB = (L, P)$. Let k_0 be the arity of p and let each a_i be of the form $p_i(B_{i1}, \ldots, B_{ik_i})$ or $p_{DL[\lambda;Q]}(t)$[3]. For all i, $1 \leq i \leq n$, let R_i be any relation on scheme Γ_{k_i}, such that if for any i, j, $p_i = p_j$, then $R_i = R_j$. Then, the relation R on scheme Γ_{k_0} obtained by evaluating D_p by interpreting each p_i as the relation R_i is*

$$T_{KB}(\langle \bigcup_{i=1}^{n} p_i \lfloor R_i \rfloor \rangle) \rhd p,$$

Proof. The proof essentially involves the definitions of the relation operators defined earlier. Here we give an easy to understand sketch. Let

$$I = (\langle \bigcup_{i=1}^{n} p_i \lfloor R_i \rfloor \rangle).$$

We divide the proof in the following two parts:

1. ($\rightarrow$) Suppose for any $t \in R^+$. Then, by the definition of $\dot{\cup}$, t is in the positive part of the expression

$$(\sigma_{F_0} \dot{\pi}_{V_1}(E))[B_{01} \ldots B_{0k_0}]$$

   output by step 3 of the algorithm *SERIALIZE*, for some rule (*dl-rule*) in P with symbol p in its head. Let Σ be the scheme of the relation E. Then, for some tuple $t' \in (\delta_{v_1 \ldots v_{k_0} \to B_{01} \ldots B_{0k_0}}(t))^{V' \cup \Sigma}$ is in E^+. Thus, for each Q_i in E, there is a tuple $t_i \in Q_i^+$ such that for each variable $X \in V_i$, $t'(X) = t_i(X)$. If Q_i is a *dl-relation*, then the tuple (t_i) is in the positive part of Q. By step 2 of the algorithm,
   (a) if the corresponding atom l_i in the rule is positive, then $t_i \in Q_i^+$
   (b) if the corresponding atom l_i is a *dl-atom* in the rule, then $t_i \in Q_i^+$. Here Q_i is a *dl-relation*.
   Therefore, due to the ground instance of this rule (*dl-rule*) for the "substitution" t', we have that $t \in T_{KB}(I)$.
2. ($\leftarrow$) Suppose $t \in (T_{KB}(I) \rhd p)^+$. Then, for some ground instance,

$$p(t(B_{01}) \ldots t(B_{0k_0})) \leftarrow l_1 \ldots l_z$$

   of a clause in P, we have that the atom of each l_i is in the correct part of I. For that clause of P, let

$$(\dot{\sigma}_{F_0} \dot{\pi}_{V'}(E))[B_{01} \ldots B_{0k_0}]$$

   be the expression output by step 3 of the algorithm *SERIALIZE*, and let Σ be the scheme of E. So, for each Q_i in E, there is a tuple $t_i \in Q_i^+$ such that for all $X \in V_i$, $t_i(X) = t'(X)$ for some $t' \in (\delta_{v_1 \ldots v_{k_0} \to B_{01} \ldots B_{0k_0}}(t))^{V \cup \Sigma}$. Hence, $t \in R^+$. □

---

[3] $\lambda = S_1 op_1 p_1, \ldots, S_m op_m p_m$.

Example 5. *Consider* $KB = (L, P)$, *where* $L = \{S \sqsubseteq C \sqcap D, D(b)\}$ *and* P *is as follows:*

$$r(X) \leftarrow DL[S \uplus q; D](X);$$
$$r(X) \leftarrow DL[S \uplus q; C](X), w(X);$$
$$q(X) \leftarrow p(X);$$
$$p(a) \leftarrow$$
$$w(a) \leftarrow$$

Solution. We construct an equation for every rule (*dl-rule*) in the *KB*. Since we have *dl-rules* in the *KB*, we need to replace *dl-atoms* with a new predicate.

$$r(X) \leftarrow f_{DL[S \uplus q; D]}(X);$$
$$r(X) \leftarrow g_{DL[S \uplus q; C]}(X), w(X);$$
$$q(X) \leftarrow p(X);$$

Now, $f_{DL[S \uplus q; D]}$ and $g_{DL[S \uplus q; C]}$ are two new predicate symbols. Then, we convert *KB* into a system of equations.

1. $r = \dot{\pi}_{\{X\}}(f_{DL[S \uplus \dot{\pi}_{\{X\}}(q)^+; D]}(X))[X]$
2. $r = (\dot{\pi}_{\{X\}}(g_{DL[S \uplus \dot{\pi}_{\{X\}}(q)^+; C]}(X) \bowtie w(X)))[X]$
3. $q = \dot{\pi}_{\{X\}}(p(X))[X]$

The LHS expression of the first and second equation are the same. Therefore,

1. $r = \dot{\pi}_{\{X\}}(f_{DL[S \uplus \dot{\pi}_{\{X\}}(q)^+; D]}(X))[X] \dot{\cup}$
   $(\dot{\pi}_{\{X\}}(g_{DL[S \uplus \dot{\pi}_{\{X\}}(q)^+; C]}(X) \bowtie w(X)))[X]$
2. $q = \dot{\pi}_{\{X\}}(p(X))[X]$

The second step is to construct the model by incrementally constructing the relation values in P. For any P in *dl-program* $KB = (L, P)$, P_E are the facts (rules in P without bodies), and P_I are the rules (rules in P with bodies). P_E^* refers to a set of all ground instances of rules in P_E. Without the loss of generality, we assume that no predicate symbol occurs both in P_E and in P_I.

ALGORITHM. MODEL CONSTRUCTION
Input. A *dl-program* $(KB = (L, P))$
Output. Relation values for the predicate symbols in P.
Method: The following steps compute the values:

1. (Initialization)
   (a) Compute EQN(P_I) using the algorithm *SERIALIZE* for each clause in P_I.
   (b) For each predicate symbol p in P_E, set
   $p^+ = \{\langle a1 \ldots ak \rangle \mid p(a1 \ldots, ak) \in P_E^*\}$, and
   $p^- = \emptyset$
   (c) For each predicate symbol p in P_I, set $p^+ = \emptyset$ and $p^- = \emptyset$.
2. For each equation of the form $p = D_p$ in $EQN(P_I)$, compute the expression D_p and set p to the following relation. If the expression contains a *dl-relation*, then perform query answering in the given description logic knowledge base (L).

3. If step 2 involved a change in the value of some p, goto 2.
4. Output the final values of all predicate symbol in P_E and P_I.

Now, we prove the termination of the second step of the algorithm.

Proposition 5 (Termination). *Algorithm* **MODEL CONSTRUCTION** *terminates for all dl-programs.*

Proof. By Proposition 3, step 1 always terminates. By Propositions 2 and 4, the loop in step 2–3 always terminates.   □

Next, we prove that the algorithm MODEL CONSTRUCTION is correct.

Theorem 1 (Correctness). *A tuple* $\langle a_1, \ldots a_k \rangle$ *is in* p^+ *computed by the algorithm MODEL CONSTRUCTION iff* $p(a_1, \ldots, a_k) \in T_{KB} \uparrow \omega$.

Proof. Following from the fact that $T_{KB} \uparrow 1$ is set up by the initialization step, and by Proposition 4, step 2 mimics the T_{KB} operator, whose power always converges by Proposition 2.   □

The following example consolidates our work presented in this paper. Here we represent relations in the form of tables in which the positive and negative parts are separated by a double line.

Example 6. *Using the same KB from Example 5.*

Solution. By step 1(a), $EQN(P_I)$ returns two equations:

1. $r = \dot{\pi}_{\{X\}}(f_{DL[S \uplus \dot{\pi}_{\{X\}}(q)^+;D]}(X))[X] \dot{\cup}$
   $(\dot{\pi}_{\{X\}}(g_{DL[S \uplus \dot{\pi}_{\{X\}}(q)^+;C]}(X) \bowtie w(X)))[X]$
2. $q = \dot{\pi}_{\{X\}}(p(X))[X]$

The domain value of every relation's attribute is $\{a\}$. By step 1(b),

$$w = \frac{\{X\}}{\langle a \rangle} \quad \text{and} \quad p = \frac{\{X\}}{\langle a \rangle}$$

Step 1 mimics the $T_{KB} \uparrow 1$.

In step 2, we have two equations. After applying the second equation,

$$w = \frac{\{X\}}{\langle a \rangle}, \quad p = \frac{\{X\}}{\langle a \rangle} \quad \text{and} \quad q = \frac{\{X\}}{\langle a \rangle}$$

Now, it is important to observe that the first equation has two *dl-relations*. So, it is necessary to perform query answering on the description logic knowledge base (L).

$$f_{DL[S \uplus \dot{\pi}_{\{X\}}(q)^+;D]} = \frac{\{X\}}{\langle a \rangle}$$

In the above relation, the tuples in q are inserted into concept S, and query answering $(D(X))$ is performed. The description logic knowledge base (L) already contains an assertion $D(b)$ but the domain values of *dl-relation* scheme does not contain b. Hence, the above relation has only one tuple. Next,

$$g_{DL[S \uplus \check{\pi}_{\{X\}}(q)^+;C]} = \dfrac{\{X\}}{\langle a \rangle}$$

After computing the second equation, we have the following:

$$r = \dfrac{\{X\}}{\langle a \rangle}$$

Finally, we have the following:

$$r = \dfrac{\{X\}}{\langle a \rangle}, \; w = \dfrac{\{X\}}{\langle a \rangle}, \; p = \dfrac{\{X\}}{\langle a \rangle} \; \text{and} \; q = \dfrac{\{X\}}{\langle a \rangle}$$

Further iterations of step 2 do not change the values of relations. Step 2 mimics the T_{KB} operator.

In other words, $T_{KB} \uparrow \omega = \{r(a), w(a), p(a), q(a)\}$.

6   Conclusion

In this paper, we took Eiter et al.'s *dl-program* [12–16] and represented it in terms of the paraconsistent relational model. We also introduced the *dl-relation* to represent the *dl-atom*, which gets its tuples from description logic knowledge base. We then determined the fixed-point semantics of positive *dl-programs* using paraconsistent algebraic operators and proved the correctness of it.

It is important to note that we can use the paraconsistent relations that were obtained at the end of the algorithm for querying using paraconsistent tuple relational calculus [2]. Thus, expressive queries can be given to paraconsistent relations. Even though we correctly find the fixed-point semantics of *dl-programs*, the given algorithm in this paper is not complete. We notice that we have not proven the complexities of the algorithm. An interesting direction for future work would be to determine the complexities of the algorithm and then to compare the complexities of the algorithm with the complexities of the Eiter et al.'s *dl-programs* [16]. There are two more possible directions of future works for this paper. The first work would be extending the algorithm to accommodate default negation (*not*) and to determine the well-found semantics of *dl-programs* in the paraconsistent relation model. Moreover, we are currently working in this direction. The second work would be representing different formalisms (as mentioned in the Introduction section) for integration of description logic and rules in the paraconsistent relation model to find its model.

References

1. Baader, F., Calvanese, D., McGuinness, D.L., Nardi, D., Patel-Schneider, P.F. (eds.): The Description Logic Handbook: Theory, Implementation, and Applications. Cambridge University Press, New York (2010)
2. Bagai, R.: Tuple relational calculus for paraconsistent databases. In: Monard, M.C., Sichman, J.S. (eds.) AI 2000. LNCS, vol. 1952, pp. 409–416. Springer, Heidelberg (2000)
3. Bagai, R., Sunderraman, R.: A paraconsistent relational data model. Int. J. Comput. Math. **55**(1–2), 39–55 (1995)

4. Bagai, R., Sunderraman, R.: Bottom-up computation of the fitting model for general deductive databases. J. Intell. Inf. Syst. **6**(1), 59–75 (1996)
5. Bagai, R., Sunderraman, R.: Computing the well-founded model of deductive databases. Int. J. Uncertainty Fuzziness Knowl. Based Syst. **4**(02), 157–175 (1996)
6. Belnap Jr., N.D.: A useful four-valued logic. In: Dunn, J.M., Epstein, G. (eds.) Modern Uses of Multiple-Valued Logic, pp. 5–37. Springer, Amsterdam (1977)
7. Boley, H., Hallmark, G., Kifer, M., Paschke, A., Polleres, A., Reynolds, D.: RIF core dialect. W3C Recommendation **22** (2010)
8. Boley, H., Kifer, M.: RIF basic logic dialect. In: W3C Working Draft, July 2009
9. Da Costa, N.C., et al.: On the theory of inconsistent formal systems. Notre Dame J. Formal Logic **15**(4), 497–510 (1974)
10. Donini, F.M., Lenzerini, M., Nardi, D., Schaerf, A.: A hybrid system with datalog and concept languages. In: Ardizzone, E., Gaglio, S., Sorbello, F. (eds.) Trends in Artificial Intelligence. LNCS, vol. 549, pp. 88–97. Springer, Heidelberg (1991)
11. Donini, F.M., Lenzerini, M., Nardi, D., Schaerf, A.: Al-log: integrating datalog and description logics. J. Intell. Inf. Syst. **10**(3), 227–252 (1998)
12. Eiter, T., Ianni, G., Lukasiewicz, T., Schindlauer, R.: Well-founded semantics for description logic programs in the semantic web. ACM Trans. Comput. Logic (TOCL) **12**(2), 11 (2011)
13. Eiter, T., Ianni, G., Lukasiewicz, T., Schindlauer, R., Tompits, H.: Combining answer set programming with description logics for the semantic web. Artif. Intell. **172**(12), 1495–1539 (2008)
14. Eiter, T., Ianni, G., Polleres, A., Schindlauer, R., Tompits, H.: Reasoning with rules and ontologies. In: Barahona, P., Bry, F., Franconi, E., Henze, N., Sattler, U. (eds.) Reasoning Web 2006. LNCS, vol. 4126, pp. 93–127. Springer, Heidelberg (2006)
15. Eiter, T., Lukasiewicz, T., Schindlauer, R., Tompits, H.: Combining answer set programming with description logics for the semantic web. In: Principles of Knowledge Representation and Reasoning: Proceedings of the Ninth International Conference (KR 2004), Whistler, Canada, 2–5 June 2004, pp. 141–151 (2004). http://www.aaai.org/Library/KR/2004/kr04-017.php
16. Eiter, T., Lukasiewicz, T., Schindlauer, R., Tompits, H.: Well-founded semantics for description logic programs in the semantic web. In: Antoniou, G., Boley, H. (eds.) RuleML 2004. LNCS, vol. 3323, pp. 81–97. Springer, Heidelberg (2004)
17. Fitting, M.: Fixpoint semantics for logic programming a survey. Theoret. Comput. Sci. **278**(1), 25–51 (2002)
18. Grosof, B.N., Horrocks, I., Volz, R., Decker, S.: Description logic programs: combining logic programs with description logic. In: Proceedings of the 12th International Conference on World Wide Web, pp. 48–57. ACM (2003)
19. Hitzler, P., Krötzsch, M., Parsia, B., Patel-Schneider, P.F., Rudolph, S.: Owl 2 web ontology language primer. W3C Recommendation **27**(1), 123 (2009)
20. Horrocks, I., Patel-Schneider, P.: Reducing owl entailment to description logic satisfiability. Web Semant. Sci. Serv. Agents World Wide Web **1**(4), 345–357 (2004)
21. Horrocks, I., Patel-Schneider, P.F.: A proposal for an owl rules language. In: Proceedings of the 13th International Conference on World Wide Web, pp. 723–731. ACM (2004)
22. Horrocks, I., Patel-Schneider, P.F., Bechhofer, S., Tsarkov, D.: Owl rules: a proposal and prototype implementation. Web Semant. Sci. Serv. Agents World Wide Web **3**(1), 23–40 (2005)

23. Horrocks, I., Patel-Schneider, P.F., Boley, H., Tabet, S., Grosof, B., Dean, M., et al.: SWRL: A semantic web rule language combining owl and ruleml. In: W3C Member Submission 21, 79 (2004)
24. Hustadt, U., Motik, B., Sattler, U.: Data complexity of reasoning in very expressive description logics. In: IJCAI, vol. 5, pp. 466–471 (2005)
25. Krisnadhi, A., Maier, F., Hitzler, P.: OWL and rules. In: Polleres, A., d'Amato, C., Arenas, M., Handschuh, S., Kroner, P., Ossowski, S., Patel-Schneider, P. (eds.) Reasoning Web 2011. LNCS, vol. 6848, pp. 382–415. Springer, Heidelberg (2011)
26. Krötzsch, M., Rudolph, S., Hitzler, P.: Complexity boundaries for horn description logics. In: AAAI, vol. 7, pp. 452–457 (2007)
27. Levy, A.Y., Rousset, M.C.: Carin: A representation language combining horn rules and description logics'. In: ECAI, pp. 323–327. Citeseer (1996)
28. Levy, A.Y., Rousset, M.C.: Combining horn rules and description logics in carin. Artif. Intell. **104**(1), 165–209 (1998)
29. Lukasiewicz, T.: A novel combination of answer set programming with description logics for the semantic web. In: Franconi, E., Kifer, M., May, W. (eds.) ESWC 2007. LNCS, vol. 4519, pp. 384–398. Springer, Heidelberg (2007)
30. McGuinness, D.L., Van Harmelen, F., et al.: Owl web ontology language overview. In: W3C Recommendation 10(10), 2004 (2004)
31. Motik, B.: Reasoning in description logics using resolution and deductive databases. Ph.D. thesis, Karlsruhe Institute of Technology (2006)
32. Motik, B., Cuenca Grau, B., Sattler, U.: Structured objects in owl: representation and reasoning. In: Proceedings of the 17th International Conference on World Wide Web, pp. 555–564. ACM (2008)
33. Motik, B., Grau, B.C., Horrocks, I., Sattler, U.: Modeling ontologies using owl, description graphs, and rules. In: OWLED (2008)
34. Motik, B., Grau, B.C., Horrocks, I., Sattler, U.: Representing structured objects using description graphs. In: KR, pp. 296–306 (2008)
35. Motik, B., Grau, B.C., Horrocks, I., Sattler, U.: Representing ontologies using description logics, description graphs, and rules. Artif. Intell. **173**(14), 1275–1309 (2009)
36. Motik, B., Horrocks, I., Rosati, R., Sattler, U.: Can OWL and logic programming live together happily ever after? In: Cruz, I., Decker, S., Allemang, D., Preist, C., Schwabe, D., Mika, P., Uschold, M., Aroyo, L.M. (eds.) ISWC 2006. LNCS, vol. 4273, pp. 501–514. Springer, Heidelberg (2006)
37. Motik, B., Rosati, R.: Closing semantic web ontologies. Technical report, University of Manchester, UK (2006)
38. Motik, B., Rosati, R.: A faithful integration of description logics with logic programming. In: IJCAI, vol. 7, pp. 477–482 (2007)
39. Motik, B., Rosati, R.: Reconciling description logics and rules. J. ACM (JACM) **57**(5), 30 (2010)
40. Motik, B., Sattler, U., Studer, R.: Query answering for OWL-DL with rules. In: McIlraith, S.A., Plexousakis, D., van Harmelen, F. (eds.) ISWC 2004. LNCS, vol. 3298, pp. 549–563. Springer, Heidelberg (2004)
41. Motik, B., Sattler, U., Studer, R.: Query answering for OWL-DL with rules. Web Semant. Sci. Serv. Agents World Wide Web **3**(1), 41–60 (2005)
42. Paschke, A.: Rules and logic programming for the web. In: Polleres, A., d'Amato, C., Arenas, M., Handschuh, S., Kroner, P., Ossowski, S., Patel-Schneider, P. (eds.) Reasoning Web 2011. LNCS, vol. 6848, pp. 326–381. Springer, Heidelberg (2011)
43. Rosati, R.: Towards expressive KR systems integrating datalog and description logics: preliminary report. In: Description Logics, vol. 22 (1999)

44. Rosati, R.: On the decidability and complexity of integrating ontologies and rules. Web Semant. Sci. Serv. Agents World Wide Web **3**(1), 61–73 (2005)
45. Rosati, R.: Semantic and computational advantages of the safe integration of ontologies and rules. In: Fages, F., Soliman, S. (eds.) PPSWR 2005. LNCS, vol. 3703, pp. 50–64. Springer, Heidelberg (2005)
46. Rosati, R.: Dl+ log: Tight integration of description logics and disjunctive datalog. In: KR, vol. 6, pp. 68–78 (2006)
47. Rosati, R.: Integrating ontologies and rules: semantic and computational issues. In: Barahona, P., Bry, F., Franconi, E., Henze, N., Sattler, U. (eds.) Reasoning Web 2006. LNCS, vol. 4126, pp. 128–151. Springer, Heidelberg (2006)
48. Volz, R.: Web ontology reasoning with logic databases. Ph.D. thesis, Karlsruhe, Univ., Diss. (2004)

A Branch & Bound Algorithm to Derive a Direct Construction for Binary Covering Arrays

Jose Torres-Jimenez[1]($\boxtimes$), Idelfonso Izquierdo-Marquez[1],
Aldo Gonzalez-Gomez[1], and Himer Avila-George[2,3]

[1] Information Technology Laboratory, CINVESTAV-Tamaulipas, Ciudad Victoria,
Tamaulipas, Mexico
jtj@cinvestav.mx, {iizquierdo,ajgonzalez}@tamps.cinvestav.mx
[2] HARAMARA TIC-LAB, CICESE-UT3, Andador 10, Ciudad Del Conocimiento,
Tepic, Nayarit, Mexico
himerag@cicese.mx
[3] Cátedras CONACyT, Avenida Insurgentes Sur 1582, Benito Juárez,
Crédito Constructor, 03940 Mexico, D.F., Mexico

Abstract. Covering arrays are used in testing deterministic systems where failures occur as a result of interactions among subsystems. The goal is to reveal if any interaction induces a failure in the system. Application areas include software and hardware testing. A binary covering array CA(N;t,k,2) is an $N \times k$ array over the alphabet $\{0,1\}$ with the property that each set of t columns contains all the 2^t possible t-tuples of 0's and 1's at least once. In this paper we propose a direct method to construct binary covering arrays using an specific interpretation of binomial coefficients: a binomial coefficient with parameters k and r will be interpreted as the set of all the k-tuples from $\{0,1\}$ having r ones and $k-r$ zeroes. For given values of k and t, the direct method uses an explicit formula in terms of both k and t to provide a covering array CA(N;t,k,2) expressed as the juxtaposition of a set of binomial coefficients; this covering array will be of the minimum size that can be obtained by any juxtaposition of binomial coefficients. In order to derive the formula, a Branch & Bound (B&B) algorithm was first developed; the B&B algorithm provided solutions for small values of k and t that allowed the identification of the general pattern of the solutions. Like others previously reported methods, our direct method finds optimal covering arrays for $k = t + 1$ and $k = t + 2$; however, the major achievement is that nine upper bounds were significantly improved by our direct method, plus the fact that the method is able to set an infinite number of new upper bounds for $t \geq 7$ given that little work has been done to compute binary covering arrays for general values of k and t.

1 Introduction

Combinatorial testing has been applied in many research areas as: materials design, medicine, agriculture, biology, software testing [1,3,13,23] and it has

G. Sidorov and S.N. Galicia-Haro (Eds.): MICAI 2015, Part I, LNAI 9413, pp. 158–177, 2015.
DOI: 10.1007/978-3-319-27060-9_13

been used recently in hardware Trojan detection [15]. Hardware Trojan detection is considered NP-hard problem [21]. To fully guarantee the quality of hardware products all possible configurations must be tested, but this exhaustive approach is not always a viable option (the number and combinations of possible inputs and internal states is intractable) [10]. A reduced set of input patterns that maximizes the probability of activating the Trojan is thus desirable. An alternative technique to accomplish this goal is the binary Covering Array CAs [15].

A covering array (CA), denoted by CA(N;t,k,v), is an $N \times k$ array where each $N \times t$ subarray contains each of the combinations of symbols from the set $\{0, 1 \ldots, v-1\}^t$ at least once. The value of N is the number of rows, t is called the strength and represents the interaction size, k is called the degree (or columns), and v is the order (or alphabet). When v equals 2, the array is called binary CA. The minimum value of N is called the *Covering Array Number (CAN)* and is defined by:

$$CAN(t, k, v) = min\{N : \exists CA(N; t, k, v)\}.$$

Covering arrays (CAs) can be classified based on their order. A covering array of order two is a *binary CA* because it only contains two different symbols, 0 and 1. If the order is three the CA is a *ternary CA*, and so on. In this paper we are dealing with binary CAs, the hardness of the construction of optimal binary covering arrays is such that there is no polynomial time algorithm for general values of k and t.

There exists more restrictive versions of the CAs called *orthogonal arrays (OA)*, or rather the CAs are relaxed versions of the OAs. In an orthogonal array every t-tuple appears exactly λ times. When $\lambda = 1$ every t-tuple arises exactly one time, and therefore the OA is an optimal CA. These types of orthogonal arrays are denominated orthogonal arrays of index unity.

The binomial coefficients $\binom{k}{r}$ are used to represent several things, and in this work they are used to represent the subset of the rows of size k having $k - r$ zeroes and r ones, and we reference this by $\{^k_r\}$. For a given k there are $k + 1$ row subsets $\{^k_0\}$, $\{^k_1\}$, ..., $\{^k_k\}$ which form a partition of the set of all the 2^k binary rows of size k. Given $k \geq 2$ an easy way to construct a binary CA with k columns and strength t, $2 \leq t \leq k$, is to take the juxtaposition of the entire collection of row subsets $\{^k_0\}$, $\{^k_1\}$, ..., $\{^k_k\}$. However, when $k > t$ it is possible to construct a CA of strength t by taking only a proper subset of these row subsets. Then, given the parameters k and t the problem is to find the subset of binomial coefficients with the minimum total number of rows that form a CA for the given parameters.

For small values of k and t it was possible to find these subsets by means of an exact algorithm based on branch and bound (B&B) that uses a clever structure called kt in order to construct only the subset of binomial coefficients that are CA, i.e. the subset of binomial coefficients that are not CA are not constructed by the algorithm. With the results produced by the exact algorithm it was possible to identify regular patterns in the optimal solutions for some values of k and t. Finally these regular patterns were summarized in a formula that for general values of k and t produces in linear time the subset of binomial coefficients that make an optimal CA for the parameters k and t.

In the case $k = t$ the only solution is to take the entire set of binomial coefficients $\binom{k}{j}$ for $j = 0, 1, \ldots, k$, and the CA generated is the OA(2^k;k,k,2). In addition to the trivial case the construction of CAs using binomial coefficients also gives the optimal solution for the cases $k = t+1$ and $k = t+2$. The formula we developed correctly finds the binomial coefficient subset that constructs the optimal CAs in these two cases. When $k > t+2$ the construction is not as good as other algorithms for small values of t such as $t \leq 7$, but for larger values of t the direct method sets an infinite number of new upper bounds given that little work has been done for $t \geq 7$.

The remaining of the document is organized as follow: Sect. 2 is a review of the relevant work related with the construction of CAs; Sect. 3 is the central part of the document, where the proposed construction is explained and the formula is derived based on the results of the B&B algorithm; Sect. 4 shows the computational results obtained for $t = 2, 3 \ldots, 26$ and $k = t+1, t+2, \ldots, t+25$, highlighting the lower bounds improved and the ones proposed for the first time; Finally, Sect. 5 summarizes the relevant contributions of this work.

2   Related Work

Given that in this work we deal only with binary covering arrays we recommend to the reader the review of the work by Lawrence et al. [17], and in this section we give a brief review of some general methods to construct covering arrays. There are several methods to construct covering arrays. According to the strategy to generate the CAs they can be classified into direct, algebraic, recursive, greedy or metaheuristic [19].

Direct methods are capable to construct a CA based on a mathematical formulation without doing any search or using other auxiliary components. The method proposed in this work is a direct method that is closely related with the idea of *constant weight vectors* [28, 29], but the two approaches are totally different, and we develop in greater depth all the implications of using binomial coefficients for building CAs.

For binary CAs, the case $t = 2$ was solved independently by Katona [14] and Kleitman and Spencer [16]. For a given $k > 1$ the method first compute the CAN$(k, 2, 2) = N$ where N is the smallest integer such as $k \leq \binom{N-1}{\lceil \frac{N}{2} \rceil}$. Then an $N \times k$ matrix is created and its first row is filled with zeroes. The columns of the remaining $N - 1$ rows are filled with all the combinations of $\lceil \frac{N}{2} \rceil$ ones and $N - 1 - \lceil \frac{N}{2} \rceil$ zeroes. Another of the most classical direct methods is the Bush's construction [2] that uses Galois finite fields to obtain orthogonal arrays of index unity OA(v^t;t,v+1,v) where $v = p^n$ is a primer power.

Algebraic constructions are those that follow a mathematical formulation to construct a CA but they use, in addition, auxiliary combinatorial components such as vectors and other CAs [19]. One of these methods is the technique of cyclotomy developed by Colbourn [6]. Given a vector $\alpha_{q,v}$ with entries from v symbols and size q, one type of construction is doing all the rotations of the vector α in order to obtain a $q \times q$ matrix. Under certain conditions, such as the vector α is derived from Galois finite fields and $q \equiv 1 \pmod{v}$ is a prime power, the matrix will be a covering array CA(q;t,q,v). Other important algebraic constructions are construction by groups used by Chateauneuf et al. [4] and Meagher and Stevens [20]; the power of a covering array [12]; the Roux-type constructions [25]; and the difference covering arrays used by Yin [32].

The *recursive methods* start with a CA and obtain other CAs with more columns in polynomial time using the operations of product and powering of other CAs. The product of two covering arrays of strength two by Stevens and Mendelsohn [27] is described next: let $A = (a_{i,j})$ be a CA(N;2,k,v) and let $B = (b_{i,j})$ be a CA(M;2,1,v), the product of these two CAs is the CA(N+M,2,kl,v) given by the array $C = (c_{i,j})$ of size $(N + M) \times kl$ constructed as follow: (a) $c_{i,(f-1)k+g} = a_{i,g}$ for $1 \leq i \leq N$, $1 \leq f \leq l$ and $1 \leq g \leq k$; (b) $c_{N+i,(f-1)k+g} = b_{i,f}$ for $1 \leq i \leq M$, $1 \leq f \leq l$ and $1 \leq g \leq k$. This work was extended after by Colbourn et al. [9].

In the category of the *greedy algorithms* the IPOG of Lei et al. [18] is one of the best known. The IPOG algorithm is the generalization to greater strengths of the IPO (In-Parameter-Order) algorithm which construct strength two CAs. The purpose of the IPOG is to construct a t-way test set for all the k parameters of the system to be tested, which is in essence the construction of CAs with strength t. For a system with t or more parameters, the IPOG strategy starts by building a t-way test set for the first t parameters, then it extends the test set for one more parameter at a time until it builds a t-way test set for all the parameters. The extension of an existing t-way test set for an additional parameter is done in two steps: *horizontal growth* which extends each existing test by adding one value for the new parameter, and *vertical growth* which adds new tests, if needed, to the test set produced by horizontal growth. Other very important greedy algorithm is the DDA (Deterministic Density Algorithm) of Colbourn and Cohen [7].

Metaheuristic algorithms are also been developed to construct CAs. These algorithms does not guarantee the construction of the optimal CA but in practice they give good results in a reasonable amount of time. Among the most used metaheuristics are simulated annealing [5,30], Tabu search [22,31] and genetic algorithms [24,26].

3 Proposed Solution

In this section the method to construct binary CA from binomial coefficients is fully explained. Also we give a B&B algorithm to find the best solution in terms of the binomial coefficients to construct a CA with k columns and strength t. A number of regular patterns were observed in the solutions provided by the exact algorithm which were exploited to obtain the general formula.

3.1 Generation of Covering Arrays Using Binomial Coefficients

In the expansion of the binomial $(x + y)^n = \sum_{r=0}^{n} \binom{n}{r} x^{n-r} y^r$ the binomial coefficient $\binom{n}{r}$ is the numeric coefficient of the term with x^{n-r} or equivalently the numeric coefficient of the term with y^r, this is the main interpretation of a binomial coefficient $\binom{n}{r}$. However, a binomial coefficient $\binom{n}{r}$ may represent several other things like the number of subsets with r different elements that can be formed from a set of n elements. For example, a binomial coefficient $\binom{n}{r}$ can represent the set of binary sequences of length n that have exactly r ones. As a concrete example, the binomial coefficient $\binom{4}{2}$ can be used to represent the six different binary sequences of length four with exactly two ones, they are: 1100, 1010, 1001, 0110, 0101 and 0011.

These six binary sequences of length four with exactly two ones may be considered as a block of six binary rows of length four in the construction of a CA. This is the basic idea in the method of construction we are proposing, i.e. the method constructs CAs by juxtaposing blocks of rows given by binomial coefficients. The key concept for the method of generating CAs from binomial coefficients is the concept of *row subset*, which is formalized next.

Definition 1. *Let k and r be two integers such as $0 \leq r \leq k$. The row subset $\left\{ {k \atop r} \right\}$ is defined to be the set of the $\binom{k}{r}$ rows having $k - r$ zeroes and r ones.*

Note that in this definition we use the notation $\left\{ {k \atop r} \right\}$ instead of the binomial notation $\binom{k}{r}$ to represent a row subset.

For a given $k \geq 2$ the set of all the 2^k binary k-column rows may be partitioned in the $k + 1$ row subsets $\left\{ {k \atop 0} \right\}, \left\{ {k \atop 1} \right\}, \ldots, \left\{ {k \atop k} \right\}$. The juxtaposition of these $k + 1$ binomial coefficients produces the orthogonal array $\mathtt{OA(2^k;k,k,2)}$ which is also a covering array for $t = 2, 3, \ldots, k - 1$. Figure 1(a) shows an example of this, the binary orthogonal array $\mathtt{OA(16;4,4,2)}$ results from the juxtaposition of the row subsets $\left\{ {4 \atop 0} \right\}, \left\{ {4 \atop 1} \right\}, \left\{ {4 \atop 2} \right\}, \left\{ {4 \atop 3} \right\}$ and $\left\{ {4 \atop 4} \right\}$; but the juxtaposition of these row subsets is also a covering array for $t = 3$ and $t = 2$. However, when $t < k$ no all the $k + 1$ binomial coefficients are required to form a CA of strength t, i.e. it is sufficient with a proper subset of the $k + 1$ binomial coefficients. For example, Fig. 1(b) and (c) shows that the two binary CAs of five rows for $k = 4$ and $t = 2$ are obtained by juxtaposing only two of the five row subsets.

Therefore, given the parameters k and t the problem of construct binary covering arrays using binomial coefficients is reduced to find a collection $\mathscr{C}$ of row subsets $\left\{ {k \atop r} \right\}$ such that the juxtaposition of its elements form a CA for the parameters k and t and whose total number of rows is minimum. Formally:

Definition 2. *Given the parameters k and t, the problem of the construction of a binary covering array $CA(N; t, k, 2)$ using binomial coefficients consists in finding a subcollection $\mathscr{C} = \left\{ {k \atop r_1} \right\}, \left\{ {k \atop r_2} \right\}, \ldots, \left\{ {k \atop r_i} \right\}$ of the row subsets $\left\{ {k \atop r} \right\}$ for $r = 0, \ldots, k$ such that the juxtaposition of all the rows subsets in $\mathscr{C}$ covers all the 2^t different binary t-tuples in any group of t columns and such that $|\mathscr{C}| \leq |\mathscr{C}'|$ for any other subcollection $\mathscr{C}'$ of row subsets that also covers the 2^t binary tuples in any group of t columns ($|\mathscr{C}|$ indicates the size in number of rows o the resulting CA).*

(a) OA(16,4,4,2)

$\left\{{4 \atop 0}\right\}$	0	0	0	0
$\left\{{4 \atop 1}\right\}$	1	0	0	0
	0	1	0	0
	0	0	1	0
	0	0	0	1
$\left\{{4 \atop 2}\right\}$	1	1	0	0
	1	0	1	0
	1	0	0	1
	0	1	1	0
	0	1	0	1
	0	0	1	1
$\left\{{4 \atop 3}\right\}$	1	1	1	0
	1	1	0	1
	1	0	1	1
	0	1	1	1
$\left\{{4 \atop 4}\right\}$	1	1	1	1

(b) CA(5;2,4,2)

$\left\{{4 \atop 0}\right\}$	0	0	0	0
$\left\{{4 \atop 3}\right\}$	1	1	1	0
	1	1	0	1
	1	0	1	1
	0	1	1	1

(c) CA(5;2,4,2)

$\left\{{4 \atop 1}\right\}$	1	0	0	0
	0	1	0	0
	0	0	1	0
	0	0	0	1
$\left\{{4 \atop 4}\right\}$	1	1	1	1

Fig. 1. (a) The binary orthogonal array $OA(16; 4, 4, 2)$ constructed by juxtaposing the row subsets $4; r$, $r = 0, 1, \ldots, 4$. (b) The binary covering array with $k = 4$ and $t = 2$ can be formed with the juxtaposition of the row subsets $4; 0$ and $4; 3$ or (c) with the juxtaposition of the row subsets $4; 1$ and $4; 4$.

The juxtaposition of two row subsets $\left\{{k \atop i}\right\}$ and $\left\{{k \atop j}\right\}$ will be denoted by $\left\{{k \atop i}\right\} + \left\{{k \atop j}\right\}$. In this way the juxtaposition of a collection of row subsets $\left\{{k \atop r_1}\right\}$, $\left\{{k \atop r_2}\right\}, \ldots \left\{{k \atop r_i}\right\}$ will be denoted by $\sum_{j=1}^{i} \left\{{k \atop r_j}\right\}$.

The set of the 2^t binary t-tuples that have to be covered in any group of t columns can also be partitioned in $t + 1$ classes, each of them represented by a binomial coefficient or row subset $\left\{{t \atop s}\right\}$, $0 \leq s \leq t$. The binomial coefficient $\left\{{t \atop s}\right\}$ contributes with the t-tuples in which there are $t - s$ zeroes and t ones. Continuing with the example in which $k = 4$ and $t = 2$, the four $(2^t = 2^2 = 4)$ 2-tuples 00, 01, 10 and 11 can be grouped in $t + 1 = 3$ classes: $\left\{{2 \atop 0}\right\} = \{00\}$, $\left\{{2 \atop 1}\right\} = \{01, 10\}$ and $\left\{{2 \atop 2}\right\} = \{11\}$.

Any row subset $\left\{{k \atop r}\right\}$ covers the same t-tuple an equal number of times in any group of t columns. For example the row subset $\left\{{4 \atop 3}\right\}$, showed in Fig. 1(a) and (b), covers the 2-tuples 01, 10 and 11 the same number of times in any two columns. As an specific case, the 2-tuple 11 is covered two times in the columns one and two, and it is covered this number of times in any other combination of two columns, i.e. in columns one and three, one and four, two and three, two and four, and three and four. This property implies that if a row subset $\left\{{k \atop r}\right\}$ covers a particular set $\left\{{t \atop s}\right\}$ of t-tuples, then the row subset covers it in any combination of t columns.

At this point we are using binomial coefficients to represent the row subsets in which the binary rows of k columns must be partitioned, and to represent the classes in which the t-tuples may be partitioned. From here, we will use the term $kClass$ to refer to the row subset $\left\{{k \atop r}\right\}$ representing the row subset with $k - r$

zeroes and r ones, and the term *tClass* to refer to the binomial coefficient $\left\{ {t \atop s} \right\}$ representing the subset of the t-tuples that have $t - s$ zeroes and s ones.

It is very easy to know which *tClass* is covered by which *kClass*: a *tClass* is covered by a *kClass if and only if* the *kClass* has at least as many zeroes as the *tClass* has, and has at least as many ones as the *tClass* has. In other words, a *kClass* $\left\{ {k \atop r} \right\}$ covers a *tClass* $\left\{ {t \atop s} \right\}$ *if and only if* the conditional expression $[(t-s) \leq (k-r)] \;\wedge\; (s \leq r)$ is true.

With the introduction of the concepts of *kClass* and *tClass* the problem of construct binary CAs using binomial coefficients is now expressed as the problem of finding the set of *kClass* with minimum cardinality that covers all the *tClass*. The computation of this subset of *kClass* is simplified by the introduction of a $(k+1) \times (t+1)$ binary matrix that summarizes which *tClass* is covered by which *kClass*, we called this matrix the *kt structure*. The *kt structure* has one row for each *kClass* and one column for each *tClass*. In each cell i, j the matrix has an 1 *if and only if* the i-th *kClass* covers the j-th *tClass* and has a 0 in other case. Figure 2 shows the *kt* structure for general values of k and t, and Fig. 2(b) shows the *kt* structure for the concrete case $k = 4$ and $t = 2$.

(a)

kClass	*tClass*			
	$\left\{ {t \atop 0} \right\}$	$\left\{ {t \atop 1} \right\}$	$\cdots$	$\left\{ {t \atop t} \right\}$
$\left\{ {k \atop 0} \right\}$	0|1	0|1	$\cdots$	0|1
$\left\{ {k \atop 1} \right\}$	0|1	0|1	$\cdots$	0|1
$\vdots$	$\vdots$	$\vdots$	$\ddots$	$\vdots$
$\left\{ {k \atop k} \right\}$	0|1	0|1	$\cdots$	0|1

(b)

kClass	*tClass*		
	$\left\{ {2 \atop 0} \right\}$	$\left\{ {2 \atop 1} \right\}$	$\left\{ {2 \atop 2} \right\}$
$\left\{ {4 \atop 0} \right\}$	1	0	0
$\left\{ {4 \atop 1} \right\}$	1	1	0
$\left\{ {4 \atop 2} \right\}$	1	1	1
$\left\{ {4 \atop 3} \right\}$	0	1	1
$\left\{ {4 \atop 4} \right\}$	0	0	1

Fig. 2. (a) The *kt structure* is a $(k+1) \times (t+1)$ binary matrix in which the cell i, j has an 1 *if and only if* the *tClass* j is covered by the *kClass* i. (b) A concrete example of the *kt structure* for $k = 4$ and $t = 2$.

One way to solve the problem of construct CAs using binomial coefficients is testing the 2^{k+1} subsets of *kClass* (i.e. all possible solutions) and selects the subset that produce a CA with minimum number of rows. To test whether or not a candidate solution generates a CA it is sufficient to verify that for each *tClass* s there exists at least one *kClass* r that covers it, i.e. if the *kt* structure has 1 in the cell corresponding to the classes r and s. According to Fig. 2(b) the solution $\{\left\{ {4 \atop 0} \right\}, \left\{ {4 \atop 3} \right\}\}$ produces a valid CA because the *kClass* $\left\{ {4 \atop 0} \right\}$ covers the *tClass* $\left\{ {2 \atop 0} \right\}$, and the *kClass* $\left\{ {4 \atop 3} \right\}$ covers the the *tClass* $\left\{ {2 \atop 1} \right\}$ and $\left\{ {2 \atop 2} \right\}$. Also the solution $\{\left\{ {4 \atop 2} \right\}\}$ produces a valid CA because the *kClass* $\left\{ {4 \atop 2} \right\}$ covers the three *tClass*.

3.2   A Branch and Bound Algorithm

With the *kt structure* given a particular solution or subset of *kClass* it is possible to test in linear time, with respect to the number of *tClass*, if the candidate solution generates a valid CA. However, since there are 2^{k+1} possible solutions or subsets of *kClass* the exhaustive approach of testing all the solutions to find the best one is impractical because the number of solutions grows exponentially with respect to k and t. But the *kt structure* provides the required information to develop a branch and bound algorithm which produces the same results as the exhaustive search.

The basic idea of a B&B algorithm is to explore only the combinations of *kClass* s.t. any *kClass* covers at least one *tClass* not covered by other *kClass* in the solution. In other words, one *kClass* is added to the partial solution *if and only if* it covers at least one *tClass* not covered by any other *kClass* in the partial solution. In this way the number of the *kClass* in one solution is at most $t + 1$.

In addition to the *kt structure* the B&B algorithm requires an auxiliary matrix, called *aux*, of $t + 1$ rows and $k + 1$ columns. In each row s the *aux* matrix stores all the *kClass* that cover the *tClass* s, where s is an integer used to identify the particular *kClass*. There are $k + 1$ *kClass* for a given value of k and any of them may be uniquely identified by an integer $0 \leq i \leq k$, with i meaning the number of 1's in the rows of the *kClass*. For example, all the rows in the *kClass* $\left\{ {k \atop 3} \right\}$ have three 1's, and therefore we identify this *kClass* by the number 3 in the B&B algorithm.

If the *tClass* s is covered by the *kClass* $\left\{ {k \atop r_{s,0}} \right\}$, $\left\{ {k \atop r_{s,1}} \right\}$, ..., $\left\{ {k \atop r_{s,m-1}} \right\}$, then the row s of the *aux* matrix contains in the first position the number $r_{s,0}$, in the second position the number $r_{s,1}$, and so on until in the position m it contains the number $r_{s,m-1}$. From the position $m + 1$ to position k the *aux* matrix stores a null value to indicate these positions are not in use (Fig. 3).

The B&B algorithm starts by adding the first *kClass* in row 0 of the *aux* matrix to the partial solution. Next the algorithm searches in the *kt structure* the *tClass* covered by the newly added *kClass*. An auxiliary vector *covered* is required to check out all the *tClass* covered by the actual solution. If the partial solution does not cover all the *tClass*, then it is necessary to add one more *kClass*

rows	cols					
	0	1	...	$m - 1$	...	k
0	$r_{0,0}$	$r_{0,1}$	...	$r_{0,m-1}$	...	—
⋮	⋮	⋮	⋱	⋮	⋱	⋮
s	$r_{s,0}$	$r_{s,1}$	...	$r_{s,m-1}$	...	—
⋮	⋮	⋮	⋱	⋮	⋱	⋮
t	$r_{t,0}$	$r_{t,1}$	...	$r_{t,m-1}$	...	—

Fig. 3. The *aux* matrix in the B&B algorithm. According to the matrix, the *tClass* s is covered by the *kClass* k; $r_{s,o}$, k; $r_{s,1}$, ..., k; $r_{s,m-1}$.

that covers at least one *tClass* not covered yet. If *tClass* j is the lesser[1] *tClass* not covered by the partial solution, then the first *kClass* stored in row j of the *aux* matrix is added to the partial solution. The algorithm proceed in this way until all the *tClass* are covered.

The first complete solution will be formed by elements in the first column of the *aux* matrix, possible not all of them. Because of this, it is necessary to know at any time to which row and column of the *aux* matrix a *kClass* in the current solution belongs, because the algorithm works by replacing the last added *kClass* by the next *kClass* in its row (the row of the last added *kClass*).

Having the first complete solution, what follows is to replace in the current solution the last added *kClass* by the next *kClass* in its row. There are two possibilities: (1) The next *kClass* covers all the *tClass* covered by the replaced *kClass*. In this case the new subset of *kClass* is tested to verify whether or not it improves (has less rows) the current best solution; (2) The next *kClass* does not cover all the *tClass* covered by the replaced *kClass*. Here the solution is not completed and has to be completed in the same way as the first solution was found.

When the row of the currently last added *kClass* is exhausted, the last added class is removed from the solution and the second from last added *kClass* is replaced by the following *kClass* in its row. If this *kClass* does not cover all the *tClass* covered by the previously two last added *kClass*, then one more *kClass* is added until all the *tClass* are covered; but if the *kClass* covers all the remaining *tClass* then no other *kClass* is added to the current solution, and the combinations containing redundant[2] *kClass* are never tested. In any case the process of replacing the last added *kClass* by the next *kClass* in its row starts again.

The algorithm works in this way, going up and down in the rows of the *aux* matrix and making bounds whenever possible. Every time a row is exhausted the *kClass* previously added is replaced by the next *kClass* in its row. Let r be this next *kClass*, then the following *kClass* added in order to complete a valid solution must be greater than r, because all the *kClass* less than r were already considered or will be considered late when the backtrack reaches the *kClass* lesser than r. In this way, all the *kClass* lesser than the last added *kClass* r are ignored in the bound phase. The algorithm ends when the first row of the *aux* matrix is exhausted.

For the example in Fig. 2(b) the *aux* matrix is showed in Fig. 4. In this example the first solution constructed is $\{0, 1, 2\}$ which is formed by the *kClass* in the first column of the *aux* matrix (not by the *kClass* in the first row). Next, the algorithm explores the solutions: $\{0, 1, 3\}$, $\{0, 1, 4\}$, $\{0, 2\}$, $\{0, 3\}$, $\{1, 2\}$, $\{1, 3\}$, $\{1, 4\}$ and $\{2\}$.

---

[1] By identifying the $t + 1$ *tClass* in the same way as the *kClass*, i.e. by the number of 1's in its rows.

[2] One *kClass* is redundant with respect to the other *kClass* in the current solution if it does not cover at least one *tClass* not covered by any *kClass* in the solution.

rows	cols				
	0	1	2	3	4
0	0	1	2	–	–
1	1	2	3	–	–
2	2	3	4	–	–

Fig. 4. *aux* matrix for the *kt structure* of the Fig. 2(b).

3.3   The Explicit Formula

The B&B algorithm was developed with the purpose of finding all the optimal solutions (in the sense of juxtaposing the interpretation of binomial coefficients) for given values of k and t. Table 1 shows the results found with the B&B algorithm for $k = 3, \ldots, 10$ and $t = 2, \ldots, 9$.

The case $k = t$ is trivial because the only solution is to take all the *kClass* $\{^k_r\}$, $0 \le r \le k$. Other patterns easy to see is that there are two solutions when t is even, except for $t = k$, and there is only one solution when t is odd, except for $t = k - 1$.

When $t = k - 1$ there are always two solutions regardless if t is even or odd. The two solutions make one partition of the *kClass* with the *kClass* whose rows have an even number of 1's in one solution and the *kClass* whose rows have an odd number of 1's in the other solution. Because the two solutions are optimal they have the same number of rows, so this solutions are isomorphic orthogonal arrays of index unity $OA(2^{k-1}; k - 1, k, 2)$.

However, the more important pattern is when the number of 1's in the rows of the *kClass* in the solutions are separated by a distance of $k - t + 1$. For example, for $k = 6$ and $t = 5$ the solutions are $\{\{^6_0\}, \{^6_2\}, \{^6_4\}, \{^6_6\}\}$ and $\{\{^6_1\}, \{^6_3\}, \{^6_5\}\}$, in both cases the number of 1's in the rows of the *kClass* are separated by one distance of $k - t + 1 = 6 - 5 + 1 = 2$. When $k = 9$ and $t = 3$, the solution is $\{\{^9_1\}, \{^9_8\}\}$, and the classes in the solution are separated by a distance of $9 - 3 + 1 = 7$. Therefore the number of 1's in the rows of the *kClass* in the solution(s) for $k = a$ and $t = b$ are separated by a distance of $a - b + 1$.

The key to derive the general formula is to determine one of the *kClass* in the solution. Because of knowing one *kClass* in the solution the others *kClass* may be inferred easily, since the number of 1's in their rows are separated by a distance of $k - t + 1$.

Again, the results in Table 1 allows to find the answer. We found that one *kClass* always present in at least one of the solutions for general values of k and t is the *kClass* whose rows have $\lfloor \frac{t}{2} \rfloor$ 1's. This *kClass* is not necessarily the class whose rows have the minimum number of 1's among all the *kClass* in the solution, but since the separation between the number of 1's in the rows of the *kClass* is known, the *kClass* with rows having less than $\lfloor \frac{t}{2} \rfloor$ 1's are obtained by subtracting $k - t + 1$ from $\lfloor \frac{t}{2} \rfloor$ while the resulting number is greater than or equal to zero.

Table 1. Optimal solutions found by the B&B algorithm for $k = 3,\ldots,10$ and $t = 2\ldots,9$. The null symbol $-$ is placed in the cells where $k < t$.

k	2	3	4	5	6	7	8	9
3	$\binom{3}{0}+\binom{3}{2}$ $\binom{3}{1}+\binom{3}{3}$	$\binom{3}{0}+\cdots+\binom{3}{3}$	–	–	–	–	–	–
4	$\binom{4}{0}+\binom{4}{3}$ $\binom{4}{1}+\binom{4}{4}$	$\binom{4}{0}+\binom{4}{2}+\binom{4}{4}$ $\binom{4}{1}+\binom{4}{3}$	$\binom{4}{0}+\cdots+\binom{4}{4}$	–	–	–	–	–
5	$\binom{5}{0}+\binom{5}{4}$ $\binom{5}{1}+\binom{5}{5}$	$\binom{5}{0}+\binom{5}{3}$ $\binom{5}{1}+\binom{5}{4}$	$\binom{5}{0}+\binom{5}{2}+\binom{5}{4}$ $\binom{5}{1}+\binom{5}{3}$	$\binom{5}{0}+\cdots+\binom{5}{5}$	–	–	–	–
6	$\binom{6}{0}+\binom{6}{5}$ $\binom{6}{1}+\binom{6}{6}$	$\binom{6}{0}+\binom{6}{5}$ $\binom{6}{1}+\binom{6}{6}$	$\binom{6}{0}+\binom{6}{4}$ $\binom{6}{1}+\binom{6}{5}$	$\binom{6}{0}+\binom{6}{4}+\binom{6}{6}$ $\binom{6}{1}+\cdots+\binom{6}{5}$	$\binom{6}{0}+\cdots+\binom{6}{6}$	–	–	–
7	$\binom{7}{0}+\binom{7}{6}$ $\binom{7}{1}+\binom{7}{7}$	$\binom{7}{0}+\binom{7}{6}$ $\binom{7}{1}+\binom{7}{6}$	$\binom{7}{0}+\binom{7}{5}$ $\binom{7}{1}+\binom{7}{6}$	$\binom{7}{2}+\binom{7}{5}$ $\binom{7}{1}+\binom{7}{5}$	$\binom{7}{0}+\binom{7}{2}+\binom{7}{4}+\binom{7}{6}$ $\binom{7}{1}+\cdots+\binom{7}{7}$	$\binom{7}{0}+\cdots+\binom{7}{7}$	–	–
8	$\binom{8}{0}+\binom{8}{7}$ $\binom{8}{1}+\binom{8}{8}$	$\binom{8}{0}+\binom{8}{7}$ $\binom{8}{1}+\binom{8}{7}$	$\binom{8}{0}+\binom{8}{6}$ $\binom{8}{1}+\binom{8}{7}$	$\binom{8}{0}+\binom{8}{6}$ $\binom{8}{1}+\binom{8}{6}$	$\binom{8}{0}+\binom{8}{3}+\binom{8}{5}$ $\binom{8}{1}+\binom{8}{4}+\binom{8}{5}$	$\binom{8}{0}+\binom{8}{2}+\binom{8}{4}+\binom{8}{6}+\binom{8}{8}$ $\binom{8}{1}+\binom{8}{3}+\binom{8}{5}+\binom{8}{7}$	$\binom{8}{0}+\cdots+\binom{8}{8}$	–
9	$\binom{9}{0}+\binom{9}{8}$ $\binom{9}{1}+\binom{9}{9}$	$\binom{9}{0}+\binom{9}{8}$ $\binom{9}{1}+\binom{9}{8}$	$\binom{9}{1}+\binom{9}{7}$ $\binom{9}{2}+\binom{9}{8}$	$\binom{9}{2}+\binom{9}{7}$ $\binom{9}{2}+\binom{9}{7}$	$\binom{9}{2}+\binom{9}{6}$ $\binom{9}{3}+\binom{9}{7}$	$\binom{9}{0}+\binom{9}{3}+\binom{9}{6}+\binom{9}{9}$ $\binom{9}{1}+\binom{9}{4}+\binom{9}{5}+\binom{9}{9}$	$\binom{9}{0}+\binom{9}{2}+\binom{9}{4}+\binom{9}{6}+\binom{9}{8}$ $\binom{9}{1}+\cdots+\binom{9}{9}$	$\binom{9}{0}+\cdots+\binom{9}{9}$
10	$\binom{10}{0}+\binom{10}{9}$ $\binom{10}{1}+\binom{10}{10}$	$\binom{10}{0}+\binom{10}{9}$ $\binom{10}{1}+\binom{10}{9}$	$\binom{10}{1}+\binom{10}{8}$ $\binom{10}{2}+\binom{10}{9}$	$\binom{10}{2}+\binom{10}{8}$ $\binom{10}{3}+\binom{10}{8}$	$\binom{10}{2}+\binom{10}{7}$ $\binom{10}{3}+\binom{10}{8}$	$\binom{10}{3}+\binom{10}{7}$	$\binom{10}{0}+\binom{10}{2}+\binom{10}{4}+\binom{10}{6}+\binom{10}{8}$ $\binom{10}{1}+\cdots+\binom{10}{9}$	$\binom{10}{0}+\binom{10}{2}+\binom{10}{4}+\binom{10}{6}+\binom{10}{8}+\binom{10}{10}$ $\binom{10}{1}+\binom{10}{3}+\binom{10}{5}+\binom{10}{7}+\binom{10}{9}$

t

For example, when $k = 9$ and $t = 8$ the $kClass$ with minimum number of 1's it its rows is obtained by repeatedly subtracting $d = 9 - 8 + 1 = 2$ from $\lfloor \frac{t}{2} \rfloor = \lfloor \frac{8}{2} \rfloor = 4$ while the resulting number is not negative. In this way the $kClass$ with less number of 1's in its rows is the $kClass$ $\left\{ \begin{smallmatrix} 9 \\ 0 \end{smallmatrix} \right\}$ because $4 - 2 = 2$ and $2 - 2 = 0$.

Successive subtractions are better expressed by a module operation. Then for given values of k and t the least number of 1's in the rows of a $kClass$ $\left\{ \begin{smallmatrix} k \\ r_0 \end{smallmatrix} \right\}$ in the solution for k and t is:

$$ r_0 = \left\lfloor \frac{t}{2} \right\rfloor \bmod (k - t + 1). $$

Thus, for $k = 9$ and $t = 8$ the $kClass$ with less number of 1's in its rows is the $kClass$ $\left\{ \begin{smallmatrix} 9 \\ \lfloor \frac{8}{2} \rfloor \bmod (9-8+1) \end{smallmatrix} \right\} = \left\{ \begin{smallmatrix} 9 \\ 4 \bmod 2 \end{smallmatrix} \right\} = \left\{ \begin{smallmatrix} 9 \\ 0 \end{smallmatrix} \right\}$. The last thing necessary for the general formula is to determine how many $kClass$ are in the solution. This number is determined as follows: the first $kClass$ in the solution is the $kClass$ whose rows have $r_0 = \lfloor \frac{t}{2} \rfloor \bmod (k - t + 1)$ 1's, then the strategy is to determine how many times the value $k - t + 1$ may be added to r_0 without exceed k, and this number of times will be the number of $kClass$ the solution has in addition to $kClass$ $\left\{ \begin{smallmatrix} k \\ r_0 \end{smallmatrix} \right\}$. So the formula to obtain the number of $kClass$ in the solution for given values of k and t is:

$$ \left\lfloor \frac{k - r_0}{k - t + 1} \right\rfloor + 1. $$

At this point we know the initial $kClass$, or the $kClass$ whose rows have less 1's, $\lfloor \frac{t}{2} \rfloor \bmod (k - t + 1)$, and the length of the separation between the number of 1's in the $kClass$, $k - t + 1$. Therefore given any values of k and t with $t \leq k$ the explicit formula to construct a binary CA is the Eq. 1.

$$ \sum_{j=0}^{\left\lfloor \frac{k - (\lfloor \frac{t}{2} \rfloor \bmod (k-t+1))}{k-t+1} \right\rfloor} \left\{ \begin{smallmatrix} k \\ (k - t + 1) j + (\lfloor \frac{t}{2} \rfloor \bmod (k - t + 1)) \end{smallmatrix} \right\} \tag{1} $$

In fact, Eq. 1 is not a formula to construct a CA rather it is the CA itself, because it denotes the juxtaposition of the row subsets that form the CA.

For example let $k = 8$ and $t = 7$ be, the first $kClass$ in the solution is the $kClass$ $\left\{ \begin{smallmatrix} 8 \\ \lfloor \frac{7}{2} \rfloor \bmod (8-7+1) \end{smallmatrix} \right\} = \left\{ \begin{smallmatrix} 8 \\ 3 \bmod 2 \end{smallmatrix} \right\} = \left\{ \begin{smallmatrix} 8 \\ 1 \end{smallmatrix} \right\}$. The total number of $kClass$ in the solution is $\lfloor \frac{8-1}{8-7+1} \rfloor + 1 = \lfloor \frac{7}{2} \rfloor + 1 = 3 + 1 = 4$. Thereby the CA for $k = 8$ and $t = 7$ is given by $\sum_{j=0}^{3} \left\{ \begin{smallmatrix} 8 \\ 2j+1 \end{smallmatrix} \right\} = \left\{ \begin{smallmatrix} 8 \\ 1 \end{smallmatrix} \right\} + \left\{ \begin{smallmatrix} 8 \\ 3 \end{smallmatrix} \right\} + \left\{ \begin{smallmatrix} 8 \\ 5 \end{smallmatrix} \right\} + \left\{ \begin{smallmatrix} 8 \\ 7 \end{smallmatrix} \right\}$.

For the cases in which two solutions exists, the Eq. 1 only provides one of them, the one that contains the $kClass$ with $\lfloor \frac{t}{2} \rfloor$ 1's in its rows, but since both solutions have an equal number of rows the Eq. 1 provides the optimal construction (for this method) of binary covering arrays from the interpretation we gave to binomial coefficients.

4   Computational Results

In order to get insight into the characteristics of the solutions provided by our direct method we will present a set of computational results derived of the use of Eq. 1 to find binary CAs for given values of k and t tables.

Equation 1 provides the row subsets which form the small CA that can be obtained with this method of construction. As mentioned in Sect. 3.3 the length of separation between the amount of 1's in the $kClass$ is equal to $k-t+1$, which in this case is $(t+1)-t+1=2$. In this and several other tables the value of k does not appear explicitly in the tables, instead a value called s appears in the tables. The value of k can be deduce from the values of t and s by adding them, for example consider $t=4$ and $s=1$, then the value of k is equal to $4+1=5$.

This case $k=t+1$ is one of the two cases in which the CA provided by the direct method is optimal with respect to any method of construction and not only with respect to our direct method, i. e. there not exist better CAs for $k=t+1$. The reason is that these CAs are orthogonal arrays of index unity $OA(2^{k-1}, k-1, k, 2)$.

Since the number of rows in a row subset $\left\{ {k \atop r} \right\}$ is given by the binomial coefficient $\binom{k}{r}$ interpreted as a number, it follows that the total number of rows (the size) of the CA $\sum_{j=0}^{m} \left\{ {k \atop r_j} \right\}$ provided by Eq. 1[3] is equal to $\sum_{j=0}^{m-1} \binom{k}{r_j}$. In this way replacing the row subsets by its corresponding binomial coefficient in Eq. 1 the size of the CA is obtained by accumulating the value of the binomial coefficients. Therefore the size of the CA generated by the direct method for certain values of k and t can be computed as easily as the generation of the CA itself.

Tables 2 and 3 contain the size of the CAs generated by the direct method for $k=t+1, t+2, \ldots, t+25$ and $t=2, 3, \ldots, 26$. The tables have three different text presentation: normal, bold and italic. Normal text is used for the result values which did not improve the previous bound reported; text in bold is used for highlight the result which improve the previous best bound reported; and the text in italic is used for the bounds proposed by first time.

In total nine previously reported upper bounds were improved by the direct method, these are extracted in Table 4 for better clarity. The previous better bounds used for comparing were the reported by Colbourn et al. [8]. The last column of Table 4 shows the improvement achieved with the direct method, i.e. the number of rows lowered with respect to the previous bound. In all cases the new upper bound given by the direct method is considerably better than the previous one. For example, the case in which less rows were lowered is the case $s=5$, $t=8$, the previous best bound was of 1051 rows while the bound given by our direct method is 1001 rows, which is an improvement of 50 rows. In the same way, the case in which more rows were lowered is the case $s=3$, $t=11$ in which the improvement was of 1158 rows because the previous best bound was of 5190 rows and the new bound given by the direct method is 4032 rows.

---

[3] Being $m = \left\lfloor \frac{k - \left(\lfloor \frac{t}{2} \rfloor \bmod d \right)}{d} \right\rfloor$ and $r = dj + (\lfloor \frac{t}{2} \rfloor \bmod d)$ with $d = k - t + 1$.

Table 2. Size of the CAs generated by the direct method for $k = t+1, t+2, \ldots, t+25$ and $t = 2, 3, \ldots, 26$. The improved upper bounds are in boldface, the not improved ones are in normal text, and new bounds are in italic.

s										t							
	2	3	4	5	6	7	8	9	10	11	12	13	14	15	16	17
1	4	8	16	32	64	128	256	512	1024	2048	4096	8192	16384	32768	65536	131072
2	5	10	21	42	85	170	341	682	1356	2730	5461	10922	21845	43690	87381	174762
3	6	12	28	56	120	240	496	992	2016	4032	8128	16256	32640	65280	130816	261632
4	7	14	36	72	165	330	715	1430	3004	6008	12393	24786	50559	101118	204820	409640
5	8	16	45	90	220	440	1001	2002	4368	8736	18565	37130	77540	155080	320001	640002
6	9	18	55	110	286	572	1356	2730	6188	12376	27132	54264	116281	232562	490337	980674
7	10	20	66	132	364	728	1820	3640	8568	17136	38760	77520	170544	341088	735472	1470944
8	11	22	78	156	455	910	2380	4760	11628	23256	54264	108528	245157	490314	1081575	2163150
9	12	24	91	182	560	1120	3060	6120	15504	31008	74613	149226	346104	692208	1562275	3124550
10	13	26	105	210	680	1360	3876	7752	20349	40698	100947	201894	480700	961400	2220075	4440150
11	14	28	120	240	816	1632	4845	9690	26334	52668	134596	269192	657800	1315600	3108105	6216210
12	15	30	136	272	969	1938	5985	11970	33649	67298	177100	354200	888030	1776060	4292145	8584290
13	16	32	153	306	1140	2280	7315	14630	42504	85008	230230	460460	1184040	2368080	5852925	11705850
14	17	34	171	342	1330	2660	8855	17710	53130	106260	296010	592020	1560780	3121560	7888725	15777450
15	18	36	190	380	1540	3080	10626	21252	65780	131560	376740	753480	2035800	4071600	10518300	21036600
16	19	38	210	420	1771	3542	12650	25300	80730	161460	475020	950040	2629575	5259150	13884156	27768312
17	20	40	231	462	2024	4048	14950	29900	98280	196560	593775	1187550	3365856	6731712	18156204	36312408
18	21	42	253	506	2300	4600	17550	35100	118755	196560	736281	1472562	4272048	8544096	23535820	47071640
19	22	44	276	552	2600	5200	20475	40950	142596	237510	906192	1812384	5379616	10759232	30260340	60520680
20	23	46	300	600	2925	5850	23751	47502	169911	285012	1107568	2215136	6724520	13449040	38608020	77216040
21	24	48	325	650	3276	6552	27405	54810	201376	339822	1344904	2689808	8347680	16695360	48903492	97806984
22	25	50	351	702	3654	7308	31465	62930	237336	402752	1623160	3246320	10295472	20590944	61523748	123047496
23	26	52	378	756	4060	8120	35960	71920	278256	474672	1947792	3895584	12620256	25240512	76904685	153809370
24	27	54	406	812	4495	8990	40920	81840	324632	649264	2324784	4649568	15380937	30761874	95548245	191096490
25	28	56	435	870	4960	9920	46376	92752	376992	753984	2760681	5521362	18643560	37287120	118030185	236060370

Table 3. Size of the CAs generated by the direct method for $k = t+1, t+2, \ldots, t+25$ and $t = 2, 3, \ldots, 26$. The improved upper bounds are in boldface, the not improved ones are in normal text, and new bounds are in italic.

s	t								
	18	19	20	21	22	23	24	25	26
1	262144	524288	1048576	2097152	4194304	8388608	16777216	33554432	67108864
2	349525	699050	1398101	2796202	5592405	11184810	22369621	44739242	89478485
3	523776	1047552	2096128	4192256	8386560	16773120	33550336	67100672	134209536
4	826045	1652090	3321891	6643782	13333932	26667864	53457121	106914242	214146295
5	1309528	2619056	5326685	10653370	21572460	43144920	87087001	174174002	350739488
6	2043275	4086550	8439210	16878420	34621041	69242082	141290436	282580872	574274008
7	3124576	6249152	13123488	26246976	54631360	109262720	225828800	451657600	928262016
8	4686826	9373652	20030078	40060078	84672780	169345560	354822776	709645552	1476390160
9	6906900	13813800	30045016	60090032	129024512	258049024	548854601	1096709202	2310796740
10	10015005	20030010	44352165	88704330	193536721	387073442	834451835	1668903670	3562467966
11	14307150	28614300	64512240	129024480	286097760	572195520	1251677701	2503955240	5414450334
12	20160075	40320150	92561040	185122080	417225900	834451800	1852482996	3704965992	8122425445
13	28048800	56097600	131128140	262256280	600805296	1201610592	2707475148	5414950296	12033222880
14	38567100	77134200	183579396	367158792	854984304	1709968152	3910797436	7821594872	17620076360
15	52451256	104902512	254186856	508373712	1203322288	2406644576	5586853480	11173706960	25518731280
16	70607460	141214920	348330196	696660272	1676056044	3352112088	7898654920	15797309840	36576848168
17	94143280	188286560	472733756	945467512	2311801440	4623602880	11058116888	22116233776	51915526432
18	124403620	248807240	635745396	1271490792	3159461968	6318923936	15338678264	30677356528	73006209045
19	163011640	326023280	847660528	1695321056	4280561376	8561122752	21090682613	42181365226	101766230790
20	211915132	423830264	1121099408	2242918816	5752004349	11504008698	28760021745	57520043490	140676848445
21	273438880	546877760	1471442973	2942885946	7669339132	15338678264	38910617655	77821235910	192928242996
22	350343565	700687130	1917334783	3834669566	10150595910	20901191820	52251400851	104502801702	262596783764
23	445891810	891783620	2481256778	4962513556	13340783196	26681566392	69668534468	139337068936	354860518600
24	563921995	1127843990	2481256778	6380374572	17417193617	34834267234	92263734896	184527469672	476260169700
25	708930508	1417861016	2481256778	8152700842	22595200368	45190400736	121399651100	242799302200	453013559600

Table 4. Comparison table between the previous best bound and the new upper bound found by the direct method for specific values of s and t. In total nine upper bounds were improved.

s	t	Previous best bound	New bound	Improvement
3	8	563	**496**	-67
3	9	1230	**992**	-238
3	10	2491	**2016**	-475
3	11	5190	**4032**	-1158
4	8	795	**715**	-80
4	9	2002	**1430**	-572
4	10	4081	**3004**	-1077
5	8	1051	**1001**	-50
5	9	3014	**2002**	-1012

Table 5. Cases in which the direct method provides a better solution than the IPOG algorithm.

s	t	IPOG	Direct method	Improvement
1	3	9	**8**	-1
1	4	22	**16**	-6
1	5	42	**32**	-10
1	6	79	**64**	-15
2	2	6	**5**	-1
2	3	11	**10**	-1
2	4	26	**21**	-5
2	5	57	**42**	-15
2	6	118	**85**	-33
3	3	14	**12**	-2
3	4	32	**28**	-4
3	5	68	**56**	-12
3	6	142	**120**	-22
4	3	16	**14**	-2
4	5	77	**72**	-2
5	3	17	**16**	-1

We also compare the proposed direct method with the IPOG algorithm, one of the best known greedy algorithm for construction covering arrays. In the Table 5 are showed the cases in which the direct method provides better results than the IPOG algorithm. In general terms the direct method outperforms the IPOG algorithm for small values of k, but as k grows the IPOG algorithm

Table 6. Polynomials that describe in terms of k the size of the CAs generated by the direct method for $s = 1, 2, 3$. The last column indicates the value of k from which the polynomial is valid, i.e. correctly gives the size of the CA.

t	Polynomial	Valid for k ≥ t
2	$k+1$	3
3	$2k$	4
4	$\frac{1}{2}k(k-1)$	7
5	$k(k-1)$	8
6	$\frac{1}{6}k(k-1)(k+1)$	9
7	$\frac{1}{3}k(k+1)(k-2)$	10
8	$\frac{1}{24}k(k-1)(k-2)(k+1)$	12
9	$\frac{1}{12}k(k-1)(k-2)(k-3)$	13
10	$\frac{1}{120}k(k-1)(k-2)(k-3)(k+1)$	15
11	$\frac{1}{60}k(k-1)(k-2)(k-3)(k-4)$	16
12	$\frac{1}{720}k(k-1)(k-2)(k-3)(k-4)(k+1)$	18
13	$\frac{1}{360}k(k-1)(k-2)(k-3)(k-4)(k-5)$	19
14	$\frac{1}{5040}k(k-1)(k-2)(k-3)(k-4)(k-5)(k+1)$	21
15	$\frac{1}{2520}k(k-1)(k-2)(k-3)(k-4)(k-5)(k-6)$	22
16	$\frac{1}{40320}k(k-1)(k-2)(k-3)(k-4)(k-5)(k-6)(k+1)$	23
17	$\frac{1}{201160}k(k-7)(k-1)(k-2)(k-3)(k-4)(k-5)(k-6)$	24
18	$\frac{1}{362880}k(k-1)(k-2)(k-3)(k-4)(k-5)(k-6)(k-7)(k+1)$	27
19	$\frac{1}{181440}k(k-1)(k-2)(k-3)(k-4)(k-5)(k-6)(k-7)(k-8)$	28
20	$\frac{1}{3628800}k(k-1)(k-2)(k-3)(k-4)(k-5)(k-6))(k-7)(k-8)(k+1)$	30
21	$\frac{1}{181440}k(k-1)(k-2)(k-3)(k-4)(k-5)(k-6))(k-7)(k-8)(k-9)$	31
22	$\frac{1}{39916800}(k-1)(k-2)(k-3)(k-4)(k-5)(k-6))(k-7)(k-8)(k-9)(k+1)$	33
23	$\frac{1}{19958400}k(k-1)(k-2)(k-3)(k-4)(k-5)(k-6))(k-7)(k-8)(k-9)(k-10)$	34
24	$\frac{1}{479001600}k(k-1)(k-2)(k-3)(k-4)(k-5)(k-6))(k-7)(k-8)(k-9)(k-10)(k+1)$	36
25	$\frac{1}{239500800}k(k-1)(k-2)(k-3)(k-4)(k-5)(k-6))(k-7)(k-8)(k-9)(k-10)(k-11)$	37
26	$\frac{1}{6227020800}k(k-1)(k-2)(k-3)(k-4)(k-5)(k-6))(k-7)(k-8)(k-9)(k-10)(k-11)(k\ a\ 1)$	39

provides better results than the direct method. Because of the results of the IPOG algorithm are only available for $t \leq 6$ in the case of binary covering arrays, it was not possible to compare our direct method with the IPOG for greater values of t. The tables with the published CAs generated with the IPOG algorithm may be found in [11].

Analysing the results by columns in Tables 2 and 3 it was observed that the growth in size of the CAs generated by the direct method has some kind of particular behaviour. By analysing these results we found the growth in size of the CAs for a particular value of t may be described by a polynomial in terms of k after a certain value of k. The polynomials found are listed in Table 6.

To map the problem to the graph domain each *kClass* is a node of the graph and an edge exists between two *kClass* if both may be part of a solution according to the criteria of the B&B algorithm described in Sect. 3.2. In this algorithm a *kClass* is added to the partial solution if and only if it covers at least one *tClass* not covered by any other *kClass* in the partial solution. Then, the pair of *kClass* such as one of them covers at least one *tClass* not covered by the other *kClass* and reciprocally, are the *kClass* that may be part of a same solution and between them will be an edge in the graph.

In this way the problem now is to find the clique that makes the CA with the minimum number of rows. The size of the clique found for each combination of the values of s and t can be represented by the Eq. 2. Replacing the variables with values, we can know the size of the clique to these values; *e.g.* if the t has a value 8 and the s is 3 substituting these values in (Eq. 2), the result will be 3, which represents the size of the clique formed by the $kClass$ in the solution.

$$2 + \left\lfloor \frac{t}{2 + 2 \times s} \right\rfloor + \left\lfloor \frac{t - 1}{2 + 2 \times s} \right\rfloor \tag{2}$$

As done for t in terms of k the growth in size of the CAs generated by the direct method may be described in terms of t for fixed values of s. Table 7 shows the polynomials that describe the growth in size of the CAs for $s = 1, 2, 3$.

Table 7. Polynomials that describe the size of the CAs in terms of t for $s = 1, 2, 3$.

s	Polynomial
1	2^t
2	$\lfloor \frac{4}{3} 2^t \rfloor$
3	$2^{t+1} - 2^{\lfloor \frac{t+1}{2} \rfloor}$

5   Conclusions

Hardware Trojans has emerged as a serious security threat to many critical systems. Detection techniques are needed to ensure trust in hardware systems. Covering arrays are used in testing deterministic systems where failures occur as a result of interactions among subsystems. The goal is to reveal if any interaction induces a failure in the system. Given the complexity of the problem, it is needed to create experimental designs with high degree of interaction, the proposed approach provides the Covering Arrays of higher strengths needed.

In this work we used binomial coefficients such as $\binom{k}{r}$ to represent the set of rows with k columns and having $k - r$ zeroes and r ones using the notation $\{_r^k\}$. The main result of our proposal is a formula that given the values of k and t we provide a collection of row subsets, represented by binomial coefficients, that juxtaposed forms a CA for the given values k and t.

Given the parameters k and t the method of construction of binary CAs from this interpretation of binomial coefficients consists in finding a subcollection

$$\mathscr{C} = \left\{ \left\{ \begin{matrix} k \\ r_1 \end{matrix} \right\}, \left\{ \begin{matrix} k \\ r_2 \end{matrix} \right\}, \dots \left\{ \begin{matrix} k \\ r_m \end{matrix} \right\} \right\}, 0 \leq r_i \leq k,$$

and making the juxtaposition of all the member of $\mathscr{C}$. The result is a covering array for the given values of k and t, and the total number of rows from all row subsets must be the minimum possible, i.e. $|\mathscr{C}| \leq |\mathscr{C}'|$ for any other subcollection of row subsets $|\mathscr{C}'|$ which is a CA for k and t.

An exact algorithm was developed to obtain the subcollection of row subsets with the above characteristics for several values of k and t. Analysing which row subsets constitutes the solutions found by the exact algorithm a set of regular patterns were detected. All of these patters were summarized in a formula that provides the optimum (with respect to this method of construction) covering arrays for general values of k and t expressed as the juxtaposition of a subcollection of row subsets. The formula is:

$$\sum_{j=0}^{\lfloor \frac{k-r_0}{d} \rfloor} \left\{ {}_{dj+r_0}^{k} \right\}, \text{ where } d = k - t + 1 \text{ and } r_0 = \left\lfloor \frac{t}{2} \right\rfloor \bmod d.$$

This direct method of construction in general provides good CAs for general values of k and t but has the advantage of generating the CA in time $O(m)$ where $m = \lfloor \frac{k-r_0}{d} \rfloor + 1 \le k$ is the number of row subsets juxtaposed to form the CA. This make feasible the computation of CAs for large values of k and t such as $k = 50$ and $t = 25$ or $k = 100$ and $t = 30$ for example.

In total nine previously reported upper bounds were improved with this direct method, being the CA we found in all cases considerably better than the previous best known CA. For example, the case in which less rows were lowered is the case $k = 13$, $t = 8$, the previous best known CA has 1051 rows and the CA given by our direct method has 1001 rows, which is an improvement of 50 rows. In the same way, the case in which more rows were lowered is the case $k = 14$, $t = 11$ in which the improvement was of 1158 rows because the CA we found has 4032 rows and the previously best known CA has 5190 rows. In addition to the upper bounds improved, we are proposing bounds for great number of cases for which none upper bound was reported, specifically for $t \ge 7$. They can be used as experimental designs in Hardware Trojan detection.

Acknowledgements. The authors acknowledge General Coordination of Information and Communications Technologies (CGSTIC) at CINVESTAV for providing HPC resources on the Hybrid Cluster Supercomputer "Xiuhcoatl", that have contributed to the research results reported. The following projects have funded the research reported in this paper: 238469 - CONACyT Métodos Exactos para Construir Covering Arrays Óptimos; 2143 - Cátedras CONACyT.

References

1. Avila-George, H., Torres-Jimenez, J., Gonzalez-Hernandez, L., Hernández, V.: Metaheuristic approach for constructing functional test-suites. IET Softw. **7**(2), 104–117 (2013)
2. Bush, K.A.: Orthogonal arrays of index unity. Ann. Math. Stat. **23**(3), 426–434 (1952)
3. Cawse, J.N.: Experimental Design for Combinatorial and High Throughput Materials Development. John Wiley & Sons, Hoboken (2003)
4. Chateauneuf, M., Colbourn, C.J., Kreher, D.: Covering arrays of strength three. Des. Codes Crypt. **16**(3), 235–242 (1999)
5. Cohen, M.B., Colbourn, C.J., Ling, A.C.H.: Constructing strength three covering arrays with augmented annealing. Discrete Math. **308**(13), 2709–2722 (2008)

6. Colbourn, C.J.: Covering arrays from cyclotomy. Des. Codes Crypt. **55**, 201–219 (2010)
7. Colbourn, C.J., Cohen, M.B.: A deterministic density algorithm for pairwise interaction coverage. In: Proceedings of the IASTED - International Conference on Software Engineering, pp. 345–352 (2004)
8. Colbourn, C.J., Kéri, G., Rivas Soriano, P.P., Schlage-Puchta, J.C.: Covering and radius-covering arrays: constructions and classification. Discrete Appl. Math. **158**(11), 1158–1180 (2010)
9. Colbourn, C.J., Martirosyan, S.S., Mullen, G.L., Shasha, D., Sherwood, G.B., Yucas, J.L.: Products of mixed covering arrays of strength two. Comb. Designs **14**(2), 124–138 (2006)
10. Flottes, M.L., Dupuis, S., Ba, P.S., Rouzeyre, B.: On the limitations of logic testing for detecting hardware Trojans horses. In: 2015 10th International Conference on Design Technology of Integrated Systems in Nanoscale Era (DTIS), pp. 1–5, April 2015
11. Forbes, M., Lawrence, J., Lei, Y., Kacker, R.N., Kuhn, D.R.: Covering arrays generated by IPOG-F (2012). http://math.nist.gov/coveringarrays/ipof/ipof-results.html
12. Hartman, A.: Software and hardware testing using combinatorial covering suites. Graph Theory. Combinatorics and Algorithms. Operations Research/Computer Science Interfaces Series, pp. 237–266. Springer, US (2005)
13. Hedayat, A.S., Sloane, N.J.A., Stufken, J.: Orthogonal Arrays: Theory and Applications. Springer-Verlag, New York (1999)
14. Katona, G.O.H.: Two applications (for search theory and truth functions) of sperner type theorems. Periodica Mathematica Hungarica **3**(1–2), 19–26 (1973)
15. Kitsos, P., Dimitris, E.S., Torres-Jimenez, J., Voyiatzis, A.G.: Exciting FPGA cryptographic Trojans using combinatorial testing. In: Proceedings of the 26th IEEE International Symposium on Software Reliability Engineering (accepted 2015)
16. Kleitman, D.J., Spencer, J.: Families of k-independent sets. Discrete Math. **6**(3), 255–262 (1973)
17. Lawrence, J., Kacker, R.N., Lei, Y., Kuhn, D.R., Forbes, M.: A survey of binary covering arrays. Electron. J. Comb. **18**(1), 1–30 (2011)
18. Lei, Y., Kacker, R.N., Kuhn, D.R., Okun, V., Lawrence, J.: IPOG: a general strategy for T-way software testing. In: Proceedings of the 14th Annual IEEE International Conference and Workshops on the Engineering of Computer-Based Systems, pp. 549–556 (2007)
19. Martinez-Pena, J.: Construction of covering arrays of ternary alphabet and variable strength. Master's thesis, CINVESTAV-Tamaulipas, Information Technology Laboratory, January 2011
20. Meagher, K., Stevens, B.: Group construction of covering arrays. J. Comb. Designs **13**(1), 70–77 (2005)
21. Mingfu, X., Aiqun, H., Yi, H., Guyue, L.: Monte Carlo based test pattern generation for hardware Trojan detection. In: IEEE 11th International Conference on Dependable, Autonomic and Secure Computing (DASC 2013), pp. 131–136, December 2013
22. Nurmela, K.J.: Upper bounds for covering arrays by tabu search. Discrete Appl. Math. **138**(1–2), 143–152 (2004)
23. Shasha, D.E., Kouranov, A.Y., Lejay, L.V., Chou, M.F., Coruzzi, G.M.: Using combinatorial design to study regulation by multiple input signals: a tool for parsimony in the post-genomics era. Plant Physiol. **127**(4), 1590–1594 (2001)

24. Shiba, T., Tsuchiya, T., Kikuno, T.: Using artificial life techniques togenerate test cases for combinatorial testing.In: Proceedings of the 28th Annual International Computer Softwareand Applications Conference, vol. 01, pp. 72–77 (2004)

25. Sloane, N.J.A.: Covering arrays and intersecting codes. J. Comb. Designs **1**(1), 51–63 (1993)

26. Stardom, J.: Metaheuristics and the search for covering and packing arrays. Master's thesis, Simon Fraser University (2001)

27. Stevens, B., Mendelsohn, E.: New recursive methods for transversal covers. J. Comb. Designs **7**(3), 185–203 (1999)

28. Tang, D.T., Chen, C.L.: Iterative exhaustive pattern generation for logic testing. IBM J. Res. Dev. **28**(2), 212–219 (1984)

29. Tang, D.T., Woo, L.S.: Exhaustive test pattern generation with constant weight vectors. IEEE Trans. Comput. **32**(12), 1145–1150 (1983)

30. Torres-Jimenez, J., Rodriguez-Tello, E.: New bounds for binary covering arrays using simulated annealing. Inf. Sci. **185**(1), 137–152 (2012)

31. Walker II, R.A., Colbourn, C.J.: Tabu search for covering arrays using permutation vectors. J. Stat. Plann. Infer. **139**(1), 69–80 (2009)

32. Yin, J.: Constructions of difference covering arrays. J. Comb. Theor. Ser. A **104**(2), 327–339 (2003)

On the Model Checking of the Graded μ-calculus on Trees

Everardo Bárcenas[1,2]([✉]), Edgard Benítez-Guerrero[2], and Jesús Lavalle[3,4]

[1] Consejo Nacional de Ciencia Y Tecnología (CONACYT), Mexico City, México
ebarcenaspa@conacyt.mx
[2] Facultad de Estadística E Informática, Universidad Veracruzana, Xalapa, México
[3] Benemérita Universidad Autónoma de Puebla, Puebla, México
[4] Instituto Nacional de Astrofísica, Óptica Y Electrónica, Puebla, México

Abstract. The μ-calculus is an expressive propositional modal logic augmented with least and greatest fixed-points, and encompasses many temporal, program, dynamic and description logics. The model checking problem for the μ-calculus is known to be in NP ∩ Co-NP. In this paper, we study the model checking problem for the μ-calculus extended with graded modalities. These constructors allow to express numerical constraints on the occurrence of accessible nodes (worlds) satisfying a certain formula. It is known that the model checking problem for the graded μ-calculus with finite models is in EXPTIME. In the current work, we introduce a linear-time model checking algorithm for the graded μ-calculus when models are finite unranked trees.

1 Introduction

The μ-calculus is a well-known propositional modal logic augmented with least and greatest fixed-point operators. This logic generalizes several temporal, program, dynamic and description logics. In this paper, we study an extension of μ-calculus with graded modalities. These constructors allow to express existential and universal quantification, with respect to a non-negative integer, on the occurrence of accessible nodes (worlds) satisfying a certain formula. Graded modalities can be seen as a generalization of the well-known counting quantifiers $\forall^{\leq k}$ and $\exists^{>k}$ of classical logics [1]. In the knowledge representation community, graded modalities are known as number restrictions in description logics [2].

The extension of the μ-calculus with graded modalities, known as graded μ-calculus, has been previously studied in the setting of the decidability problem [3–5]. In this paper, we study the model checking problem for the graded μ-calculus with finite unranked tree models. In general, the model checking problem concerns the evaluation of a system specification, in this case written as a logic formula, against a formal model of a given system, in this case a finite unranked tree structure. The model checking problem have found applications in a wide range of areas in computer science [6,7]. For instance, the path planning problem, which concerns the automatic generation of agents paths, satisfying certain constraints, has been recently studied in the setting of the model

© Springer International Publishing Switzerland 2015
G. Sidorov and S.N. Galicia-Haro (Eds.): MICAI 2015, Part I, LNAI 9413, pp. 178–189, 2015.
DOI: 10.1007/978-3-319-27060-9_14

checking of linear temporal logic with great success [8]. With graded modalities, for example, one may express the existence of at least k paths ($\langle\downarrow, k\rangle\,\phi$) satisfying a certain property ϕ. Since we consider tree models, paths are collision-free and may be navigated by a team of agents. In the current work, we provide a linear-time algorithm for the model checking problem of the graded μ-calculus.

1.1   Motivations and Related Works

The model checking problem for the μ-calculus is known to be in NP $\cap$ Co-NP [9]. A linear-time algorithm for the model checking of the alternation-free fragments of the μ-calculus is reported in [10]. This result is replicated in [11] for an extension of the logic with inverse modalities on tree models. An extensive study of the model checking problem for the μ-calculus extended with combinations of graded and inverse modalities, and nominals, can be found in [12]. In particular, in this work is provided an exponential time algorithm for the model checking of the graded μ-calculus with finite models. In the current work, we provide a linear-time model checking algorithm for the graded μ-calculus with finite unranked tree models.

There are several recent studies about the representation of numerical restrictions on tree structures [5,13–17]. However, all those works focus on the study of reasoning problems only. In [18], there is an extensive study of the Computation Tree Logic (CTL) extended with numerical restrictions. In particular, this work provides several complexity results regarding the model checking problem for CTL counting extensions, which ranges from polynomial-time to undecidable. In [19], it is provided a linear-time model checking algorithm for an extension of CTL with graded paths. In contrast with these works [18,19], in the current paper we study the model checking problem of a counting extension of the μ-calculus, which is known to be more expressive than CTL.

1.2   Contributions and Outline

In Sect. 2, we introduce an extension of the μ-calculus with graded modalities. We also describe some examples in the usage of the logic. We present a model checking algorithm for the graded μ-calculus on trees in Sect. 3. The algorithm is based on a Fischer-Ladner representation of nodes, where graded modalities are coded in binary notation. We show the algorithm takes linear-time with respect the product of the sizes of the input formula and tree. We provide conclusions in Sect. 4, together with a discussion of further related research perspectives.

2   Graded μ-calculus for Trees

In this section, we introduce the μ-calculus for trees extended with graded modalities. This formalism is a propositional multi-modal logic with least and greatest fixed-points, augmented with graded modalities. These constructors constrain, with respect to a non-negative integer in binary notation, the occurrence of children nodes satisfying a certain formula.

Definition 1 (Syntax). *The syntax of the graded μ-calculus is defined by the following grammar:*

$$\phi := p \mid x \mid \neg\phi \mid \phi \vee \phi \mid \langle m \rangle \, \phi \mid \mu x.\phi \mid \langle \downarrow, k \rangle \, \phi$$

Formulas are interpreted over tree models as subset nodes. More precisely, propositions p are used as node labels. Negation and disjunction are interpreted as set complement and union, respectively. Modal formulas $\langle m \rangle \, \phi$ hold in nodes where there is *at least one* accessible node through m such that ϕ is true. Modalities $m \in \{\downarrow, \rightarrow\}$ are interpreted as the children $\downarrow$ and right siblings $\rightarrow$ relations. Formulas $\mu x.\phi$ are interpreted as least fixed-points and they are used as constructors for finite recursive navigation. Graded modalities $\langle \downarrow, k \rangle \, \phi$ hold in nodes where there are *at least $k + 1$ children* nodes where ϕ is true.

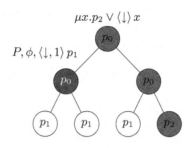

Fig. 1. A tree model for $\langle \downarrow, 1 \rangle \, p_1$ and $\mu x.p_2 \vee \langle \downarrow \rangle \, x$.

For instance, in a given tree, the following formula holds in nodes with at least 2 children named p_1:

$$\langle \downarrow, 1 \rangle \, p_1$$

In Fig. 1 is depicted a graphical representation of a model for this formula. The formula holds in the root of the left subtree, the only node with two p_1 children. To illustrate the usage of the least fixed-point operator as finite recursion, consider the following example formula:

$$\mu x.p_2 \vee \langle \downarrow \rangle \, x$$

This formula holds in nodes with at least 1 *descendant* (including itself) labeled by p_2. A graphical model for this formula is depicted in Fig. 1. This formula holds in the root, its right child and its rightest descendant.

In order to provide a precise semantics of logic formulas, we first introduce a formal notion of trees. A tree structure is defined as tuple $K = (N, R, L)$, where

- N is a finite set of nodes;
- R is family of binary relations $R^m : N \times N$, associating nodes through modalities forming a tree, written $n \in R(n, m)$; and
- $L : N \mapsto 2^P \setminus \emptyset$ is a left-total labeling function naming nodes with propositions.

Before defining formula semantics, we need the notion of a valuation V, which is a function from variables to a set of nodes of a given tree. A substitution in a valuation $V\left[^{x}/_{N}\right]$ stands for another valuation V' such that $V'(x) = N$ and $V'(x') = V(x')$ when $x \neq x'$.

Definition 2 (Semantics). *Formulas are interpreted with respect to a tree structure $K = (N, R, V)$ and a valuation V as follows:*

$$[p]_V^K = \{n \mid p \in L(n)\}$$
$$[x]_V^K = V(x)$$
$$[\neg \phi]_V^T = N \setminus [\phi]_V^K$$
$$[\phi \vee \psi]_V^K = [\phi]_V^K \cup [\psi]_V^K$$
$$[\langle m \rangle\, \phi]_V^K = \{n \mid R(n, m) \in [\phi]_V^K\}$$
$$[\mu x.\phi]_V^K = \bigcap \left\{ N' \subseteq N \mid [\phi]_{V[^{x}/_{N'}]}^K \subseteq N' \right\}$$
$$[\langle m, k \rangle\, \phi]_V^K = \{n \mid |[\phi]_V^K \cap R(n, \downarrow)| > k\}$$

If the interpretation of a formula ϕ is not empty with respect to a tree T, we say ϕ is satisfied by T, moreover, if $n \in [\phi]_V^T$, we say ϕ is satisfied by T in n. A formula is valid, if and only if, it is satisfied by any tree. The model checking of a formula with respect to a tree consists in finding the nodes in the tree where the formula is satisfied.

Definition 3 (Model checking). *Given a formula ϕ, a tree structure K, and a valuation V, the model checking problem is defined by the set of nodes in K satisfying ϕ under V, that is, $[\phi]_V^K$.*

We also use the following syntactic sugar: $\phi \wedge \psi \equiv \neg(\neg \phi \vee \neg \psi)$, $[m, k]\, \phi \equiv \neg \langle m, k \rangle\, \neg \phi$, $[m]\, \phi \equiv \neg \langle m \rangle\, \neg \phi$ and $\nu x.\phi \equiv \neg \mu x.\phi$. Conjunction follows the traditional De Morgan's laws, $[\downarrow, k]\, \phi$ holds in nodes with *all but k* children nodes where ϕ is true, nodes where $[m]\, \phi$ is true have all m-accessible neighbors witnessing ϕ, and $\nu x.\phi$ is interpreted as a greatest fixed-point.

3   Model Checking

In this Section, we describe a model checking algorithm for the graded μ-calculus for trees, that is, given a formula ϕ and a tree K, the algorithm computes the set of nodes in K, if any, where ϕ is satisfied. The algorithm is based on a Fischer-Ladner representation of trees. Intuitively, in a Fischer-Ladner tree, a node is defined as a set containing the propositions and modal subformulas satisfied by that particular node, then the satisfaction of the input formula can be tested by a boolean evaluation. In order to test graded formulas, we introduce counters, which are also contained in the nodes. Since numerical bounds in graded formulas are coded in binary, counters are also coded in binary. The algorithm test the input formula in a bottom-up manner, that is, first the formula is tested in the leaves, then, iteratively, the formula is tested in the parents. The process is bottom-up in order to guarantee the correct saturation of nodes with counters. Nodes satisfying the input formula are saved at each step. Finally, the stop condition is at the root node.

3.1   Preliminaries

There is a well-known relation between binary and n-ary unranked trees [17]. Hence, without loss of generality, we consider binary trees only (see Fig. 2). For this purpose, at the logic level, modal formulas are reinterpreted as follows:

- $\langle\downarrow\rangle\,\phi$ denotes the nodes where ϕ holds in the *first* child; and
- $\langle\rightarrow\rangle\,\phi$ stands for nodes where ϕ is true in the *following right* sibling.

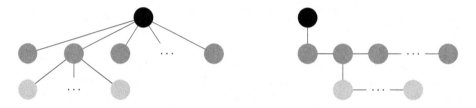

Fig. 2. Binary and n-ary correspondence on trees.

For the model checking algorithm, we consider cycle-free formulas only, that is, formulas where the fixed-point does not perform recursion in a cyclic manner. For instance, the following formula is not allowed: $\mu x.\,\langle\downarrow\rangle\,x\wedge\langle\uparrow\rangle\,x$. An interesting observation about cycle-free formulas on tree models is that the least and greatest fixed-points collapse [20].

Negation symbols in formulas in negation normal form occurs only immediately in front of propositions, modal subformulas $\langle m\rangle\top$, and $\top$. The negation normal form of a formula is obtained by replacing each occurrence of a negated subformula $\neg\phi$ by $nnf(\phi)$, where:

$$nnf(p) = \neg p \qquad\qquad nnf(\top) = \neg\top$$
$$nnf(x) = x \qquad\qquad nnf(\phi\vee\psi) = nnf(\phi)\wedge nnf(\psi)$$
$$nnf(\langle m\rangle\,\phi) = \langle m\rangle\,nnf(\phi)\vee\neg\,\langle m\rangle\top \quad nnf(\langle\downarrow,k\rangle\,\phi) = [\downarrow,k]\,nnf(\phi)$$
$$nnf(\mu x.\phi) = \mu x.nnf(\phi)$$

Considering the obvious semantics of conjunctions and graded box formulas, it is easy to see that a formula and its negation normal form are equivalent. Hence, without loss of generality, we consider formulas in negation normal form only.

We now introduce the notion of a counter, which is a boolean combination of propositions representing a binary number. For instance, given four propositions, the constant 2, which is coded as 0010 in binary, is represented by the following formula: $\neg p_1 \wedge \neg p_2 \wedge p_3 \wedge \neg p_4$. Then, for a graded formula $\langle \downarrow, k \rangle \phi$ or $[\downarrow, k]\phi$, we associate a finite set of fresh propositions, written $\phi^{k'}$, representing the occurrence of ϕ k'-times. The number of propositions, associated to some formula ϕ, is bounded by $maxK(\phi) = n * (b+1)$ (or simply $maxK$ when clear from context), where is the number of graded subformulas $\langle \downarrow, k \rangle \psi$ occurring in ϕ and b is the greatest constant occurring in those graded subformulas. The consistency of this bound comes from the following theorem.

Theorem 1 ([3,5]). *If a formula ϕ is satisfiable, then there is model for ϕ with at most $maxK(\phi)$ children of each node.*

We now define the lean set of a formula, which intuitively contains the propositions, modal subformulas, and graded subformulas together with their corresponding counters.

Definition 4 (Lean). *The lean set of a formula ϕ is inductively defined by the fixed-point of the following function:*

$$lean(\top) = \emptyset$$
$$lean(p) = \{p\}$$
$$lean(\neg \psi) = lean(\psi)$$
$$lean(\psi \circ \varphi) = lean(\psi) \cup lean(\varphi) \qquad\qquad \circ \in \{\wedge, \vee\}$$
$$lean(\langle m \rangle \psi) = \{\langle m \rangle \psi\} \cup lean(\psi)$$
$$lean(\circ \psi) = \left\{ \circ \psi, \psi^{maxK(\phi)}, \langle \downarrow \rangle \mu x.\psi \vee \langle \rightarrow \rangle x \right\} \cup lean(\psi) \quad \circ \in \{\langle \downarrow, k \rangle, [\downarrow, k]\}$$
$$lean(\mu x.\psi) = lean \left(\psi \left[{}^x / {}_{\mu x.\psi} \right] \right)$$

In addition, the lean set also considers the following formulas $\langle m \rangle \top$ for any m.

Due to fact that the lean function is monotone and to the Fixed-Point Theorem, it is clear there is a fixed-point.

Another straightforward observation is that the lean set of a formula is of linear size.

Proposition 1. *Given a formula ϕ, the size of $lean(\phi)$ is linear with respect to the size of ϕ.*

Example 1. Consider for instance the following formula:

$$\phi := p_0 \wedge (\langle \downarrow \rangle \mu x.p_1 \vee \langle \rightarrow \rangle x) \wedge \langle \downarrow, 2 \rangle p_2$$

The lean of this formula is then defined as follows:

$$lean(\phi) = \{p_0, p_1, p_2, \langle \downarrow \rangle \mu x.p_1 \vee \langle \rightarrow \rangle x, \langle \rightarrow \rangle \mu x.p_1 \vee \langle \rightarrow \rangle x,$$
$$\langle \downarrow, 2 \rangle p_2, p_2^3, \langle \downarrow \rangle \mu x.p_2 \vee \langle \rightarrow \rangle x, \langle \rightarrow \rangle \mu x.p_2 \vee \langle \rightarrow \rangle x, \langle \downarrow \rangle \top, \langle \rightarrow \rangle \top\}$$

We now define the notion of a pre-model, which is the syntactic version of a tree structure, where each node is a subset of the input formula lean.

Definition 5 (Pre-model). *Given a tree structure $K = (N, R, L)$ and a formula ϕ, a pre-model is defined as a tuple $T = (N', R', b)$, such that:*

- *each node of the pre-model is a subset of the lean of ϕ, that is, $N' \subseteq 2^{lean(\phi)}$;*
- *$b : N \mapsto N'$ is a partial bijection; and*
- *$R' : N' \times M \times N'$, such that $b(n') \in R'(b(n), m)$ whenever $n' \in R(n, m)$.*

Notice that a pre-model is not necessarily a tree. This is because the algorithm evaluates the input tree in a bottom-up manner, hence the pre-model is also constructed in a bottom-up manner. This implies the pre-model may take the form of a forest (set of trees). We also define the function $root(T)$ which outputs the root nodes of the pre-model T. Abusing of notation, function $root(K)$ denotes the set with the root node of K.

Example 2. Consider for instance the following tree structure $K = (N, R, L)$, where:

- $N = \{n_i \mid i = 0, \ldots, 6\}$;
- $n_1 \in R(n_0, \downarrow)$, $n_2 \in R(n_1, \downarrow)$, $n_3 \in R(n_1, \rightarrow)$, $n_4 \in R(n_3, \downarrow)$, $n_5 \in R(n_4, \rightarrow)$, and $n_6 \in R(n_5, \rightarrow)$; and
- $L(n_0) = \{p_0\}$, $L(n_1) = \{p_1\}$, $L(n_2) = \{p_1\}$, $L(n_3) = \{p_2\}$, $L(n_4) = \{p_2\}$, $L(n_5) = \{p_1\}$, and $L(n_6) = \{p_1\}$.

A graphical representation of this tree is depicted in Fig. 3. Now consider ϕ as defined in Example 1: $p_0 \wedge (\langle \downarrow \rangle \mu x.p_1 \vee \langle \rightarrow \rangle x) \wedge \langle \downarrow, 2 \rangle p_2$. We then define a pre-model $T = (N', R', b)$ of ϕ and K as follows:

- $N' = \{b(n_i) \mid i = 0, 1, \ldots, 6\}$, such that

$$b(n_0) = \{p_0, \langle \downarrow \rangle \mu x.p_1 \vee \langle \rightarrow \rangle x, \langle \downarrow, 2 \rangle p_2, \langle \downarrow \rangle \mu x.p_2 \vee \langle \rightarrow \rangle x, \langle \downarrow \rangle \top\}$$

$$b(n_1) = \{p_2, \langle \downarrow \rangle \mu x.p_1 \vee \langle \rightarrow \rangle x, \langle \rightarrow \rangle \mu x.p_1 \vee \langle \rightarrow \rangle x, \langle \downarrow \rangle \top, \langle \rightarrow \rangle \top, p_2^3,$$
$$\langle \rightarrow \rangle \mu x.p_2 \vee \langle \rightarrow \rangle x\}$$

$$b(n_2) = \{p_1\}$$

$$b(n_3) = \{p_1, \langle \downarrow \rangle \top, \langle \rightarrow \rangle \top, p_2^2, \langle \downarrow \rangle \mu x.p_2 \vee \langle \rightarrow \rangle x, \langle \rightarrow \rangle \mu x.p_2 \vee \langle \rightarrow \rangle x\}$$

$$b(n_4) = \{p_2, p_2^1\}$$

$$b(n_5) = \{p_2, \langle \rightarrow \rangle \top, p_2^2, \langle \rightarrow \rangle \mu x.p_2 \vee \langle \rightarrow \rangle x\}$$

$$b(n_6) = \{p_2, p_2^1\}$$

We also need to define a notion of syntactic satisfaction of formulas (entailment), which is binary relation of nodes in a pre-model and formulas.

Algorithm 1. Model checking algorithm

Input: (K, ϕ)

$T \leftarrow Init(K)$
$T \leftarrow Saturate(T)$
$Sat \leftarrow \emptyset$
$Sat \leftarrow Sat \cup satisfiables(T)$
while $root(T) \neq root(K)$ **do**
    $T \leftarrow Update(T)$
    $T \leftarrow Saturate(T)$
    $Sat \leftarrow Sat \cup satisfiables(T)$
end while
return Sat

Definition 6 (Entailment). *We define entailment as a binary relation as follows:*

$$\frac{}{n \vdash \top} \qquad \frac{p \in n}{n \vdash p} \qquad \frac{\phi \notin n}{n \vdash \neg\phi} \qquad \frac{\langle m \rangle \phi \in n}{n \vdash \langle m \rangle \phi}$$

$$\frac{n \vdash \phi \quad n \vdash \psi}{n \vdash \phi \wedge \psi} \qquad \frac{n \vdash \phi}{n \vdash \phi \vee \psi} \qquad \frac{n \vdash \psi}{n \vdash \phi \vee \psi} \qquad \frac{n \vdash \phi\,[^x/_{\mu x.\phi}]}{n \vdash \mu x.\phi}$$

$$\frac{\langle \downarrow, k \rangle \phi \in n}{n \vdash \langle \downarrow, k \rangle \phi} \qquad \frac{[\downarrow, k] \phi \in n}{n \vdash [\downarrow, k] \phi}$$

Relation $\nvdash$ is defined as expected: when not $\vdash$ and $n \nvdash \neg\top$ for any n.

We will distinguish leaf nodes in tree structures. Given a tree structure $K = (N, R, L)$, we define the set of leaves as follows:

$$Leaves(K) = \{n \in N \mid R(n, \downarrow) \cup R(n, \rightarrow) = \emptyset\}$$

3.2 The Algorithm

The algorithms builds a pre-model from the input tree in a bottom-up manner: starting from the leaves, the algorithm iteratively adds the corresponding parents. At each step, the input formula is tested using the entailment relation. In case the root node satisfies (entails) the formula, then the node is saved. The algorithm stops at the root node of the input tree. Finally, the (possibly empty) set of nodes satisfying the input formula is returned. In Fig. 1, the algorithm is depicted.

We now give a precise description of each component of the algorithm. The leaf nodes are the first ones to be considered in the construction of the pre-model.

Definition 7 (Init). *Given a tree structure K, we define the initial pre-model $Init(K) = (N, R, b)$ as follows:*

- *if* $n \in Leaves(K)$, *then* $b(n) \in N$; *and*
- $R = \emptyset$

Consider for instance the formula ϕ and tree of Fig. 3. It is easy to see the *Init* pre-model is composed by the leaves $b(n_2)$, $b(n_4)$ and $b(n_6)$, defined in Example 2. Notice that, at this point, counters in the leaves are set to zero.

The second step in the algorithm consists in the saturation of leaves in the pre-model. In general, the saturation of a node consists in the addition of formulas, in the lean, satisfied by the node itself. Counter are also updated in the saturation process.

Definition 8 (Saturate). *Given a a pre-model* $T = (N', R', b)$ *of a formula* ϕ *and a tree structure* $K = (N, R, L)$, *we define the saturation of* T, *in particular, for each* $b(n) \in root(T)$, *as follows:*

- *for each* $p \in lean(\phi)$, *if* $p \in L(n)$, *then* $p \in b(n)$;
- *for each* $\langle m \rangle \, \psi \in lean(\phi)$, *if* $n' \in R'(b(n), m)$ *and* $n' \vdash \psi$, *then* $\langle m \rangle \, \psi \in b(n)$;
- *for each* $\circ \psi \in lean(\phi)$ ($\circ \in \{ \langle \downarrow, k \rangle, [\downarrow, k] \}$), *if* $n' \in R'(b(n), \to)$ *and* $\psi^k \in n'$, *we distinguish two cases, one when* $b(n) \vdash \psi$, *in which case* $\psi^{k+2} \in b(n)$, *the other when* $b(n) \nvdash \psi$, *which implies* $\psi^{k+1} \in b(n)$;
- *for each* $\langle \downarrow, k \rangle \, \psi \in lean(\phi)$, *if* $n' \in R'(b(n), \downarrow)$, $\psi^{k'} \in n'$, *and* $k' > k$, *then* $\langle \downarrow, k \rangle \, \psi \in b(n)$; *and*
- *for each* $[\downarrow, k] \, \psi \in lean(\phi)$, *if* $n' \in R'(b(n), \downarrow)$, $\psi^{k'} \in n'$, *and* $k' \leq k$, *then* $[\downarrow, k] \, \psi \in b(n)$.

As an example of saturation consider again the formula and tree structure of Fig. 3. Notice leaves $b(n_2)$, $b(n_4)$ and $b(n_6)$ as defined in Example 2 corresponds to the saturation process. In subsequent evaluation steps of the model checking algorithm, once the parents are considered in the pre-model, notice how the counters are updated in nodes $b(n5)$, $b(n_3)$ and $b(n_1)$. Since counter p_2^3 is in $b(n_1)$, then in the last of step of the algorithm, subformula $\langle \downarrow, 2 \rangle \, p_2$ is thus added to $b(n_0)$.

Once the leaves are saturated, the algorithm saves the ones satisfying the input formula.

Definition 9 (satisfiables). *Given a pre-model* $T = (N', R', b)$ *of a formula* ϕ *and tree structure* $K = (N, R, L)$, *we define the set of nodes satisfying the formula as follows:*

$$satisfiables(T) = \{ n \in N \mid b(n) \vdash \phi, b(n) \in root(T) \}$$

Considering the example of Fig. 3, and the pre-model as defined in Example 2, node $b(n_0)$ satisfies the input formula ϕ.

The next step of the algorithm is the iterative addition of parents to the previously built pre-model. This is performed by the *Update* function.

Definition 10 (Update). *Given a pre-model* $T = (N', R', b)$ *of a formula* ϕ *and tree structure* $K = (N, R, L)$, *we define the pre-model* $Update(T) = (N'', R'', b')$ *of* ϕ *and* K *as follows:*

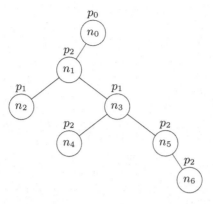

Fig. 3. (Pre)-model for $\phi := p_0 \wedge (\langle\downarrow\rangle\, \mu x.p_1 \vee \langle\rightarrow\rangle\, x) \wedge \langle\downarrow, 2\rangle\, p_2$

– $N' \subseteq N''$, $R' \subseteq R''$, and $b \subseteq b'$; and
– for each $b(n) \in root(T)$, if $b(n) \in R(n', m)$ for any m, then $b'(n') \in N''$ and $b'(n) \in R''(b'(n'), m)$.

It is not hard to see the *Update* process resulting in the pre-model defined in Example 2 for the formula and tree of Fig. 3.

The stop condition in the loop of the algorithm $root(T) \neq root(K)$ does not hold, if and only if, $root(T) = \{b(n)\}$ and n is the root of K.

Theorem 2. *Given a tree structure K and a formula ϕ, for any valuation V, we have that*

– $Sat = [\phi]_V^K$, *where Sat is produced by the model checking algorithm; and*
– *the model checking algorithm takes linear time with respect to the product of the sizes of the input formula and the input tree structure.*

Proof. We first show that the algorithm builds a pre-model of ϕ and K. This is achieved by induction on the height of K. The base case is trivial, and the inductive step is straight forward by noticing the *Update* function is monotone.

We now show that $b(n) \vdash \phi$, if and only if, $n \in [\phi]_V^K$. The if direction is shown by induction on the derivation of $\vdash$. The only interesting case is for the fixed-point, which is guaranteed to be fixed by the Knaster-Tarsky Theorem on fixed-points and by a reduction from the graded μ-calculus to the simple μ-calculus [5]. The only if direction is shown by structural induction on the input formula ϕ. Most cases are straightforward. For the cases of graded formulas, it is required to guarantee that the bound on the counters is correct. This was proven in Theorem 1.

We now prove the second item of the Theorem. It is easy to see that computing the leaves takes linear times with respect to the size of K. For the saturation process, first recall from Proposition 1 that the size of the lean set is linear. It then takes linear time the evaluation of the entailment relation $\vdash$. This evaluation is applied to each node of the pre-model. Finally, it is not hard to see that the *Update* function takes linear time with respect to $|K|$.

4   Conclusions

In this paper, we studied the model checking problem for the μ-calculus for finite unranked trees extended with graded modalities. These constructors constrain the occurrence, with respect to a non-negative integer coded in binary, of children nodes satisfying a certain formula. Current model checking algorithms for the graded μ-calculus, in the case of finite models, are known to take exponential time [12]. In this paper, we provide a linear-time algorithm for the case of finite unranked tree models. We are currently exploring symbolic techniques [6] for the implementation of the model checking algorithm.

An immediate application of the algorithm is in XML typing [21]. This consists in the evaluation of XML documents (tree models) against XML schemas with numerical constraints, which are known to be captured by the graded μ-calculus [5].

Another source of application of the current work is in the path planning problem [8]. This problem consists in the generation of paths, from an initial to a final goal in a known environment and under certain constraints, and it is known to be reducible to the model checking problem. In this context, current ubiquitous computer systems demands more expressive languages with efficient associated algorithms, such as the graded μ-calculus, in the specification of path constraints.

Acknowledgment. This work was partially developed under the support of the Mexican National Science Council (CONACYT) in the scope of the Cátedras CONACYT project Infraestructura para Agilizar el Desarrollo de Sistemas Centrados en el Usuario (Ref 3053).

References

1. Grädel, E., Otto, M., Rosen, E.: Two-variable logic with counting is decidable. In: Proceedings, 12th Annual IEEE Symposium on Logic in Computer Science, pp. 306–317. IEEE Computer Society (1997)
2. Hollunder, B., Baader, F.: Qualifying number restrictions in concept languages. In Allen, J.F., Fikes, R., Sandewall, E. (eds.) Proceedings of the 2nd International Conference on Principles of Knowledge Representation and Reasoning (KR 1991), pp. 335–346. Morgan Kaufmann (1991)
3. Kupferman, O., Sattler, U., Vardi, M.Y.: The complexity of the graded μ-calculus. In: Voronkov, A. (ed.) CADE 2002. LNCS (LNAI), vol. 2392, pp. 423–437. Springer, Heidelberg (2002)
4. Bonatti, P.A., Lutz, C., Murano, A., Vardi, M.Y.: The complexity of enriched mu-calculi. Logical Methods in Computer Science 4(3) (2008)
5. Bárcenas, E., Genevès, P., Layaïda, N., Schmitt, A.: Query reasoning on trees with types, interleaving, and counting. In: Walsh, T. (ed.) IJCAI. IJCAI/AAAI (2011)
6. Burch, J.R., Clarke, E.M., McMillan, K.L., Dill, D.L., Hwang, L.J.: Symbolic model checking: $10^2 0$ states and beyond. Inf. Comput. **98**(2), 142–170 (1992)
7. Clarke Jr., E.M., Grumberg, O., Peled, D.A.: Model Checking. MIT Press, Cambridge (1999)

8. Fainekos, G.E., Girard, A., Kress-Gazit, H., Pappas, G.J.: Temporal logic motion planning for dynamic robots. Automatica **45**(2), 343–352 (2009)
9. Emerson, E.A., Jutla, C.S., Sistla, A.P.: On model checking for the μ-calculus and its fragments. Theor. Comput. Sci. **258**(1–2), 491–522 (2001)
10. Cleaveland, R., Steffen, B.: A linear-time model-checking algorithm for the alternation-free modal mu-calculus. Formal Methods Syst. Des. **2**(2), 121–147 (1993)
11. Calvanese, D., Giacomo, G.D., Lenzerini, M., Vardi, M.Y.: Node selection query languages for trees. In: Fox, M., Poole, D. (eds.) AAAI. AAAI Press (2010)
12. Ferrante, A., Murano, A., Parente, M.: Enriched μ-calculi module checking. Logical Methods in Computer Science 4(3) (2008)
13. Seidl, H., Schwentick, T., Muscholl, A.: Counting in trees. In Flum, J., Grädel, E., Wilke, T. (eds.) Logic and Automata. Texts in Logic and Games, vol. 2, pp. 575–612. Amsterdam University Press (2008)
14. Demri, S., Lugiez, D.: Complexity of modal logics with Presburger constraints. J. Applied Logic **8**(3), 233–252 (2010)
15. Bianco, A., Mogavero, F., Murano, A.: Graded computation tree logic. ACM Trans. Comput. Log. **13**(3), 25 (2012)
16. Bárcenas, E., Lavalle, J.: Expressive reasoning on tree structures: recursion, inverse programs, Presburger constraints and nominals. In: Castro, F., Gelbukh, A., González, M. (eds.) MICAI 2013, Part I. LNCS, vol. 8265, pp. 80–91. Springer, Heidelberg (2013)
17. Bárcenas, E., Lavalle, J.: Global numerical constraints on trees. Logical Methods in Computer Science 10(2) (2014)
18. Laroussinie, F., Meyer, A., Petonnet, E.: Counting CTL. Logical Methods Comput. Sci. **9**(1), 1–34 (2012)
19. Ferrante, A., Napoli, M., Parente, M.: Model checking for graded CTL. Fundam. Inform. **96**(3), 323–339 (2009)
20. Genevès, P., Layaïda, N., Schmitt, A., Gesbert, N.: Efficiently deciding μ-calculus with converse over finite trees. ACM Trans. Comput. Logic **16**(2), 16:1–16:41 (2015)
21. Gottlob, G., Koch, C., Pichler, R., Segoufin, L.: The complexity of XPath query evaluation and XML typing. J. ACM **52**(2), 284–335 (2005)

Lifelong Learning Selection Hyper-heuristics for Constraint Satisfaction Problems

José Carlos Ortiz-Bayliss$^{(\boxtimes)}$, Hugo Terashima-Marín,
and Santiago Enrique Conant-Pablos

Tecnológico de Monterrey National School of Engineering and Sciences,
Av. Eugenio Garza Sada 2501 Sur Col. Tecnológico,
64849 Monterrey, Nuevo Leon, Mexico
{jcobayliss,terashima,sconant}@itesm.mx

Abstract. Selection hyper-heuristics are methods that manage the use of different heuristics and recommend one of them that is suitable for the current problem space under exploration. In this paper we describe a hyper-heuristic model for constraint satisfaction that is inspired in the idea of a lifelong learning process that allows the hyper-heuristic to continually improve the quality of its decisions by incorporating information from every instance it solves. The learning takes place in a transparent way because the learning process is executed in parallel in a different thread than the one that deals with the user's requests. We tested the model on various constraint satisfaction problem instances and obtained promising results, specially when tested on unseen instances from different classes.

Keywords: Heuristics · Selection hyper-heuristics · Constraint satisfaction · Lifelong learning

1 Introduction

A constraint satisfaction problem (CSP) contains a set of variables V, each with a domain D_v of possible values and a set of constraints C that restricts the values that can be assigned to those variables. When using backtracking-based algorithms to solve CSPs [1], the ordering in which the variables are considered for instantiation affects the way the solution space is explored and also, the cost of the search. If this ordering is poor, the risk of taking the search into long unpromising branches increases and, as a consequence, the time required to find one solution also increases. Then, bad choices in the ordering in which the variables are instantiated represent a huge amount of unnecessary work. Various heuristics have been proposed to tackle the variable ordering problem in CSPs and they have proven to be efficient for specific classes of instances, but usually to fail when tested on distinct classes. As a consequence, applying the same heuristic to every instance rarely produces good results. This drawback in the performance of such methods arises mainly from the vast range of parameters or algorithm

© Springer International Publishing Switzerland 2015
G. Sidorov and S.N. Galicia-Haro (Eds.): MICAI 2015, Part I, LNAI 9413, pp. 190–201, 2015.
DOI: 10.1007/978-3-319-27060-9_15

choices involved, and the lack of guidance on how to properly tune them when the problems change. Also, the understanding of how heuristics work on different situations is not fully understood yet, making it difficult to decide, only based on what we currently know about them, which one is the best option for a certain instance. For these reasons it seems reasonable to rely on an automatic method to produce the mapping between features and heuristics.

The idea of selecting from a set of algorithms the most suitable one to solve one specific problem is usually referred to as the algorithm selection problem [18]. This problem has been addressed in the literature by using different strategies, but two of the most used terms include algorithm portfolios and selection hyper-heuristics. Algorithm portfolios attempt to allocate a period for running a chosen algorithm from a set of algorithms in a time-sharing environment [8,12], while selection hyper-heuristics [5,19] are high-level methodologies that select among different heuristics given the properties of the instance at hand.

This paper is organized as follows. In Sect. 2 we present related works on hyper-heuristics for CSPs. Section 3 describes the features used to characterize the instances and the ordering heuristics considered for this investigation. The main contribution of this investigation, the lifelong learning selection hyper-heuristic model for CSP, is described in Sect. 4. Section 5 presents the experiments conducted, their analysis and the discussion of the results. Finally, in Sect. 6 we present our conclusion and future work.

2   Related Work

Regarding algorithm portfolios for CSPs, the work conducted by O'Mahony et al. [15] collects a set of solvers and decides which solver is the most suitable one according to the features of the instance to solve. Their approach aims at solving the instances as well as the best possible solver from the set does. More recent studies on the combination of heuristics for CSPs include the work done by Petrovic and Epstein [17], who studied the idea of combining various heuristics to produce mixtures that work well on particular classes of CSP instances. Their approach bases their decisions on random sets of what they call advisers, which are basically the criteria used by the variable and value ordering heuristics to make their decisions. The advisers are weighted according to their previous decisions: good decisions increase their weights, while bad ones decrease them. This approach has proven to be able to adapt to a wide range of instances but it requires to define the size of the sets of advisers. There is a trade-off that must be considered: the larger the set of advisers, the larger the amount of computational resources required to evaluate the criteria of the different advisers but the fewer the number of instances to train the system.

With regard to selection hyper-heuristics, Bittle and Fox [2] worked on a symbolic cognitive architecture to produce variable ordering hyper-heuristics for map colouring and job shop scheduling problems represented as CSPs. Their approach produces small 'chunks' of code that serve as the components of rules for variable ordering. As a result, hyper-heuristics composed by a large set of rules operate to solve the instances by selectively applying the most suitable heuristic for the instance being solved. The last two years include some important developments regarding hyper-heuristics for CSPs. Autonomous search was applied to replace bad performing strategies by more promising ones during the search, producing competent variable ordering strategies for CSPs [23]. The authors used a choice function that evaluates some indicators of the search progress and dynamically ranks the ordering heuristics according to their quality to exclude those that exhibit a low performance. Ortiz-Bayliss et al. [16] proposed a learning vector quantization framework to tackle the dynamic selection of heuristics on different sets of CSP instances. Although their approach proved to be useful for the instances where it was tested, the model requires the expertise of the user for tuning the parameters in the framework in order to produce reliable hyper-heuristics.

An area of opportunity regarding all the hyper-heuristic strategies proposed in the past for CSP involves the learning approach. Most of the hyper-heuristic methods previously proposed for CSP require a training phase and, only after the training process is over, the hyper-heuristic can be used to solve as many instances as wished. Once the hyper-heuristic is trained, no further learning is done and then, the hyper-heuristics are unable to incorporate additional information to improve their decisions. The main limitation derived from this situation is that such hyper-heuristics usually fail to generalize well on instances from unseen classes of instances.

Lifelong learning [20,21] was recently introduced as an alternative learning approach that responds to the constant changes in the nature of the instances being solved and the available solvers. As Silver suggests [21], systems that use lifelong learning have the ability to learn, retain and use knowledge over a life time. Lifelong learning is more than just extending the learning phase or executing it various times: it requires the use of a suitable knowledge representation that allows the system to modify only small parts of what it knows to improve its further performance. The concept of lifelong learning was recently introduced to the field of hyper-heuristics, specifically for the Bin Packing problem with exceptional results [11,13,22]. The lifelong learning mechanism in those models was implemented by using an artificial immune system [6].

3   Problem Characterization and Ordering Heuristics

In this section we describe the features used to characterize the instances and the variable ordering heuristics considered for this investigation.

3.1   Problem State Characterization

Four commonly used features are considered to characterize the instances in this investigation:

- **Problem size (N).** The problem size is defined as the number of bits required to represent the whole solution space. N is calculated as $\sum_{v \in V} \log_2(|D_v|)$, where $|D_v|$ is the domain size of variable v.

- **Constraint density** (p_1). The constraint density of an instance is defined as the number of constraints in which the variables participate divided by the maximum number of possible constraints in the instance.
- **Constraint tightness** (p_2). A conflict is a pair of values $\langle a, b \rangle$ that is not allowed by a particular constraint. Thus, the tightness of a constraint is the number of forbidden pairs over the total number of pairs that may occur between the two variables involved in the constraint. The tightness of a CSP instance is calculated as the average tightness over all the constraints within the instance.
- **Clustering coefficient** (C). The clustering coefficient estimates how close the neighbours of a variable are to being a complete graph. Thus, the clustering coefficient of a CSP instance is calculated as the average of the clustering coefficient of all the variables within the instance.

All the previous features lie in the range $[0, 1]$ (the values of N have been normalized to lie in the same range as the rest of the features).

3.2   Ordering Heuristics

Although various heuristics for variable ordering are available in the literature, we have selected a representative set of five of them for this investigation:

- **Domain (DOM).** DOM [10] prefers the variable with the fewest values in its domain.
- **Degree (DEG).** The degree of a variable is calculated as the number of edges incident to that variable. Thus, DEG selects the variable with the largest degree [7].
- **Domain Over Degree (DOM/DEG).** DOM/DEG tries first the variable with that minimizes the quotient of the domain size over the degree of the variable [4].
- **Kappa (K).** The value of κ is suggested in the literature as a general measure of how restricted a combinatorial problem is. If κ is small, the instances usually have many solutions with respect to their size. When κ is large, instead, the instances often have few solutions or do not have any at all [9]. κ is defined as $\kappa = \frac{-\sum_{c \in C} \log_2(1 - p_c)}{\sum_{v \in V} \log_2(|D_v|)}$, where p_c is the fraction of unfeasible tuples on constraint c. K prefers the variable whose instantiation produces the less constrained subproblem (the subproblem with the smallest value of κ).
- Weighted degree (WDEG). WDEG assigns a counter to each constraint, and every time such constraint is unsatisfied, the corresponding counter is increased by one [3]. WDEG prefers the variable with the largest weighted degree. This is, the variable with the largest sum of weights over its constraints.

In all cases, ties are broken by using the lexical ordering of the variables. Once a variable is selected, the value that participates in the fewest conflicts (forbidden pairs of values between two variables) will be tried before the others [14]. In case of ties, the minimum value will always be preferred.

4   A Lifelong Learning Selection Hyper-heuristic Model for CSPs

The motivation behind the lifelong learning selection hyper-heuristic (LLSHH) model for CSP is the lack of continuous learning in current hyper-heuristic models for CSP. The proposed hyper-heuristic model keeps learning with every instance it solves, improving its decisions. The system uses the information from previous instances solved with different heuristics to predict one suitable heuristic to apply once a similar instance appears.

In order to describe the LLSHH model for CSP we will introduce two important concepts: scenarios and predictors. A scenario attempts to answer the question "How is the performance of heuristic h on instance p?". Then, a scenario is the time required by a specific heuristic to solve a CSP instance. Every time an instance is solved, a new scenario is created and, during the training, the scenario is analyzed –instance p is solved by using heuristic h and the time consumed by the solving process is recorded. A predictor, on the other hand, gathers information from different scenarios to allow the system to predict the performance of a given heuristic on a new instance. A predictor contains a vector of features that characterize a point in the problem space, and a collection of scenarios associated to such a point. A scenario cannot belong to more than one predictor.

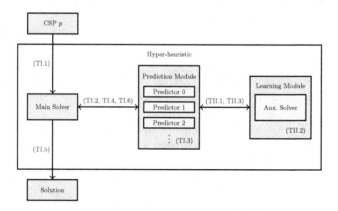

Fig. 1. The lifelong learning selection hyper-heuristic model for solving CSPs.

As shown in Fig. 1, the LLSHH model consists of three main components: a solver, a prediction module and a learning module. The solver is exclusively devoted to solving the instances presented to the system. It requests the prediction module for one suitable heuristic given the properties of the current instance under exploration. The prediction module has two tasks: it first recommends a heuristic and then, it communicates with the learning module to improve further decisions. The solver and the learning module run in parallel, each on its own thread. Because both the solver and the prediction module can read from and write to the prediction module, the access to the prediction module is synchronized to avoid problems due to concurrency. A detailed view of the model is described in the following lines. Please note that two descriptions are provided as the solver and learning module run in parallel in different threads.

The main thread of the model (TI) runs as follows:

(TI.1) The user requests the hyper-heuristic to solve instance p.

(TI.2) The main solver requests the prediction module one suitable heuristic to apply for instance p.

(TI.3) The prediction module analyzes instance p by using the features described in Sect. 3.1. The characterization of instance p locates it on a specific point of the problem space. The prediction module analyzes all the available predictors and selects the one whose problem state is closest to the characterization of p. The closeness of the problem state to the characterization of instance p is calculated by using the Euclidean distance. For a predictor to be considered, there is a minimum acceptance distance d_{min}. This minimum distance is needed to allow the system to create new predictors and avoid using predictors with little relation to the current characterization of p.

  (TI.3a) The predictor r with the closest problem state to the characterization of p (if the distance is smaller than d_{min}) is selected. By using the information from the scenarios in predictor r, the system selects the heuristic with the smallest median recorded time among these scenarios. Let the selected heuristic be referred to as h.

  (TI.3b) If the prediction module cannot find a predictor with distance smaller than d_{min}, the module creates a new predictor r with a problem state equal to the characterization of p. One heuristic h from the ones described in Sect. 3.2 is randomly chosen.

(TI.4) The prediction module returns the heuristic selected from the previous step, h, and instance p is solved with that heuristic.

(TI.5) A solution is returned to the user.

(TI.6) A new scenario is created to register the performance of h on instance p. The scenario is assigned to predictor r.

As we already mentioned, the learning process is executed in a different thread. The learning process runs as follows:

(TII.1) The prediction module sends instance p, the selected predictor r and the selected heuristic h to the learning module.

(TII.2) With a probability α, each available heuristic (except for h, which is used and evaluated in thread T1 when the system solves the instance for the user) may be selected for the generation of new scenarios. For all the heuristics selected, a new scenario is created and analyzed.

(TII.3) The scenarios analyzed are sent to the prediction module to incorporate them to their respective predictors.

4.1   Benchmark Instances

In this investigation we have incorporated instances taken from a public repository available at http://www.cril.univ-artois.fr/~lecoutre/benchmarks.html. All the instances in this work are binary CSPs coded in XCSP 2.1 format (http://www.cril.univ-artois.fr/CPAI08/XCSP2_1.pdf). In the following lines we briefly describe the classes of instances considered for this investigation:

- **RAND**. This class contains 50 random instances from the set `frb30-15.tgz` listed in the public repository.
- **QRND**. This class contains 140 random instances containing a small structure. The instances correspond to the sets `geom.tgz`, `composed-25-10-20.tgz` and `composed-75-1-2.tgz` in the public repository.
- **PATT**. The 52 instances in this class follow a regular pattern and involve a random generation. The instances were taken from sets `coloring.tgz`, `QCP-10.tgz` and `QCP-15.tgz` from the public repository.
- **REAL**. This class contains 18 instances taken from real world applications. The instances correspond to the sets `driver.tgz` and `rlfapScens.tgz` in the repository.

Although the proposed model is able to start from scratch (with no previous information), we recommend to conduct a training phase to provide some initial information about the heuristics and the instances that may be updated later when the test instances are solved. In this investigation, around 50 % of the instances of each class were used for training and the rest exclusively for testing.

5   Experiments

We conducted two main experiments in this investigation. In total, five hyper-heuristics were produced and tested. The first experiment is related to the ability of the hyper-heuristics to solve specific classes of instances. The second experiment explores the idea of a more general use of the hyper-heuristic where only one general method is capable of overcoming the use of a single heuristic for all the classes.

In both experiments we used a maximum running time of 25 seconds per instance, a minimum acceptance distance (d_{min}) equal to 0.1 and a probability of scenario generation (α) equal to 0.75.

5.1   Producing Hyper-heuristics for Specific Classes of Instances

We used the training instances from each class to produce one hyper-heuristic for the specific class used for training. In total, four hyper-heuristics were produced in this experiment: RAND-HH, QRND-HH, PATT-HH and REAL-HH. For each class, all the training instances were solved by using the corresponding hyper-heuristic. Once the system provided a solution to all the training instances, we used the hyper-heuristics produced to solve only the test instances from their respective class. The idea of this experiment is to observe whether it is possible to produce hyper-heuristics that perform better than the heuristics applied in isolation for specific classes of instances.

Table 1 presents the success rate of the four hyper-heuristics on their respective classes of instances. The success rate in this investigation refers to the percentage of instances in each class where the hyper-heuristic required no more time than one specific heuristic. For example, the results shown in Table 1 indicate that for instances in class RAND, the hyper-heuristic RAND-HH is almost always at least as good as DOM, DEG, DOM/DEG and WDEG, but only in 12 % of the test instances for that class it was able to perform at least as well as K.

Table 1. Success rate of RAND-HH, QRND-HH, PATT-HH and REAL-HH on their respective class of instances with respect to each heuristic.

	DOM	DEG	DOM/DEG	K	WDEG
RAND	84.00 %	84.00 %	84.00 %	12.00 %	88.00 %
QRND	88.33 %	81.67 %	80.00 %	63.33 %	66.67 %
PATT	96.00 %	100.00 %	76.00 %	88.00 %	96.00 %
REAL	100.00 %	75.00 %	50.00 %	62.50 %	62.50 %

Table 2 complements the information of the performance of the four hyper-heuristics, as it shows the average gain/loss of each hyper-heuristic on instances from their respective classes of instances. For example, we know that the hyper-heuristic RAND-HH is almost always at least as good as DOM, DEG, DOMDEG and WDEG, but with the results from Table 2 we also know that when such hyper-heuristic was used, the average time required to solve a test instance in the class RAND decreased by 32.06 %, 23.57 % and 27.68 % with respect to DOM, DEG and WDEG, respectively. The result for DOM/DEG is interesting, as it shows that although the hyper-heuristic RAND-HH is in 84.00 % of the instances at least as good as DOM/DEG, there is no real benefit from using this hyper-heuristic (in average, 0.38 % time less per instance with respect to DOM/DEG). When we compared hyper-heuristic RAND-HH against K, we observed that, in average, it requires 56.09 % more time per instance than K.

The behaviour of hyper-heuristics QRND-HH, PATT-HH and REAL-HH shows that these hyper-heuristics are good solving options for the classes of instances they were trained for. In all cases, important savings in time were obtained by using hyper-heuristics on their corresponding classes of instances.

5.2   Producing a Hyper-heuristic for Multiple Classes of Instances

In the previous experiment we produced and tested hyper-heuristics for each specific class. Now, in this experiment we were interested in showing that there

Table 2. Average time gain/loss per instance of RAND-HH, QRND-HH, PATT-HH and REAL-HH on their respective class of instances when compared against each heuristic.

	DOM	DEG	DOM/DEG	K	WDEG
RAND	−32.06 %	−23.57 %	−0.38 %	+56.09 %	−27.68 %
QRND	−45.47 %	−52.12 %	−30.96 %	−8.35 %	−40.05 %
PATT	−17.17 %	−58.84 %	−14.37 %	−14.84 %	−51.60 %
REAL	−71.61 %	−23.66 %	−15.57 %	−56.17 %	−1.24 %

is a benefit from using hyper-heuristic as we can produce only one general method and then, use it on instances from different classes with acceptable results. In this section, we focused on producing one single hyper-heuristic (MC-HH) that could perform well on the four classes of instances.

The training process for MC-HH was conducted in the same way we did for training the four hyper-heuristics from the previous experiment but this time, we constructed only one set of training instances that includes the training instances from the four classes into a single training set.

Tables 3 and 4 show the results obtained for MC-HH when compared against each heuristic.

Table 3. Success rate of MC-HH on each class of instances.

	DOM	DEG	DOM/DEG	K	WDEG
RAND	80.00 %	84.00 %	48.00 %	8.00 %	88.00 %
QRND	88.33 %	80.00 %	86.66 %	56.66 %	68.33 %
PATT	68.00 %	88.00 %	60.00 %	76.00 %	84.00 %
REAL	75.00 %	75.00 %	75.00 %	87.50 %	62.50 %

Table 4. Average time gain/loss per instance of MC-HH on each class of instances when compared against each heuristic.

	DOM	DEG	DOM/DEG	K	WDEG
RAND	−40.94 %	−34.42 %	+0.70 %	+65.96 %	−39.37 %
QRND	−45.61 %	−52.23 %	−31.14 %	−8.40 %	−40.22 %
PATT	−11.33 %	−56.57 %	−7.26 %	−7.09 %	−48.72 %
REAL	−78.54 %	−45.96 %	−41.24 %	−70.24 %	−29.59 %

In general, MC-HH is not as good as the hyper-heuristics trained for each particular class of instances with regard to the success rate. But, its ability to reduce the average time for solving the instances improved for some classes, specially for the instances from REAL. An important consideration is that K was the best performing heuristic for classes RAND, QRND and PATT, but for REAL the best heuristic was WDEG. MC-HH is capable of performing as well as K and WDEG in each of these classes (except for RAND), showing that one hyper-heuristic can combine the strengths of single heuristics to perform well on different classes of instances.

5.3   Discussion

There is an important observation that needs to be discussed about the running time of the proposed hyper-heuristic model. First, assuming that a hyper-heuristic always selects the same heuristic h, it will always require more time than h applied directly to solve the problems. The additional time is the result of revising the predictors to find one that is close to the characterization of the current instance. The benefit of using a hyper-heuristic in this model occurs when the hyper-heuristic changes the heuristic to apply based on the features of each instance being solved. When that happens, its performance can be superior to the one of a single heuristic applied to solve the same instances.

Finally, we observed that classes QRND, PATT and REAL are suitable to be solved by the model proposed. But, RAND is difficult to solve by the hyper-heuristic because of its lack of structure. It seems that the learning strategy in the hyper-heuristic is unable to properly characterize the instances by using the features described in Sect. 3.1. For this reason, we think that more features should be considered in the future.

6   Conclusion

In this paper we have described a lifelong learning hyper-heuristic model for solving CSPs. The hyper-heuristic learns from a set of scenarios that represent the historical performance of heuristics on previously solved instances. Then, the system creates predictors that group those scenarios and, when the system deals with a new instance, it predicts one suitable heuristic for such instance based on what the system knows about the heuristics and previously solved instances. Every instance the hyper-heuristic solves can produce, with probability α, a new scenario to increase the system's knowledge about the heuristics and the instances. Those scenarios are analyzed in a different thread, making the learning process transparent for the user. With this model, the system is continually learning from new instances it solves.

Although we observed promising results with this hyper-heuristic model, it is clear for us that some elements might be improved. For example, the minimum acceptance distance was introduced as a way to allow the hyper-heuristic to discard some predictors, the ones which are "not similar enough" to the current instance being solved. Despite this idea is something we found important to include (it allows the creation of new predictors), we think that should work in a different way. Having one d_{min} for the distance worked well for this investigation but ignores the fact that some features may have a larger effect on the time required to solve an instance. For example, two instances with the same values of p_1, p_2 and C but different N may require completely different running times, as the number of variables increases the size of the search space. For this reason, we think that d_{min} should represent a vector, where each feature has its own minimum acceptance distance. Also, this value should be automatically updated according to the scenarios analyzed for each predictor. At this moment we only have preliminary ideas on how to achieve this, but we still need to figure out how to implement it in an efficient way.

Another important aspect to consider is that the order in which the instances are solved by the hyper-heuristic may affect the way the predictors are created. This may not seem like an issue for the experiments conducted in this investigation but opens the door for a future and important development of the model: predictor segmentation and integration. With segmentation, a predictor that has evidence that two instances with similar features require considerably different solving times may be split into two different predictors. On the other hand, integration deals with the idea of creating one new predictor by merging two or more existing ones.

Finally, we would like to include more features and heuristics to our model and compare the proposed model against other existing hyper-heuristic models for CSP to better estimate its quality.

Acknowledgments. This research was supported in part by ITESM Research Group with Strategic Focus in Intelligent Systems and CONACyT Basic Science Project under grant 241461.

References

1. Bitner, J.R., Reingold, E.M.: Backtrack programming techniques. Commun. ACM **18**, 651–656 (1975)
2. Bittle, S.A., Fox, M.S.: Learning and using hyper-heuristics for variable and value ordering in constraint satisfaction problems. In: Proceedings of the 11th Annual Conference Companion on Genetic and Evolutionary Computation Conference: Late Breaking Papers, pp. 2209–2212. ACM (2009)
3. Boussemart, F., Hemery, F., Lecoutre, C., Sais, L.: Boosting systematic search by weighting constraints. In: European Conference on Artificial Intelligence (ECAI 2004), pp. 146–150 (2004)
4. Brelaz, D.: New methods to colour the vertices of a graph. Commun. ACM **22**, 251–256 (1979)
5. Burke, E., Hart, E., Kendall, G., Newall, J., Ross, P., Shulenburg, S.: Hyper-heuristics: an emerging direction in modern research technology. In: Handbook of metaheuristics, pp. 457–474. Kluwer Academic Publishers (2003)
6. Capodieci, N., Hart, E., Cabri, G.: Artificial immune systems in the context of autonomic computing: integrating design paradigms. In: Proceedings of the 2014 Conference Companion on Genetic and Evolutionary Computation Companion, GECCO Comp 2014, pp. 21–22. ACM, New York (2014)

7. Dechter, R., Meiri, I.: Experimental evaluation of preprocessing algorithms for constraint satisfaction problems. Artif. Intell. **38**(2), 211–242 (1994)
8. Gagliolo, M., Schmidhuber, J.: Dynamic algorithm portfolios. Ann. Math. Artif. Intell. **47**, 3–4 (2006)
9. Gent, I., MacIntyre, E., Prosser, P., Smith, B., T.Walsh: An empirical study of dynamic variable ordering heuristics for the constraint satisfaction problem. In: Proceedings of the International Conference on Principles and Practice of Constraint Programming (CP 1996), pp. 179–193 (1996)
10. Haralick, R.M., Elliott, G.L.: Increasing tree search efficiency for constraint satisfaction problems. Artif. Intell. **14**, 263–313 (1980)
11. Hart, E., Sim, K.: On the life-long learning capabilities of a NELLI*: a hyper-heuristic optimisation system. In: Bartz-Beielstein, T., Branke, J., Filipič, B., Smith, J. (eds.) PPSN 2014. LNCS, vol. 8672, pp. 282–291. Springer, Heidelberg (2014)
12. Huberman, B.A., Lukose, R.M., Hogg, T.: An economics approach to hard computational problems. Science **27**, 51–53 (1997)
13. Sim, K.E.H., Paechter, B.: A lifelong learning hyper-heuristic method for bin packing. Evol. Comput. **23**(1), 37–67 (2015)
14. Minton, S., Johnston, M.D., Phillips, A., Laird, P.: Minimizing conflicts: a heuristic repair method for CSP and scheduling problems. Artif. Intell. **58**, 161–205 (1992)
15. O'Mahony, E., Hebrard, E., Holland, A., Nugent, C., O'Sullivan, B.: Using case-based reasoning in an algorithm portfolio for constraint solving. In: Proceedings of the 19th Irish Conference on Artificial Intelligence and Cognitive Science (2008)
16. Ortiz-Bayliss, J.C., Terashima-Marín, H., Conant-Pablos, S.E.: Learning vector quantization for variable ordering in constraint satisfaction problems. Pattern Recogn. Lett. **34**(4), 423–432 (2013)
17. Petrovic, S., Epstein, S.L.: Random subsets support learning a mixture of heuristics. Int. J. Artif. Intell. Tools **17**, 501–520 (2008)
18. Rice, J.R.: The algorithm selection problem. Adv. Comput. **15**, 65–118 (1976)
19. Ross, P., Marín-Blázquez, J.: Constructive hyper-heuristics in class timetabling. In: Proceedings of the 2005 IEEE Congress on Evolutionary Computation (CEC 2005), vol. 2. IEEE Press (2005)
20. Silver, D.L.: Machine lifelong learning: challenges and benefits for artificial general intelligence. In: Schmidhuber, J., Thórisson, K.R., Looks, M. (eds.) AGI 2011. LNCS, vol. 6830, pp. 370–375. Springer, Heidelberg (2011)
21. Silver, D.L., Yang, Q., Li, L.: Lifelong machine learning systems: beyond learning algorithms. In: Lifelong Machine Learning, Papers from the 2013 AAAI Spring Symposium, Palo Alto, California, USA, 25–27 March 2013
22. Sim, K., Hart, E.: An improved immune inspired hyper-heuristic for combinatorial optimisation problems. In: Proceedings of the 2014 Conference on Genetic and Evolutionary Computation, GECCO 2014, pp. 121–128. ACM, New York (2014)
23. Soto, R., Crawford, B., Monfroy, E., Bustos, V.: Using autonomous search for generating good enumeration strategy blends in constraint programming. In: Murgante, B., Gervasi, O., Misra, S., Nedjah, N., Rocha, A.M.A.C., Taniar, D., Apduhan, B.O. (eds.) ICCSA 2012, Part III. LNCS, vol. 7335, pp. 607–617. Springer, Heidelberg (2012)

A Parametric Polynomial Deterministic Algorithm for #2SAT

J. Raymundo Marcial-Romero[1]([⊠]), Guillermo De Ita Luna[2],
J. Antonio Hernández[1], and Rosa María Valdovinos[1]

[1] Facultad de Ingeniería, UAEM, Toluca, Mexico
{jrmarcialr,rvaldovinosr}@uaemex.mx, xoseahernandez@gmail.com
[2] FCC, Benémerita Universidad Autónoma de Puebla, Puebla, Mexico
deita@ccc.inaoep.mx

Abstract. Counting models for two Conjunctive Normal Form formulae (2-CFs), known as the #2SAT problem, is a classic #P complete problem. It is known that if the constraint graph of a 2-CF F is acyclic or contains loops and parallel edges, $\#2SAT(F)$ can be computed efficiently. In this paper we address the cyclic case different from loops and parallel edges.

If the constraint graph G of a 2-CF F is cyclic, T a spanning tree plus loops and parallel edges of G and $\overline{T} = G \setminus T$, what we called its cotree, we show that by building a set partition $\cup T_i$ of $\overline{T}$, where each T_i of the partition is formed by the frond edges of the cycles that are chained via other intersected cycles, then a parametric polynomial deterministic procedure for computing #2SAT with time complexity for the worst case of $O(2^k \cdot poly(|E(T)|))$ can be obtained, where $poly$ is a polynomial function, and k is the cardinality of the largest set in the partition.

This method shows that #2SAT is in the class of fixed-parameter tratable (FPT) problems, where the fixed-parameter k in our proposal, depends on the number of edges of a subcotree of a decomposition of the constraint graph (tree+loops+parallel:cotree) associated to the formula.

Keywords: #SAT problem · Counting models in 2-CF formulae · Parameterized complexity · FPT complexity class

1 Introduction

Counting combinatorial objects is an interesting and important area of research in Mathematics, Physics, and Computer Sciences. Counting problems, being mathematically relevant by themselves, are closely related to practical problems. Several relevant counting problems are hard time-complexity problems, for example, the maximum polynomial class recognized for #2SAT is the class $(\leq 2, 2\mu)$-CF (2-CF where each variable appears twice at most) [3,5].

#SAT (the problem of counting models for a Boolean formula) is of special concern to Artificial Intelligence (AI), and it has a direct relation with Automated Theorem Proving, as well as to approximate reasoning [1,5,7].

© Springer International Publishing Switzerland 2015
G. Sidorov and S.N. Galicia-Haro (Eds.): MICAI 2015, Part I, LNAI 9413, pp. 202–213, 2015.
DOI: 10.1007/978-3-319-27060-9_16

#SAT can be reduced from several problems in approximate reasoning. For example, estimating the degree of belief in propositional theories, the generation of explanations to propositional queries, repairing inconsistent databases, Bayesian inference and truth maintenance systems [1–3, 5, 7]. The previous problems come from several AI applications such as planning, expert systems, approximate reasoning, among others.

#SAT is at least as hard as the SAT problem, however in some cases, even when SAT is solved in polynomial time, no computationally efficient method is known for #SAT. For instance, 2-SAT (SAT restricted to consider ($\leq$ 2)-CF's) can be solved in linear time. However, the corresponding counting problem #2SAT is a #P-complete problem.

Recently, new upper bounds for exact deterministic exponential algorithms for #2SAT have been found by Dahllöf [6], Fürer [10], and Angelsmark [2].

Parameterized complexity theory relaxes the classical notion of tractability and allows to solve some classically hard problems in a reasonably efficient way. It turned out that many intractable problems can be solved efficiently "by the slice", that is, in time $O(f(k) \cdot n^c)$ where f is a function of some parameter k, n is the size of the instance, and c is a constant independent from k. In this case the problem is called fixed-parameter tractable (FPT). If a problem is FPT, then some instances of large size can be solved efficiently [14].

There are parameterized algorithms to solve #SAT based on a k-tree decomposition of the constraint graph of the input formula. Furthermore, the time complexity on the fixed-parameter for those algorithms has been doubly exponential on k [11] and 4^k in another case [9].

In this proposal, we present a parameterized algorithms to solve #SAT in a different way. We show that building a set partition $\cup T_i$ of the cotree of the constraint graph of the input formula as follows: each T_i of the partition is formed by the frond edges of the cycles that are chained via other intersected cycles, then a parametric polynomial deterministic procedure for computing #2SAT with time complexity in the worst case of $O(2^k \cdot poly(|E(T)|))$ can be obtained, where $poly$ is a polynomial function and k is the cardinality of coarsest partition. The algorithm extends the results presented in [7] for the #2SAT problem.

In Sect. 2 we present the preliminaries to understand the rest of the paper. In Sect. 3 previous results for computing #SAT when its constraint graph is acyclic with loops and parallel edges are presented. In Sect. 4 we show how to compute #2SAT of a formula F based on its constraint graph and our main result. Finally, the conclusions of the paper are established.

2   Preliminaries

Let $X = \{x_1, \ldots, x_n\}$ be a set of n Boolean variables. A literal is either a variable x_i or a negated variable $\overline{x}_i$. As usual, for each $x_i \in X$, we write $x_i^0 = \overline{x}_i$ and $x_i^1 = x_i$. A clause is a disjunction of different literals (sometimes, we also consider a clause as a set of literals). For $k \in N$, a k-clause is a clause consisting of exactly k literals and, a ($\leq k$)-clause is a clause with at most k literals. A variable $x \in X$ appears in a clause c if either x^1 or x^0 is an element of c.

A Conjunctive Normal Form (CF) F is a conjunction of clauses (we also call F a Conjunctive Form). A k-CF is a CF containing clauses with at most k literals.

We use $\nu(Y)$ to express the set of variables involved in the object Y, where Y could be a literal, a clause or a Boolean formula. $Lit(F)$ is the set of literals which appear in a CF F, i.e. if $X = \nu(F)$, then $Lit(F) = X \cup \overline{X} = \{x_1^1, x_1^0, \ldots, x_n^1, x_n^0\}$. We also denote $\{1, 2, \ldots, n\}$ by $[[n]]$.

An assignment s for F is a Boolean function $s : \nu(F) \to \{0, 1\}$. An assignment can be also considered as a set which does not contain complementary literals. If $x^\epsilon \in s$, being s an assignment, then s turns x^ϵ true and $x^{1-\epsilon}$ false, $\epsilon \in \{0, 1\}$. Considering a clause c and assignment s as a set of literals, c is satisfied by s if and only if $c \cap s \neq \emptyset$, and if for all $x^\epsilon \in c$, $x^{1-\epsilon} \in s$ then s falsifies c.

If $F_1 \subset F$ is a formula consisting of some clauses of F, then $\nu(F_1) \subset \nu(F)$, and an assignment over $\nu(F_1)$ is a partial assignment over $\nu(F)$.

Let F be a Boolean formula in Conjunctive Form (CF), F is satisfied by an assignment s if each clause in F is satisfied by s. F is contradicted by s if any clause in F is contradicted by s. A model of F is an assignment for $\nu(F)$ that satisfies F. We will denote as $SAT(F)$ the set of models for the formula F.

Given a CF F, the SAT problem consists of determining if F has a model. The #SAT problem consists of counting the number of models of F defined over $\nu(F)$. #2-SAT denotes #SAT for formulas in 2-CF.

2.1   The Constraint Graph of a 2-CF

There are some graphical representations of a conjunctive form (see e.g. [14]), we use here the signed primal graph of a two conjuctive form.

Let F be a 2-CF, its constraint graph (signed primal graph) is denoted by $G_F = (V(F), E(F))$, with $V(F) = \nu(F)$ and $E(F) = \{\{\nu(x), \nu(y)\} : \{x, y\} \in F\}$, that is, the vertices of G_F are the variables of F, and for each clause $\{x, y\}$ in F there is an edge $\{\nu(x), \nu(y)\} \in E(F)$. For $x \in V(F)$, $\delta(x)$ denotes its degree, i.e. the number of incident edges to x. Each edge $c = \{\nu(x), \nu(y)\} \in E$ is associated with an ordered pair (s_1, s_2) of signs, assigned as labels of the edge connecting the variables appearing in the clause. The signs s_1 and s_2 are related to the variables x and y, respectively. For example, the clause $\{x^0, y^1\}$ determines the labelled edge: "$x \overset{-}{\underset{+}{}} y$" which is equivalent to the edge "$y \overset{+}{\underset{-}{}} x$".

Formally, let $S = \{+, -\}$ be a set of signs. A graph with labelled edges on a set S is a pair (G, ψ), where $G = (V, E)$ is a graph, and ψ is a function with domain E and range S. $\psi(e)$ is called the label of the edge $e \in E$. Let $G = (V, E, \psi)$ be a constraint graph with labelled edges on $S \times S$. Let x and y be nodes in V, if $e = \{x, y\}$ is an edge and $\psi(e) = (s, s')$, then $s(resp.s')$ is called the adjacent sign to $x(resp.y)$. We say that a 2-CF F is a path, cycle, or a tree if its signed constraint graph G_F represents a path, cycle, or a tree, respectively.

Notice that a constraint graph of a 2-CF can be a multigraph since two fixed variables can be involved in more than one clause of the formula forming so parallel edges. Furthermore, a unitary clause is represented by a loop in the constraint graph (an edge to join a vertex to itself). A polynomial time algorithm to process parallel edges and loops to solve #SAT has been shown in [7].

Let $\rho : 2\text{-CF} \rightarrow G_F$ be the function whose domain is the space of Boolean formulae in 2-CF and codomain the set of multi-graphs, ρ is a bijection. So any 2-CF formula has a unique signed constraint graph associated via ρ and viceversa, any signed constraint graph G_F has a unique formula associated.

3   Computing #2SAT According to the Topology of the Constrained Graph

The results of this section can be consulted at [7], they are included in the article for completeness. We show simple topologies on a graph representing a 2-CF and how to compute the value #2SAT for the formulas represented by those graphs. We start with simple topologies as acyclic graphs.

3.1   #2SAT for 2-CF Representing a Path

We said that a graph G_F represents a path for a 2-CF F, if

$$F = \{C_1, C_2, \ldots, C_m\} = \{\{x_1^{\epsilon_1}, x_2^{\delta_1}\}, \{x_2^{\epsilon_2}, x_3^{\delta_2}\}, \ldots, \{x_m^{\epsilon_m}, x_{m+1}^{\delta_m}\}\},$$

where $\delta_i, \epsilon_i \in \{0,1\}$, $i \in [\![m]\!]$. Let f_i be a family of clauses of the formula F built as follows: $f_1 = \emptyset$; $f_i = \{C_j\}_{j<i}$, $i \in [\![m]\!]$. Notice that $n = |v(F)| = m+1$, $f_i \subset f_{i+1}$, $i \in [\![m-1]\!]$. Let $SAT(f_i) = \{s : s \text{ satisfies } f_i\}$, $A_i = \{s \in SAT(f_i) : x_i \in s\}$, $B_i = \{s \in SAT(f_i) : \overline{x}_i \in s\}$. Let $\alpha_i = |A_i|$; $\beta_i = |B_i|$ and $\mu_i = |SAT(f_i)| = \alpha_i + \beta_i$.

For every node $x \in G_F$ a pair (α_x, β_x) is computed, where α_x indicates how many times the variable x is 'true' and β_x indicates the number of times that the variable x can take value 'false' into the set of models of F. The first pair is $(\alpha_1, \beta_1) = (1,1)$ since x_1 can be true or false in order to satisfy f_1. The pairs (α_x, β_x) associated to each node x_i, $i = 2, \ldots, m$ are computed according to the signs (ϵ_i, δ_i) of the literals in the clause c_i by the following recurrence equation:

$$(\alpha_i, \beta_i) = \begin{cases} (\beta_{i-1} & , \alpha_{i-1} + \beta_{i-1}) \text{ if } (\epsilon_i, \delta_i) = (-,-) \\ (\alpha_{i-1} + \beta_{i-1}, \beta_{i-1} &) \text{ if } (\epsilon_i, \delta_i) = (-,+) \\ (\alpha_{i-1} & , \alpha_{i-1} + \beta_{i-1}) \text{ if } (\epsilon_i, \delta_i) = (+,-) \\ (\alpha_{i-1} + \beta_{i-1}, \alpha_{i-1} &) \text{ if } (\epsilon_i, \delta_i) = (+,+) \end{cases} \qquad (1)$$

Note that as $F = f_m$ then $\#SAT(F) = \mu_m = \alpha_m + \beta_m$.

3.2   #2SAT for 2-CF Whose Graph Contains Parallel Edges

Consider the case where in a Conjunctive Form there are two 2-clauses involving the same variables. In this case, the constrained graph has a pair of edges between the same endpoints, and the computation has to consider four different signs to compute #SAT as in the path case.

Suppose, the two clauses are $c_k = (x_{i-1}^{\epsilon_k}, x_i^{\delta_k})$ and $c_j = (x_{i-1}^{\epsilon_j}, x_i^{\delta_j})$, which involve variables x_{i-1} and x_i. Then, we compute the values for (α_i, β_i) associated to the node x_i, according to the signs (ϵ_k, δ_k) and (ϵ_j, δ_j) as:

$$(\alpha_i, \beta_i) = \begin{cases} (\alpha_{i-1}, \alpha_{i-1}) & \text{if } (\epsilon_k, \delta_k) = (1,1) \ and \ (\epsilon_j, \delta_j) = (1,0) \\ (\mu_{i-1}, 0\ \ ) & \text{if } (\epsilon_k, \delta_k) = (1,1) \ and \ (\epsilon_j, \delta_j) = (0,1) \\ (\beta_{i-1}, \alpha_{i-1}) & \text{if } (\epsilon_k, \delta_k) = (1,1) \ and \ (\epsilon_j, \delta_j) = (0,0) \\ (\alpha_{i-1}, \beta_{i-1}) & \text{if } (\epsilon_k, \delta_k) = (1,0) \ and \ (\epsilon_j, \delta_j) = (0,1) \\ (0\ \ \ , \mu_{i-1}) & \text{if } (\epsilon_k, \delta_k) = (1,0) \ and \ (\epsilon_j, \delta_j) = (0,0) \\ (\beta_{i-1}, \beta_{i-1}) & \text{if } (\epsilon_k, \delta_k) = (0,1) \ and \ (\epsilon_j, \delta_j) = (0,0) \end{cases} \tag{2}$$

Let F be a 2-CF such that three clauses in F involve the same variables then the value of (α_i, β_i) is computed by recurrence (3).

$$(\alpha_i, \beta_i) = \begin{cases} (0\ \ \ , \alpha_{i-1}) & \text{if } \{(x_{i-1}, x_i), (x_{i-1}, \overline{x}_i), (\overline{x}_{i-1}, \overline{x}_i)\} \subseteq F \\ (\mu_{i-1}, 0\ \ ) & \text{if } \{(x_{i-1}, x_i), (x_{i-1}, \overline{x}_i), (\overline{x}_{i-1}, x_i)\} \subseteq F \\ (\beta_{i-1}, \alpha_{i-1}) & \text{if } \{(x_{i-1}, x_i), (\overline{x}_{i-1}, x_i), (\overline{x}_{i-1}, \overline{x}_i)\} \subseteq F \\ (\alpha_{i-1}, \beta_{i-1}) & \text{if } \{(\overline{x}_{i-1}, x_i), (x_{i-1}, \overline{x}_i), (\overline{x}_{i-1}, \overline{x}_i)\} \subseteq F \end{cases} \tag{3}$$

Of course, four parallel edges among the same endpoints indicate that the 2-CF F is unsatisfiable and then #2SAT$(F) = 0$.

Processing Unitary Clauses: A unitary clause represents a loop in the constrained graph of a 2-CF. When (α_i, β_i) is computed over a node x_i which has a loop edge, recurrence (4) is being applied.

$$(\alpha_i, \beta_i) = \begin{cases} (0, \beta_i) & \text{if } (\overline{x}_i) \in U \\ (\alpha_i, 0) & \text{if } (x_i) \in U \end{cases} \tag{4}$$

Since an unitary clause uniquely determines the values of its variable. Furthermore when both $(x_i) \in U$ and $(\overline{x}_i) \in U$ then the original formula is unsatisfiable. Both parallel edges and unitary clauses can be considered in a preprocessing of the formula before applying the general algorithm presented at Sect. 4.

3.3   Processing Acyclic Graphs

Let F be a 2-CF where its associated constrained graph G_F is acyclic which may contain loops and parallel edges, then we can assume that G_F as a rooted tree, a traversal of the graph allows to built a rooted tree. A rooted tree has three kinds of nodes: a root node, interior nodes and leaf nodes. We denote with (α_v, β_v) the pair associated with the node v ($v \in G_F$). We compute #$SAT(F)$ while we are traversing G_F in post-order with the following algorithm.

Algorithm Count_Models_for_trees_loops_parallel(G_F)
Input: G_F - a tree graph which may contain parallel edges and loops.
Output: The number of models of F
Procedure:
Traversing G_F in post-order, and when a node $v \in G_F$ is left, assign:

1. $(\alpha_v, \beta_v) = (1, 1)$ if v is a leaf node in G_F.
2. If v is a parent node with a list of child nodes associated, i.e., $u_1, u_2, ..., u_k$ are the child nodes of v, as we have already visited all child nodes, then each pair $(\alpha_{u_j}, \beta_{u_j})$ $j = 1, ..., k$ has been determined. Let $e_1 = v^{\epsilon_1} u_1^{\delta_1}, e_2 = v^{\epsilon_2} u_2^{\delta_2}, ..., e_k = v^{\epsilon_k} u_k^{\delta_k}$ be the edges connecting v with each of its child nodes. A pair $(\alpha_{e_j}, \beta_{e_j})$ is computed for each edge e_j based on recurrence (1) where $\alpha_{e_j - 1}$ is α_{u_j} and $\beta_{e_j - 1}$ is β_{u_j} for $j = 1, ... k$. Then, let $\alpha_v = \prod_{j=1}^{k} \alpha_{e_j} + \beta_v$ and $\beta_v = \prod_{j=1}^{k} \beta_{e_j}$. Notice that this step includes the case when v has just one child node.
3. if v has parallel edges apply recurrence (2) or (3).
4. if v has a loop apply recurrence (4)
5. If v is the root node of G_F then return $(\alpha_v + \beta_v)$.

This procedure returns the number of models for F in time $O(n + m)$ which is the necessary time for traversing G_F in post-order.

4 Formulas with Constraint Cyclic Graph

In this section we show how to compute $\#2SAT(F)$ when the signed constraint graph G_F of F represents a graph which contains cycles. Although parallel edges and loops are cycles in graphs, they can be treated by the polynomial time algorithm presented at Sect. 3, so our splitting procedure presented below is applied for cycles different from parallel edges and loops.

The following lemma shows that if a 2-CF formula F has a clause C_i whose variables are contained in a pair of clauses C_j and C_k of F where $i \neq j$, $j \neq k$ then an upper bound for $\#SAT(F)$ can be established.

Lemma 1. If $F = \{C_i\}_{i=1}^{m} \cup \{\{x_a^{\epsilon_a}, x_b^{\delta_b}\}\}$ is such that

- $x_a^{\epsilon_a}$ or $x_a^{1-\epsilon_a} \in C_j$ for some $j = 1, ... m$ and
- $x_b^{\delta_b}$ or $x_b^{1-\delta_b} \in C_k$ for some $k = 1, ... m$

  then $\#SAT(\{C_i\}_{i=1}^{m}) \geq \#SAT(F)$.

Proof. Let s be a satisfying assignment of $\{C_i\}_{i=1}^{m}$. Then either $x_a^{\epsilon_a}$ or $x_a^{1-\epsilon_a} \in s$ and also $x_b^{\delta_b}$ or $x_b^{1-\delta_b} \in s$. If $x_a^{\epsilon_a}$ & $x_b^{\delta_b} \in s$ then s is also a satisfying assignment of F. Similarly, if $(x_a^{\epsilon_a}$ & $x_b^{1-\delta_b} \in s)$ or $(x_a^{1-\epsilon_a}$ & $x_b^{\delta_b} \in s)$ then s is also a satisfying assignment of F. If $x_a^{1-\epsilon_a}$ & $x_b^{1-\delta_b} \in s$ then the clause $\{x_a^{\epsilon_a}, x_b^{\delta_b}\}$ does not hold, so this assignment is not a model of F. □

It is obvious that a model of $F \cup \{\{x_a^{\epsilon_a}, x_b^{\delta_b}\}\}$ is not a model of $F \cup \{\{x_a^{1-\epsilon_a}\}, \{x_b^{1-\delta_b}\}\}$ since $\overline{(x_a^{\epsilon_a} \vee x_b^{\delta_b})} = x_a^{1-\epsilon_a} \wedge x_b^{1-\delta_b}$.

The following lemma shows how to split the computation of the models of a 2-CF formula F when the conditions of Lemma 1 are satisfied.

Lemma 2. *If $F = \{C_i\}_{i=1}^m \cup \{\{x_a^{\epsilon_a}, x_b^{\delta_b}\}\}$ is such that*

- *$x_a^{\epsilon_a}$ or $x_a^{1-\epsilon_a} \in C_j$ for some $j = 1, \ldots m$ and*
- *$x_b^{\delta_b}$ or $x_b^{1-\delta_b} \in C_k$ for some $k = 1, \ldots m$ and $j \neq k$*

then $\#SAT(F) = \#SAT(\{C_i\}_{i=1}^m) - \#SAT(\{C_i\}_{i=1}^m \cup \{\{x_a^{1-\epsilon_a}\}, \{x_b^{1-\delta_b}\}\})$.

Proof. It is equivalent to prove that

$$\#SAT(\{C_i\}_{i=1}^m) = \#SAT(F) + \#SAT(\{C_i\}_{i=1}^m \cup \{\{x_a^{1-\epsilon_a}\}, \{x_b^{1-\delta_b}\}\})$$

Let s be a satisfying assignment of $\{C_i\}_{i=0}^m$. By Lemma 1 if $x_a^{1-\epsilon_a}$ & $x_b^{1-\delta_b} \in s$ then s is not a model of F. Adding to $\{C_i\}_{i=1}^m$ the unitary clauses $\{x_a^{1-\epsilon_a}\}$ and $\{x_b^{1-\delta_b}\}$ keeps s as a model of $\{C_i\}_{i=1}^m \cup \{\{x_a^{1-\epsilon_a}\}, \{x_b^{1-\delta_b}\}\}$. Then a model of $\{C_i\}_{i=1}^m$ is either a model of F or a model of $\{C_i\}_{i=1}^m \cup \{\{x_a^{1-\epsilon_a}\}, \{x_b^{1-\delta_b}\}\}$ $\square$.

Then the constraint graph of a formula that satisfies the conditions of Lemma 2 contains at least one cycle (different from a parallel edge or a loop).

Proposition 1. *Let $H = \{C_i\}_{i=1}^m$ be a 2-CF such that $\rho(H)$ represents a connected graph. Let $F = H \cup \{\{x_a^{\epsilon_a}, x_b^{\delta_b}\}\}$ such that*

- *$x_a^{\epsilon_a}$ or $x_a^{1-\epsilon_a} \in C_j$ for some $j = 1, \ldots m$ and*
- *$x_b^{\delta_b}$ or $x_b^{1-\delta_b} \in C_k$ for some $k = 1, \ldots m$ and $j \neq k$*

then $\rho(F)$ contains at least one cycle.

Proof. Since $\rho(H)$ is connected, there is a path from x_a to x_b in $\rho(H)$. Then $\rho(\{x_a^{\epsilon_a}, x_h^{\delta_b}\})$ adds an edge which makes a cycle $\square$.

We want to define a function $Models(G_F)$ on graphs such that

$$Models(G_F) = \#2SAT(F)$$

Since G_F is connected, a spanning tree together with parallel edges and loops T_{G_F} can be built, i.e., $V(G_F) = V(T_{G_F})$, for the sake of simplicity we just call *tree* to this subgraph. Let $\overline{T}_{G_F}$ be the *cotree* associated i.e., $G_F = T_F \cup \overline{T}_{G_F}$. if $\overline{T}_{G_F}$ is empty means that G_F is a tree.

The base cycles of G_F with respect to T_{G_F} form a basis for the cycle space of G_F and also $\overline{T}_{G_F}$ contains no edge-cuts for G_F [13].

Let $e = (v, w) \in E(\overline{T}_{G_F})$, since ρ is a bijection it comes out that the split $F = \rho^{-1}(G_F \setminus e) \cup \rho^{-1}(e)$ satisfies the conditions of Lemma 2.

Let $e = (v, w) \in E(\overline{T}_{G_F})$, we denote as $cycle(e)$ the path from v to w in the spanning tree of T_{G_F} plus the edge e itself, and $e\_cycle(e) = E(cycle(e))$.

Thus, $Models(G_F)$ can be computed as:

$$Models(G_F) = Models(G_F \setminus e) - Models(G_F \setminus e \cup \{e_1, e_2\})$$

where $e_1 = (v, v)$ and $e_2 = (w, w)$.

That means that the computation of $Models(G_F)$ when G_F is cyclic can be reduced to the computation of $Models(G') - Models(G'')$ where G' has one basic cycle less than G_F and G'' additionally of having one cycle less than G_F, has two loops more than G_F.

The following recurrence establishes how split the computation of $Models(G_F)$, where G_F is a graph which contains cycles, until acyclic graphs (with loops and possibly parallel edges) are obtained. We use $Models(G_F) = M(T, \overline{T})$ where T and $\overline{T}$ are a tree, cotree decomposition of G_F respectively.

$$M(T, \overline{T}) = \begin{cases} M(T, \overline{T} \setminus e) - M(T \cup \{(v,v), (w,w)\}, \overline{T} \setminus e) & \text{if } e = (v, w) \in \overline{T} \\ Count\_Models\_for\_trees\_loops\_parallel(T) & \text{if } \overline{T} = \emptyset \end{cases}$$

$$(5)$$

Theorem 1. *Let G_F be the constraint graph of a 2-CF formula F. Let T and $\overline{T}$ be a spanning tree (with the parallel edges and loops of G_F added) and cotree of G_F respectively then $\#2SAT(F) = M(T, \overline{T})$.*

Proof. Consequence of Lemma 2.   □

Theorem 2. *Let F be a 2-CF formula, let $G = \rho(F)$ be its constraint graph. If T and $\overline{T}$ are a spanning tree (with the parallel edges and loops of G added) and its cotree for G respectively, then the time complexity to compute $M(T, \overline{T})$ is $O(2^{|E(\overline{T})|} \cdot poly(|E(T)|))$, where poly is a polynomial function.*

Proof. By Eq. 5 each element of $\overline{T}$ doubles the computation without reducing the number of elements of the tree. The computation of $M(T, \emptyset)$ can be done in polynomial time.   □

Let F be a formula whose constraint connected graph $G_F = \rho(F)$ represents a cyclic graph. Let T be a spanning tree (with the parallel edges and loops added) of G_F and $\overline{T}$ its cotree.

Definition 1. *Let $e \in \overline{T}$, we say that $cycle(e)$ is independent in G_F if for any other cycle $cycle(e') \in G_F, e\_cycle(e) \cap e\_cycle(e') = \emptyset$. If two distinct fundamental cycles $cycle(e_i)$ and $cycle(e_j)$ from G_F have common edges then we say that both cycles are intersected.*

An improvement of the time complexity for our proposal can be achieved in the following way.

Definition 2. *A family of sets T_i of $\overline{T}$ is built as follows: two different edges $e_1, e_2 \in \overline{T}$ belong to the same set T_i iff $\exists S \subseteq T_i, e_1 \notin S, e_2 \notin S$ and $e\_cycle(e1) \cap (\bigcup_{e \in S} e\_cycle(e)) \cap e\_cycle(e_2) \neq \emptyset$. In fact, S could be the emptyset.*

Note that each $T_i \in \overline{T}$ is formed by the frond edges of the cycles that can be chained via one or more intersected cycles.

Definition 3. *As for any independent cycle cycle(e) of G_F there is not any other edge $e' \in \overline{T}$ holding Definition 2, then a unitary set $T_i = \{e\}$ is formed. In this way, there are as much unitary sets T_i as independent cycles in G_F.*

According to Definitions 2 and 3, two different sets T_a, T_b of the partition $\cup T_i$ have not any common cycles. So, all the cycles determined by T_a are independent with all the cycles determined by T_b.

Lemma 3. *The family of sets $\cup T_i$ of Definitions 2 and 3 is a set partition of $\overline{T}$.*

Proof. Let $X, Y \in \cup T_i$, $X \neq Y$, then $X \cap Y = \emptyset$. If X or Y are unitary, assuming $X = \{e\}$, e is not member of Y because $cycle(e)$ is independent in G_F and has not common edges with any other cycle in G_F. If X and Y are not unitary then they have not common elements because in other case, we can build S with the common edges of X and Y and S holds the condition in Definition 2, and then $X = Y$.

Due to each element $e \in \overline{T}$ belong to a unique partition then $\cup T_i = \overline{T}$. □

Definition 4.   *1. For each $P \in \cup T_i$, build a subgraph as follows: $\forall e \in P$,*

$$G_P(V(path(e)), e\_cycle(e))$$

2. Define $G_R = G_F \setminus \bigcup G_{P \in \cup T_i}$.

Lemma 4. *The sets $E(G_P), P \in \cup T_i$ together with $E(G_R)$ forms a set partition of $E(G_F)$.*

Proof. The union of the subgraphs generated from the paths of the elements of the cotree $\overline{T}$ form the cyclic part of the graph, whose set of edges are disjoint, the rest of the edges comes from G_R as stated in Definition 4. □

Lemma 5. *For each pair of graphs G_{P_1}, G_{P_2}, from Lemma 4, either $V(G_{P_1}) \cap V(G_{P_2}) = \emptyset$ or $V(G_{P_1}) \cap V(G_{P_2}) = \{v\}$ e.g. is a singleton.*

Proof. By contradiction suppose that $V(G_{P_1}) \cap V(G_{P_2}) \neq \emptyset$ and $V(G_{P_1}) \cap V(G_{P_2}) \neq \{v\}$ it means that there are at least two vertices, let say v_1, v_2 in the intersection, meaning that the edge $e = (v_1, v_2)$ belongs to the intersection contradicting the hypothesis that G_{P_1} and G_{P_2} have a set of disjoint edges. □

Theorem 3. *For each pair of graphs G_{P_1}, G_{P_2} from Lemma 4*

1. If $G_{P_1} \cap G_{P_2} = \emptyset$ then the models which represents G_{P_1} are independent of the models which represents G_{P_2} e.g. $Models(G_{P_1} \cup G_{P_2}) = Models(G_{P_1}) \times Models(G_{P_2})$.

2. *If $G_{P_1} \cap G_{P_2} = \{v\}$ then*

$$Models(G_{P_1} \cup G_{P_2}) = Models(G_{P_1}|_{v^1}) \times Models(G_{P_2}|_{v^1})$$
$$+$$
$$Models(G_{P_1}|_{v^0}) \times Models(G_{P_2}|_{v^0})$$

Proof. 1. If $G_{P_1} \cap G_{P_2} = \emptyset$ neither edges nor vertices are shared. Since each vertex of the graphs represents a variable of the input formula, $\rho^{-1}(G_{P_1}) \cap \rho^{-1}(G_{P_2}) = \emptyset$, e.g. there are no common variables of the formulas represented by each subgraph. It is well known that the models of formulas without common variables can be computed by the product of the models of the formulas.

2. If $|G_{P_1} \cap G_{P_2}| = 1$, means that if $F_1 = \rho^{-1}(G_{P_1})$ and $F_2 = \rho^{-1}(G_{P_2})$ then $\nu(F_1) \cap \nu(F_2) = \{x_1\}$, e.g. there is a single variable common to both sub formulas. A classical branch and bound strategy can be used, where one branch counts the models where x_1 is fixed to be true and the other branch counts the models where x_1 is fixed to be false in both sub formulas and then add them. Once x_1 has been fixed either to true or false, no common variable exists between the sub formulas, so by 1, their models can be computed independently by their product. □

From Theorem 3 we can conclude that the number of models of each of the $G_{P \in \cup T_i}$ can be computed independently.

Due to G_F is a connected graph, if there are subgraphs G_{P_1} and G_{P_2} such that $V(G_{P_1}) \cap V(G_{P_1}) = \emptyset$ there should exists a path in G_R joining them. Fortunately, the model of a path can be computed in polynomial time, see Sect. 3.

Theorem 4. *Let F be a 2-CF, let $G = \rho(F)$ be its constraint graph. If P is a set partition of G as in Definition 2 and $\cup T_i, i = 1, \ldots r$ are those partitions which contain edges of the cotree $\overline{T}$, then the time complexity to compute $M(T, \overline{T})$ is $O(2^{max\{|T_i|\}} \cdot poly(|E(T)|))$, where poly is a polynomial function.*

Proof. Recurrence 5 doubles the computation of a given tree T based on the elements of the cotree associated. By Theorem 3 each T_i can be computed independently. So the maximum number of times that Recurrence 5 is applied is given by $k = max\{| T_i|\}$. While the computation of $M(T, \emptyset)$ is done in polynomial time. □

4.1 Example

Let $F = \{\{v_1, v_2\}, \{v_1, v_7\}, \{v_2, v_4\}, \{v_2, v_3\}, \{v_3, v_7\}, \{v_3, v_{10}\}, \{v_4, v_5\}, \{v_4, v_9\}, \{v_5, v_6\}, \{v_7, v_{10}\}, \{v_6, v_8\}, \{v_6, v_9\}\}$. The constraint graph $\rho(F)$ is (we ommited the signs since all variables are positive):

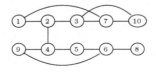

The partition of G is G_{p_1}, G_{p_2} and G_R whose elements are respectively:

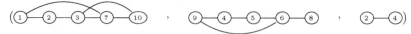

The computation of each partition is:

$$G_{p_1} = M \begin{bmatrix} \begin{smallmatrix}2\\3\\7\\10\end{smallmatrix} & , & \begin{smallmatrix}1\\2\\3\\10\end{smallmatrix} \end{bmatrix} = MA \begin{bmatrix} \begin{smallmatrix}2\\3\\(5,4)\\(2,1)\\10\end{smallmatrix}(9,5) \\ (2,1)\\1 \end{bmatrix} - MA \begin{bmatrix} \begin{smallmatrix}2\\3\\(1,0)\\10\end{smallmatrix}(2,0)(0,2)(2,2)(2,1)(0,1)\\1 \end{bmatrix} - MA \begin{bmatrix} \begin{smallmatrix}2\\3\\(2,1)\\10\end{smallmatrix}(0,2)(4,2)(2,2)(1,0)(0,1)\\1 \end{bmatrix}$$

$$+ MA \begin{bmatrix} \begin{smallmatrix}2\\(1,0)\\3\\(1,0)\\10\end{smallmatrix}(0,0)(1,0)(0,1)(1,1)(1,0)(0,1)(0,1)\\1 \end{bmatrix} = (9,5) - (2,0) - (0,2) + (0,0) = (7,3)$$

$$G_{p_2} = M \begin{bmatrix} \begin{smallmatrix}4\\5\\6\\9\end{smallmatrix} & , & \begin{smallmatrix}4\\9\\8\end{smallmatrix} \end{bmatrix} = MA \begin{bmatrix} \begin{smallmatrix}4\\5\\(5,4)\\(2,1)\\9\end{smallmatrix}(9,5)(2,1)\\8 \end{bmatrix} - MA \begin{bmatrix} \begin{smallmatrix}4\\5\\(2,2)\\(1,0)\\9\end{smallmatrix}(0,2)(4,2)(2,1)(0,1)\\8 \end{bmatrix} = (9,5) - (0,2) = (9,3)$$

$$G_R = M \begin{bmatrix} \begin{smallmatrix}2\\4\end{smallmatrix}(7,3)\\(9,3) \end{bmatrix} = M \begin{bmatrix} 2 & (7,3)\times(12,9) \end{bmatrix} = 84 + 27 = 111$$

The time complexity $O(2^{max\{|T_i|\}} \cdot poly(|E(T)|))$ of our algorithm results in a polynomial time for computing #2SAT for several classes of graphs. For example, for *Cactus Graphs* which are acyclic or when they are cyclic then each cycle is independent to any other of the graph. So, for this class of graphs $k = max\{|T_i|\} = 1$.

The Cactus Graphs appeared in the scientific literature more than half a century ago under the name of *Husimi trees*, dealing with cluster integrals in the theory of condensation in statistical mechanics. Besides statistical mechanics, where Husimi trees and their generalizations serve as simplified models of real lattices, the concept has also found applications in the theory of electrical and communication networks [4] and in chemistry [8, 12].

5   Conclusion

#SAT problem for the class of Boolean formulas in 2-CF is a classical #P-complete problem. However, there are several instances of 2-CF's for which #2SAT can be solved efficiently.

If the constraint graph G of an input 2-CF F is cyclic, T a spanning tree of G and $\overline{T}$ its cotree, we show that by building a set partition $\cup T_i$ of $\overline{T}$, we show a parametric polynomial deterministic method to compute #2SAT with time complexity of order $O(2^{max\{|E(\overline{T_i})|\}} \cdot poly(|E(T)|))$, where *poly* is a polynomial function, and each T_i is formed by the frond edges of the cycles that are chained via intersected cycles.

This is a novel method which shows that #2SAT is in the complexity class FPT, and where the fixed-parameter k depends on the maximum number of frond edges chained via intersected cycles in a subcotree, and of a decomposition (tree:cotree) of the constraint graph associated to the formula.

References

1. Darwiche, A.: On the tractability of counting theory models and its application to belief revision and truth maintenance. J. Appl. Non-Class. Logics **11**(1–2), 11–34 (2011)
2. Angelsmark, O., Jonsson, P.: Improved algorithms for counting solutions in constraint satisfaction problems. In: Rossi, F. (ed.) CP 2003. LNCS, vol. 2833, pp. 81–95. Springer, Heidelberg (2003)
3. Russ, B.: Randomized Algorithms: Approximation, Generation, and Counting. Distingished Dissertations. Springer, Heidelberg (2001)
4. Zmazek, B.: Estimating the traffic on weighted cactus networks in linear time. In: 9th International Conference on Information Visualization, pp. 536–541 (2005)
5. Roth, D.: On the hardness of approximate reasoning. J. Artif. Intell. **82**, 273–302 (1996)
6. Wahlström, M., Dahllöf, V., Jonsonn, P.: Counting models for 2SAT and 3SAT formulae. Theor. Comput. Sci. **332**(1–3), 265–291 (2005)
7. De Ita G., C.M., Bello, P.: New polynomial classes for #2sat established via graph-topological structure. Eng. Lett. **15**(2), 250–258 (2007)
8. Mäloy, F., Došlič, V.: Chain hexagonal cacti: matchings and independent sets. Discrete Math. **310**, 1676–1690 (2010)
9. Ravve, E.V., Fischer, E., Makowsky, J.A.: Counting truth assignments of formulas of bounded tree-width or clique-width. Discrete Appl. Math. **156**(4), 511–529 (2008)
10. Prasad, S.K., Fürer, M.: Algorithms for counting 2-sat solutions and coloring with applications. Technical report 33, Electronic Colloqium on Comp. Complexity (2005)
11. Makowsky, J.A.: Algorithmic uses of the feferman-vaught theorem. Ann. Pure Appl. Logic **126**, 1–3 (2004)
12. Kalyani, D.: Design of Algorithms on Some Problems on Cactus Graphs: Algorithms on Graphs. Lambert Acad. Pub., Germany (2012)
13. Kreher, D.L., Kocay, W.: Graphs, Algorithms, and Optimization. Chapman & Hall, NewYork (2004)
14. Szeider, S.: On fixed-parameter tractable parameterizations of SAT. In: Giunchiglia, E., Tacchella, A. (eds.) SAT 2003. LNCS, vol. 2919, pp. 188–202. Springer, Heidelberg (2004)

A Performative-Based Information Capacity Calculation Metric for MultiAgent Interaction Protocols

Dogus Bebek[1] and Hurevren Kilic[2(✉)]

[1] Business Intelligence and Datawarehouse Systems Department,
Akbank T.A.S, Istanbul, Turkey
dbebek@gmail.com
[2] Computer Engineering Department, Engineering and Architecture Faculty,
Gediz University, Menemen, Izmir, Turkey
hurevren.kilic@gediz.edu.tr, hurevren@gmail.com

Abstract. A performative-based information capacity calculation metric for MultiAgent Interaction Protocols is developed. The metric uses Shannon's L-channel combinatorial information capacity calculation idea. In the approach, MultiAgent System (MAS) protocol is modeled as a discrete noiseless channel and provides not data level but language specific information capacity calculation for high level performative-based protocols. The amount of information that flow in MAS due to FIPA-ACL performatives used in given communication protocol is measured and figured out. The unit of measurement is bits per performative. Since the metric is a design time metric, it gives the system designer an opportunity to evaluate his/her design without implementing and testing it. In the application of the proposed metric to FIPA contract net protocol and its iterated versions, we observed a correlation between iteration counts and metric values.

Keywords: Agent communication protocol · Metric for multiagent systems · L-channel · Shannon language · Discrete noiseless channel · Combinatorial capacity calculation · Agent communication language performatives

1 Introduction

A common requirement of today's distributed computing systems is to handle intensive data and communication among units via well-designed communication languages and protocols. Clearly, the system's performance is directly affected by the expressive power of designed communication language and efficiency of the protocol. Specific to agent systems, languages like KQML [1] and FIPA-ACL [2] based on speech-act theory [3] provide us useful well-defined standards in agent communication. In [4], criteria to evaluate agent communication languages for an appropriate use have been defined.

While the role of communication language in computing is becoming more important, accessibility to encapsulated internal designs of computing units is either becoming more limited or impossible as in the case of MultiAgent Systems (MAS). Separate ownership of agents and their adopted autonomous nature are two factors

G. Sidorov and S.N. Galicia-Haro (Eds.): MICAI 2015, Part I, LNAI 9413, pp. 214–224, 2015.
DOI: 10.1007/978-3-319-27060-9_17

fostering such trend. On the other side, we know that successful operation in MAS environments requires development of efficient measurement tools and techniques for their designers [5]. As a consequence, communication-based modeling became a critical and challenging issue for realizing better MAS products operating in large, complex, dynamic environments [6]. Such an effort needs quantified assessment of inter-agent communication protocols via some formal measurement approach. This is also true for self-diagnosis and/or self-healing purposes. In [7], a communication-based performance measure for MAS has been proposed. Their approach includes measurement of task achievement performances of agents through pattern-based examination of agent communication. In [8], it has been pointed out that measuring the size of communication and the level of conversation is useful for sustaining agent activities. Therefore, figuring out MAS agent communication via some metric is a problem whose solution may affect the system's run-time task achievement performance.

In [9], the effect of communication protocols and organizational structure on the performance of MAS has been studied. Specifically, they have considered the Contract-Net [10] and auction protocols implemented in KQML agent communication language over mesh and hierarchical organizational structures. They have shown that protocol and organizational structure are two key factors in predicting MAS perfor-mance. In [11], alternative metrics based on graph theory are proposed to analyze agent organizational structures. They present an evaluation approach to measure general but not topic and/or application dependent characteristics of MAS. In [12], a metric for calculating maximum rate of information that can be transmitted over peer-to-peer organizational structure using Gnutella protocol has been proposed. Similarly, in [13], an information capacity calculation metric for component-based software systems has been developed. Different from peer-oriented organizational structure aware approach of [12], they focused on the system level information capacity calculation due to traditional messaging among software components. In their nature, MAS protocols are different from traditional distributed system protocols; however, we know that the agent communication research can borrow ideas from distributed systems [14] and we should still have metrics to measure qualitative aspects of MAS protocols [6]. We or an agent in a MAS environment must be able to compare two MAS protocols at design or run-time for the purpose of better design or task achievement or possible agreement.

In this study, we propose a performative-based information capacity calculation metric for MAS by adapting Shannon's traditional L-channel combinatorial informa-tion capacity calculation [15]. In our approach, MAS is modeled as a discrete noiseless channel whose performative level agent communications define a Shannon language. Note that existence of a performative level noise in communication among software agents simply implies a non-working system for which information capacity calcula-tion is meaningless. To the best of our knowledge, there is no study in the MAS literature that attacks to development of a metric for information capacity calculation of multiagent interaction protocols. According to the classification developed for the software measurement of agent-based systems by [8], our proposal is a product metric characterizing systems at runtime working level. The amount of information that flow in MAS due to FIPA-ACL performatives used in given communication protocol is measured and figured out. The unit of measurement is bit per performative. In Sect. 2, we describe discrete noiseless channel modeling of MAS and give formal description of the metric. Section 3 includes the details application of the metric to an example agent communication protocol. The results & discussions and conclusions are given in Sects. 4 and 5, respectively.

2   Discrete Noiseless Channel Modeling of MAS Communication and the Metric

In the following, we give definitions related to the discrete noiseless channel [15] and after each definition we explain its meaning in MAS protocol context.

Definition 1: A discrete noiseless channel is a channel which allows the noiseless transmission of a sequence of symbols chosen from a finite alphabet A (called q-letter alphabet), each symbol, say $a \in A$, having a certain value $\tau(a)$ from a parameter of interest (e.g. duration for time parameter), possibly different for different symbols.

In our case, a MAS protocol is a noiseless channel and discrete alphabet symbols are coded FIPA-ACL performatives of the agent communication language of the MAS. For example, i for inform, b for broadcast, r for request etc. So, A is the set of performatives. Also, $\tau(a)$ is assumed to be performative value due to use performative a that causes state change of the MAS. Note that performative sender and/or receiver identities are not important.

Definition 2: A word of length k over A is a finite string of k letters from A. If $\alpha = a_1 a_2 \ldots a_k$ is such a word, its value is defined to be $\tau(\alpha) = \tau(a_1) + \tau(a_2) + \ldots + \tau(a_k)$.

A word of length k defined over performative alphabet A is a sequence of performatives $\alpha = a_1 a_2 \ldots a_k$ where each symbol a_i changes state of the global MAS. The total performative value generated by a word of length k is the sum of each value generated by corresponding performative during inter-agent communication.

Definition 3: A language L over A is a collection of words defined over A. The discrete noiseless channel associated with L, the L-*channel* for short, is the channel which is only allowed to transmit sequences from L, where it transmits them without error.

Language defined by an agent communication protocol is a set of valid interaction or state change sequences (i.e. words of the language) defined by different executions of the protocol and L-*channel* is the protocol itself.

The basic question answered by Shannon is: "What is the capacity of such L-*channel* to transmit information?" Note that, in its original definition, the capacity (also called combinatorial capacity) is the maximum rate (in bits per second) that information can be transmitted over the channel. The parameter of interest in the Shannon's original work is associated with duration (in seconds) of single letter in spend in the channel. In our agent communication protocol capacity calculation case, the parameter of interest is supposed to be unit value generated by the use of performative sent from sender agent to receiver agent defined by the protocol under consideration. As a consequence, the unit of the calculated capacity is bits per performative.

Simply, Shannon language can be represented by a directed graph $G = (V, B)$ whose vertices are defined by V and branches/edges B are labeled with letters from the alphabet A. The corresponding language L is then defined to be the set of words that result by reading off the edge labels on paths of the graph. Analogously, we define a given protocol in terms of states of the MAS as the graph vertices and performatives as the directed edges labeled by mapping $\lambda : B \rightarrow A$ where B is the set of edges and A is the set of performatives. Edge weight $\tau(a)$ on the other hand, defines unit performative value generated due to performative a.

Based on the Shannon's work [15], we define performative-based combinatorial capacity of a MAS protocol as:

$$C_{comb} = \lim_{t \to \infty} sup \frac{1}{t} \log(N(t)) \tag{1}$$

where $N(t)$ is the total number of interaction or state change sequences defined by MAS protocol of total value generated due to performative sequence of length t.

In Shannon's original work, an algebraic method of computing C_{comb} has been given. In [16], a relatively simpler alternative C_{comb} computation has also been given. Below, we prefer to continue with definitions from [16] that are finalized by a theorem defining the C_{comb} calculation in an alternative way.

Definition 4: Let $\lambda : B \rightarrow A$ be a labeling. λ is right-resolving iff for each vertex v, the labels on all branches having the same source vertex v are distinct.

Simply, right resolving property of labeling implies deterministic behavior of MAS communication in terms of used performatives. Therefore, non-deterministic protocol instances require a conversion to corresponding deterministic instances as a pre-processing step before metric calculation. The performative value partition function for set of all possible performative sequences defining language $L_{G,\lambda}$ generated by protocol graph G, and labeling λ together with given performative values $\tau(a)$ for each performative a is defined below.

Definition 5: Let s be nonnegative real number, and for a given pair of protocol state vertices (v, w), performative edge partition function is defined by

$$P_{v,w}(s) = \sum_{b \in B_{v,w}} e^{-s\tau(b)} \tag{2}$$

where $B_{v,w}$ is a performative edge having source state v and destination state w.

The functions $P_{v,w}(s)$ can be considered as the entries of a $M \times M$ matrix $P(s)$ where M is the number of vertices. The spectral radius (the magnitude of the largest eigenvalue) of matrix $P(s)$ is represented by $\rho(s)$ and it is also called the partition function for the language $L_{G,\lambda}$.

Theorem: The combinatorial capacity of the language is given by

$$C_{comb} = \ln(s_0) \tag{3}$$

where s_0 is the unique solution to the equation $\rho(s) = 1$.

Alternatively, C_{comb} is the greatest positive solution of the equation (in nats),

$$q(s) = \det(I - P(s)) = 0 \tag{4}$$

where I is the identity matrix and $P(s)$ is the performative edge partition function.

3 Application of the Metric to Agent Communication Protocols

In a typical data-oriented low level approach, communication between units is identified at message-data level and the effect of communication due to higher level outer language primitives and designed protocol is not considered. Traditionally, protocols specify a flow of messages however recent approaches also ascribe meanings to the messages [17]. In the context of MAS, outer languages like KQML and FIPA-ACL define an envelope for messages, using which an agent can explicitly state the intended illocutionary force of a message. In both languages, the illocutionary effect is mainly characterized by the use of primitives called performatives (e.g. inform, request, ask-one, broadcast etc.). The term performative is defined as: "Being or relating to an expression that serves to effect a transaction or that constitutes the performance of the specified act by virtue of its utterance" [18]. Performatives are the main sources of illocutionary effect generation in MAS. There are 40 different performatives defined in the original KQML and 20 around different performatives in FIPA-ACL. Two core primitives of FIPA-ACL are inform and request. All other performatives in FIPA-ACL can be defined in terms of these performatives. Therefore, one can assume inform and request performatives as the basic units of communication.

In order to illustrate the application of Shannon's combinatorial capacity calculation metric to the agent communication protocols at performatives level, we will use two known protocols: Contract Net [19] and Iterated Contract Net [20].

3.1 FIPA Contract Net Protocol

Contract Net protocol is developed to carry out negotiations between participants in distributed environments. It allows the distribution of tasks among a group of agents. Also, a user in marketplace specifies his/her goods (call for proposal act) and among the bids received (proposal act) chooses the winner. In the e-Bay example winner is the highest bidder. In contract net, one agent (the Initiator) takes the role of manager which wishes to have some task performed by one or more other agents (the Participants) and, further wishes to optimize a function that characterizes the task. This characteristic is commonly expressed as the price, in some domain specific way, but could also be soonest time to completion, fair distribution of tasks, etc.

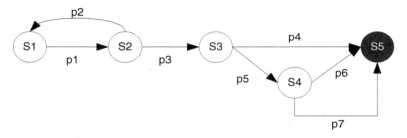

Fig. 1. Graph-based representation of contract net protocol.

In FIPA contract net protocol, initiator agent starts the communication by sending Call for Proposal (CFP) to the participants in the environment. Participants can reply the CFP either with refuse or propose performative. Communication continues with the participants that replies with propose performative. After initiator agent collects proposals from the participants, it can accept one of them and refuse the rest or refuse all of the proposals. If a proposal accepted then related participant informed with the accept-proposal act. After the given task is executed by the participant, initiator is going to be informed according to the result of the execution with inform or failure performative. See [19] for UML representation of the protocol. Corresponding graph representation of Contract Net protocol that forms the basis for Shannon Language is in Fig. 1. In the figure, S_1 is the initial state where initiator agent sends the Call for Proposal performative. S_2 is the state where participants reply call for proposal either by refuse or propose performative. In state S_3, initiator either accepts or rejects one of the proposals sent by participants. If the proposal accepted by the initiator, in state S_4 participant informs the initiator with the result. If the result is done then system goes to the final state S_5 In case of failure system also goes to final state S_5 and communication ends.

If proposal rejected by the initiator then initiator sends the reject performative to the participant and system goes to the final state S_5. Performatives that realize the communication are labeled as p_1 to p_7. Description of the performatives can be found in Table 1.

Table 1. Symbol vs. performative descriptions.

Symbol	Performative
p_1	Call for proposal
p_2	Refuse
p_3	Propose
p_4	Reject proposal
p_5	Accept proposal
p_6	Inform (result/done)
p_7	Failure

$$P(s) = \begin{bmatrix} 0 & e^{-s} & 0 & 0 & 0 \\ e^{-s} & 0 & e^{-s} & 0 & 0 \\ 0 & 0 & 0 & e^{-s} & e^{-s} \\ 0 & 0 & 0 & e^{-s} & e^{-s} \\ 0 & 0 & 0 & 0 & 0 \end{bmatrix}$$

Fig. 2. Performative edge partition function obtained for the example protocol.

FIPA-ACL performatives can be represented in terms of two primitive performatives: *inform* and *request*. So, for each performative, one can determine its value $\tau(a)$ based on count of the primitive performatives in its formal definition, recursively. Note that alternative (even cognitive) metrics other than simple primitive counting can further be defined for their more suitable handling. In this study, we supposed $\tau(a_i) = 1$ for all performatives a_i occur in the protocol without any further elaboration. Based on Eq. 2, first we obtain performative edge partition function in Fig. 2. Then, the performative-based information capacity of the contract net protocol as: 0.2406 bits/performative.

3.2   FIPA Iterated Contract Net Protocol

Iterated Contract Net Protocol is the modified version of the Contract Net Protocol. Different from the Contract Net protocol, negotiation is iterated for a fixed number of times by the initiator agent to get better bids. During the iterations, according to the proposals received initiator agent revises its call for proposal and starts the negotiation process over the participants replied with propose act in the previous iteration. See [20], for sequence diagram defining Iterated Contract Net protocol. Graph-based representations of FIPA Iterated Contract Net protocols for two, three, and four iterations and their corresponding performative edge partition functions are given in Fig. 3. The obtained performative-based information capacity values are: 0.2812, 0.2992 and 0.3094 bits/performative, respectively. From the obtained results, we can say that as the number of iterations of FIPA contract net protocol increases, performative-based information capacity of the protocol also increases.

4   Results and Discussions

The proposed metric is a product metric usable at design time. Since agent cooperation in a multiagent system is a very complex process, it is valuable to have a clue about the product at design time. Empirical criterion for the metric is: Higher performative-based communicative capacity of the protocol provides more robust and flexible MAS design. Capacity maximization is supposed to be MAS design goal. Note that usage of an alternative agent communication languages or changing MAS organizational structure are still two possible design decisions that can be taken for obtaining higher communicative capacity achievement.

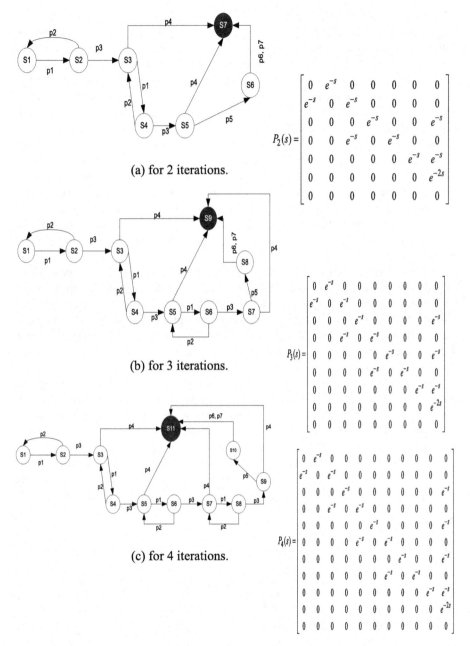

Fig. 3. Graph-based representation and performative edge partition functions obtained for the iterated contract net protocol (a) for 2 iterations (b) for 3 iterations and (c) for 4 iterations.

Protocol designer can model; his/her protocol and test it against various predefined communication protocols (if they are alternative to designed protocol). Or for any possible modifications in the protocol, designer can compare the existing protocol with the modified one by means of efficiency at design time. Having designed two protocols being alternative to each other, instead of developing software with implementing protocols and testing them, using proposed metric, one can conclude which protocol is more useful in terms of information generated/passed per unit performative at run-time. As we pointed out higher the value is expected to result in more robust MAS design (compare with bit per second measure in traditional data communication networks). From that sense, the proposed metric provides not data level but language specific information capacity calculation for high level performative-based protocols.

Clearly, the metric value is shaped by how the cost value $\tau(a_i)$ for performatives are defined. Even though we assumed fixed $\tau(a_i)= 1$ values for all performatives, one can develop alternative valuations for different performatives based on their formal definitions. This may range from simple counting of primitives inform and request occurrences in the definition to performative's occurrences in the other performative (simple their level of primitiveness). In [21], for example, a weight is associated with each six type of KQML performatives based on its state change impact on sender and receiver agents.

Specific to the results that we have obtained for application of the metric to the iterated and non-iterated versions of FIPA contract net protocol in Sect. 3, there exist a correlation between the metric application results and iteration count of the protocol (see Fig. 4). It would be interesting to make an asymptotic analysis of possible upper bound of the attained capacity when the number of iterations goes to infinity. Existence of such correlation seems a consequence of increased number of alternative paths that brings MAS communication into its final state.

The metric can also be used for dynamic reorganization of MAS organizational structure at run-time. By this way a centralized authority like directory facilitator can decide on the neighborhood of new created agent in the organizational structure for which the performative-based combinatorial information capacity value of MAS is maximized. However, in our experiments, we observed that run-time metric computation is a performance demanding task especially when the number of agents in MAS becomes high. Note that this is not an issue for protocol level application of the metric whose graph-based representation generates matrices with small size and sparse.

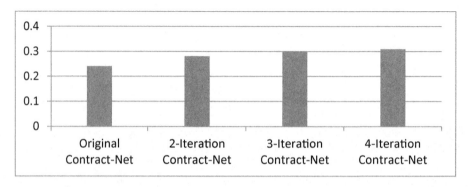

Fig. 4. Performative-based information capacity calculation results (in bits/performative) for FIPA contract net and iterated contract net protocols.

5 Conclusions

Paradigm shift in software development from independent single body design to integration of communicating autonomous agents residing in complex, dynamically changing, distributed environments enforces communication-based metrics to be developed. A new design time product metric that measures performative-based run-time information capacity of MAS protocols in bits per performative is proposed. The metric is based on Shannon's classical work of combinatorial capacity calculation of discrete noiseless channels. The metric is easily applicable to agent communication languages other than FIPA ACL. In the application of the proposed metric to FIPA contract net protocol and its iterated versions, we observed a correlation between increased iteration counts and their increased metric values.

The metric can also be used for dynamic reorganization of MAS organizational structure at run-time. However, it becomes rather performance demanding especially when the number of agents is exceeds 25. In application to MAS protocol capacity calculation, on the other hand, relatively small size and sparse nature of the performative edge partition function does not result in high computational time demand, relatively. Finally, since the metric is applicable to any performative based communication forms of communication between agents, an empirical study that investigates potential correlation(s) among the metric and known software metrics in literature would contribute to provide stronger evidence(s) for benefits of the proposed metric, in future.

References

1. Finin, T., Fritzon, R., McKay, D., McEntire, R.: KQML as an agent communication language. In: Proceedings of Third International Conference on Information and Knowledge Management, CIKM 1994, pp. 456–463. ACM Press, New York (1994)
2. FIPA Communicative Act Library Spec. http://www.fipa.org/specs/fipa00037/
3. Austin, J.L.: How to Do Things With Words, 2nd edn. Oxford Univ. Press, Oxford (1976)
4. Singh, M.P.: Agent communication languages: rethinking the principles. IEEE Comput. **31** (12), 40–47 (1998)
5. Helsinger, A., Lazarus, R., Wright, W., Zinky, J.: Tools and techniques for performance measurement of large distributed multiagent systems. In: Proceedings of Second International Joint Conference on Autonomous Agents and Multiagent Systems, AAMAS 2003, pp. 843–850. ACM, New York (2003)
6. Chopra, A.K., Artikis, A., Bentahar, J., Colombetti, M., Dignum, F., Fornara, N., Jones, A.J. I. Singh, M.P., Yolum, P.: Research directions in agent communication. ACM Trans. Intell. Syst. Technol. (TIST), 1–26 (2011)
7. Rovatsos, M., Schillo, M., Fischer, K., Weiss, G.: Indicators for self-diagnosis: communication-based performance measures. In: Schillo, M., Klusch, M., Müller, J., Tianfield, H. (eds.) MATES 2003. LNCS (LNAI), vol. 2831, pp. 25–37. Springer, Heidelberg (2003)

8. Dumke, R., Koeppe, R., Wille, C.: Software agent measurement and self-measuring agent-based systems. In: Preprint no. 11. Fakultatfur Informatik, Otto-von-Guericke-Universitat, Magdeburg (2000)

9. Lee, L.C., Nwana, H.S., Ndumu, D.T., De Wilde, P.: The stability, scalability and performance of multi-agent systems. BT Technol. J. **13**(3), 94–103 (1998)

10. Davis, R., Smith, R.G.: Negotiation as a metaphor for distributed problem solving. Artif. Intell. **20**(1), 63–109 (1983)

11. Hmida, F.B., Chaari, W.L., Dupas, R., Seguy, A.: Graph-based evaluation of organization in multiagent systems. In: Proceedings of 9th International Conference of Modeling, Optimization and Simulation, MOSIM 2012, Bordeaux, France (2012)

12. Oztoprak, K., Kilic, H.: Protocol and connectivity based overlay level capacity calculation of P2P networks. In: Proceedings of IEEE/WIC/ACM International Workshop on P2P Computing and Autonomous Agents (IEEE/WIC/ACM P2PAA 2006), Hong Kong/China, pp. 447–450 (2006)

13. Seker, R., Tanik, M.M.: An information-theoretical framework for modeling component-based systems. IEEE Trans. Syst. Man Cybern. Part C Appl. Rev. **34**(4), 475–484 (2004)

14. Yolum, P.: Design time analysis of multiagent protocols. Data Knowl. Eng. J. **63**(1), 137–154 (2007)

15. Shannon, C.E.: A mathematical theory of communication. Bell Syst. Tech. J. **27**, 379–423 (1948)

16. Khandekar, A., McEliece, R., Rodemich, E.: The discrete noiseless channel revisited. In: Farrel, P., Darnell, M., Honary, B. (eds.) Coding, Communications, and Broadcasting, Baldock, pp. 115–137. Research Studies Series Ltd., UK (2000)

17. Yolum, P., Singh, M.P.: Flexible protocol specification and execution: applying event calculus planning using commitments. In: Proceedings of 1st International Joint Conference on Autonomous Agents and MultiAgent Systems, pp. 527–534. ACM Press (2002)

18. Merriam-Webster Dictionary. http://www.merriam-webster.com/dictionary/performative

19. FIPA Contract Net Interaction Pro. http://www.fipa.org/specs/fipa00029/SC00029H.html

20. FIPA Iterated Contract Net Interaction Pro. www.fipa.org/specs/fipa00030/SC00030H.pdf

21. Bouslimi, I., Hanachi, C., Ghedira, K.: An experimental evaluation of communication in an organization-based multi-agent system. In: Proceedings of International Joint Conference on Web Intelligence & Intelligent Agent Technology, IEEE/WIC/ACM, Poland, vol. 3, pp. 72–78 (2014)

Bioinspired Algorithms

Bio-Inspired Optimization Algorithm Based on the Self-defense Mechanism in Plants

Camilo Caraveo[✉], Fevrier Valdez, and Oscar Castillo

Division of Graduate Studies Tijuana Institute of Technology Tijuana,
Tijuana, Mexico
Camilo.caraveo@Gmail.com,
{fevrier,Ocastillo}@tectijuana.mx

Abstract. In this paper the application of a new method of bio-inspired optimization based on the self-defense mechanism of plants is presented. Through time the planet has gone through changes, so plants have had to adapt to these changes and adopt new techniques to defend from natural predators (herbivores). Several works have shown that plants have mechanisms of self-defense to protect themselves from predators. When the plants detect the presence of invading organisms this triggers a series of chemical reactions that are released to air and attract natural predators of the invading organism [1, 9, 10]. For the development of this algorithm we consider as a main idea the predator prey mathematical model of Lotka and Volterra, where two populations are considered and the objective is to maintain a balance between the two populations.

Keywords: Predator prey model · Plants · Self-defense · Mechanism

1 Introduction

Several meta-heuristic algorithms have been developed to solve various combinatorial optimization problems. These can be classified into different groups based on the criteria that are, for example, deterministic, iterative, population based, stochastic, etc. While an algorithm works with a set of solutions and the use of multiple iterations to approach the desired solution is called as iterative algorithm based on populations.

Throughout history there have been developed and tested multiple methods of search and optimization inspired by natural processes. This with the goal of solving particular problems in the area of computer science and several different bio-inspired methods have been tried, such as ACO, PSO, BCO, GA etc. [7, 8, 11]. Trying in all cases to get the solution of a specific problem with a smaller error.

In this work a new optimization algorithm inspired in the self-defense mechanisms of plants is presented. This in order to compete against the existing optimization methods. In nature, plants are exposed to many different pathogens in the environment. However, only a few can affect them. If a particular pathogen is unable to successfully attack a plant, it is said that it is resistant to it, in other words, cannot be affected by the pathogen.

The proposed approach takes as its main basis the Lotka and Volterra predator-prey model, which is a system formed by a pair of first order differential equations, nonlinear

© Springer International Publishing Switzerland 2015
G. Sidorov and S.N. Galicia-Haro (Eds.): MICAI 2015, Part I, LNAI 9413, pp. 227–237, 2015.
DOI: 10.1007/978-3-319-27060-9_18

for moderating the growth of two populations that interact with each other (predator and prey) [6].

2 Self-defense Mechanisms of the Plants

In nature, plants as well as animals are exposed to a large number of invading organisms such as insects, fungi, bacteria and viruses that can cause various types of diseases, and even death [10, 14].

Defense mechanisms (or coping strategies) are automatic processes that protect the individual against external or internal threats. The plant is able to react to external stimuli. When it detects the presence or attack of an organism triggers a series of chemical reactions that are released into the air that attracts natural predator of the assailant or cause internal damage to the aggressor [9]. In Fig. 1 a general scheme is shown to illustrate the behavior of the plant when it detects the presence or attack by a predator.

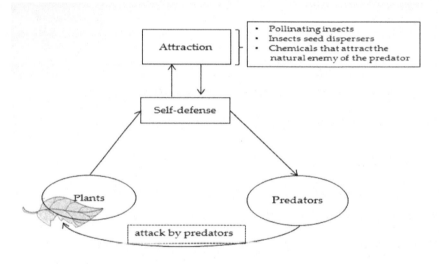

Fig. 1. Representation of the process of self-defense of the plant

The leaves normally release into the air small amounts of volatile chemicals, but when a plant is damaged by herbivorous insects, the amount of chemicals tends to grow. Volatile chemicals vary depending on the plant species and species of herbivorous insects [12]. These chemicals attract both predators and parasitic insects that are natural enemies of herbivores see Fig. 1. Such chemicals, which work in the communication between two or more species, as well as those who serve as messengers between members of the same species are called semi-chemicals [1, 2, 5, 10].

Although in nature, this type of immunity stops almost all parasites, has received little investigation. Some scientists have uncovered the molecular components of the first line of defense. In their findings, they conclude parallels between plant and animal immune systems.

3   Predator-Prey Model

The organisms live in communities, forming intricate relationships of interaction, where each species directly or indirectly dependent on the presence of the other. One of the tasks of Ecology is to develop a theory of community organization for understanding the causes of diversity and mechanisms of interaction. In this paper, we consider the interaction of two whose population size at time t is x (t) and y (t) species [2, 3]. Furthermore, we assume that the change in population size can be written as:

$$\frac{dy}{dt} = I(x,y) \tag{1}$$

$$\frac{dx}{dt} = P(x,y) \tag{2}$$

There are different kinds of biological interaction can be represented mathematically with this system of equations [3]. As $P(x, y)$ and $I(x, y)$ determining the growth rate of each of the populations; there is the case where one of these species is fed from the other, then the system of survival is given by: Eq (3)

$$
\begin{aligned}
P_y(x, y) &< 0 \\
I_x(x, y) &> 0
\end{aligned}
\tag{3}
$$

That is, the change of the prey population relative to the predator decreases and the change of the predator population relative to the prey increases. These are some of the conditions that must meet a set of predator prey equations [3, 13].

3.1   Analysis of the Lotka and Volterra Model

This model is based on the following assumptions.

1. The population grows proportionally to its size, and has enough space and food. If this happens and x (t) represents the prey population (in the absence of predators), then the population growth is given by:

$$
\begin{aligned}
\frac{dx}{dt} &= ax, a > 0, \\
x(t) &= x_0 e^{at}.
\end{aligned}
\tag{4}
$$

The population of prey in the absence of the predator grows exponentially.

2. The predator y (t) only feeds on the prey x (t). Thus, if there is no prey, their size decreases with a rate proportional to its population is represented by. Equation (5)

$$\frac{dy}{dt} = -dy, d > 0,$$

$$y(t) = y_0 e^{-dt}$$

(5)

The population of predators in the absence of prey decreases exponentially to extinction.

3. The number of encounters between predator and prey is proportional to the product of their populations. Each of the number of encounters favor predators and reduces the number of prey.

The presence of prey helps the growth of the predator and is represented by Eq. (6)

$$cxy, c > 0.$$

(6)

While the interaction between them, reduces the growth of prey is represented by Eq. (7)

$$-bxy, b > 0.$$

(7)

Under the above hypothesis, we have a model of interaction between x (t) and y (t) is given by the following system: Eqs (8),(9)

$$\frac{dx}{dt} = Ax - Bxy$$

(8)

$$\frac{dy}{dt} = -Cxy + Dy$$

(9)

X: is the number of prey
Y: is the number of predators
$\frac{dx}{dt}$ Is the growth of the population of prey time t
$\frac{dy}{dt}$ Is the growth of the population of predator at time t
A: It represents the birth rate of prey in the absence of predator
B: It represents the death rate of predators in the absence of prey.
C: Measures the susceptibility of prey.
D: Measures the ability of predation.

4   Proposed Optimization Algorithm Based on the Self-defense Mechanisms of Plants

The proposed approach takes as its main basis the Lotka and Volterra predator-prey model, which is a system formed by a pair of first order nonlinear differential equations for moderating the growth of two populations that interact with each other

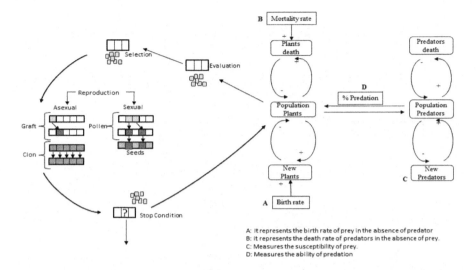

Fig. 2. General illustration of our proposal

(predator and prey). In Fig. 2 a general scheme of our proposal was taken as the base the traditional model of predator prey shows, using the principle of the dynamics of both populations the evolutionary process of plants is generated to develop the techniques of self-defense.

In nature, plants have different methods of reproduction, in our approach we consider only the most common: clone, graft and pollen. **Clone:** the offspring identical to the parent plant. **Graft:** it takes a stem of a plant and is encrusted on another to generate an alteration in the structure of the plant. **Pollen:** one plant pollinates other flowers and generates a seed and the descent is a plant with characteristics of both plants.

To generate the initial population of the algorithm we use the equations of the model of Lotka and Volterra, the mathematical representation is shown in Sect. 3.1 Eqs. (8) (9). Equation 8 is used to generate the population of prey (plants), and Eq. 9 is used to generate the population of predators (herbivores), as mentioned above functions predator prey model is used to model our proposed model variables adapted to the proposal.

Figure (3) describes the steps of the optimization algorithm inspired by the defense mechanisms of plants.

The initial sizes of both populations (prey, predators) are defined by the user, the parameters (a, b, c, d) are also defined by the user, the model of Lotka and Volterra recommended the following parameter values a = 0.4, b = 0.37, c = 0.3, d = 0.05. Both populations that initiated these populations interact with each other prey and predator, use this method to generate new offspring of plants, these plant reproduction in biological processes are applied. The population is re-evaluated and if the stop criterion is not satisfied, return the iterative cycle of the algorithm.

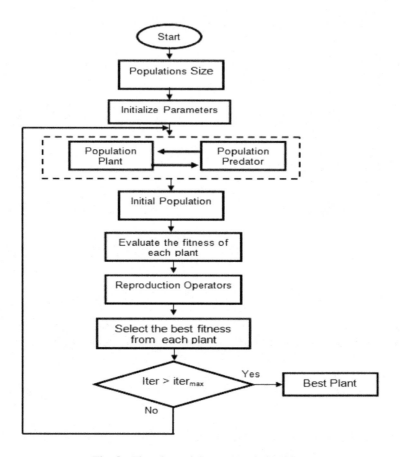

Fig. 3. Flowchart of the proposed algorithm

5   Results

In this section the results obtained are shown to the test the performance of the algorithm, we used a set of five benchmark functions, where the goal is to approximate the value of the function to zero. In this case, 30 experiments were performed for the following mathematical functions, and the evaluation is for 10, 30, 50 variables, see Table 1.

Table 1 shows the definitions of the mathematical functions used in this work.

Parameters Settings for the Algorithm. The common parameters in the control of algorithms are the population size and the maximum number of iterations and some others, but in this case the algorithm uses many parameters compared to other bio-inspired methods. We are planning to find a way to optimize the parameters setting of the algorithm using intelligent computing techniques.

Table 1. Mathematical functions

Function	Mathematical Representation
Sphere	$$f(x) = \sum_{i=1}^{n} x_i^2$$
Griewank	$$f(x) = \sum_{i=1}^{d} \frac{x_i^2}{4000} - \prod_{i=1}^{d} \cos\left(\frac{x_i}{\sqrt{i}}\right) + 1$$
Rastrigin	$$f(x) = 10n + \sum_{i=1}^{n}[x_i^2 - 10\cos(2\pi x_i]$$
Ackley	$$f(x) = -a \cdot \exp(-b \cdot \sqrt{\frac{1}{n}\sum_{i=1}^{n} x_i^2}) - \exp(\frac{1}{n}\sum_{i=1}^{n}\cos(cx_i)) + a + \exp(1)$$
Rosenbrock	$$f(x) = \sum_{i=1}^{n-1}[100(x_{i+1} - x_i^2)^2 + (1 - x_i)^2]$$

The proposal uses more parameters than other traditional algorithms, it is difficult to find the optimal parameters to achieve acceptable results. The parameters of the algorithm are usually moved manually by trial and error to observe and determine the range of parameters used. The configuration of parameters are defined below: the parameters (a, b, c, d), $a = 0 - 1$, $b = 0 - 1$, $c = 0 - 1$, $d = 0.0 - 0.1$. We also need to define the size of prey populations (plants) and predators (herbivores), the model does not recommend optimal values for populations, and we use plants = 250, Herbivores = 200, must also define the time and maximum number of iterations, and we use the iteration in the range of 200–500 to observe the results.

Tables 2, 3, and 4 show the experimental results for the benchmark mathematical functions used in this work and optimized with the proposed method. The Tables show the results of the evaluations for each function with 10, 30, and 50 dimensions; where we can find the best, worse, standard deviation, average, values shown was obtained from 30 experiments performed by moving the parameters a, b, c, d in the above ranges established.

Table 2. Experimental results with 10 dimensions

Function	Algorithm performance with 10 dimensions			
	Best	*Worse*	*σ*	*Average*
Sphere	3.62E-308	4.994E-23	1.2628E-23	3.700E-24
Ackley	8.88E-16	3.21E-09	6.8865E-10	2.06E-10
Rosenbrock	0.0339	8.9300	2.16266548	1.4421
Rastrigin	3.94E-09	2.32E-05	4.2294E-06	8.42E-07
Griewank	1.90E-10	2.23E-09	3.8869E-10	8.23E-10

Table 3. Experimental results with 30 dimensions

Function	Algorithm performance with 30 dimensions			
	Best	*Worse*	*σ*	*Average*
Sphere	1.523E-252	3.427E-07	6.4224E-08	1.529E-08
Ackley	8.88E-16	3.78E-03	0.00069861	1.94E-04
Rosenbrock	0.0494	37.2144	7.53849331	4.9807
Rastrigin	1.57E-07	7.97E-03	0.00160841	4.22E-04
Griewank	5.07E-10	2.45E-08	4.0204E-09	4.92E-09

Table 4. Experimental results with 50 dimensions

Function	Algorithm performance with 50 dimensions			
	Best	*Worse*	*σ*	*Average*
Sphere	2.136E-214	3.938E-04	7.2512E-05	1.594E-05
Ackley	8.88E-16	3.27E-01	0.05971378	1.13E-02
Rosenbrock	0.2656	41.0000	8.79412663	6.4178
Rastrigin	1.86E-05	3.78E-02	0.00959503	3.01E-03
Griewank	8.10E-09	3.23E-04	5.8959E-05	1.09E-05

The results presented in the previous tables show that we are on track in the development of the bio-inspired optimization algorithm sbased on the self-defense mechanisms of plants. With all the experiments we deduce a pattern of behavior of the data by moving the a, b, c, d parameters manually by trial and error for optimization problems of mathematical functions. This shows that when the variables are in the following ranges a = 0.3 − 0.7, b = 0.1 − 0.4, c = 0.2 − 0.3, d = 0.01 − 0.05, we can maintain a best balance between the two populations managing to obtain less dispersion of data to model them in the mathematical functions used.

5.1 Statistical Comparison

To conclude, in this work is necessary statistical comparison between the proposed method vs Artificial Bee Colony (ABC) [4] for this problems studieds. The statistical test used for comparison is the z-test, whose parameters are defined in Table 5. With the parameters of the tables above (Tables 2, 3, 4), we applied the statistical z-test for all the cases shown in this study, giving the following results shown in the Table 6. In applying the statistic z-test, with a significance level of 0.05, and the alternative hypothesis says that the average of the proposed method is lower than the average of ABC, and of course the null hypothesis tells us that the average of the proposed method is greater than or equal to the average of ABC, with a rejection region for all values fall below −1.699. So the statistical test results are that: for the proposed method, there is significant evidence to reject the null hypothesis −1.8798.

Table 5. Parameters for the statistical z-test.

Parameters	Values
Level of significance	95 %
Alpha	0.05 %
Ha	$\mu_1 < \mu_2$
H0	$\mu_1 \geq \mu_2$
Critical values	−1.699

Table 6. Results of applying statistical z-tests.

Function	N. Variables	Our method	ABC	Z-Value	Evidence
Griewank	10	8.23E-10	0.00087	−1.8798	Significant
	30	4.92E-09	2.87E-08	−31.7664	Significant
Rastrigin	10	8.42E-07	0.0	1.09424	Not significant
	30	4.22E-04	0.033874	−1.0091	Not significant
Rosenbrock	10	1.4421	0.034072	3.56522	Not significant
	30	4.9807	0.219626	3.4585	Not significant
Ackley	10	2.06E-10	7.8E-11	0.5157	Not significant
	30	1.94E-04	6.0E-12	1.5250	Not significant

Analyzing the results of the statistical test shows that the proposed algorithm needs some improvements and consider other biological processes in plants. In Table 6 it shows that the proposed algorithm exceeds some published results of the bee colony algorithm.

6 Conclusions

The proposal is to create, develop and test a new optimization algorithm inspired by the bio-defense mechanism of plants, the first challenge is to adapt the predator-prey model and test the algorithm in an optimization problem, in this case, we decided to test the performance in mathematical functions and we have achieved acceptable results. When we move the parameters manually observe that the algorithm has better performance when the values are in a range of values, these observations are only for this problem, we need to apply it to other optimization problems to analyze the behavior. This algorithm is in the early stages, but we are working on the necessary information about the natural processes of plants to add adaptations of biological processes to the algorithm, this in order to improve results and achieve a proposal that can be make a competitive algorithm against methods bio-inspired existing.

References

1. Bennett, R.N., Wallsgrove, R.M.: Secondary metabolites in plant defense mechanisms. New Phytol. **127**(4), 617–633 (1994)
2. Berryman, A.A.: The origins and evolution of predator-prey theory. Ecology **73**, 1530–1535 (1992)
3. Cruz, J.M.L., González, G.B.: Modelo depredador-presa. Revista de Ciencias Básicas UJAT **7**(2), 25–34 (2008)
4. García-Garrido, J.M., Ocampo, J.A.: Regulation of the plant defense response in arbuscular mycorrhizal symbiosis. J. Exp. Bot. **53**(373), 1377–1386 (2002)
5. Karaboga, D., Basturk, B.: A powerful and efficient algorithm for numerical function optimization: artificial bee colony (ABC) algorithm. J. Global Optim. **39**(3), 459–471 (2007)
6. Law, J.H., Regnier, F.E.: Pheromones. Ann. Rev. Bio-Chem. **40**(1), 533–548 (1971)
7. Lez-Parra, G.G., Arenas, A.J., Cogollo, M.R.: Numerical-analytical solutions of predator-prey models. WSEAS Trans. Biol. Biomed. **10**(2), 1–7 (2013)
8. Melin, P., Olivas, F., Castillo, O., Valdez, F., Soria, J., Valdez, M.: Optimal design of fuzzy classification systems using PSO with dynamic parameter adaptation through fuzzy logic. Expert Syst. Appl. **40**(8), 3196–3206 (2013)
9. Neyoy, H., Castillo, O., Soria, J.: Dynamic fuzzy logic parameter tuning for ACO and its application in TSP problems. In: Castillo, O., Melin, P., Kacprzyk, J. (eds.) Recent Advances on Hybrid Intelligent Systems. SCI, vol. 451, pp. 259–272. Springer, Heidelberg (2013)
10. Ordeñana, K.M.: Mecanismos de defensa en las interacciones planta-patógeno. Revista Manejo Integrado de Plagas. Costa Rica **63**, 22–32 (2002)
11. Paré, P.W., Tumlinson, J.H.: Plant volatiles as a defense against insect herbivores. Plant Physiol. **121**(2), 325–332 (1999)
12. Teodorović, D.: Bee colony optimization (BCO). In: Lim, C.P., Jain, L.C., Dehuri, S. (eds.) Innovations in Swarm Intelligence. SCI, vol. 248, pp. 39–60. Springer, Heidelberg (2009)
13. Tollsten, L., Müller, P.M.: Volatile organic compounds emitted from beech leaves. Phytochemistry **43**, 759–762 (1996)
14. Vivanco, J.M., Cosio, E., Loyola-Vargas, V.M., Flores, H.E.: Mecanismos químicos de defensa en las plantas. Investigación y ciencia **341**(2), 68–75 (2005)

15. Xiao, Y., Chen, L.: Modeling and analysis of a predator–prey model with disease in the prey. Math. Biosci. **171**(1), 59–82 (2001)
16. Yoshida, T., Jones, L.E., Ellner, S.P., Fussmann, G.F., Hairston, N.G.: Rapid evolution drives ecological dynamics in a predator–prey system. Nature **424**(6946), 303–306 (2003)

On the Use of Ant Colony Optimization for Video Games

José Luis Estrada Martínez, Abraham Sánchez López[✉],
and Miguel Angel Jara Maldonado

Pue-México Computer Science Department,
Benemérita Universidad Autónoma de Puebla, Puebla, Mexico
dirus.umbratrox@gmail.com, asanchez@cs.buap.mx, mikejm92@gmail.com

Abstract. Traditionally, games and video games have provided a framework for the study of Artificial Intelligence approaches. The main objective of this work is to verify whether the optimization method based on ant colonies can be applied to the development of a competitive agent in the environment of videogames in real time. One of the important characteristics of the presented work is the optimization calculations to void losing the game fluidity. In addition, another aim of the work is to obtain an architecture for the development of educational type videogames to encourage inexperienced users to interact with artificial intelligence algorithms. The game allows the user to experience the changes in the algorithm given certain changes in the parameters and variables used by the Ant Colony Optimization algorithm itself.

1 Introduction

The video game industry is flourishing for more than three decades now, with revenues surpassing even those of the movie and music industries. Due to their high popularity and huge computational demands, video games would always introduce leading technologies and pioneering methods in the field of human-computer interaction at large. Today's technologies have reached a point where new add-ons can boost the gameplay experience, altering and guiding game content and evolution following affect-dependent strategies [1,2].

Despite the huge advances made in processor power and associated resources in both the PC and console gaming world, over the past two decades, AI in games has not advanced. 99 % of commercial games on the market in 2008 use a combination of the basic AI techniques from games of the 1980s namely, state machines, rule-based systems, and planning techniques [3].

AI in games has become the most interesting element in actual games from the player's point of view, once the technical components (graphics, sound, human-computer interaction) have reached almost an upper bound. They mostly request opponents exhibiting intelligent behavior, or just better human-like behaviors.

There is no research indicating the use of ACO (Ant Colony Optimization) in video game artificial intelligence (AI). Pheromone trails in ACO are essentially a way for independent ants to communicate with each other. This style of

© Springer International Publishing Switzerland 2015
G. Sidorov and S.N. Galicia-Haro (Eds.): MICAI 2015, Part I, LNAI 9413, pp. 238–247, 2015.
DOI: 10.1007/978-3-319-27060-9_19

communication can be incorporated into a game AI allowing separate AI agents to communicate with each other.

The basics of the ant colony optimization approach is presented in Sect. 2. The main ideas of this proposal about the development of a video game are detailed in Sect. 3. Implementation details are discussed in Sect. 4. Finally, results and conclusions are discussed in Sects. 5 and 6.

2 Ant Colony Optimization

Swarm intelligence studies the collective behavior of unsophisticated agents that interact locally through their environment [4].

In nature, ants usually wander randomly, and upon finding food they return to their nest while laying down pheromone trails. The other ants will find the path (pheromone trail), and follow the trail, returning and reinforcing it if they eventually find food. The pheromone starts to evaporate as time passes. If the time taken for an ant to travel down the path and back again to the nest is very large, the pheromone evaporates thereby making the path less prominent. A shorter path, in comparison will be visited by more ants (can be described as a loop of positive feedback) and thus the pheromone density remains high for a longer time.

Ant colony optimization (ACO) is implemented as a collective group of intelligent agents, which simulate the ants behavior, walking around the graph representing the problem to solve using mechanisms of cooperation and adaptation.

ACO algorithm requires the following definitions:

1. The problem needs to be represented appropriately, which would allow the ants to incrementally update the solutions through the use of a probabilistic transition rules, based on the amount of pheromone in the trail and other problem specific knowledge. It is also important to enforce a strategy to construct only valid solutions corresponding to the problem definition.
2. A problem-dependent heuristic function η that measures the quality of components that can be added to the current partial solution.
3. A rule set for pheromone updating, which specifies how to modify the pheromone value π.
4. A probabilistic transition rule based on the value of the heuristic function η and the pheromone value π that is used to iteratively construct a solution.

2.1 Mathematical Model of ACO

ACO was first introduced using the Traveling Salesman Problem (TSP). Starting from the first node, an ant iteratively moves from one node to another. When being at a node, an ant chooses to go to a unvisited node at time t with a probability given by

$$P_{i,j}^k(t) = \frac{[\tau_{i,j}(t)]^\alpha [\eta_{i,j}(t)]^\beta}{\sum_{t \in N_i^k} [\tau_{i,j}(t)]^\alpha [\eta_{i,j}(t)]^\beta} j \in N_i^k \tag{1}$$

where N_i^k i is the feasible neighborhood of the ant_k, that is, the set of cities which ant_k has not yet visited; $\tau_{i,j}(t)$ is the pheromone value on the edge (i,j) at the time t, α is the weight of the pheromone; $\eta_{i,j}(t)$ is a priori available heuristic information on the edge (i,j) at the time t, β is the weight of heuristic information. Two parameters α and β determine the relative influence of pheromone trail and heuristic information. $\tau_{i,j}(t)$ is determined by

$$\tau_{i,j}(t) = \rho\tau_{i,j}(t-1) + \sum_{k=1}^{n} \Delta\tau_{i,j}{}^k \forall (i,j) \tag{2}$$

$$\Delta\tau_{i,j}{}^k(t) = \begin{cases} \frac{Q}{L_k(t)} & \text{if the edge } (i,j) \text{ chosen by } ant_k, \\ 0 & \text{otherwise.} \end{cases} \tag{3}$$

where ρ is the pheromone trail evaporation rate $(0 < \rho < 1)$, n is the number of ants, Q is a constant for pheromone updating.

3 Algorithm Development for the Video Game

The mathematical model of the algorithm presented above constitutes the most important organ. This is responsible for controlling the iterations which updates nodes and pheromones; it allows the ants to choose the direction to be taken; and can even modify the intelligence of each of the agents to find food and return to the colony faster (through its parameters).

Traditionally, the algorithm is focused on finding a solution to some problem. For this project, the ants are programmed to look for food; and thus bring well-being to their colony. Using a mathematical model to implement the ACO algorithm in a video game facilitated the gameplay, where players can modify the values of intelligence of their ants to experience changes in their behavior.

To use such a wide formula as the one that will be presented later; it was necessary to divide its elements into different components and analyze them at different stages of the code, to guarantee both the fluidity of the video game as the operation of the formula guarantee.

In the traditional ACO algorithm, the ants travel through a graph where each "turn" they change of node, this means that the traditional algorithm time measurement is based on shifts and not on measurements of real time, which is far away from the video game behavior that was implemented. By that time the new representation of the mathematical model of ACO was the first contribution of this work. For the video game presented in this work, updates are generated in real time, which means that the ants are in constant motion and are not subject to "shift", but state changes.

The algorithm proposes changes of position in relation to meters to measure these changes of state (a yes and a not), this means that instead of a graph, the ants of this games are guided by a matrix, and in that matrix each box is separated by a meter away from its center to the center of the next box. These boxes are coordinates x, z within a 3D world. When an ant approaches a midpoint of a square grid (for example: 3.4,1 approximates 3,1 if the ant was in that position 3.6,1; the ant is considered in the table 4,1 by approximation), it is considered that there has been a state change and at this point, the formula is recalculated to determine which direction should take the ant (North, Northeast, East, Southeast, South, Southwest, West, Northwest).

Returning to the equations presented in the previous section, and for purposes of this paper, it was determined that the best heuristic η priori for the game should be the distance from the node with respect to the origin, which is the colony (where the ants deposit food once they have found it). Thanks to this heuristic, the ants can find food closer to the colony and, once they have obtained food, these ants will determine the shortest path back to the colony (sometimes ignoring the travelled path to get that node).

During this work, ACO approach was modified in different ways to achieve an optimization to increase the intelligence of ants and improve the entertainment that the game offers the player. One of the most important improvements to be mentioned with respect to the traditional formula presented above, was that ants have a preference for certain directions and different types of pheromone.

The formula $[\tau_{i,j}(t)]^\alpha [\eta_{i,j}(t)]^\beta$ is changed as follows during the selection of the next node to travel:

1. If the analyzed node is in the same direction that the ant travelled, the formula changes to:
$$[\tau_{i,j}(t)]^\alpha [\eta_{i,j}(t)]^\beta \times 2 \tag{4}$$

2. If the analyzed node contains a successful path to go, i.e., priority is added to nodes where the ant has walked to carry food, the formula is:
$$[\tau_{i,j}(t)]^\alpha [\eta_{i,j}(t)]^\beta \times 15 \tag{5}$$

3. If the ant loads food, heuristics is enhanced and the ant increases its preference for nodes near the colony, according to the intelligence value I (there are buildings that can improve the ants intelligence):
$$[\tau_{i,j}(t)]^\alpha [\eta_{i,j}(t)]^{\beta+I} \tag{6}$$

4. Finally, to select the next direction that the ant will take, a random tournament is performed, where the probability (obtained by the above formula) to be a useful node increases the possibility of taking certain direction. This tournament will be made only between three different nodes (this reduced the analysis of nodes and also allows to simulate a more realistically the ants travel). For example: If an ant walks to the north, the nodes will analyze the Northeast, North and Northwest, for being closest to the north.

The above data depends on a value τ of the pheromone that is constantly updated. For this value of pheromone in each node, the traditional ACO method uses the formulae (2, 3) and assigns each node in each "turn".

However, in an application such as a video game, where operations must be performed constantly; calculating all values of pheromone in each level of nodes, is very expensive in computing resources. Therefore, a solution which consists of calculating the value of the pheromone in the node is implemented, only at the moment that intends to analyze if the node will be occupied or not (when ants change position). In this way, each node has a personal variable that stores the last time that the pheromone of the node was assessed. When the ant requires to use the node, the elapsed time from that update is estimated, and to simulate the pheromone evaporation, time is submitted to the proposed exponential formulae which is expressed as follows:

$$(1 - \rho)^{current\ time-last\ updated} * \tau_{i,j} + \frac{Q}{L_k} \tag{7}$$

Thus, the update variable is subject to time and its updating can be postponed until the moment in which it is used.

4   Video Game Implementation

Once established the necessary changes to implement ACO in a 3D environment, the next step taken was to create the necessary elements to transform the algorithm into an entertaining video game. To achieve this goal, a series of rules were designed to establish all the limits of the game and to define the goals that the player must reach. The goal of the video game is to ensure the anthill's survival. This implies that at least one of the ants must stand for the player to continue playing. The ants (agents in the game) work for the player, they collect food scattered over the map and take these food back to the anthill, see the Fig. 1.

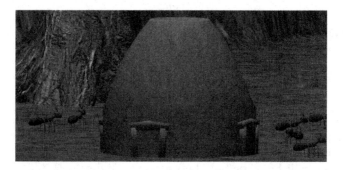

Fig. 1. Ants must return to the anthill to deposit food.

Each ant has the modified ACO algorithm, which implies that each ant can be modified and upgraded by using the algorithm's parameters. Thanks to this, the creation of buildings was added to the rules of the game, where the player can create buildings to upgrade its ants. Some of these upgrades are:

- Modify the ant's movement speed.
- Increase the intelligence of the ants: The intelligence is measured as the efficiency to get back to the anthill once the ant has gathered food (by modifying the heuristic formula).
- Improve the ant's strength/food carry capacity. This particular variable is not related to the algorithm but to the game's mechanics, each food has a limit of waste and every ant can carry an X quantity of food, depending on their carry capacity. Strength also helps ants to battle against the enemies, taking off a certain amount of life to the spiders when combat is enhanced. The total life taken from enemies is counted as food for the anthill and thus can be returned to the ant's base.
- Enhance the ant's life: The ants will sometimes face combat against spiders, to avoid them to die quickly, it is important to improve the ant's total life.

Over time, the player will face several challenges within the map; for this reason, it is important for him to plan the distribution of the buildings carefully. Some buildings that help to upgrade ants may be desirable to be more distanced from the anthill than those which provide of food, so the distance from the food source to the anthill is reduced (Fig. 2).

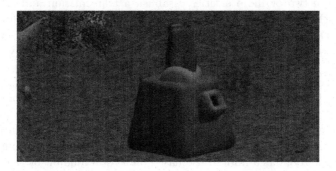

Fig. 2. The player must think strategically before placing his buildings.

Another challenge that the ant population will face within time are the spiders. All over the game, there is a corner in which a spider inhabits, this spider is capable of damaging ants and will in fact pursuit them once they reach its cobweb. The spider has the ability to generate aleatory raids of small spiders that will invade the entire map (not only their mother's cobweb) and will reduce the population of ants.

Further, it is possible to manipulate the pheromone trail by using the right button of the mouse over a visible pheromone trail. By doing so, the existing trail will be erased and the ants will no more prefer to follow that path. This can avoid ants to walk towards the spider or to move over a place where food has been already finished (Fig. 3).

As time goes by, and depending on the number of ants that the player has, the amount of food will be consumed and if the amount of food reaches zero,

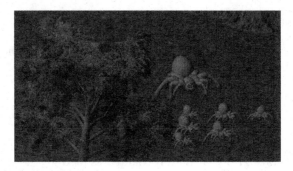

Fig. 3. The spiders will difficult the growth of the ants' population, making it harder for the player to care for the ant's wealth.

the ants will begin to starve. The player must then take care of several aspects to avoid the dangers that the environment has for the anthill like real life.

To offer the right interaction between the player and the game, it is necessary to count with a mediator which helps to transmit the information, achieving like a good communication (in the understanding of communication on a global context, where two or more entities establish a transmission and reception of information through a medium). In the case of this project, the medium is a User Interface (UI) that will allow us to transmit information between the system and the player, by using a visual and user friendly screen. This screen will provide the user with the necessary tools and information to manipulate the video game and have a better understanding of ACO.

The visualization of the pheromone among the game is very important, it is like this that we can observe the pheromone trail and evaluate how useful it is. By evaluating the pheromone trail, the player can determine which directions are taking his ants, and it will be easier for him to use the pheromone erase tool. The erase tool has a limited use based on a total amount of "energy" that will be wasted each time the player uses the right button of the mouse, and this same energy bar will be restored over time if the user is not using the tool. This energy bar is displayed at the top left corner of the screen so the player can see at all time the current amount of energy available and make a good use of this resource.

The player's higher priority is the ants, making the anthill grow is one of the main objectives of the game and thus it is important for the player to know at every time:

- The birthrate of the ants.
- The actual amount of living ants.
- The amount of storage food.
- The consume of food per minute. (Very important considering that the fee for buildings and upgrades is based on food).

Both birthrate status and actual amount of ants are displayed in the bottom left corner of the screen, and the food concerning data is displayed on the right bottom corner of the screen (Fig. 4).

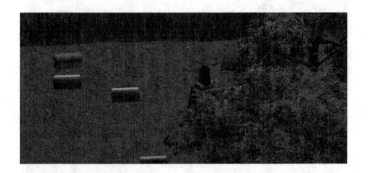

Fig. 4. Player must care for the well-being of your ants.

5   Results

AI research and video games are a mutually beneficial combination. On the one hand, AI technology can provide solutions to an increasing demand to add realistic, intelligent behavior to the virtual creatures that populate a game world. On the other hand, as game environments become more complex and realistic, they offer a range of excellent testbeds for fundamental AI research [5–7].

A remarkable improvement to ACO has been reached over this Project, this amelioration has been implemented for a 3D environment (which required more calculations than the traditional ACO algorithm) and also permitted to optimize the time and resources invested on the calculation of pheromone evaporation and direction decision making of the ants. These will ease users comprehend the algorithm even if they are not related to artificial intelligence at all, adding a playful bonus to the lesson.

The most important elements that the game contributed with, have been the improvement of the ACO algorithm, because it models the ants' behavior within the whole software. A whole world of mechanics and rules has been created so the game can be enjoyed by the players, teaching them how to use the ACO algorithm to find the solution of a problem (Fig. 5).

Video games have different design considerations and usability issues than other types of software. The ISO 9241-11 definition of usability includes three independent measures including efficiency, effectiveness, and satisfaction. In the case of video game usability, effectiveness and efficiency are secondary considerations in relation to satisfaction. A consumer may need to purchase or use other software to perform necessary tasks, but a game is bought on a voluntary basis purely for entertainment value. If a game is not fun to play, it will not sell in the marketplace. To ensure the satisfaction of game players, considerable care

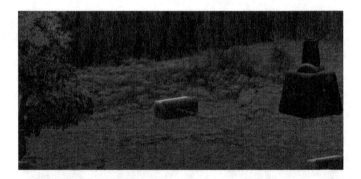

Fig. 5. Screenshot of the video game, the blue items show the current quantity of pheromone trail on each node (Color figure online).

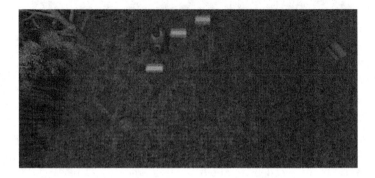

Fig. 6. Screenshot of the video game.

is required in the game design process and could be better guaranteed with the use of formal usability evaluation procedures by game developers (Fig. 6).

Video games can be designed for very large and diverse audiences. Running video game usability testing sessions with each segment of the audience is the best way to ensure that the final product delivers the best possible video gaming experience. Identifying a video game's different audience segments can, however, be challenging. Some of the parameters that we have found to be very useful in helping identify audience segments for video game usability testing include: name, age, sex, occupation, education level, city where the respondent lives, do you like video games?, are you familiar with video games on PC?, previous experience, select video games that you have played, global reactions of the user. Select the number that most closely reflects their views on the system use, display, performance and appearance. We conducted these tests with 10 persons and we can summarize that the video game seems appropriate to 95 %.

6   Conclusions

The traditional ACO algorithm has been improved to the point that its relation
to the real ants behavior has been modelled and demonstrated on a 3D video
game. This means that the algorithm has been modelled correctly even though
it has suffered adaptations like the time modification. For the realization of this
project it was necessary to fulfill the three main rules of the algorithm:

1. Defining the problem correctly: The problem is to obtain the higher amount
   of food and return it to the colony as soon as possible.
2. Posing the correct η heuristic: To look for the nodes that are closer to the
   anthill.
3. Defining a τ that lets the pheromone to be updated: With the suggested
   exponential formula, it was possible to model the elapsed time between one
   and another actualization of the pheromone.

Thanks to these three points, it was easier to define the video game rules.
To obtain the higher amount of food within the less possible time, so the ant
population can develop successfully. At first, the time factor was a great limiting,
because when updating the pheromone values at every frame, the application
consumed a great amount of resources from the computer; and it was very difficult and stressful to play the video game. Later, this limiting became the game's
rule to update the pheromone trail, by maintaining it on a controlled frame
with a scheme in which, the pheromone evaporation exponentially depends on
the elapsed time since the last update of the node's pheromone (Nodes are not
necessarily update at each frame).

The combination between artificial intelligence and video games has demonstrated that we can mix both, as long as the number of calculations and resources
consumed are taken in mind, and carefully controlled to avoid the video game
frame rate and gameplay to be affected.

References

1. Yannakakis, G.N.: Game AI revisited. In: Proceedings of ACM Computing Frontiers
   Conference, pp. 285–292 (2012)
2. Yannakakis, G.N., Togelius, J.: Experience-driven procedural content generation.
   IEEE Trans. Affect. Comput. **2**(3), 147–161 (2011)
3. Lecky-Thompson, G.W.: AI and Artificial Life in Video Games. Cengage Learning,
   Course Technology, Boston (2008)
4. Dorigo, M., Stützle, T.: Ant Colony Optimization, 1st edn. Bradford Books,
   Cambridge (2004)
5. Algfoor, Z.A., Sunar, M.S., Kolivand, H.: A comprehensive study on path-finding
   techniques for robotics and video games. Int. J. Comput. Games Technol. **2015**, 11
   (2015). Article ID 736138. http://dx.doi.org/10.1155/2015/736138
6. Anguelov, B.: Video game pathfinding and improvements to discrete search on grid-
   based maps, Master Thesis, University of Pretoria (2011)
7. Martin, E., Martinez, M., Recio, G., Saez, Y.: Pac-mAnt: optimization based on ant
   colonies applied to developing an agent for Ms. Pac-Man. In: IEEE Symposium on
   Computational Intelligence and Games (CIG), pp. 458–464 (2010)

A System for Political Districting
in the State of Mexico

Eric Alfredo Rincón García[1]([⊠]), Miguel Ángel Gutiérrez Andrade[2],
Sergio Gerardo de-los-Cobos-Silva[2], Antonin Ponsich[1],
Roman Anselmo Mora-Gutiérrez[1], and Pedro Lara-Velázquez[2]

[1] Dpto. de Sistemas, Universidad Autónoma Metropolitana,
Unidad Azcapotzalco, 02200 Mexico D.F., Mexico
{rigaeral,aspo,mgra}@correo.azc.uam.mx
[2] Dpto. de Ing. Eléctrica, Universidad Autónoma Metropolitana,
Unidad Iztapalapa, 09340 Mexico D.F., Mexico
{gamma,cobos,plara}@xanum.uam.mx

Abstract. Districting is the redrawing of the boundaries of legislative
districts for electoral purposes in such a way that the Federal or state
requirements, such as contiguity, population equality, and compactness,
are fulfilled. The resulting optimization problem involves the former
requirement as a hard constraint while the other two are considered
as conflicting objective functions. The solution technique used for many
years by the Mexican Federal Electoral Institute was an algorithm based
on Simulated Annealing. In this article, we present the system proposed
for the electoral districting process in the state of Mexico. This system
included, a geographic tool to visualize and edit districting plans, and for
first time in Mexico, the use of an Artificial Bee Colony based algorithm
that automatically creates redistricting plans.

Keywords: Districting system · Simulated annealing · Artificial Bee
Colony

1 Introduction

The zone design problem arises from the need of aggregating small geographical
units (GUs) into regions, in such a way that one (or more) objective function(s)
is (are) optimized and some constraints are satisfied. The GUs can be cities,
postal code regions, blocks or geographic areas specially designed for the studied
problem. The constraints can include, for example, the construction of connected
zones, with the same amount of population, clients, mass media, public services,
etc. [9,15]. The zone design is used in diverse problems like school districting
[6,8], police district [7], service and maintenance zones [25,26], sales territory
[28] and land use [19,23].

The design of electoral zones or electoral districting is the best known case,
due to its influence in the results of electoral processes and its computational

© Springer International Publishing Switzerland 2015
G. Sidorov and S.N. Galicia-Haro (Eds.): MICAI 2015, Part I, LNAI 9413, pp. 248–259, 2015.
DOI: 10.1007/978-3-319-27060-9_20

complexity, which has been shown to be NP-Hard [12]. In this framework, the GUs are grouped into a predetermined number of zones or districts, and democracy must be guaranteed through the satisfaction of restrictions that are imposed by law [13,20]. As a matter of fact, this problem has been studied by researchers coming from different areas, such as computer [24], social [1], political sciences [10] or operations research [4,21].

The automated political districting began in the sixties, when Vickrey [27] in 1961, propagated that the human element should be removed from the political districting process, and proposed that mechanical rules without human influence could solve these problems. In 1965 Hess et al. [14] proposed a heuristic districting method to solve the legislative districting problem of Delaware. In 1970 Garfinkel and Nemhauser [11] proposed an exact technique, but the computational complexity of the problem restricted the application of this technique to small instances. These papers were the starting point for a wide set of models, algorithms and techniques, proposed to formulate and solve the political districting problem. Nowadays, different meta-heuristics have been reported in specialized literature, such as local search [4,19,20], Genetic [2], Evolutionary [5] and Swarm Intelligence [22] algorithms.

In Mexico, the algorithm used by the Federal Electoral Institute[1] (IFE), in the federal districting processes in 2006 and 2013, was a Simulated Annealing (SA) based algorithm. However, in 2014 the Electoral Institute of the State of Mexico (IEEM) carried out its state districting. In this case, the process included the implementation of a software with tools for creating and editing districting plans. The resulting system is a novel proposal that includes a geographic system to visualize and edit districting plans, and two automated districting algorithms: a Simulated Annealing based algorithm, and, for the first time in Mexico, a population based technique was used: an Artificial Bee Colony (ABC) algorithm.

The primary purpose of this paper is to describe the main characteristics of the IEEM's system. To address this issue, we provide a description of the problem in Sect. 2, a brief overview of the inner working mode of the SA, and ABC algorithms are presented in Sect. 3. The description of the IEEM's system is presented in Sect. 4. Some computational results are detailed in Sect. 5. Finally, some conclusions and perspectives for future work are drawn in Sect. 6.

2 Problem Description

In the Mexican Republic, the state of Mexico is the most populated entity, with 15,175,845 inhabitants, and has the mayor number of GU, 6462. Due to its large population, this state holds 45 representatives or seats in the Congress. Thus, 45 contiguous electoral districts must be designed, in such a way that population equality and compactness are promoted.

---

[1] The National Electoral Institute, INE, since April 4, 2014.

2.1 Population Equality

In order to handle population equality the IEEM used the following measure:

$$C_1(P) = \sum_{s=1}^{45} \left(\left(1 - \frac{P_s}{A_P} \right) \left(\frac{1}{0.15} \right) \right)^2 \tag{1}$$

Where $P = \{Z_1, Z_2, ..., Z_{45}\}$ is a districting plan. Each district Z_s is defined through a set of binary variables x_{is} such that $x_{is} = 1$ if the ith GU belongs to district s and $x_{is} = 0$ otherwise. P_s is the population of district s, and A_P is the expected number of inhabitants in each district. For the state of Mexico $A_P = 337{,}241$, the maximum percentage of deviation allowed is 15 % and 45 electoral districts must be generated in the state.

Thus, the lower the cost C_1, the better the population equality of a solution. Indeed, the perfect population equality is achieved when all districts have 337,241 inhabitants, and in this case the measure assigns a value of zero to C_1.

2.2 Compactness

To measure compactness, the IEEM used a metric that can be easily computed, in order to improve the runtime performance. This measure of compactness compares the perimeter of each district with that of a square having the same area.

$$C_2(P) = \sum_{s=1}^{45} \left(\frac{PC_s}{\sqrt{AC_s}} - 1 \right) \tag{2}$$

Where PC_s and AC_s are the perimeter and the area of the considered district s, respectively. Thus, districts with a good compactness will have a compactness value close to 0.

2.3 Indigenous Districts

According to the 2010 census, the state of Mexico has 376,830 indigenous inhabitants that represent the 5.63 % of the national indigenous population. Besides, there are 14 municipalities with at least 20 % of indigenous population, including the municipalities of San Felipe del Progreso and Temoaya, where more than 40 % of the population is indigenous. Hence, the IEEM established that:

(a) These municipalities could not be fragmented, thus the algorithms should consider them as GU.
(b) San Felipe del Progreso and Temoaya should belong to different districts.
(c) The algorithms should promote the design of two districts with large percentages of indigenous population.

Requirements (b) and (c) were satisfied with a probability density function, that was used when the algorithms have to decide if a GU should be moved into a neighboring district. The higher the percentage of indigenous population in a GU, the higher the probability of being included in a district with GUs with similar characteristics. However, if the GU was San Felipe del Progreso (resp., Temoaya) the probability of being included in the same district as Temoaya (resp., San Felipe del Progreso) was low.

2.4   Geographical Features

The state of Mexico is located in the central part of the Anahuac Mesa. Most of the state consists of the Mexico and Toluca Valleys. The east of the state is dominated by the Sierra Nevada, which divides the state from Puebla, and contains the Popocatépetl and Iztaccíhuatl volcanos. The Sierra de las Cruces divides the west side of the Distrito Federal from the state. The Sierra de Xinantécatl is to the south of the Toluca Valley. At northern edge of this mountain range is the Nevado de Toluca volcano.

The IEEM used this information to avoid the design of districts traversed by geographical features, since their administration can be more complicated. Therefore, the GUs on the frontier of 4 neighboring municipalities divided by the Nevado de Toluca volcano, and 11 municipalities divided by the Sierra de las Cruces, were considered as not adjacent. The IEEM considered that the remaining geographical features did not justify more modifications, since the time required to travel between the divided municipalities was not seriously affected.

2.5   Objective Function

Therefore, population equality and compactness were considered as objectives to be optimized. The design of districts with large indigenous population was promoted by a probability density function, and geographical features were considered as constraints of the problem. Finally, to handle the multi-objective nature of the problem, the IEEM used a weight aggregation function strategy:

$$Minimize \ f(P) = \lambda_1 C_1(P) + \lambda_2 C_2(P) \tag{3}$$

The weighting factors were established after a discussion between political parties and IEEM's authorities. Both sectors agreed that the main objective in this process was to preserve the principle "one man one vote", even above the shape of the districts. Besides, compactness was included in order to avoid the gerrymandering manipulation, but the automated process and the open code, that could be revised by all parties, were considered a guaranty of transparency and legality. Thus, population equality was considered twice as important as compactness, and the weighting factors were set to $\lambda_1 = 1$ and $\lambda_2 = 0.5$ respectively.

The minimization is subjected to constraints that guarantee that (**R1**) each district is connected, (**R2**) the number of districts is equal to 45, and (**R3**) each GU is assigned to exactly one district. This problem formulation therefore seeks for a districting plan that represents the best balance between population equality and compactness, a balance obviously biased by the weighting factors.

3   Heuristic Algorithms

Since the design of electoral zones is an NP-Hard problem, the automated heuristic algorithms are an appropriate strategy to design electoral districting plans. In Mexico, since 1995, the IFE has used a SA algorithm to carry out the federal districting processes. However, new heuristic techniques have proven to get better solutions for this kind of problems. Therefore, the IEEM decided to propose a system implementing a new strategy, based on Artificial Bee Colony, for districting the state of Mexico. Nevertheless, the system also includes a traditional SA algorithm. The selection of these techniques was motivated by previous results obtained in academic instances inspired from previous electoral processes, but this work is the first application of such techniques, integrated in a single software application developed and used in a real political districting process. In this section, a brief description of the Simulated Annealing and Artificial Bee Colony strategies used in the districting system is provided.

3.1   Simulated Annealing

Simulated Annealing is a metaheuristic introduced by Kirkpatrick in [18]. The SA algorithm starts with an initial solution P and generates, in each iteration, a random neighbor solution Q. If this neighbor improves the current value of the objective function, it is accepted as the current solution. If the neighbor solution does not improve the objective's value, then it is accepted as the current solution according to a probability η based on the Metropolis criterion:

$$\eta = \exp\left(\frac{f(P) - f(Q)}{T}\right) \qquad (4)$$

Where $f(P)$ and $f(Q)$ represent the objective value of the current and neighbor solutions, respectively. T is a parameter called temperature, which is controlled through a cooling schedule that defines initial and final temperature, temperature decrease and the (finite) number of iterations for each temperature value.

For large temperature values, virtually all proposed solutions are accepted and the algorithm can explore the search space, in order to avoid premature convergence. However, during the execution, the temperature and, as a consequence, the probability of deterioration of the objective function, gradually decrease. The algorithm then reduces to a classical local search process. The algorithm finishes when the final temperature is reached.

3.2   Simulated Annealing Adaptation

A classical implementation of SA was used in the IEEM's system, with a geometric decreasing cooling schedule. The initial solution is created using the following strategy. All GUs are labeled as available. The algorithm then selects randomly 45 GUs, assigns them to different zones and labels them as not available. At this moment, each zone has therefore only one GU. Finally, each zone is iteratively extended by adding an available GU having a frontier with the zone in its current shape. Every time a GU is incorporated to a zone, it is labeled as not available in order to avoid the construction of overlapping zones. The latter step is performed until all the GUs are labeled as not available. This process ensures that the initial solution consists of 45 connected zones that include all GUs. Note that SA and ABC use the same procedure to create initial solutions.

Regarding now the construction of a neighbor solution, a random zone is chosen and a GU in this zone is moved to a neighbor zone in such way that the new solution satisfies constraints (**R1–R3**). Therefore, the neighbor solution is identical to the current one, except that one GU is reassigned to an adjacent zone. The new solution is evaluated and accepted or rejected according to the Metropolis criterion. If the neighbor solution is rejected, another GU is randomly selected; this process is repeated until the temperature reaches a predefined lower bound.

3.3 Artificial Bee Colony

Artificial Bee Colony (ABC) is a bio-inspired metaheuristic, originally proposed by Karaboga [16,17] and it is based on the natural behavior of honey bees when searching for food resources. In the ABC algorithm, each solution to the problem under consideration is called a food source and represented by an D-dimensional real-valued vector. The objective value of a solution is associated to the fitness or amount of nectar in the food source. Artificial bees are classified into three groups of bees: employed, onlookers, and scouts. In the initialization phase, the algorithm starts with a population of randomly generated food sources, each one representing a feasible solution.

The algorithm cycle begins with an improvement phase, which is carried out by employed bees. For each solution $Y_i = [y_{i,1}, y_{i,2}, ..., y_{i,D}]$ in the population, a solution $Y_k = [y_{k,1}, y_{k,2}, ..., y_{k,D}]$ ($i \neq k$) is randomly chosen to produce a new solution $V_i = [v_{i,1}, v_{i,2}, ..., v_{i,D}]$ according to the following equation:

$$v_{i,j} = y_{i,j} + r * (y_{i,j} - y_{k,j}) \tag{5}$$

Where j is an index randomly generated in $\{1, ..., D\}$ and r is a uniformly distributed real random number in the range (-1,1). Each produced solution V_i is subsequently evaluated by the employed bees and passes through a greedy selection process: if the new food source has a nectar amount equal to or better than the employed bee's current food source, it replaces the current solution; otherwise, the old food source is kept.

When the employed bees searching phase is over, each onlooker bee evaluates the nectar information provided by the employed bees and chooses a food source according to a probability p_i, computed on the basis of its nectar amount (i.e., the corresponding fitness):

$$p_i = \frac{fit_i}{\sum_{j=1}^{M} fit_j} \tag{6}$$

Where fit_i is the fitness value of the food source Y_i and M is the number of food sources. Once the food source is chosen, the onlooker tries to improve the corresponding solution generating a new one, in the same way the employed bees do, i.e. through Eq. 5. The new solution is then evaluated by the onlooker bee, its quality is compared with that of the current one and the best solution is selected applying a greedy selection process.

If a solution cannot be further improved through a predetermined number of trials, the solution is abandoned and a scout bee produces a new random solution. The termination criterion is, typically, a fixed number of computed iterations, or generations, of the previously described cycle.

3.4   Artificial Bee Colony Adaptation

The ABC heuristic was originally designed for continuous optimization problems, and cannot directly be used for discrete cases. For the IEEM's system, in order to handle discrete decision variables, we proposed some modifications to the ABC algorithm based on a recombination strategy.

First, M food sources are generated using the strategy described in Sect. 3.2, in such a way that each solution satisfies constraints **R1–R3**. The number of onlooker and employed bees is set equal to the number of food sources, and exactly one employed bee is assigned to each food source.

According to Eq. (5), employed and onlooker bees generate new solutions by combining two food sources. However, after some experiments, we found that the performance of the algorithm was improved if employed and onlooker bees used different strategies to explore the solution space. Thus, we decided that each employed bee must apply a local search, similar to the strategy used by SA described in Sect. 3.2, while onlooker bees use a recombination technique inspired in Eq. (5).

First, each employed bee, i, modifies its food source, P_i, using the following strategy. A random zone is chosen and a GU in this zone is moved to a neighbor zone in such way that the new solution, V_i, satisfies constraints (**R1–R3**). If the new solution V_i has a nectar amount better than or equal to that of P_i, V_i replaces P_i and becomes a new food source exploited by the hive. In other case, V_i is rejected and P_i is preserved.

As soon as the employed bees process has been completed, each onlooker bee chooses two solutions. The first solution, P_1, is selected depending on the probability given by (6), where the fitness value of the food source is given by (3). The second solution, P_2, is randomly selected from the food sources exploited by the hive. A new food source, V_1, is produced through a recombination technique described straightforward.

A GU k is randomly selected. Thus, there is a zone $Z_i \in P_1$ and a zone $Z_j \in P_2$ such that $k \in Z_i \cap Z_j$. Let us now consider the following sets:

$$H_1 = \{l : x_{li} = 0, x_{lj} = 1\} \tag{7}$$

$$H_2 = \{l : x_{li} = 1, x_{lj} = 0\} \tag{8}$$

Then a GU in H_1 is inserted into Z_i, and a GU in H_2 is extracted from Z_i, and inserted into any randomly chosen zone contiguous to Z_i.

Note that these moves can produce a disconnection in zone Z_i, so that a repair process must be applied. The number of connected components in Z_i is counted after the moves previously described. If the number of connected components equals 1, then the zone is connected. Otherwise, the algorithm defines the connected component that includes GU k (i.e., the GU used within the above-described recombination strategy) as zone Z_i; subsequently, the remaining components are assigned to other adjacent zones. In this way, properties **R1–R3** are preserved.

This way, an onlooker bee modifies a food source P_1. If the new solution V_1 has a nectar amount better than or equal to that of P_1, V_1 replaces P_1 and becomes a new food source exploited by the hive. In other case, V_1 is rejected and P_1 is preserved.

4   IEEM's Districting System

The IEEM's districting system is a software that includes:

- Two algorithms based on SA and ABC to generate districting plans for the state of Mexico.
- A geographic visualization system to view, edit and evaluate districting plans.

4.1   Geographic Visualization System

The visualization system displays a map of the state of Mexico in a web page. This tool can be used to: visualize districting plans, edit or modify districting plans. Moreover the user can move GUs to neighbouring districts in order to explore different solutions, compute the objective function after changes, and save new solutions.

When the user opens a previously created plan, each GU is colored to indicate the zone to which it belongs, see Fig. 1. Also, the following information is provided: (a) cost of the solution, and sum of population equality and compactness over the 45 districts, (b) cost of each district including population equality, compactness, given by Eqs. (1) and (2) respectively, as well as the number of inhabitants.

4.2   Simulated Annealing Module

The simulated annealing and artificial bee colony modules were designed in such a way that the user can introduce different parameters required by the algorithms. For the SA algorithm the user can set the following parameters:

- Initial temperature: a real positive number.
- Final temperature: a real positive value smaller than the initial temperature.

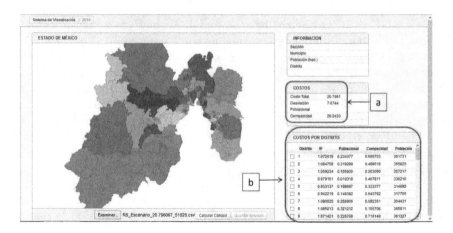

Fig. 1. Solutions and costs.

- Number of iterations: an integer number higher than 100.
- Cooling factor: a real value in the range (0,1).

These fields have default values, which were found after a brute force tuning process [3], but the user can modify them, respecting the above-mentioned conditions.

Also, a field called "Seed" is included. In this field the user can write an integer, between 1 and 2,147,483,647 ($2^{31} - 1$), that will be the seed for the random number generator used in the algorithm. A different option is to select the "Seedbed". In this case, a predefined set of 100 seeds is used, and the algorithm is executed once for each seed.

When all fields have been filled in, the user can execute the algorithm. When the stopping criterion is met, in this case when the final temperature is reached, the algorithm saves the best solution found, and the user can analyze it using the geographic visualization system. If the user selects the seedbed option, the algorithm realizes a new search, for each number in this set, and a new districting plan is constructed. This process finishes when all seeds have been used.

4.3   Artificial Bee Colony Module

The Artificial Bee Colony module includes 3 fields, where the user can set the operating parameters of the ABC based algorithm.

- Number of food sources: an integer number between 3 and 500. Based in previous experiments more than 500 food sources do not provide significant improvement.
- Number of generations: an integer value higher than zero.
- Generation number without improvement: an integer value higher than 3.

As in the previous case, the user can modify these parameters, and select a seed, or the seedbed, for the random number generator used by the algorithm.

When all fields have been filled in, the user can execute the algorithm. When the stopping criterion is met, in this case when the number of generations is reached, the algorithm saves the best solution found.

5   Experimental Results and Discussion

The two algorithms described in the previous section were tested with the tuned parameters. In order to deal with the stochastic effect inherent to heuristic techniques, 100 independent executions were performed for each algorithm. Additionally, the same seeds were used for both algorithms, thus both techniques started with the same initial solution. Each run produced a single solution, an electoral districting plan. The resulting 100 solutions were feasible according to restrictions **R1–R3**, and the number of inhabitants in each district was under the 15 % deviation allowed. Thus, all solutions were analyzed just in terms of their cost and execution time. Both algorithms were run with an Intel Pentium D processor.

Computational results are summarized in Table 1. They highlight that the ABC algorithm outperforms the SA version, since it was able to determine, on average, higher quality solutions than SA. In addition, a Wilcoxon rank sum test was performed in order to prove that populations of solutions produced by both algorithms are significantly different. The p-value obtained is equal to 8.75×10^{-165}, so the null hypothesis (there is no significant difference between both solution sets) can be rejected: ABC indeed robustly outperforms SA for this test case. These conclusions are confirmed by the observation of Fig. 2, where the superiority of ABC is indisputable. Finally, the average runtime per run used by the ABC algorithm was marginally higher (30 s.) than the time used by SA.

Table 1. Costs for both algorithms.

Algorithm	Best cost	Mean cost	Std. deviation	Average runtime (min.)
SA	21.13	22.15	1.72	11.31
ABC	19.89	20.35	2.3721	12.12

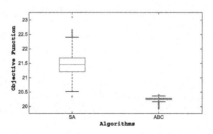

Fig. 2. Solutions and costs.

However, this difference can be omitted since the districting plans produced will be used for 3 years.

6   Conclusions

In this paper, we presented the districting system used by the Electoral Institute of the state of Mexico, for the 2014 electoral districting process. This system includes three modules: (a) a geographic visualization system, (b) a Simulated Annealing based algorithm, and (c) an Artificial Bee Colony based algorithm. Both heuristic algorithms solve the optimization problem corresponding to the districting process, promoting the design of districts with an indigenous population majority.

The system was designed in such a way that the user can set the algorithm operating parameters and the seed initializing the random numbers generator. However, some default values found through a brute force tuning strategy [3] are proposed, allowing the design of high quality districting plans, in an acceptable amount of computational time. On the other hand, the geographic visualization system was designed to show, edit, evaluate and save existing districting plans.

The resulting system is a novel proposal that combines automated and manual techniques to produce electoral districting plans. Furthermore, a population based algorithm (ABC) is used in an electoral districting process for the first time in Mexico, producing better solutions than the SA algorithm, the heuristic technique used by IFE in the last two Federal districting processes. It is worth noting that the results of this work were presented to INE, who adapted and applied this application for the 2015 districting process.

References

1. Ardanaz, M., Leiras, M., Tommasi, M.: The politics of federalism in Argentina and its implications for governance and accountability. World Dev. **53**, 26–45 (2014)
2. Baçao, F., Lobo, V., Painho, M.: Applying genetic algorithms to zone design. Soft Comput. **9**, 341–348 (2005)
3. Birattari, M.: Tuning Metaheuristics: A Machine Learning Perspective. Studies in Computational Intelligence, vol. 197. Springer, Heidelberg (2009)
4. Bozkaya, B., Erkut, E., Laporte, G.: A tabu search heuristic and adaptive memory procedure for political districting. Eur. J. Oper. Res. **144**, 12–26 (2003)
5. Chung-I, C.: A knowledge-based evolution algorithm approach to political districting problem. Comput. Phys. Commun. **182**(1), 209–212 (2011)
6. Caro, F., Shirabe, T., Guignard, M., Weintraub, A.: School redistricting: embedding GIS tools with integer programming. J. Oper. Res. Soc. **55**, 836–849 (2004)
7. Dell'Amico, S., Wang, S., Batta, R., Rump, C.: A simulated annealing approach to police district design. Comput. Oper. Res. **29**, 667–684 (2002)
8. DesJardins, M., Bulka, B., Carr, R., Jordan, E., Rheingans, P.: Heuristic search and information visualization methods for school redistricting. AI Mag. **28**(3), 59–72 (2006)
9. Duque, J.C., Ramos, R., Suriach, J.: Supervised regionalization methods: a survey. Int. Reg. Sci. Rev. **30**(3), 195–220 (2007)

10. Forest, B.: Redistricting and the elusive ideals of representation. Polit. Geogr. **32**, 15–17 (2013)
11. Garfinkel, R.S., Nemhauser, G.L.: Optimal political districting by implicit enumeration techniques. Manag. Sci. **16**, 495–508 (1970)
12. Gilbert, K.C., Holmes, D.D., Rosenthal, R.E.: A multiobjective discrete optimization model for land allocation. Manag. Sci. **31**, 1509–1522 (1985)
13. Andrade, M.A.G., García, E.A.R.: Redistricting by square cells. In: Aguirre, A.H., Borja, R.M., Garciá, C.A.R. (eds.) MICAI 2009. LNCS, vol. 5845, pp. 669–679. Springer, Heidelberg (2009)
14. Hess, S.W., Weaver, J.B., Siegfeldt, H.J., Whelan, J.N., Zitlau, P.A.: Nonpartisan political redistricting by computer. Oper. Res. **13**(6), 998–1006 (1965)
15. Kalcsics, J., Nickel, S., Schrder, M.: Towards a unified territorial design approach: applications, algorithms and GIS integration. Top **13**(1), 1–74 (2005)
16. Karaboga, D., Basturk, B.: A powerful and efficient algorithm for numerical function optimization: artificial bee colony (ABC) algorithm. J. Global Optim. **39**, 459–471 (2007)
17. Karaboga, D., Basturk, B.: On the performance of artificial bee colony (ABC) algorithm. Appl. Soft Comput. **8**, 687–697 (2008)
18. Kirkpatrick, S., Gellat, C.D., Vecchi, M.P.: Optimization by simulated annealing. Science **220**, 671–680 (1983)
19. Macmillan, W.: Redistricting in a GIS environment: an optimisation algorithm using switching-points. J. Geogr. Syst. **3**, 167–180 (2001)
20. Ricca, F., Simeone, B.: Local search algorithms for political districting. Eur. J. Oper. Res. **189**(3), 1409–1426 (2008)
21. Ricca, F., Scozzari, A., Simeone, B.: Political districting: from classical models to recent approaches. J. Oper. Res. **204**(1), 271–299 (2011)
22. Rincón-García, E.A., Gutiérrez-Andrade, M.A., de-los-Cobos-Silva, S.G., Lara-Velázquez, P., Mora-Gutiérrez, R.A., Ponsich, A.: A discrete particle swarm optimization algorithm for designing electoral zones. In: Methods for decision making in an uncertain environment, pp. 174–197. World Scientific Proceedings Series on Computer Engineering and Information Science, Reus (2012)
23. Shirabe, T.: A model of contiguity for spatial unit allocation. Geogr. Anal. **37**, 2–16 (2005)
24. Shirabe, T.: Prescriptive modeling with map algebra for multi-zone allocation with size constraints. Comput. Environ. Urban Syst. **36**, 456–469 (2012)
25. Shortt, N.K., Moore, A., Coombes, M., Wymer, C.: Defining regions for locality health care planning: a multidimensional approach. Soc. Sci. Med. **60**, 2715–2727 (2005)
26. Tavares-Pereira, F., Rui, J., Mousseau, V., Roy, B.: Multiple criteria districting problems: the public transportation network pricing system of the Paris region. Ann. Oper. Res. **154**, 69–92 (2007)
27. Vickrey, W.: On the prevention of gerrymandering. Polit. Sci. Q. **76**(1), 105–110 (1961)
28. Zoltners, A.A., Sinha, P.: Sales territory design: thirty years of modeling and implementation. Mark. Sci. **24**(3), 313–331 (2005)

Particle Swarm Optimization Algorithm for Dynamic Environments

Sadrollah Sadeghi[1], Hamid Parvin[1,2(✉)], and Farhad Rad[1]

[1] Department of Computer Engineering, Yasooj Branch,
Islamic Azad University, Yasooj, Iran
parvin@iust.ac.ir
[2] Young Researchers and Elite Club, Nourabad Mamasani Branch,
Islamic Azad University, Nourabad Mamasani, Iran

Abstract. Particle Swarm Optimization (PSO) algorithm is considered as one of the crowd intelligence optimization algorithms. Dynamic optimization problems in which change(s) may happen over the time are harder to manage than static optimization problems. In this paper an algorithm based on PSO and memory for solving dynamic optimization problems has been proposed. The proposed algorithm uses the memory to store the aging best solutions and uses partitioning for preventing convergence in the population. The proposed approach has been tested on moving peaks benchmark (MPB). The MPB is a suitable problem for simulating dynamic optimization problems. The experimental results on the moving peaks benchmark show that the proposed algorithm is superior to several other well-known and state-of-the-art algorithms in dynamic environments.

Keywords: Swarm intelligence · Dynamic environment · Optimization

1 Introduction

In recent years, evolutionary algorithms have attracted much interest among researchers for solving dynamic optimization problems. An evolutionary algorithm suitable for dynamic optimization problems should not only be able to locate the optimum, as it does in the static optimization problems, but also be capable of detecting the time when the changes in the positions of optima occur and also tracking the newly relocated optima. In the static environments for the reason that optima are not moved in the environment and each of them remains in a fixed position passing the time, it is easy for evolutionary algorithms to find the global optimum, but in an environment that is subject to change it is not an easy task to find the optimum following every changes that occur in the environment. Thus strong heuristic mechanisms are needed to solve dynamic optimization problems. One of the weaknesses in evolutionary algorithms for solving dynamic optimization problems is that they can't single-handedly solve them. Thus they should employ some appropriate strategies that make them able to manage dynamic optimization problems. One of the proper strategies for dynamic environments is to use a combination of some auxiliary elements, for example using of the memory element in evolutionary algorithms can be very useful. Some of these auxiliary elements are presented in [1–3]. The main weakness of using standard evolutionary

© Springer International Publishing Switzerland 2015
G. Sidorov and S.N. Galicia-Haro (Eds.): MICAI 2015, Part I, LNAI 9413, pp. 260–269, 2015.
DOI: 10.1007/978-3-319-27060-9_21

algorithms in a dynamic environments is that, once the algorithm starts to converge around some optimal or near optimal solution, it will highly likely lose its ability to continue the search for new optima, when the environment changes. Thus, one key point in optima tracking approaches is the need to increase or maintain diversity in the middle of the individuals in the population, so that the algorithm keeps its ability to explore the new optima when the environments change, even after when the population has incompletely converged to an optimum or close to optimal solution. In recent years, several methods have been expanded for solving dynamic optimization problems with the aim of increasing and maintaining diversity as the generations go forward during the entire run [4–6]. Ramsey and Grefenstette [7] have introduced a case-based method for initializing the genetic algorithm when a change is detected. Louis and Xu [8] have applied the same idea to the open shop scheduling problem. They have used an Evolutionary Algorithm combined with case-based reasoning. Yang and Tinos [9] have used a hybrid immigrant scheme. This method has combined the concepts of elitism, dualism and random immigrants. The best individual from the previous generation and its dual individual is retrieved in order to create immigrants via mutation. These elitism-based and dualism based immigrants together with some random immigrants were substituted into the current population, replacing the worst individuals in the population. This paper involves a comprehensive experimental study based on the moving peaks benchmark (MPB) problem [11]. In order to show whether the proposed technique effects on increasing convergence speed the examinations will be conducted on MPB. We compare the performance of proposed approach with other well-known and state-of-the-art approaches in dynamic environments. Other algorithms selected to be compared with proposed approach are some state-of-the-art traditional algorithms that the most researchers use them as their competent methods. This paper is organized as follows. Section 1 includes memory definition. It also defines strategies for updating and retrieving of the memory in ABC algorithm. Section 1 also describes dynamic environments and offline error. The proposed method is presented in sufficient details in Sect. 2 along with its algorithmic pseudo-code. Section 3 first presents MPB problem. Then experimental results and the analysis of assimilated results have been presented in the rest of Sect. 3. Finally, the paper is concluded in Sect. 4 with a discussion on the possible future works of the research.

2 Proposed Method

In this article we have proposed an particle based optimization algorithm based on memory and clustering for dynamic environments. In this method we use an explicit memory to store the optimum solution to use it in the new environment, because in a dynamic environment for the reason that of cyclic form of the environment, it is probable that a optimum which has been appeared in past generations, reappears at the same point and in that condition the memory can detect the optimum point and increase the convergence rate in the algorithm and use a replacement strategy (strategy 1) to update memory to maintain diversity when implementing the algorithm. One of the main challenges in dynamic environments is to maintain the diversity when implementing the algorithm and in this method we have maintained diversity in the population using clustering of memory and the population. In this method the memory and the population in the first phase are initialized based on Eq. 11. So memory and the population are clustered after being initialized. Each person needs to be placed in his cluster for insertion and retrieval. Clustering is an unsupervised learning branch in which the samples are divided into a series of clusters as the samples in a cluster are similar and they are different than the samples in other clusters. There are many criteria to measure the similarities one of which is Euclidean distance between the two samples. Similar samples have lower Euclidean distance and they are placed in a cluster. This clustering is called distance-based clustering. One of the distance-based clustering is k-means clustering. In k-means clustering the center of a cluster is the average amount of data within each cluster. Then the data are clustered based on the Euclidean distance to cluster centers. This method in each iteration improves the inside cluster changes of the model which is done by estimating the new cluster center in iteration phase. In this way the data are allocated to different clusters based on updated average. This work will continue until the center of the cluster is fixed and the value will remain unchanged in successive iterations and the clusters are stable.

Imagine a space that helps to explain the proposed approach. Assume the problem space is divided into three clusters and in each cluster, the position of the particles is defined by a small star, the center of cluster is defined by the plus, the position of the memory is determined by a circle, the center of cluster of memory population is defined by the square, the center of each peak is marked by a diamond and the new center of the peal is marked by a bug star sign. As discussed before the worst individual of the population is the one who has the greatest distance from the center of the peak and in fact it can be said that the worst person has the least efficiency. If the environment changes and the peak center is changed then the efficiency of the members can be changed.

The closest memory to the new peak is considered as the best memory and this memory after the change and displacement of the optimum peak can lead members of the population toward the new peak. The question that arises here is that how a memory understands is close or far from the new peak center. In response to this question, we can say that, if the efficiency of a memory after the change of environment is increased the memory understands that it is closer to the peak and if the efficiency is lowered the memory understands that is far from it. The best individual of the population is the closest one to the center of the peak center.

3   Experiments

In order to perform the tests on the proposed algorithm and its comparison with other algorithms in a dynamic environment moving peaks benchmark [10] is used to test the efficiency of the proposed method.

3.1   Moving Peaks Benchmark Problem

Moving peaks benchmark problem [11] is a good simulator for simulating the dynamic environment. This problem includes n peaks in an m dimension space with real value parameters and the height, width and position of peaks may change over time which is the dynamic problem simulation. Moving peaks benchmark function is formulated based on Eq. (1):

$$F(\vec{x}, t) = max(B(\vec{x}), \max_{i=1...m} P(\vec{x}, h_i(t), w_i(t), \vec{p}_i(t)))$$ (1)

where, $B(\vec{x})$ is the base value of the environment that is independent of time and P is a function that defines the shape of the peak, that each m peak has their time variable parameters, height (h), width (w), and their own position (p). In each ΔE evaluating height), width and position of each peak are changed. The height and width of each peak changes by adding a Gaussian random variable. The change frequency parameter indicates when the environment is changed or when the algorithm must respond to changes in the environment. Moving peaks benchmark function has various parameters that by changing each one of these parameters change may result. Figure 1 presents the change of the peaks in this problem with multiple peaks.

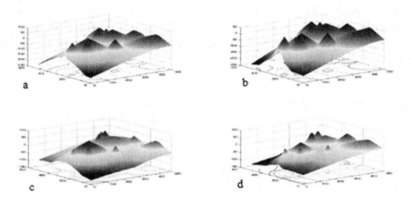

Fig. 1. The changes in the peaks in moving peaks benchmark function.

Therefore the parameter s controls the amount of variation, ΔE determines the frequency of changes, the parameter λ determines how the position of a peak is changed based on its previous motion.

If $\lambda = 0$ every motion is random and for $\lambda = 1$ peaks move in a determined path. Whenever a change occurs in the environment this change is mention on the location, height and width of a peak as the equations mentioned in (2).

$$h_i(t) = h_i(t-1) + height_{severity} \cdot \sigma$$
$$w_i(t) = w_i(t-1) + width_{severity} \cdot \sigma$$
$$\vec{p}_i(t) = \vec{p}_i(t-1) + \vec{v}_i(t)$$ (2)
$$\sigma \in N(0, 1)$$

Transmission vector $\vec{v}_i(t)$ combines a random vector $\vec{r}$ with the previous transmission vector $\vec{v}_i(t-1)$. The random vector $\vec{v}_i(t)$ is generated by producing the random numbers in [0, 1] for each dimension and normalizing it as s. Vector $\vec{v}_i(t)$ can be created based on the previous change where the position of the peaks is align the previous changes or it is created randomly which changes the position of the peaks and they would have no dependence to the last change. Vector $\vec{v}_i(t)$ is calculated based on Eq. (3):

$$\vec{v}_i(t) = \frac{s}{|\vec{r} + \vec{v}_i(t-1)|} \left((1 - \lambda)\vec{r} + \lambda \vec{v}_i(t-1) \right) \tag{3}$$

Peak function for height, width and position of each peak is calculated based on Eq. (4).

$$P(\vec{x}, h(t), w(t), \vec{p}(t)) = h(t) - w(t) \cdot \sqrt{\sum_{j=1...n} (x_j - p_j)^2} \tag{4}$$

The part related to radical mentions the distance between the point and the position of each peak. Numerical experiments concerning the moving peaks benchmark (MPB), scenario 2, as proposed by Branke (2001) were performed in order to test the behavior of proposed method. The default settings and definition of the benchmark used in the experiments of this paper can be found in Table 1. Parameter settings for proposed algorithm presented in Table 2.

Table 1. The standard configuration parameters for the dynamic peaks.

Parameter	Value
peaks (number of peaks)	10
Change frequency *(U)*	5000
Height severity	7.0
Width severity	1.0
Peak shape	Con
Basic function	No
Shift length s	1.0
Number of dimensions D	5
Correlation coefficient λ	0
S	[0, 100]
H	[30.0, 70.0]
W	[1, 12]
I	50.0

3.2   Varying Shift Severity

The shift severity parameter of the MPB controls the severity of the change in height, width and position of peaks. From Table 3, it can be seen that the results achieved by proposed algorithm are much better than the results of the other 11 algorithms on the MPB problems with different shift severity. As we know, the peaks are more and more

Table 2. The proposed algorithm parameters.

Parameter	Value
Lower bound	0
Upper bound	100
Total population	100
Memory Size	10
The possibility of intersection	0.6
The possibility of mutation	0.2
Number of main population clusters	2.0
The number of population clusters Memory	2.0

difficult to track with the increasing of the shift severity. Of course, the performance of all algorithms degrades when the shift severity increases. However, the offline error of proposed algorithm is better than in comparison with the other 11 algorithms. These results indicate proposed algorithm to adapt better than others algorithm to more severe changes in the landscape.

Table 3. Average Offline Errors for Different Algorithms on the MPB Problem with Different Shift Severities.

Algorithm	Shift Severity(s)						
	0	1	2	3	4	5	6
Proposed algorithm	**0.0853**	**0.0995**	**0.1473**	**0.8629**	**0.9933**	**1.017**	**1.1096**
CPSO [12]	0.465	0.715	0.843	0.911	0.997	1.08	1.23
mQSO [13]	1.17	1.75	2.40	3.0	3.59	4.24	4.79
rSPSO [14]	0.74	1.50	1.87	2.4	2.90	3.25	3.87
ESCA [15]	1.72	1.53	1.57	1.67	1.72	1.78	1.79
CESO [16]	0.58	1.38	1.78	2.03	2.23	2.52	2.74
mCPSO [14]	1.18	2.05	2.80	3.57	4.18	4.89	5.53
SPSO [17]	0.95	2.51	3.78	4.96	2.56	6.76	7.68
CGAR [18]	1.48	2.62	2.76	2.96	3.16	3.46	3.8
CDER [18]	2.56	2.52	7.47	8.62	9.81	10.7	11.4
PSO-CP [19]	0.87	1.31	1.98	2.21	2.61	3.20	3.93
CPSOR [18]	0.418	0.599	0.849	0.964	1.38	1.69	2.07

3.3   Varying Number of Peaks

Table 4 presents the experimental results in terms of the offline error of 19 algorithms, where the results of the other 18 algorithms are provided by the corresponding papers with their optima configuration that enables them to achieve their best performance. In Table 4, mCPSO* and mQSO* denote mCPSO without anti-convergence and mQSO without anti-convergence, respectively. From Table 4, it can be seen that the performance of proposed algorithm is not influenced too much when the number of peaks is increased.

Table 4. Average offline errors for different algorithms on the MPB problem with different numbers of peaks, where the suggested configuration for the framework and the default settings for the MPB problem in Table 1.

Algorithm	Peak number									
	1	2	5	7	10	20	30	50	100	200
Proposed algorithm	**0.0595**	**0.0645**	**0.0635**	**0.0952**	**0.0995**	**0.1938**	**0.1871**	**0.2842**	**0.6922**	**0.5434**
CGAR	2.02	1.88	2.56	2.98	2.62	3.66	3.12	3.26	2.68	2.39
CDER	0.903	2.6	8.02	6.74	5.52	7.49	5.51	5.79	4.12	3.71
CPSO	2.29	0.005	0.361	0.675	0.715	1.18	1.34	1.42	1.09	0.955
mCPSO	4.93	3.36	2.07	2.11	2.08	2.64	2.63	2.65	2.49	2.44
mQSO	5.07	3.47	1.81	1.77	1.80	2.42	2.48	2.50	2.36	2.26
mCPSO*	4.93	3.36	2.07	2.11	2.05	2.95	3.38	3.68	4.07	3.97
mQSO*	5.07	3.47	1.81	1.77	1.75	2.74	3.27	3.65	3.93	3.86
CESO	1.04	-	-	-	1.38	1.72	1.24	1.45	1.28	-
rSPSO	1.42	1.10	1.04	1.21	1.50	2.20	2.62	2.72	2.93	2.79
SPSO	2.64	2.31	2.15	1.98	2.51	3.21	3.64	3.86	4.01	3.82
ESCA	0.98	-	-	-	1.54	1.89	1.52	1.67	1.61	-
PSO-CP	3.41	-	-	-	-	1.31	202	2.14	2.04	-
HmSO [20]	0.87	-	1.18	-	1.42	1.5	1.65	1.66	1.68	1.71
RVDEA [21]	1.02	-	-	-	3.54	3.87	3.92	3.87	3.37	3.54
FMSO [22]	3.44	-	2.94	-	3.11	3.36	3.28	3.22	3.06	2.84
Cellular PSO [23]	2.55	-	1.68	-	1.78	2.60	2.93	3.26	3.41	3.40
rPSO [24]	0.56	-	12.58	-	12.98	12.79	12.35	11.34	9.73	8.90
Adaptive mQSO [25]	0.51	-	1.01	-	1.51	2.00	2.19	2.43	2.68	2.62

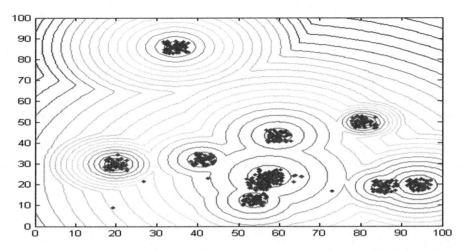

Fig. 2. Cover peaks via particles for 10 peaks and default setting MPB derived in 2 Dimensions.

Usually, increasing the number of peaks makes it harder for algorithms to track the optima. However, the offline error decreases when the number of peaks is larger than 50 for proposed algorithm. Figure 2 show the cover of peaks via particles that is drawn in 2 dimensions.

3.4   Varying Number of Dimensions

Table 5 shows the result of the proposed method with different dimensions involving peaks number is 10, frequency of change is 5000 and shift severity is 1, in addition to those of mQSO, Adaptive mQSO, rPSO and mPSO. Result of exist in Table 5 shows with increasing dimension of the landscape space, the performance of the proposed algorithm is better than other algorithms.

Table 5. Result of the proposed method with different dimensions involving peaks number is 10, frequency of change is 5000 and shift severity is 1, in comparison with mQSO, Adaptive mQSO, rPSO and mPSO.

Algorithm	Dimension						
	2	3	4	5	10	15	20
proposed method	0.0485	0.0643	0.0731	0.0995	0.1517	0.2625	0.3547
Adaptive mQSO	0.71	1.16	1.33	1.51	3.37	4.91	5.83
mQSO	1.01	1.49	1.47	1.85	4.22	6.50	8.88
rPSO	2.62	6.61	10.43	12.98	16.87	18.48	18.48
mPSO	1.24	1.42	1.35	1.61	4.32	7.07	10.77

4 Conclusions

Intelligent optimization algorithms in dynamic environment should be designed in such a way that they could follow the intended optimum efficiently. In this article we use a combination of the memory and particle swarm optimization algorithm to maintain good solutions. We increase algorithms' efficiency by population clustering algorithms and employed an appropriate strategy to maintain diversity in population. We experimentally have shown that proposed algorithm completely outperforms the state-of-the-art algorithms in terms of convergence speed. Usage of the proposed algorithm with chaos theory can be good idea for future works.

References

1. Branke, J.: Memory enhanced evolutionary algorithms for changing optimization problems. In: Proceedings of Congress on Evolutionary Computation, vol. 3. pp. 1875–1882 (1999)
2. Yang, S.: Associative memory scheme for genetic algorithms in dynamic environments. In: Rothlauf, F., Branke, J., Cagnoni, S., Costa, E., Cotta, C., Drechsler, R., Lutton, E., Machado, P., Moore, J.H., Romero, J., Smith, G.D., Squillero, G., Takagi, H. (eds.) EvoWorkshops 2006. LNCS, vol. 3907, pp. 788–799. Springer, Heidelberg (2006)
3. Yang, S., Yao, X.: Population-based incremental learning with associative memory for dynamic environments. IEEE Trans. Evol. Comput. 12(5), 542–561 (2008)
4. Cobb, H.G., Grefenstette, J.J.: Genetic algorithms for tracking changing environments. In: Proceedings of 5th International Genetic Algorithms Conference, pp. 523–530 (1993)
5. Grefenstette, J.J.: Genetic algorithms for changing environments. In: Proceedings of 2nd International Conference Parallel Problem Solving from Nature, pp. 137–144 (1992)
6. Yang, S.: Genetic algorithms with memory and elitism-based immigrants in dynamic environment. Evol. Comput. 16(3), 385–416 (2008)
7. Ramsey, C.L., Grefenstette, J.J.: Case-based initialization of genetic algorithms. In: Forrest, S. (ed.) Proceedings of the 5th International Conference on Genetic Algorithms. Morgan Kaufmann, pp. 84–91 (1993)
8. Louis, S.J., Xu, Z.: Genetic algorithms for open shop scheduling and re-scheduling. In: Cohen, M.E., Hudson, D.L. (eds) Proceedings of the 11th International Conference on Computers and their Applications (ISCA), pp. 99–102 (1996)
9. Yang, S., Tinos, R.: A hybrid immigrants scheme for genetic algorithms in dynamic environments. Int. J. Autom. Comput. 3(4), 243–254 (2007)
10. Trojanowski, K., Michalewicz, Z.: Searching for optima in non-stationary environments. In: Proceedings of the IEEE Congress on Evolutionary Computation (CEC 1999). IEEE Press, pp. 1843–1850 (1999)
11. Branke, J.: Memory enhanced evolutionary algorithms for changing optimization problems. In: Proceedings of the IEEE Congress on Evolutionary Computation (CEC 1999). IEEE Press, pp. 1875–1882 (1999)
12. Yang, S., Li, C.: A clustering particle swarm optimizer for dynamic optimization. In: Proceedings of Congress on Evolutionary Computation, pp. 439–446 (2009)
13. Blackwell, T., Branke, J., Li, X.: Particle swarms for dynamic optimization problems. Swarm Intelligence, pp. 193–217. Springer, Berlin (2008)
14. Blackwell, T.M., Branke, J.: Multiswarms, exclusion, and anticonvergence in dynamic environments. IEEE Trans. Evol. Comput. 10(4), 459–472 (2006)

15. Lung, R.I., Dumitrescu, D.: Evolutionary swarm cooperative optimization in dynamic environments. Nat. Comput. **9**(1), 83–94 (2010)
16. Lung, R.I., Dumitrescu, D.: A collaborative model for tracking optima in dynamic environments. In: Proceedings of Congress on Evolutionary Computation, pp. 564–567 (2007)
17. Li, X.: Adaptively choosing neighborhood bests using species in a particle swarm optimizer for multimodal function optimization. In: Proceedings of Genetic Evolutionary Computation Conference, pp. 105–116 (2004)
18. Yang, S., Li, C.: A clustering particle swarm optimizer for locating and tracking multiple optima in dynamic environments. IEEE Trans. **16**(4), 556–577 (2012)
19. Liu, L., Yang, S., Wang, D.: Particle swarm optimization with composite particles in dynamic environments. IEEE Trans. Syst. Man Cybern. B Cybern. **40**(6), 1634–1648 (2010)
20. Kamosi, M., Hashemi, A.B., Meybodi, M.R.: A hibernating multiswarm optimization algorithm for dynamic environments. In: Proceedings of World Congress on Nature and Biologically Inspired Computing, pp. 363–369 (2010)
21. Woldesenbet, Y.G., Yen, G.G.: Dynamic evolutionary algorithm with variable relocation. IEEE Trans. Evol. Comput. **13**(3), 500–513 (2009)
22. Yang, S., Li, C.: Fast multi-swarm optimization for dynamic optimization problems. Proc. Int. Conf. Nat. Comput. **7**(3), 624–628 (2008)
23. Hashemi, A.B., Meybodi, M.R.: Cellular PSO: a PSO for dynamic environments. In: Cai, Z., Li, Z., Kang, Z., Liu, Y. (eds.) ISICA 2009. LNCS, vol. 5821, pp. 422–433. Springer, Heidelberg (2009)
24. Wang, H., Yang, S., Ip, W.H., Wang, D.: A memetic particle swarm optimization algorithm for dyanamic multi modal optimization problems. Int. J. Syst. Sci. **43**(7), 1268–1283 (2012)
25. Blackwell, T., Branke, J., Li, X.: Particle swarms for dynamic optimization problems. In: Yang, S.S., Li, C. (eds.) A Clustering Particle Swarm Optimizer for Locating and Intelligence, pp. 193–217. Springer, Berlin (2008)

A Migrating Birds Optimization Algorithm for Machine-Part Cell Formation Problems

Ricardo Soto[1,2,3], Broderick Crawford[1,4,5], Boris Almonacid[1(✉)],
and Fernando Paredes[6]

[1] Pontificia Universidad Católica de Valparaíso, Valparaíso, Chile
{ricardo.soto,broderick.crawford}@ucv.cl, boris.almonacid.g@mail.pucv.cl
[2] Universidad Autónoma de Chile, Santiago, Chile
[3] Universidad Científica Del Sur, Lima, Peru
[4] Universidad Central de Chile, Santiago, Chile
[5] Universidad San Sebastián, Santiago, Chile
[6] Escuela de Ingeniería Industrial, Universidad Diego Portales, Santiago, Chile
fernando.paredes@udp.cl

Abstract. Machine-Part Cell Formation Problems consists in organizing a plant as a set of cells, each one of them processing machines containing the same type of parts. In recent years, different meta-heuristic have been used to solve this problem. This paper addresses the problem of Machine-Part Cell Formation by using the Migrating Birds Optimization algorithm. The computational experiments show that in most of the benchmark problems the results obtained from the proposed approach are better than those obtained by other methods which are reported in the literature.

Keywords: Cell formation problem · Nature-inspired algorithms · Migrating birds optimization · Meta-heuristics

1 Introduction

Cellular Manufacturing is an organizational approach based on Group Technology [17]. The purpose of the manufacturing cell is to divide the plant in a set of cells. This identification process requires an effective approach to form part families so that similarity within a part family can be optimized. According to Selim et al. [23], clustering analysis is one of the most used methods for manufacturing cell design methods. The formation of cells is known to be NP-complete and there is still the challenge of creating an efficient grouping method.

This paper focuses on solving machine-part cell formation problems. We use a new nature-inspired meta-heuristic for combinatorial optimisation problems called Migrating Birds Optimization (MBO) [7], that has successfully been used to solve complex optimization problems such as: A hybrid flowshop scheduling with total flowtime minimisation [19], Closed loop layout with exact distances in flexible manufacturing systems [18], Obstacle neutralization problem [1].

© Springer International Publishing Switzerland 2015
G. Sidorov and S.N. Galicia-Haro (Eds.): MICAI 2015, Part I, LNAI 9413, pp. 270–281, 2015.
DOI: 10.1007/978-3-319-27060-9_22

We perform tests to resolve machine-part cell formation problem using MBO and compared with Simulated Annealing (SA) [4,29] and Particle Swarm Optimization (PSO) [8,9], obtaining encouraging results. This paper is organized as follows: Sect. 2 presents the related work. Section 3 describes and models the machine-part cell formation problems; Sect. 4 gives an overview of MBO; Sect. 5 presents and discuss the experimental results. Finally, we conclude and give some directions for future work.

2   Related Work

The machine-part cell formation has emerged in the last two decades as innovation for manufacturing strategy, which includes the advantages of serial production. However, the independence between cells is difficult to produce in practice, because some parts need to be processed in more than one machine. Therefore, the objective of the machine-part cell formation problems, consists on grouping machines and parts so as to minimize the flow between them.

Several investigations have been carried out for the problem. Burbidge [5] has been one of the early researchers focused on the problem of machine-part cell formation, in which he focused on the implementation of a new production strategy focused on a reduction of flows and costs. Some methods are just trying to find a family of parts, resulting in a partial solution; because the identification of part families require machines to process all parts within the same cell. This is modeled as a p-median problem or one can take advantage of the special structure of clustering matrices and solve it by the rank energy algorithm [13]. In addition, there have been other relevant research to solve the machine-part cell formation problem as a linear formulation of the problem [4], simultaneous grouping of parts and machines in cellular manufacturing systems in an integer programming approach [10] and a comparative study of similarity coefficients and clustering algorithms in cellular manufacturing [22].

The problem of machine-part cell formation has had two complementary lines of research. These are organized into two groups: Global optimization and Approximate methods. The global optimization is to analyze the entire search space, in order to guarantee a global optimum, as a result, the computational cost in terms of memory and time consumed is much higher. In this group we find research based on Linear programming [20], Goal programming [24], Constraint programming [6,26] and Boolean satisfiability [25]. By contrast, the approximate methods as meta-heuristic focus on finding an approximate solution to a given amount of time; therefore, they can not guarantee a global optimum. Duran et al. proposed to Particle Swarm Optimization algorithm enhanced with a data mining technique for manufacturing cell design [9]. Simulated Annealing Approaches for machine-part cell formation problems can be found in [4] and [29], respectively. Other research using meta-heuristics are: Tabu seach [16,28], Ant colony optimization [14], Genetic algorithms [12,27].

In this paper, we focus on solving the problem machine-part cell formation using a metaheuristic called Migrating Birds Optimization, which to our knowledge has not yet been reported.

3   Problem Description

In this work, we model the machine-part cell formation problem by using an array-based clustering approach. The main idea is to represent the processing requirements of parts on machines through an incidence matrix named machine-part (MxP). This matrix holds binary domains and is denoted as $A = a_{ij}$, where:

$$a_{ij} = \begin{cases} 1 \text{ if part } j \text{ visits machine } i \text{ for the processing;} \\ 0 \text{ otherwise.} \end{cases}$$

Let us note that when a machine-part incidence matrix is contructed, cells or part of families are easily visible. The main objective for machine-part cell formation problems is the organization of set of machines and parts in groups so that the number of intercell transportation is minimized. Figure 1 presents an example of diagonal block formation. This example corresponds to a machine-part cell formation problem with the following parameters: 5 machines, 7 parts, an incidence matrix a_{ij} (left matrix in Fig. 1), $M_{max} = 3$ for 2 cells. Finally, assignment matrices y_{ik} and z_{jk} can be observed in Fig. 2, the optimum value obtained is 0 and the new incidence matrix a_{ij} constructed from the results of y_{ik} and z_{jk}, has to be transformed into a solution matrix that has a block diagonal structure (right matrix in Fig. 1).

A mathematical formulation of machine-part cell formation problem is given by Boctor [4]. The optimization model is stated as follows, Let:

– M: the number of machines.

	P1	P2	P3	P4	P5	P6	P7
M1	0	1	0	1	1	1	0
M2	1	0	1	0	0	0	0
M3	1	0	1	0	0	0	1
M4	0	1	0	1	0	1	0
M5	1	0	0	0	0	0	1

		P1	P3	P7	P2	P4	P5	P6
Cell 1	M2	1	1	0	0	0	0	0
	M3	1	1	1	0	0	0	0
	M5	1	0	1	0	0	0	0
Cell 2	M1	0	0	0	1	1	1	1
	M4	0	0	0	1	1	0	1

Fig. 1. An example of cell formation.

	Cell 1	Cell 2
M1	0	1
M2	1	0
M3	1	0
M4	0	1
M5	1	0

	Cell 1	Cell 2
P1	1	0
P2	0	1
P3	1	0
P4	0	1
P5	0	1
P6	0	1
P7	1	0

Fig. 2. Machine-Cell matrix y_{ik} and Part-Cell matrix z_{jk}.

- P: the number of parts.
- C: the number of cells.
- i: the index of machines $(i = 1, \ldots, M)$.
- j: the index of parts $(j = 1, \ldots, P)$.
- k: the index of cells $(k = 1, \ldots, C)$.
- M_{max}: the maximum number of machines per cell.
- $A = a_{ij}$: the $M \times P$ machine-part incidence matrix.
- y_{ik}: the $M \times C$ machine-cell matrix, where:

$$y_{ik} = \begin{cases} 1 \text{ if machine } i \in \text{cell } k; \\ 0 \text{ otherwise;} \end{cases}$$

- z_{jk}: the $P \times C$ part-cell matrix, where:

$$z_{jk} = \begin{cases} 1 \text{ if part } j \in \text{cell } k; \\ 0 \text{ otherwise;} \end{cases}$$

The problem is represented by the following mathematical model:

$$\text{minimize} \sum_{k=1}^{C} \sum_{i=1}^{M} \sum_{j=1}^{P} a_{ij} z_{jk} (1 - y_{ik}) \tag{1}$$

Subject to:

$$\sum_{k=1}^{C} y_{ik} = 1 \quad \forall_i \tag{2}$$

$$\sum_{k=1}^{C} z_{jk} = 1 \quad \forall_j \tag{3}$$

$$\sum_{i=1}^{M} y_{ik} \leq M_{max} \quad \forall_k, \tag{4}$$

4   Migrating Birds Optimization

4.1   Natural Migration of Birds

The migrating birds optimization imitates the behaviour of bird migration in V-shaped flight formation when season changes. There is a bird that is the leader of the flock, which is followed by other birds, that are going after him on his right and left hand, so that in the sky you can see the classic V-formation [3]. In this formation of migrating birds, some parameters like Wing-Tip Spacing (WTS), angle of the V-formation (α), maximum width of the wing (w), depth and wing span (b) are important to form an effective V-formation (show in Fig. 4).

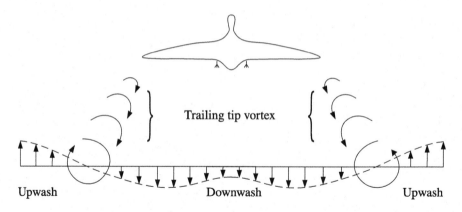

Fig. 3. Regions of upwash and downwash created by trailing vortices.

To determine the WTS some experiments [2,15] have been done, but finally the best optimal value of WTS was obtained by Hummel and Beukenberg [11], which it is formulated as $\text{WTS}_{opt} = -0.05b$. In addition to the WTS, energy saving flight can also be affected by the depth (the distance of a bird flying bird behind leader position). The vortex sheet behind a fixed wing in constant flight, level winds to form two vortices (show in Fig. 3) concentrated in two lengths of rope of the wing [21]. Therefore, the optimum depth can be formulated as $D_{opt} = -2w$.

4.2 Migrating Birds Optimization Method

The migrating birds optimization (MBO) starts with a number of initial solutions corresponding to birds in a V-formation. The initial population is composed of n solutions that are randomly generated in the feasible solution space. Starting with the first solution (corresponding to the leader bird) and progressing on the lines towards the tails. Each solution try to be improved by its neighbor solutions. If the best neighbor solution brings an improvement, the current solution is replaced, otherwise, the leader stays unchanged. Also there is a benefit, which is a mechanism for the solutions (birds) to share unused solutions. This mechanism consist in sharing with the unused neighbors the solutions that follow in the flock. In other words, a solution evaluates a number of its own neighbors and a number of neighbors of the previous solution. Subsequently, the solution is replaced with the best set of neighbors and shared solutions. Once all the solutions are improved by neighbor solutions, this procedure is repeated a number of times m (tours) after which the leader solution becomes the last one, and one of the other solutions with best value becomes leader and another loop starts. The algorithm terminates when the number of iterations reaches the limit.

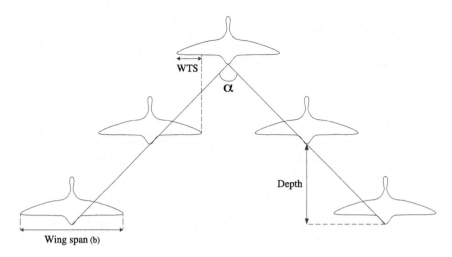

Fig. 4. The V-formation.

Table 1. Similarities of MBO meta-heuristic and V-shape natural migration of birds.

Parameter of MBO	Parameter description	Similar concept in real migration birds in V-formation
n	The number of initial solutions of the flock	Birds in V-formation
k	The number of neighboring solutions generated for each initial solution	The induced power required which is inversely proportional to the speed
x	The number of neighboring solutions shared with the next solution	Wing-Tip Spacing (WTS)
m	The number of tours	The number of wing flaps before a change occurs in the leading bird
K	The number of iterations (total number of generated neighbor solutions)	There is no conceptual relationship

The conceptual similarity between the parameters of the algorithm of MBO with the actual migration of birds in V-formation is studied in Duman et al. [7] and is summarized in Table 1.

Below, first the notation used and then the pseudocode of the MBO algorithm are given.

Algorithm 1. Pseudocode of Migrating Birds Optimization

---

1 Generate n initial solutions in a random manner and place them on an
   hypothetical V-formation arbitrarily;

2 $i = 0$;

3 **while** $(i < K)$ **do**

4   **for** $j = 0$ to $j < m$ **do**

5   Try to improve the leading solution by generating and evaluating k
   neighbors of it (for the implementation of machine-part cell
   formation problem, a neighbor solution is obtained randomly by
   choosing a machine and reassigning it to a randomly chosen cell);

6          $i = i + k$;

7   **for** *each solution S_r in the flock (except leader)* **do**

8   Try to improve S_r by evaluating $(k - x)$ neighbors of it and x
   unused best neighbors from the solution in the front;

9              $i = i + (k - x)$;

10   **end**

11   **end**

12   Move the leader solution to the end and forward one of the solutions
   following it to the leader position;

13 **end**

14 return the best solution in the flock;

---

5   Computational Experiments

The MBO algorithms for machine-part cell formation was coded in Java SE-1.7
(Java SE 7, 1.7.0_55) and was run on a computer MacBook Pro (Retina, 13-inch,
Late 2013) with an Intel Core i5 Processor 2.4 GHz, 4 GB RAM 1600 MHz DDR3
and Video Card Intel Iris 1536 MB running OS X Yosemite version 10.10.4. We
have tested 90 problems (10 instances considerering 5 values of $Mmax$ for $C = 2$
(Cells) and 10 intances considering 4 values of $Mmax$ for $C = 3$, see Tables 2
and 3).

Such 90 problems have been taken from Boctor's experiments [4] in order to
compare it with previous work. To consider the parameters used by MBO, the
best values reported by Duman et al. [7], $n = 51, k = 3, m = 10$ and $x = 1$.
In addition to the K (iteration limit) setting a value of 1020 is assigned. Each
experiment was executed 100 times.

Tables 2 and 3 contrasts the optimun value reached by using different techniques for the 90 problems. Column 1 (Instance) corresponds to the identifier
assigned to each instance, column 2 (Boctor Problem) represents the identifier
of the 10 Boctor problems [4], column 3 (Mmax) corresponds to the maximum
number of machines per cell, column 4 (Optimum Value) depicts the optimum
value for the given problem, column 5 (MBO-Optimum) the best value reached
by using Migrating Birds Optimization, column 6 (MBO-Average) the average
value of 100 executiones is depicted, column 7 (MBO-RPD%) represents the

Table 2. Experiments using $C = 2$: Optimum values for Migrating Birds Optimization (MBO), Simulated Annealing (SA), and Particle Swarm Optimization (PSO).

Instance	Boctor Problem	Mmax	Optimum Value	MBO			SA	PSO
				Optimum	Average	RPD%	Optimum	Optimum
1	1	8	11	11	12.81	0.00	11	11
2	1	9	11	11	11.42	0.00	11	11
3	1	10	11	11	11.27	0.00	11	11
4	1	11	11	11	11.65	0.00	11	11
5	1	12	11	11	12.95	0.00	11	11
6	2	8	7	7	7.82	0.00	7	7
7	2	9	6	6	7.3	0.00	6	6
8	2	10	4	4	5.43	0.00	10	5
9	2	11	3	3	3.86	0.00	4	4
10	2	12	3	3	3.73	0.00	3	4
11	3	8	4	4	5.22	0.00	5	5
12	3	9	4	4	5.29	0.00	4	4
13	3	10	4	4	5.19	0.00	4	5
14	3	11	3	3	3.95	0.00	4	4
15	3	12	1	1	2.62	0.00	4	3
16	4	8	14	14	15.1	0.00	14	15
17	4	9	13	13	13.37	0.00	13	13
18	4	10	13	13	13.47	0.00	13	13
19	4	11	13	13	13.68	0.00	13	13
20	4	12	13	13	13.65	0.00	13	13
21	5	8	9	9	9.92	0.00	9	10
22	5	9	6	6	7.1	0.00	6	8
23	5	10	6	6	6.98	0.00	6	6
24	5	11	5	5	5.9	0.00	7	5
25	5	12	4	4	5.06	0.00	4	5
26	6	8	5	5	6.69	0.00	5	5
27	6	9	3	3	3.77	0.00	3	3
28	6	10	3	3	4.08	0.00	5	3
29	6	11	3	3	4.03	0.00	3	4
30	6	12	2	2	2.74	0.00	3	4
31	7	8	7	7	7.81	0.00	7	7
32	7	9	4	4	6.02	0.00	4	5
33	7	10	4	4	5.26	0.00	4	5
34	7	11	4	4	5.32	0.00	4	5
35	7	12	4	4	5.24	0.00	4	5
36	8	8	13	13	13.7	0.00	13	14
37	8	9	10	10	11.66	0.00	20	11
38	8	10	8	8	9.19	0.00	15	10
39	8	11	5	5	6.22	0.00	11	6
40	8	12	5	5	7	0.00	7	6
41	9	8	8	8	9.9	0.00	13	9
42	9	9	8	8	9.85	0.00	8	8
43	9	10	8	8	9.64	0.00	8	8
44	9	11	5	5	6.77	0.00	8	5
45	9	12	5	5	6.91	0.00	8	8
46	10	8	8	8	8.95	0.00	8	9
47	10	9	5	5	6.31	0.00	5	8
48	10	10	5	5	6.29	0.00	5	7
49	10	11	5	5	5.84	0.00	5	7
50	10	12	5	5	6.41	0.00	5	6

difference between the best known optimun value and the best optimum value reached by MBO in terms of percentage, column 8 (SA-Optimum) the best value using Simulated Annealing [4, 29], and column 9 (PSO-Optimum) the optimun value using Particle Swarm Optimization [8, 9].

As can be observed (see Tables 2 and 3), the algorithm MBO able to find an optimal solution to all problems and takes the first place. Table 4 summarizes

Table 3. Experiments using $C = 3$: Optimum values for Migrating Birds Optimization (MBO), Simulated Annealing (SA), and Particle Swarm Optimization (PSO).

Instance	Boctor Problem	Mmax	Optimum Value	MBO			SA	PSO
				Optimum	Average	RPD%	Optimum	Optimum
51	1	6	27	27	29.44	0.00	28	-
52	1	7	18	18	20.77	0.00	18	-
53	1	8	11	11	13.22	0.00	11	-
54	1	9	11	11	12.23	0.00	11	-
55	2	6	7	7	9.08	0.00	7	-
56	2	7	6	6	7.42	0.00	6	-
57	2	8	6	6	7.01	0.00	7	-
58	2	9	6	6	7.33	0.00	6	-
59	3	6	9	9	10.08	0.00	12	-
60	3	7	4	4	6.67	0.00	8	-
61	3	8	4	4	5.51	0.00	8	-
62	3	9	4	4	4.84	0.00	4	-
63	4	6	27	27	28.03	0.00	27	-
64	4	7	18	18	20	0.00	18	-
65	4	8	14	14	15.71	0.00	14	-
66	4	9	13	13	14.42	0.00	13	-
67	5	6	11	11	12.29	0.00	11	-
68	5	7	8	8	9.55	0.00	9	-
69	5	8	8	8	9.53	0.00	9	-
70	5	9	6	6	7.82	0.00	8	-
71	6	6	6	6	6.97	0.00	8	-
72	6	7	4	4	5.72	0.00	5	-
73	6	8	4	4	5.39	0.00	5	-
74	6	9	3	3	4.64	0.00	4	-
75	7	6	11	11	13.21	0.00	11	-
76	7	7	5	5	6.37	0.00	5	-
77	7	8	5	5	7.1	0.00	5	-
78	7	9	4	4	6.35	0.00	5	-
79	8	6	14	14	15.11	0.00	14	-
80	8	7	11	11	12.71	0.00	11	-
81	8	8	11	11	13.23	0.00	11	-
82	8	9	10	10	11.69	0.00	10	-
83	9	6	12	12	14.39	0.00	12	-
84	9	7	12	12	13.42	0.00	12	-
85	9	8	8	8	10.73	0.00	13	-
86	9	9	8	8	9.68	0.00	8	-
87	10	6	10	10	13	0.00	12	-
88	10	7	8	8	9.32	0.00	14	-
89	10	8	8	8	9.14	0.00	8	-
90	10	9	5	5	7.45	0.00	8	-

the optimal amount that have reached MBO, SA and PSO for each instance of Boctor's problem. The experimental results shows that the proposed MBO provides high quality solutions and good performance within 2 and 3 cells reaching RPD% = 0 for all tested instances. Figure 5 shows the graph of convergence for instance number 55 (Boctor Problem 2 solved by MBO with $C = 3$, $Mmax = 6$ and Optimum value = 7). MBO has a rapid convergence (left graph in Fig. 5), this is because employing a mechanism neighboring solutions shared with the next solution. Therefore, the algorithm MBO found the optimum value for the instance 55 in the iteration number 2. For a more detailed view of the convergence of the algorithm MBO, a modification of pseudocode MBO was developed ignoring lines 6 and 9, subsequently increased iteration after line 12 was

Table 4. Number of optimal values reached.

Meta-heuristic	C = 2					C = 3			
	M8	M9	M10	M11	M12	M6	M7	M8	M9
MBO	10	10	10	10	10	10	10	10	10
SA	8	9	7	5	6	6	6	5	6
PSO	4	6	5	4	2	-	-	-	-

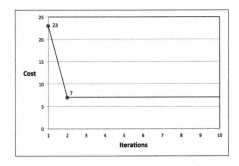 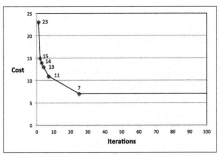

Fig. 5. Convergence chart for Instance 55.

implemented. The results of these changes can be seen in Fig. 5 (see chart right) with the best evaluations of the objective function (see Eq. 1).

6   Conclusions

In this paper, a new approach for machine-part cell formation problem based on migrating birds optimization has been proposed. The result obtained in the computational experiences carried out show that proposed algorithm can generate optimal. The comparisons between MBO and other metaheuristics indicates that our algorithm is a better algorithm for solving machine-part cell formation problem. Indeed, the global optimum was reached in all instances. This is because MBO has a rapid convergence, mainly because it uses a mechanism to share neighboring solutions to the next solution. In future steps, the algorithm will be applicate to a variety with larger problems. In addition, parameter optimization and other approaches are also topics for future research.

Acknowledgements. Boris Almonacid is supported by Postgraduate Grant Pontificia Universidad Católica de Valparaíso 2015 (INF-PUCV 2015). Ricardo Soto is supported by Grant CONICYT / FONDECYT / INICIACION / 11130459. Broderick Crawford is supported by Grant CONICYT / FONDECYT / REGULAR / 1140897. Fernando Paredes is supported by Grant CONICYT / FONDECYT / 1130455.

References

1. Alkaya, A.F., Algin, R.: Metaheuristic based solution approaches for the obstacle neutralization problem. Expert Syst. Appl. **42**(3), 1094–1105 (2015)
2. Badgerow, J.P., Hainsworth, F.R.: Energy savings through formation flight? a re-examination of the vee formation. J. Theor. Biol. **93**(1), 41–52 (1981)
3. Bajec, I.L., Heppner, F.H.: Organized flight in birds. Anim. Behav. **78**(4), 777–789 (2009)
4. Boctor, F.: A linear formulation of the machine-part cell formation problem. Int. J. Prod. Res. **29**(2), 343–356 (1991)
5. Burbidge, J.L.: Production flow analysis. Prod. Eng. **42**(12), 742–752 (1963)
6. Crawford, B., Soto, R., Zuñiga, G., Monfroy, E., Paredes, F.: Modeling manufacturing cell design problems: CP vs. MH. In: Stephanidis, C. (ed.) HCI 2014, Part I. CCIS, vol. 434, pp. 498–502. Springer, Heidelberg (2014)
7. Duman, E., Uysal, M., Alkaya, A.F.: Migrating birds optimization: a new metaheuristic approach and its performance on quadratic assignment problem. Inf. Sci. **217**, 65–77 (2012)
8. Duran, O., Rodriguez, N., Consalter, L.A.: Hybridization of PSO and a discrete position update scheme techniques for manufacturing cell design. In: Gelbukh, A., Morales, E.F. (eds.) MICAI 2008. LNCS (LNAI), vol. 5317, pp. 503–512. Springer, Heidelberg (2008)
9. Durán, O., Rodriguez, N., Consalter, L.A.: Collaborative particle swarm optimization with a data mining technique for manufacturing cell design. Expert Syst. Appl. **37**(2), 1563–1567 (2010)
10. Gunasingh, K.R., Lashkari, R.: Simultaneous grouping of parts and machines in cellular manufacturing systemsan integer programming approach. Comput. Ind. Eng. **20**(1), 111–117 (1991)
11. Hummel, D., Beukenberg, M.: Aerodynamische interferenzeffekte beim formationsflug von vögeln. J. für Ornithologie **130**(1), 15–24 (1989)
12. Joines, J.A., Kay, M.G., King, R.E., Thomas Culbreth, C.: A hybrid genetic algorithm for manufacturing cell design. J. Chin. Inst. Ind. Eng. **17**(5), 549–564 (2000)
13. Kusiak, A.: The part families problem in flexible manufacturing systems. Ann. Oper. Res. **3**(6), 277–300 (1985)
14. Li, X., Baki, M., Aneja, Y.P.: An ant colony optimization metaheuristic for machine-part cell formation problems. Comput. Oper. Res. **37**(12), 2071–2081 (2010)
15. Lissaman, P., Shollenberger, C.A.: Formation flight of birds. Science **168**(3934), 1003–1005 (1970)
16. Lozano, S., Adenso-Diaz, B., Eguia, I., Onieva, L., et al.: A one-step tabu search algorithm for manufacturing cell design. J. Oper. Res. Soc. **50**(5), 509–516 (1999)
17. Mosier, C., Taube, L.: The facets of group technology and their impacts on implementationa state-of-the-art survey. Omega **13**(5), 381–391 (1985)
18. Niroomand, S., Hadi-Vencheh, A., Şahin, R., Vizvari, B.: Modified migrating birds optimization algorithm for closed loop layout with exact distances in flexible manufacturing systems. Expert Syst. Appl. **42** (2015)
19. Pan, Q.K., Dong, Y.: An improved migrating birds optimisation for a hybrid flowshop scheduling with total flowtime minimisation. Inf. Sci. **277**, 643–655 (2014)
20. Purcheck, G.F.K.: A linear-programming method for the combinatorial grouping of an incomplete power set. J. Cybern. **5**(4), 51–76 (1975)

21. Rayner, J.: A new approach to animal flight mechanics. J. Exp. Biol. **80**(1), 17–54 (1979)
22. Seifoddini, H., Hsu, C.P.: Comparative study of similarity coefficients and clustering algorithms in cellular manufacturing. J. Manuf. Syst. **13**(2), 119–127 (1994)
23. Selim, H., Askin, R., Vakharia, A.: Cell formation in group technology: review, evaluation and directions for future research. Comput. Ind. Eng. **34**(1), 3–20 (1998)
24. Shafer, S.M., Rogers, D.F.: A goal programming approach to the cell formation problem. J. Oper. Manage. **10**(1), 28–43 (1991)
25. Soto, R., Kjellerstrand, H., Durán, O., Crawford, B., Monfroy, E., Paredes, F.: Cell formation in group technology using constraint programming and boolean satisfiability. Expert Syst. Appl. **39**(13), 11423–11427 (2012)
26. Soto, R., Kjellerstrand, H., Gutiérrez, J., López, A., Crawford, B., Monfroy, E.: Solving manufacturing cell design problems using constraint programming. In: Jiang, H., Ding, W., Ali, M., Wu, X. (eds.) IEA/AIE 2012. LNCS, vol. 7345, pp. 400–406. Springer, Heidelberg (2012)
27. Venugopal, V., Narendran, T.: A genetic algorithm approach to the machine-component grouping problem with multiple objectives. Comput. Ind. Eng. **22**(4), 469–480 (1992)
28. Wu, T.H., Low, C., Wu, W.T.: A tabu search approach to the cell formation problem. Int. J. Adv. Manuf. Technol. **23**(11–12), 916–924 (2004)
29. Wu, T.H., Chang, C.C., Chung, S.H.: A simulated annealing algorithm for manufacturing cell formation problems. Expert Syst. Appl. **34**(3), 1609–1617 (2008)

Solving Manufacturing Cell Design Problems Using an Artificial Fish Swarm Algorithm

Ricardo Soto[1,2,3], Broderick Crawford[1,4,5], Emanuel Vega[1(✉)], and Fernando Paredes[6]

[1] Pontificia Universidad Católica de Valparaíso, Valparaíso, Chile
{ricardo.soto,broderick.crawford}@ucv.cl, emanuelvm88@gmail.com
[2] Universidad Autónoma de Chile, Temuco, Chile
[3] Universidad Científica del Sur, Lima, Peru
[4] Universidad Central de Chile, Santiago, Chile
[5] Universidad San Sebastián, Santiago, Chile
[6] Escuela de Ingeniería Industrial, Universidad Diego Portales, Santiago, Chile
fernando.paredes@udp.cl

Abstract. The design of manufacturing cells is a manufacturing strategy that involves the creation of an optimal design of production plants, whose main objective is to minimize movements and exchange of material between these cells. Optimal solution of large scale manufacturing cell design problems (MCDPs) are often computationally unfeasible and only heuristic and approximate methods are able to handle such problems. Artificial fish swarm algorithm (AFSA) belongs to the swarm intelligence algorithms, which based on population search, are able to solve complex optimization problems. In this paper we present an AFSA-based approach to solve the MCDP by using the classic Boctor's mathematical model. The obtained results show that the proposed algorithm produces optimal solutions for all the 50 studied instances.

Keywords: Manufacturing cell design problem · Artificial fish swarm algorithm · Metaheuristic

1 Introduction

The design of manufacturing cells has emerged in the last two decades as innovation for manufacturing strategy, this strategy involves the creation of an optimal design of production plants. The manufacturing cell design problem (MCDP) considers grouping similar parts into part-families. Ideally, each of these families is processed by a dedicated cluster of manufacturing facilities called manufacturing cell, where the main goal is to minimize movement and exchange of material between cells. In this context, the cell formation problem has been matter of considerable research, where Burbidge with his production flow analysis in 1963, becomes one of the first to propose a process to solve this concern.

© Springer International Publishing Switzerland 2015
G. Sidorov and S.N. Galicia-Haro (Eds.): MICAI 2015, Part I, LNAI 9413, pp. 282–290, 2015.
DOI: 10.1007/978-3-319-27060-9_23

In this paper, we propose an Artificial Fish Swarm Algorithm (AFSA) to solve the MCDP. The AFSA was presented by X.L. Li in 2002 [1], it is a technique based on swarm behaviors and was inspired from social conduct of fish swarm in nature. AFSA, works based on population, random search, and behaviorism. This algorithm has been used in optimization applications, such as clustering [2,3], machine learning [4,5], PID control [6], data mining [7], and image segmentation [8]. We illustrate promising results where the proposed approach noticeable competes with previous reported techniques for solving manufacturing cell design problems.

The rest of this paper is organized as follows. In Sect. 2, we present the related work. Section 3 describes the mathematical model of the MCDP. The AFSA is explained in Sect. 4. Finally, Sect. 5 illustrates the experimental results, followed by conclusions and future work.

2   Related Work

The problem of formulating cells has been the subject of considerable research, where Burbidge, with his production flow analysis in 1963, becomes one of the first to solve this problem [9]. Other approaches try to solve the MCDP by attempting to determine the part families, finding only partial solutions [9,10]. Most of these methods are based on the incidence machine-part matrix, and can be divided into hierarchical and non-hierarchical clustering. For instance Shargal [11] presented search algorithms and clustering efficiency measures for machine-part matrix, Seifoddini and Hsu [12] work with clustering algorithms in cellular manufacturing, and Srinivasan [13] use clustering algorithm for machine cell formation in group technology using minimum spanning tree. Also, graph theoretical mathematical programming methods, for instance Deutsch [14] uses an improved p-median model for cell formation, Atmani [15] presents a mathematical programming approach to joint cell formation and operation allocation in cellular manufacturing, Adil [16] propose a mathematical model for cell formation considering investment and operational costs, Purcheck [18] presents a linear-programming method for the combinatorial grouping of an incomplete set, Olivia Lopez and Purcheck [19] works in a load balancing for group technology planning and control, and Boctor [9,20,21] presented work with cell formation. The implementation of approximate methods, such as metaheuristics, has been material of work for researchers devoted to solve cell formation problems.Durn, Rodriguez and Consalter [22] combines particle swarm optimization and discrete position update scheme techniques for manufacturing cell design. Wu, Chang, and Chung [23] present a simulated annealing (SA) approach, and Venugopal and Narendran [24] propose the use of genetic algorithms (GA), which would be used later by Gupta, Gupta, Kumar, and Sundaram [25] but focused in multiobjective optimization approach. In this paper, our goal is to employ a modern metaheuristic to report better solutions than the ones applied before to manufacturing cell design.

3   Manufacturing Cell Design Problem

Manufacturing strategy consisting in creating an optimal design of production plants, which are composed of manufacturing cells and machines that process subsets of parts forming families, determined according to the similarity of them. The objective is to minimize movement and exchange of material between cells, in order to reduce production costs and increase productivity. We represent the processing requirements of machine parts through an incidence matrix called machine-part. This matrix contains a binary domains and is denoted as A, where $a_{ij} = 1$ means that machine i is necessary to process part j and $a_{ij} = 0$ otherwise. A rigorous mathematical formulation of machine-part grouping problem with these objectives is given by Boctor [21] and its as follows:

- let M, the number of machines,
- let P, the number of parts,
- let C, the number of cells,
- let i, the index of machines (i = 1, ..., M),
- let j, the index of parts (j = 1, ..., P),
- let k, the index of cells (k = 1, ..., C),
- $A = [a_{ij}]$ the binary machine-part incidence matrix MxP,
- M_{max}, the maximum number of machines per cell. We selected as the objective function to be minimized the number of times that a given part must be processed by a machine that does not belong to the cell that the part has been assigned to. Let:

$$y_{ik} = \begin{cases} 1 & \text{if} \quad \text{machine} \quad i \in \text{cell} \quad k; \\ 0 & \text{otherwise}; \end{cases}$$

$$z_{jk} = \begin{cases} 1 & \text{if} \quad \text{part} \quad j \in \text{family} \quad k; \\ 0 & \text{otherwise}; \end{cases}$$

The problem is represented by the following mathematical model:

$$Minimize \sum_{k=1}^{C} \sum_{i=1}^{M} \sum_{j=1}^{P} a_{ij} z_{j_k} (1 - y_{i_k})$$

Subject to

$$\sum_{k=1}^{C} y_{ik} = 1 \qquad \forall i$$

$$\sum_{k=1}^{C} z_{jk} = 1 \qquad \forall j$$

$$\sum_{i=1}^{M} y_{ik} \leq M_{max} \qquad \forall k$$

4   Artificial Fish Swarm Algorithm

AFSA is an ordered and finite set of bionic operations for optimization, based on the study of intelligent behavior of the fish swarm. This means that, in an area of water, the fish can often find places that contain many nutrients by himself or following other fish. Therefore, where there is the largest number of fish is usually the place that has the most nutrients [26, 27].

4.1   Proposed Algorithm

AFSA simulates the behavior of a fish swarm, which shapes the Artificial Fish (AF) that seeks an optimal solution in the solution space. The AF perceives external concepts with sense of sight. Current position of AF is shown by vector $X = (X_1, X_2, ..., X_n)$. The visual is equal to sight field of AF and X_v is a position in visual where the AF wants to go. Then if X_v has better food consistence than current position of AF, it goes one step toward X_v which causes change in AF position from X to X_{next}, but if the current position of AF is better than X_v, it continues searching in his visual area. Food consistence in position X is the fitness value of the current position and it is shown with f(x). The step is equal to maximum length of the movement. The AF consists in two parts, variables and functions. Variables include X (current AF position), step (maximum length step), visual (sight field), *trynumber* (the maximum test interactions and tries) and crowd factor σ $(0 < \sigma < 1)$. Also his functions consist on the prey behavior, free move behavior, swarm behavior and follow behavior. In each step for the optimization process the AF search for locations with better fitness values all over the search space, the AF is behaviors are explained:

1. Prey behavior: This behavior is an individual behavior that each AF performs independently and performs a local search around itself. Every AF by performing this behavior attempts try-number times to move to a new position with better fitness.
2. Follow behavior: The best AF of the swarm locates the best found position so far by the swarm. In follow behavior, each of AF moves one step toward the best AF of swarm.
3. Swarm behavior: To ensure the security and integrity of each AF, they trend to group up. This, they follow 3 basis rules, separation, alignment and cohesion.
4. Free Move behavior: This is a special behavior where the AF search for a random position, if it is not a better one, the AF will go through a modification of the new step to ensure not to be stagated in a local optimum, otherwise the AF will move ahead.

Performing these four behaviors based on an algorithm procedure [28] it is described as follows:

1. Initialization;
2. Calculate the fitness value;
3. For each AFi, where (i = 1, 2, .., N);
   3.1 Follow behavior; determine whether the state after the follow is better than the previous state, if so, advances to step 4, otherwise we resort to step 3.2;
   3.2 Prey behavior; determine whether the search state is better than the old one *Trynumber* times, if so proceeds to step 4, otherwise we resort to Step 3.3;
   3.3 Swarm behavior; determine whether the state after grouping is better than previous state, if so, advances to step 4, otherwise we resort to step 3.4;
   3.4 Movement;
4. Refresh the current best value;
5. If it concludes the number of Iterations, out; otherwise, return to step 3;

5 Experimental Result

The effectiveness of our proposed approach has been tested using the incidence matrices [21]. In this paper these 10 problems were solved using the model presented in Sect. 2 with different sets of parameters. For the experimental evaluation, the parameters employed are defined as follows: 16 Machines, 30 Parts, and a combination between 2 Cells with 8, 9, 10, 11, 12 Mmax. Concerning the AFSA, the configuration uses 40 as initial population size, a crowd factor σ between 0.9 and 0.5 and *Trynumber* 4 and 50.000 iterations for the AFSA. The algorithm has been implemented using Java and launched on a 2.4 GHz Intel Core i7 with 8 GB RAM running Windows 8. Tables 1 and 2 show detailed information of the results obtained by our approach. Here, we compare our results with the ones reported in [21,22]. Concerning to the others values, represented as column OPT, is the Boctors values, column PSO, the best value obtained by Particle Swarm Optimization in [22], column SA, the best value obtained by Simulated Annealing reported in [21] and column AFSA, the best value obtained by our proposed AFSA. Table 3 shows the relative percentage derivation (RPD) and the average values of our AFSA in order to evaluate the quality of every solution.

According to Tables 1 and 2, results obtained by AFSA are better than or equal to those reported result by PSO and SA in all the test problems from the literature. To be more specific, the proposed AFSA has high quality solutions and good performance. Thus, shown in Fig. 1, we illustrate the convergence rate by AFSA accomplishing robust search capability in early stages. Also, it is reported by the RPD value the quality, which quantifies the deviation of the objective value that our approach has a high consistency on it is solutions.

Table 1. Results of AFSA using 2 cells

Pblm	Mmax = 8				Mmax = 9				Mmax = 10			
	Opt	SA	PSO	AFSA	Opt	SA	PSO	AFSA	Opt	SA	PSO	AFSA
1	11	11	11	11	11	11	11	11	11	11	11	11
2	7	7	7	7	6	6	6	6	4	10	5	4
3	4	5	5	4	4	4	4	4	4	4	5	4
4	14	14	15	14	13	13	13	13	13	13	13	13
5	9	9	10	9	6	6	8	6	6	6	6	6
6	5	5	5	5	3	3	3	3	3	5	3	3
7	7	7	7	7	4	4	5	4	4	4	5	4
8	13	13	14	13	10	20	11	10	8	15	10	8
9	8	13	9	8	8	8	8	8	8	8	8	8
10	8	8	9	8	5	5	8	5	5	5	7	5

Table 2. Results of AFSA using 2 cells

Pblm	Mmax = 11				Mmax = 12			
	Opt	SA	PSO	AFSA	Opt	SA	PSO	AFSA
1	11	11	11	11	11	11	11	11
2	3	4	4	3	3	3	4	3
3	3	4	4	3	1	4	3	1
4	13	13	13	13	13	13	13	13
5	5	7	5	5	4	4	5	4
6	3	3	4	3	2	3	4	2
7	4	4	5	4	4	4	5	4
8	5	11	6	5	5	7	6	5
9	5	8	5	5	5	8	8	5
10	5	5	7	5	5	5	6	5

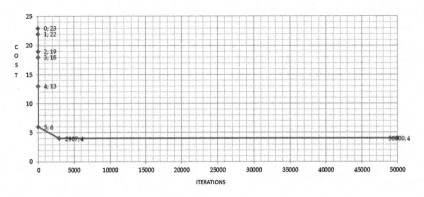

Fig. 1. Graph of Problem 7 solved by AFSA with Mmax 10

Table 3. Average and relative percentage derivation

Pblm	Mmax = 8		Mmax = 9		Mmax = 10		Mmax = 11		Mmax = 12	
	Avg	RPD (%)	Avg	RPD (%)	Avg	RPD (%)	Avg	RPD (%)	Avg	RPD (%)
1	11	0	11	0	11	0	11	0	11	0
2	7	0	6	0	4	0	3	0	3	0
3	4	0	4	0	4	0	3	0	1	0
4	14	0	13	0	13	0	13	0	13	0
5	9	0	6	0	6	0	5	0	4	0
6	5	0	3	0	3	0	3	0	2	0
7	7	0	4	0	4	0	4	0	4	0
8	13	0	10	0	8	0	5	0	5	0
9	8	0	8	0	8	0	5	0	5	0
10	8	0	5	0	5	0	5	0	5	0

6 Conclusion and Future Work

The metaheuristic usually applies to problems that have no specific algorithm or heuristic that gives a satisfactory solution. Thus, we employed the search algorithm AFSA to tackle the design of manufacturing cells, where the execution of the natural behaviors, minimizes the movement and exchange of material between cells; looking for an optimization of time and costs. The convergence rate demonstrated by AFSA, it is related to the values of its parameters. Initially high values are used, such as a crowd factor σ of 0.8 or a *Trynumber* of 20. After analyzing the results it is concluded that the use of parameters with smaller or dynamic values improve the performance. Also, parameters as crowd factor, *Trynumber*, and distance calculation were tuned from his original values, standard AFSA, and example is the use of Hamming distance. We also applied fix to possible solutions that could not satisfy the constraint and fixed the swarm behavior to be more compatible with the nature of the problem ending with better results and convergence rate.

Also, there are some relevant works to pursue in the future. First, change how we tackle the MCDP, there is some heavy initial work done to set good initialization, and for every time we generate the matrix part-cell. Second, work on a better adaptation of the swarm behavior, this will benefit also to improve the efficiency of the algorithm.

Acknowledgements. Ricardo Soto is supported by Grant CONICYT/FONDECYT/ INICIACION/11130459, Broderick Crawford is supported by Grant CONICYT/FON-DECYT/1140897, and Fernando Paredes is supported by Grant CONICYT/FON-DECYT/1130455.

References

1. Li, L.X., Shao, Z.J., Qian, J.X.: An optimizing method based on autonomous animate: fish swarm algorithm. In: Proceeding of System Engineering Theory and Practice, pp. 32–38 (2002)
2. Hi, S., Belacel, N., Hamam, H., Bouslimani, Y.: Fuzzy clustering with improved artificial fish swarm algorithm. In: International Joint Conference on Computational Sciences and Optimization 2009, Hainan, pp. 317–321 (2009)
3. Xiao, L.: A clustering algorithm based on artificial fish swarm. In: 2nd International Conference on Computer Engineering and Technology, Chengdu, pp. 766–769 (2010)
4. Yazdani, D., Golyari, S., Meybodi, M.R.: A new hybrid algorithm for optimization based on artificial fish swarm algorithm and cellular learning automata. In: 5 International Symposium on Telecommunication (IST), Tehran, pp. 932–937 (2010)
5. Yazdani, D., Nadjaran Toosi, A., Meybodi, M.R.: Fuzzy adaptive artificial fish swarm algorithm. In: 23rd Australian Conference on Artificial Intelligent, Adelaide (2010)
6. Luo, Y., Zhang, J., Li, X.: The optimization of PID controller parameters based on artificial fish swarm algorithm. In: IEEE International Conference on Automation and Logistics, Jinan, pp. 1058–1062 (2007)
7. Zhang, M., Shao, C., Li, M., Sun, J.: Mining classification rule with artificial fish swarm. In: 6 World Congress on Intelligent Control and Automation, Dalian, pp. 5877–5881 (2006)
8. Li, C.X., Ying, Z., JunTao, S., Qing, S.J.: Method of image segmentation based on fuzzy c-means clustering algorithm and artificial fish swarm algorithm. In: International Conference on Intelligent Computing and Integrated Systems (ICISS), Guilin (2010)
9. Xambre, A.R., Vilarinho, P.M.: A simulated annealing approach for manufacturing cell formation with multiple identical machines. Eur. J. Oper. Res. **151**, 434–446 (2003)
10. Kusiak, A.: The part families problem in flexible manufacturing systems. Ann. Oper. Res. **3**, 279–300 (1985)
11. Shargal, M., Shekhar, S., Irani, S.A.: Evaluation of search algorithms and clustering efficiency measures for machine-part matrix clustering. IIE Trans. **27**(1), 43–59 (1995)
12. Seifoddini, H., Hsu, C.-P.: Comparative study of similarity coefficients and clustering algorithms in cellular manufacturing. J. Manuf. Syst. **13**(2), 119–127 (1994)
13. Srinivasan, G.: A clustering algorithm for machine cell formation in group technology using minimum spanning tree. Int. J. Prod. Res. **32**(9), 2149–2158 (1994)
14. Deutsch, S.J., Freeman, S.F., Helander, M.: Manufacturing cell formation using an improved p-median model. Comput. Ind. Eng. **34**(1), 135–146 (1998)
15. Atmani, A., Lashkari, R.S., Caron, R.J.: A mathematical programming approach to joint cell formation and operation allocation in cellular manufacturing. Int. J. Prod. Res. **33**(1), 1–15 (1995)
16. Adil, G.K., Rajamani, D., Strong, D.: A mathematical model for cell formation considering investment and operational costs. Eur. J. Oper. Res. **69**(3), 330–341 (1993)
17. Kusiak, A., Chow, W.: Efficient solving of the group technology problem. J. Manuf. Syst. **6**, 117–124 (1987)

18. Purcheck, G.: A linear-programming method for the combinatorial grouping of an incomplete set. J. Cybern. **5**, 51–58 (1975)
19. Olivia-Lopez, E., Purcheck, G.: Load balancing for group technology planning and control. Int. J. MTDR **19**, 259–268 (1979)
20. Soto, R., Kjellerstrand, H., Durn, O., Crawford, B., Monfroy, E., Paredes, F.: Cell formation in group technology using constraint programming and Boolean satisfiability. Expert Syst. Appl. **39**, 11423–11427 (2012)
21. Boctor, F.F.: A linear formulation of the machine-part cell formation problem. Int. J. Prod. Res. **29**(2), 343–356 (1991)
22. Durn, O., Rodriguez, N., Consalter, L.: Collaborative particle swarm optimization with a data mining technique for manufacturing cell design. Expert Syst. Appl. **37**(2), 1563–1567 (2010)
23. Wu, T., Chang, C., Chung, S.: A simulated annealing algorithm for manufacturing cell formation problems. Expert Syst. Appl. **34**(3), 1609–1617 (2008)
24. Venugopal, V., Narendran, T.T.: A genetic algorithm approach to the machine-component grouping problem with multiple objectives. Comput. Ind. Eng. **22**(4), 469–480 (1992)
25. Gupta, Y., Gupta, M., Kumar, A., Sundaram, C.: A genetic algorithm-based approach to cell composition and layout design problems. Int. J. Prod. Res. **34**(2), 447–482 (1996)
26. Yazdani, D., Golyari, S., Reza, M.M.: A new hybrid approach for data clustering. In: 5th International Symposium on Telecommunication (IST), Tehran, pp. 932–937 (2010)
27. Wang, L., Ma, L.: A hybrid artificial fish swarm algorithm for bin-packing problem. In: International Conference on Electronic and Mechanical Engineering and Information Technology, pp. 27–29 (2011)
28. Zhang, M., et al.: Mining classification rule with artificial fish swarm, pp. 5877–5881 (2006)

Neural Networks

A Simple Bio-Inspired Model for Synaptogenesis in Artificial Neural Networks

Alexander Espinosa Garcia[(⊠)] and Jonatan Gomez Perdomo

Universidad Nacional de Colombia, Bogotá, Colombia
{aespinosag,jgomezpe}@unal.edu.co
http://www.unal.edu.co

Abstract. Neural network morphology in Artificial Neural Networks (ANN) is typically designed depending on specific learning purposes. Biological neural networks, on the contrary, generate their morphology using biochemical markers secreted by each neuron. Specific features such as molecular signalling, electrochemical alphabet and neurite propagation rules are genetically encoded. However, the environment plays also a critical role in network morphology. Neurites are propagated through tissues to reach target neurons, following paths defined by the diffusion of molecular markers. Neurite paths are affected among other phenomena by competence for synaptic resources and volumetric economy.

Along this paper we observe some of the mechanisms of biological morphogenesis and their mathematical models. We analyze neurite navigation in short distances using local random propagation rules. Then, using reaction-difussion patterns, the process of molecular signalling and its influence in network morphology is studied. Finally we combine both strategies to generate morphology in ANN's.

Keywords: Artificial neural network · Synaptogenesis · Morphogenesis · Reaction-diffusion pattern · Artificial life

1 Introduction

While the architecture of artificial neural networks is usually defined at design time, a biological neural network builds its interconnections among neurons progressively by projecting its neurites into the surrounding space. Connection patterns of these neurons are determined by a set of chemical messengers produced by each neuron. These substances act as markers between neurites and their target neurons [22].

Since morphology has great importance in the network ability to learn [16], it is important to understand the factors influencing network structure that can be used to modify artificial neural networks configuration. These factors include dendritic growth affected by environment (such as in diffusion limited aggregation) [16] and neuritic projection determined mainly by genetic rules, which

J. Gomez Perdomo—Universidad Nacional de Colombia. ALIFE research group.

G. Sidorov and S.N. Galicia-Haro (Eds.): MICAI 2015, Part I, LNAI 9413, pp. 293–305, 2015.
DOI: 10.1007/978-3-319-27060-9_24

in ANN's are simulated by using techniques such as simple rules of propagation, fractal and differential growth equations or simulation of chemoattractive concentrations [21].

Although in both neurology and in axonal growth simulation, the random interconnection model is frequently used [5], research studies in live neural tissue, state that there are elements of molecular type affecting the behavior of the neuritic cones and consequently the navigation of axon and dendrites through the interneuronal space [2,3,16]. According to these research, the morphology of biological neural networks results from both the random propagation of neurites and molecular guidance secreted by neurons themselves.

In the first section of this paper, we will study the morphogenesis conditions observed in biological nervous systems and the relevant behavior models. First, we study random behavior of neurites growth, especially in short distances among neurons where molecular markers have low effect on the trend of growth cones direction. Later we examine molecular markers as synaptogenesis mechanism and the reaction-diffusion process that produces interconnection patterns in living tissues. Particularly, we focus on the Gierer-Meinhardt reaction-diffusion model, in order to simulate characteristic patterns observed in biological nervous tissues as morphogenesis determinants.

In subsequent sections a simulation model is proposed to generate architecture of artificial neural networks using concepts and strategies presented in biological systems. The last part of this work analyzes simulation results in terms of number of synapses and time.

2   Random Neuritic Propagation

Neurons interconnect each other using body projections known as neurites. Afferent neurites are called dendrites and their work as inputs. The efferent neurites or axons are the mechanism to stimulate other neurons. Nerve morphology depends on the ability of the axon to reach other nerve cells through the extracellular medium to form a synaptic connection [23]. Neurites body is called growth cone and its distal part is a movable structure known as filopodia. This structure is responsible for guiding the axon tip through the extracellular environment [17]. The projection of the axon is the result of the generation of micro tubules formed by a globular protein called tubulin produced within the cell body [25]. The path followed by the axon is affected by the presence of molecular cues or messengers such as neurotrophins [18]. The cues are locally secreted by each cell according to its specific type within the nervous tissue [2,3].

Molecular guidance becomes less important, when the distance among neurons are in lengths shorter than 0.7 mm due to the difficulty of sustaining a steady gradient of markers [13]. In small volumes, where local distances are short, Braitenberg and Schuz propose a random approach that avoids the problems caused by the unsteady distributions of chemical cues in short distances [4].

Following these authors, Kaiser determines that a random process of neurite projection adequately mimics the average distances observed in neural living tissue [13]. Due to the properties of the neurite growth cone, projection is approximately in a straight line [1]. Forward advance changes when the filopodia detects a molecular cue or when it is obstaculized by other neurites. Thus the local interconnection is favored over the global one and competition for dendritic resources occurs. Axons unable to achieve local objectives, continue their progress depending on availability of tubulin [25]. In practice, the limitation on axonal growth results in a decrease of neurite diameter up to values below 0.5 microns [3].

3   Reaction-Difussion Mechanism in Neural Networks

Neurons produce specific neurotrophins that act as identifiers to guide the incoming axons [18]. These biochemical markers are diffused through the tissue [13], decreasing their concentration as they move away from the cell. The process of diffusion of these substances in the extracellular environment, is consistent with some of the patterns formally defined by Turing in his works about pattern generation by reaction-diffusion process [24]. Because of the diffusion of chemoattractants that identify each neuron, the network shows an emerging pattern of neuritic projections that follow these molecular clues [10]. The morphology of the interconnected network is affected not only by the reaction-diffusion between the different molecular markers, but also for competition between axons to reach the same target neuron [3]. Both the reactive and inhibitor substances are known as morphogens and determine the chemical pattern formation that axonal projections follow, as occurs in nerve regeneration described by Podhajsky as a reaction-diffusion system [20].

3.1   Reaction-Difussion Models Applied to Morphogenesis

According to models proposed by Belousov and Zhabotinsky, reaction-diffusion systems must be kept out of balance so that the generation of characteristic patterns occurs without violating the second law of thermodynamics [2,9]. Turing proposed a particular set of inestabilities to explain the occurrence of patterns present in living tissue such as skin [24]. Various models of reaction-diffusion behavior have been tested since then. Particularly in the neural network interconnection process, diverse pattern generation models are used, as in the case of research works about nerve regeneration, described by Gray-Scott [2], dendritic growth modeling using Van Der Pol-FitzHugh-Nagumo inestabilities and the models proposed by Schnakenberg, Gierer, Meinhardt and others [6,9,14].

3.2   The Gierer-Meinhardt Model of Reaction-Difussion

The reaction diffusion model proposed by Gierer and Meinhardt is an activator-inhibitor system that can be used to generate patterns similar to those of nervous tissues [2,3,9,12], this model allows the emergence of dense interconnection areas called patches, especially observed in cortex area [3]. The system consists of an autocatalytic activator denoted as u and an inhibitor v, spreading quickly.

The antagonism between the two components (u and v) leads to patterns with high and stable concentrations of each substance [3, 26]. The model studies the solution to the set of state equations [3, 8]:

$$\frac{\partial u}{\partial t} = D_u + \nabla^2 u + f_1(u, v), \frac{\partial v}{\partial t} = D_v + \nabla^2 v + f_2(u, v). \tag{1}$$

where $u(X, t)$ and $v(X, t)$ are the morphogen concetrations in position vector $X = (x, y)^T$ on a bounded domain $\mathbf{R}^2$, where D_u and D_v are the positive diffusion coefficients of each morphogen, the two-dimensional Laplacian operator has the form:

$$\nabla^2 = \frac{\partial^2}{\partial x^2} + \frac{\partial^2}{\partial y^2}. \tag{2}$$

Functions f_1 and f_2 describe the mobility behavior of concentrations due to the reaction between morphogens [8]. In the Gierer-Meinhardt model [9] these functions correspond to:

$$f_1(u, v) = \frac{ru^2}{v} - \mu u + r. \tag{3}$$

and

$$f_2(u, v) = ru^2 - \alpha v. \tag{4}$$

With r, μ and α positive constants whose values appropriately selected allow the morphogens converge to a spatial distribution pattern of concentrations in equilibrium.

3.3   The Gierer-Meinhardt Model Implementation

The simplest procedure to discretize the Laplacian of reaction-diffusion equation is finite differences method [7, 14, 15]. Assuming a space constructed in a regular grid where each point contains some degree of concentration. A distribution of discrete values in each point is calculated depending on the concentration values in neighbor points [7, 14].

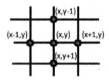

Fig. 1. Five points stencil used for gradient concentration calculation

This discretization can be obtained simply by Taylor series. In this way a five points calculation stencil, as shown in Fig. 1, is used to obtain a concentration value in each assembly point (x, y): First $f(x, y)$ concentration function is evaluated in each neighbor point according to the stencil. And with $f_1(x, y)$ defined as:

$$f_1(x, y) = f(x + 1, y) + f(x - 1, y) + f(x, y - 1) + f(x, y + 1). \tag{5}$$

Gradient is calculated using

$$\nabla^2 f(x, y) = \frac{f1(x, y)}{h^2}. \tag{6}$$

where h is the distance between each near point and the point under consideration. Finite difference method calculates the value of the Laplacian. Time related equation is calculated using the derivative definition by Euler's direct method. In the case of the two-dimensional grid, finite difference equation is:

$$f_{x,y}(t + \Delta t) = \begin{array}{l} f_{x,y}(t) + \frac{D\Delta t}{\Delta h}(f_{x-1,y}(t) + f_{x+1,y}(t) + \\ f_{x,y-1}(t) + f_{x,y-1}(t) - 4f_{x,y}(t)). \end{array} \tag{7}$$

The Eulers direct method slows down the simulation considerably because the method is stable only when the time increments Δt are very small, ($\frac{D\Delta t}{\Delta h} <$ 0.25). An alternative to it, in order to use larger intervals and thus increase the simulation speed is to use the Dufort-Frankel variant.

In this case the central difference takes into account the variation both in space and time. Thus the next step in the calculation is not directly dependent from the previous step. The difference equation can be presented as:

$$f_{x,y}(t + \Delta t) - f_{x,y}(t - \Delta t) = \begin{array}{l} \frac{D\Delta t}{\Delta h}(f_{x-1,y}(t) + f_{x+1,y}(t) + f_{x,y-1}(t) + \\ f_{x,y-1}(t) - 4f_{x,y}(t)). \end{array} \tag{8}$$

To compensate inestabilities derived from the calculations in time and space, each instance of calculated point in the right side is replaced by the average of the previous and next step:

$$f_{x,y}(t) = \frac{f_{x,y}(t + \Delta t) - f_{x,y}(t - \Delta t)}{2}. \tag{9}$$

Figure 2 shows the behavior of a reaction-diffusion system where both the activator and the inhibitor are distributed in random concentrations in a 400×400 points array. The rate of reaction and diffusion are equal in this simulation (0.5). it is possible to observe pattern generation of activator (dark grey) with stability trend over time. Stability of patterns is determined by the reaction and diffusion rates, as well as the initial concentration values for each substance.

3.4   Neuritic Branching Conditioned by Markers Concentration

In synaptogenesis process, the axon advances in an approximately lineal trajectory and is curved as it detects higher concentrations of molecular cues secreted

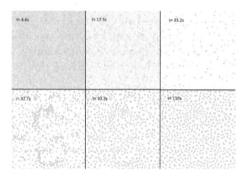

Fig. 2. Gierer - Meinhardt model evolution in time

by neurons [10]. Neurite extension occurs at an axon diameter cost, due to tubulin levels reduction in cell [3]. Along the projection occurs branching, where the concentrations of chemoattractants exceed threshold values [10]. A projection tends to make sharp bends when the tip finds higher concentrations of cues near the neurons. Once the point of greatest concentration is reached, the curvature is much less pronounced leading to a straight line for a closer approximation in the vicinity of the synapse [2,10]. Neurites not only increase their elongation but generate multiple branches as a result of a growth cone bifurcation or by interstitial branching along the neurite body [11]. Neuritic bifurcation may or may not occur and not necessarily a branch reaches a synaptic target. According to Gierer, branching occurs when the molecular guide is no longer detected in front of the neurite [10]. In this case an excitation occurs on the rear of the projecting cone, firing the projection of a new bifurcated growth cone.

4   Implementation and Results

Simulation scenario uses a 400×400 points matrix, where two values, corresponding to activator and inhibitor concentration are assigned to each point. A variable number of neurons (6 to 100 units) are located in the matrix to evaluate the effect of number of neurons in interconnection process. The maximum dendrite number in each neuron is programmable to study competence for synaptic resources. All the neurons are randomly distributed through the simulation matrix and each of them is used as activator secretion point by the reaction-difussion algorithm. Inhibitor substance represents other molecules normally present in nervous tissues, such as N-cadherins and other markers. Only one type of molecular cue is diffused through reaction diffusion matrix to keep simplicity and simulation speed, thus any neuron is able to interconnect with any other neuron present. There is no layer distribution as occurs in ANNs multi layered architectures.

4.1 Efferences Propagation Rules

Each axon initial point is located in the cartesian coordinates of corresponding neuron, from there, the axon propagates radially forward following a random straight path [13]. Efference projection algorithm analyzes activator concentration values surrounding the axon tip. If the activator concentration gradient inside detection radius around the neurite tip, is lower than a threshold then axon is projected with no deviation from the projection front. To mimic some obstacle effects, a random angle deviation (α) with low probability is introduced. This rule of propagation is showed in Fig. 3.

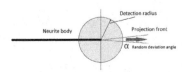

Fig. 3. Frontal propagation rule with low deviation probability due to very low activator concentration

A deviation from the line of forward propagation will occur when the sensing mechanism in the tip, detects activator concentration that exceeds the threshold for straight line projection but with a value lower than the bifurcation concentration threshold.

Deviation angle of propagation front is governed by the amount of activator near the tip. Angle will decrease as the value of gradient is closest to the threshold of straight trajectory and thus it will be greater as this value approaches the bifurcation threshold as depicted in Fig. 4. When a high activator concentration is detected behind the neurite tip, a low probability random mechanism determines whether a branch occurs or only a change in the propagation angle is calculated [10]. Probability of branching increases with the value of the concentration gradient and the angle of concentration variation respect to the neurite propagation front.

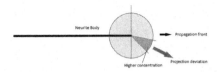

Fig. 4. Rule for deviation depending on high activator concentrations

Bifurcation angle cannot be greater than 120 degrees respect to the propagation front in order to comply with cost efficiency in volumetric branching as proposed by Murray [19]. A random value is introduced to increase the probability that the axon follows the highest concentration gradient shown in Fig. 5.

Due to progressive diameter loss, neurite projection affects its diameter. Axon is a conical structure called growth cone and its maximum elongation is determined by the neurite diameter. Loss of diameter ranges from 0.1 % to 10 % depending on whether a front projection or a bifurcation occurs [3].

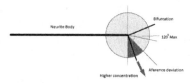

Fig. 5. Rule for axon bifurcation

Figure 6 shows the spread of axons following the rules set out above. In this picture, the marker concentration is calculated using the Gierer-Meinhardt reaction-diffusion model. Gray color indicates the concentration of activator present in each point of matrix, the axon propagation path is in red. Arborization pattern is produced from strong concentration changes behind propagation front. In low concentration variations where the neurite propagates forward, there is less than 0.1 % probability of branching.

4.2 Synaptogenesis

Synaptogenesis in live nervous tissue is a complex and little known process where not only dendrites and axons are involved, but the effect of other elements like glia and neurotransmitters flowing between neurons are important [3]. Dendritic tree projection to receive the presynaptic axons raises the complexity and the

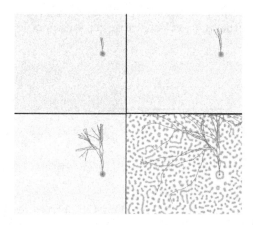

Fig. 6. Arborization pattern resulting of navigation rules and Gierer-Meinhardt model of reaction-diffusion (Color figure online)

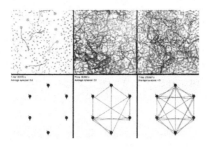

Fig. 7. Synaptogenesis process in a test with six neurons. Each neuron is color coded.

simulation time, limiting the number of neurons, axonal and dendritic branching and dendritic spaces that can be considered simultaneously.

According to the above and in order to simplify the process, the proposed model does not project dendritic afferences. Synapses is performed by using a rule of proximity between axonal tip and neuron position. Proximity measurement is carried out using the Manhattan distance algorithm, being a method best suited for matricial calculation with higher speed simulation than other computationally expensive techniques such as euclidean distance.

Figure 7 shows the evolution of the process of complete interconnection in a six neurons network. Initially, simulation spreads activator from the neurons and diffuses it through the matrix. Characteristic patterns are formed surrounding the neuron positions, stimulating mechanisms of propagation, angle deviation and axon bifurcations while mitigating the random navigation of efferences. First exploratory axon elongation occur near the 10 % of total simulation time, past 20 % of time the network is interconnected to the half the capacity of each neuron. After 50 % of simulation time, the network is nearly the full interconnection capacity for each neuron.

5 Results

Code to simulate the whole process is developed using java language. Hardware used consist of a system based on INTEL I5 first generation microprocessor with six gigabytes RAM capacity and supported by graphic hardware based on Nvidia GeForce GT435 graphics card. Space simulation is non-spherical and exclusively two-dimensional. The program calculates activator and inhibitor concentration values every twenty milliseconds and draws the reactiondiffusion patterns. Once obtained every new distribution, it analyzes the elongation paths of axonal projections from each neuron coordinates. The first set of experimentssimulate only random propagation rules of axons. Results for different populations of neurons randomly distributed in space of 400 × 400 pixels are presented.

Results establish how the propagation of molecular cues affect the neural interconnection rate. In order to study the independent effect of the random propagation rules described above, the first experiments apply such rules to a number of neuronal populations (6, 10, 50 and 100). Each set of experiments is composed of 20 simulations with different neuron position in each population. For all tests, the stop condition is reached when the average synapse number is greater than 50 % of number of neurons in the test. Figure 8 shows the behaviour of the frontal random propagation rules with no influence of molecular cues applied to the proposed neuron populations.

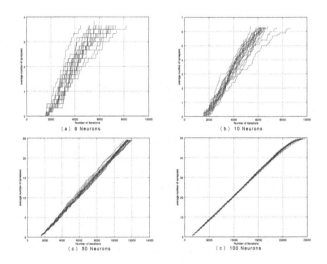

Fig. 8. Synaptogenesis using simple random frontal projection rules

Random exploration takes higher times of interconnection as is particularly showed in populations of 50 and 100 neuron. Low number of neurons populations take proportionaly more time due to low density of neurons. Axons must travel through bigger spaces where there are no clues to indicate the presence of neurons. Projections does not reach other neurons but grow until they diminish their growth cone to the minimum. In this case the program deletes the particular branch path and starts it again, delaying the interconection process.

In nervous tissues, specially in cortical areas, axon uses random propagation in order to avoid physical obstacles such as other axons and neurons before the neurite reaches its target. Clearly this type of propagation is not the main cause of morphogenesis in neuronal tissues due to this mechanism does not allows a significant number of synapses in relative short time.

In contrast, Fig. 9 shows an important decrement in time when the reaction-difussion model of molecular cues is added to the random propagation model in each population. In the Gierer Meinhardt model of reaction-diffusion, pattern and stability is affected by the rate of dispersion of the activator and the reaction rate of inhibitor. Some of the characteristic patterns like strips and spots are used in the simulation of axonal projection because of their tendency to form neurite patches near the spots obtained [2].

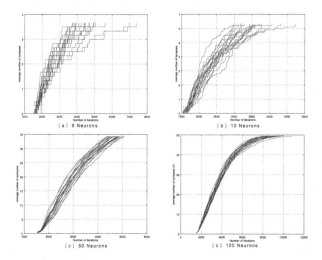

Fig. 9. Synaptogenesis applying random and pattern driven propagation strategies

In the simulated model, strips and spots pattern is obtained with stable activator reaction rates of 50 %. But other reaction rates (Dispersion rate = 0.78 %) lead to patterns similar to those studied by Turing or to a wide areas of activator diffusion (Dispersion rate = 90 %). Each set of patterns favors either random propagation rules or gradient guided propagation, each with longer times of morphogenesis as occurs in the Turing pattern case.

6   Conclusions

In relatively long inter-neuronal spaces, axons navigation is affected mainly by molecular patterns resulting of reaction-diffusion process. Random forward navigation is the main strategy when distances between neurons are short. Both strategies work together as an exploration and exploitation model with a particular intense effect when greater concentrations stimulate succesive bifurcations in one or more axons in neuron patchy areas.

The propagation mechanisms are affected by neuronal density. Network morphology is determined in short distances between neurons by random forward propagation where reaction-diffusion phenomena show no important variations in concentration. This means the morphogenesis can be accelerated by decreasing the size of simulation matrix.

As is showed by the experiments presented above, it is possible to generate morphology in articial neural networks using strategies observed in biological nervous tissues. Morphology is only a part of a more complex process that allows a network redistribute its interconnections to model different input patterns allowing to forget non used patterns and learn new ones in a more dynamic way than feedforward and other models of artificial neural networks.

This work concentrates only in neural networks morphogenesis causes. New studies are required to understand progressive synaptogenesis effects in the network learning capacity and how the emergent learning strategies can affect network morphology.

Acknowledgments. The authors wish to thank ALIFE research group at the Universidad Nacional de Colombia for their support in developing this research.

References

1. Achacoso, T.B., Yamamoto, W.S.: Ay's Neuroanatomy of C. Elegans for Computation. CRC Press, Boca Raton (1991)
2. Bauer, R.: Axon Guidance Using Turing Patterns in the Cortex. PhD thesis, Institute of Neuroinformatics (INI) (2008)
3. Bauer, R., Zubler, F., Hauri, A., Muir, D.R., Douglas, R.J.: Developmental origin of patchy axonal connectivity in the neocortex: a computational model. Cereb. Cortex **24**(2), 487–500 (2012)
4. Braitenberg, V., Schüz, A.: Cortex: Statistics and Geometry of Neuronal Connectivity. Springer, Heidelberg (1998)
5. Brunel, N.: Dynamics of sparsely connected networks of excitatory and inhibitory spiking neurons. Comput. Neurosci. **8**(3), 183–208 (2000)
6. Cartwright, J.H.E.: Labyrinthine turing pattern formation in the cerebral cortex. Theoret. Biol. **217**, 97–103 (2002)
7. Douglas, J., Russell, T.: Numerical methods for convection-dominated diffusion problems based on combining the method of characteristics with finite element or finite difference procedures. SIAM J. Numer. Anal. **19**, 871–885 (1982)
8. Garvie, M.R., Maini, P.K., Trenchea, C.: An efficient and robust numerical algorithm for estimating parameters in turing systems. Comput. Phys. **229**(19), 7058–7071 (2010)
9. Gierer, A., Meinhardt, H.: A theory of biological pattern formation. Kibernetik **12**(1), 30–39 (1972)
10. Gierer, A.: Directional cues for growing axons forming the retinotectal projection. Development **101**, 479–489 (1987)
11. Graham, B.P., van Ooyen, A.: Mathematical modelling and numerical simulation of the morphological development of neurons. BMC Neurosci. **7**, S9 (2006)
12. Grossberg, S.: On the development of feature detectors in the visual cortex with applications to learning and reaction-diffusion systems. Biol. Cybern. **21**(3), 145–159 (1976)
13. Kaiser, M., Hilgetag, C.C., van Ooyen, A.: A simple rule for axon outgrowth and synaptic competition generate realistic connection lengths and filling fractions. Cereb. Cortex **19**(12), 3001–3010 (2009)
14. Kamranian, M., Dehghan, M.: The finite point method for reaction-diffusion systems in developmental biology. CMES Comput. Model. Eng. Sci. **82**(1), 1–27 (2011)
15. Kim, T., Sewall, J., Sud, A., Lin, M.: Fast simulation of laplacian growth. IEEE Comput. Graph. Appl. **27**(2), 68–76 (2007)
16. Luczak, A.: Spatial embedding of neuronal trees modeled by diffusive growth. Neurosci. Methods **157**(1), 132–141 (2006)

17. Maskery, S.M., Buettner, H.M.: Simulation of growth cone pathfinding. In: IEEE Conference Publications (ed.) First International IEEE EMBS Conference on Neural Engineering, pp. 237–240 (2003)

18. McAllister, A.K.: Cellular and molecular mechanisms of dendrite growth. Cereb. Cortex **10**(10), 963–973 (2000)

19. Murray, C.D.: The physiological principle of minimum work. I. The vascular system and the cost of blood volume. Proc. Natl. Acad. Sci. U.S.A. **12**(3), 207–214 (1926)

20. Podhajsky, R.J., Myers, R.R.: A diffusion-reaction model of nerve regeneration. Neurosci. Methods **60**(1–2), 79–88 (1995)

21. Rust, A.G., Adams, R., Bolouri, H.: Evolutionary neural topiary: growing and sculpting artificial neurons to order (2000)

22. Tepass, U., Truong, K., Godt, D., Ikura, M., Peifer, M.: Cadherins in embryonic and neural morphogenesis. Nat. Rev. Mol. Cell Biol. **2**, 91–100 (2000)

23. Thompson, D.M., Buettner, H.M.: Simulation and analysis of nerve growth cone-target encounter. In: Twenty-Second Annual Northeast Bioengineering Conference Proceedings, pp. 34–35. IEEE (1996)

24. Turing, A.M.: The chemical basis of morphogenesis. Philos. Trans. R. Soc. Lond. B Biol. Sci. **327**, 37–72 (1952)

25. van Ooyen, A., Graham, B.P., Ramakers, G.J.A.: Competition for tubulin between growing neurites during development. Neurocomputing **38**(40), 73–78 (2001)

26. Zubler, F., Douglas, R.: An instruction language for the explicit programming of axonal growth patterns. In: The 2010 International Joint Conference on Neural Networks (IJCNN), pp. 1–4 (2010)

Control by Imitation Using a Maximum Sensibility Neural Network

Erick Ordaz-Rivas, Luis Torres-Treviño$^{(\boxtimes)}$, and Angel Rodriguez-Liñan

DIE FIME, Universidad Autónoma de Nuevo León,
San Nicolás de los Garza, Mexico
luis.torres.ciidit@gmail.com

Abstract. In this paper, a maximum sensibility neural network was implemented in an embedded system with which was performed a control by imitation of a proposed plant. The plant consists of a cooling system and temperature indicator, the learning of the neural network is given by manually adjusting of output values of the indicators and a fan while input signals are obtained by sensors of temperature and presence, the neural network in run mode is able to interpret these data to automatically adjust the output settings and imitate the process with good performance.

Keywords: Neural networks · Control by imitation · Cooling system

1 Introduction

Currently, the use of automated systems for the control of processes are required to get faster decisions, repeatability, error reduction and other advantages they offer. This requires the choice of an appropriate system otherwise the process could have a poor performance or even can become unstable [6].

The choice of a proper system require to know the dynamic model of the process, which is not always available, and solve a lot of calculations, in other cases there is needed the information of the dynamics of the process for tuning the controllers.

The neural networks are presented as a solution to these problems based on their ability to learn data patterns, in order to represent the behavior of the system autonomously [4]. With the learning ability of neural networks is the relationship posible use input - output complex systems as training data and then used to control a system even if these data are unknown underlying relationships or physical meaning is hard to explain. With this we are allowed to imitate almost all types of systems, however presents a disadvantage when required to learn new data relationships, learning must be done online.

The maximum sensibility neuronal network does not have this disadvantage because it can learn the system either offline or online, and also keep updating the behavior of the system online [3]. The advantage in using this neural network is that during training only weights of the neurons that reach a sensibility margin

© Springer International Publishing Switzerland 2015
G. Sidorov and S.N. Galicia-Haro (Eds.): MICAI 2015, Part I, LNAI 9413, pp. 306–315, 2015.
DOI: 10.1007/978-3-319-27060-9_25

are updated. This makes it easier to train the neural network without having to disengage from the system or plant [1].

This network also got calculation but these are not calculations that consume a lot of time, giving it the advantage to implement it in a embedded system, making it to not need much hardware materials and easy to use.

This paper intends to implement a maximum sensibility neuronal network in an embedded system for controlling a plant by imitation. The proposed plant consists of a cooling system with an indicator that changes color as the temperature varies, the system input data are obtained through of sensors of temperature and presence.

2   Maximum Sensibility Neural Network

The Maximum Sensibility Neural Network (MSNN) is a multilayer network composed by an input layer consisting of multiple distribution neurons, a hidden layer of Gaussian neurons, and an output layer that adds the effect of all the hidden layer neurons or selects the output of the neuron with the maximum sensibility neuron. This behavior is shown in the Fig. 1.

The first layer normalizes the data input and distributes the information to all the neurons to the second layer. The connections between these layers have weights (W) that regulates the information. The second layer uses a Gaussian function of the sum of all the inputs of each neuron. The connection between this and the output layer also has weights (AC) for each neuron. The third layer detects if any neuron has maximum sensitivity and uses the output neuron, and if no neuron with maximum sensitivity, the output approaches by calculating the values of all the neurons in the hidden layer.

2.1   Running of MSNN

This state is the first procedure of the neural net, the neuron reads an input value and verifies if a similar pattern has been learned, in this case the neuron

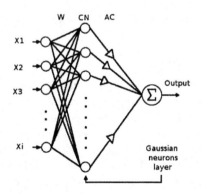

Fig. 1. Diagram of the MSNN structure.

will show the output corresponding to that input. An important parameter of the MSNN is sensibility margin (ms), which tell us if an input pattern has been already learned or if it has already a neuron with an approximated value. This parameter can be selected to be very specific to not recycle a value already learned if it is not almost equal to the new received, or it also can be loose and recycle values, even if they are not alike.

When the input does not resemble any input already learned by the network, what the network does is that it actually approximate the output value with the neuron that most resembles the input. The network shows the output corresponding to the learned pattern, according to the following equations:

$$Y = N_{ms} * AC_{ms} \tag{1}$$

where N_{ms} is the output of the maximum sensibility neuron, AC_{ms} is the weight of maximum sensibility neuron in the output layer, and Y is the actual output of the neural network.

The output of each neuron in the hidden layer is given by a Gaussian function:

$$N_{ms} = e^{-(x-cm)^2/\lambda} \tag{2}$$

where cm represents the center of mass or weights and $lambda$ represents sensibility of the neuron because controls the width of the Gaussian function. In case where the inputs are very different to the patterns learned, the neural network approximates the output using all of the hidden layer output

$$Y = \frac{\sum_{i=1}^{CN} N_i * AC_i}{\sum_{i=1}^{CN} N_i} \tag{3}$$

where CN is the number of neurons in the middle layer.

Finally the use vector values U of each neuron are established:

- Regardless of what neuron receives the settings of W and AC, it must update its value $U = 1$ to the adjusted neuron.
- And to all the neurons are subtracts a forgetting factor FU

This behavior of the *run mode* is shown in the Fig. 2.

2.2   Training of the MSNN

In the learning process the desired inputs and outputs are read, and check if there is one neuron which has a maximum sensibility value, that means there is a neuron that has already learned that pattern, and if there is one, it adjust the values of that neuron. To determine if a neuron presents maximum sensibility, the network uses the sensibility margin parameter, which can be very specific and creates new neurons, that is done to not affect all the others pattern already learned, or it can be less specific and creates groups multiple patterns in the same neuron to match the result of the new pattern learned.

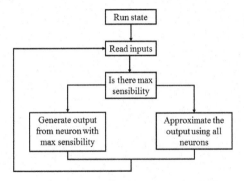

Fig. 2. Diagram of Run mode in MSNN.

The equation used to update the values of the weights that are between the first and the second layer when there is maximum sensibility is:

$$W_{ms,i} = \frac{W_{ms,i} + X_i}{2} \tag{4}$$

The equation that is used to update the values of the weights that are in the layer between the second and the third layer is:

$$AC_j = \frac{AC_j + Y_d}{2} \tag{5}$$

where X_i is the ith input, $W_{ms,i}$ is the weight of the ith input to the maximum sensibility neuron in the middle layer, AC_j is the jth weight of output layer, Y_d is the desired output.

When there is not maximum sensibility the network creates a new neuron and assigns the values of the inputs to the weights, this is

$$W_{ms,i} = X_i \tag{6}$$

$$AC_j = Y_d \tag{7}$$

In case the limit of neurons is reached, the neural network replaces the ith weight of the least used neuron by the ith input. The behavior of the *learning mode* is shown in the Fig. 3.

3   Experiments

3.1   Plant Description

The plant control consists of a cooling system, which uses an RGB LED as an indicator of temperature, where blue color indicates that the system is at room temperature while red color indicates a high temperature, also it has a fan that changes its velocity relative to the temperature of the system, and this just turns on when a presence sensor is exited this to save energy and do not turn on the fan when it is not needed although the temperature of system is high.

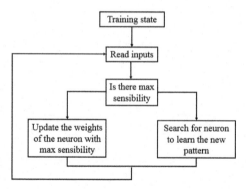

Fig. 3. Diagram of learning mode in MSNN.

3.2 Control Structure

The MSNN is trained using a manually adjusting of output values desired of the network while input signals are obtained by sensors, and the response of the plant to this values desired is used as the training input as shown in Fig. 4.

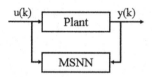

Fig. 4. Block diagram of training process of the MSNN.

In Fig. 5 is observed that after training, the desired plant output is given as input of the MSNN along with the actual plant output. Where the output of the MSNN is used as control signal of the plant.

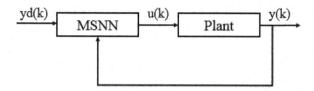

Fig. 5. Block diagram of the control process with the MSNN.

where $u(k)$ is a data vector given by the fan speed and the indicator of temperature (blue color for room temperature and red color for high temperature) and $y(k)$ is a data vector obtained by signals of sensors of presence and temperature.

3.3   Implementation in an Embedded System

The MSNN algorithm was implemented on an Arduino UNO board and was used in a control by imitation of cooling system. The hardware characteristics of the board is shown in the Table 1.

Table 1. Hardware characteristics

Characteristic	Description
Microcontroler	ATmega328
Operation voltage	5 V
Recommended alimentation voltage	7-12 V
Maximum alimentation voltage	6-20 V
Single I/O digital ports	14
Single I/O analog ports	6
Current of I/O digital ports	40 mA
Flash memory	32 KB
SRAM	2 KB
EEPROM	1 KB
Clock frequency	16 MHz

The learning process consisted in using three potentiometers as the expected to learn the values desired, and two sensors (presence and temperature) to give the pattern to learn. When the inputs were correctly selected, one button was used to tell the micro-controller to learn the pattern, and with that one learning process was run. After that the micro-controller automatically changes back to the running state [2,5].

4   Results

To obtain the results, by practicality the value of presence sensor remained constant at a high state and the MSNN was trained to regulate the fan speed

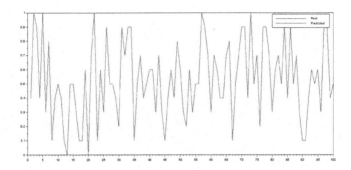

Fig. 6. MSNN performance with NTN = 20, $\lambda = 0.14$, ms $= 0.8$, error $= 0$

regarding the temperature change, the following graphs show the performance of the MSNN comparing a desired output with the actual output of the fan for different values of λ, maximum sensitivity ms and total number of neurons NTN. Plots illustrate performance of every neural network considering different parameters of sensibility (λ), margin of sensibility ms and the maximum number of available neurons NTN. The chosen values for the parameters were to lambda $= 0.14$ ms $= 0.8$ and NTN $= 20$, for the best performance in the simulations (Figs. 6, 7, 8 and 9).

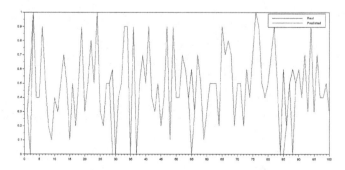

Fig. 7. MSNN performance with NTN $= 20$, $\lambda = 0.14$, ms $= 0.9$, error $= 0.0670820$

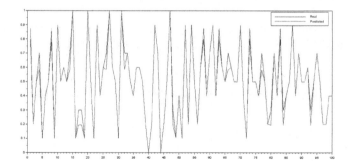

Fig. 8. MSNN performance with NTN $= 25$, $\lambda = 0.16$, ms $= 0.9$, error $= 0.0213402$

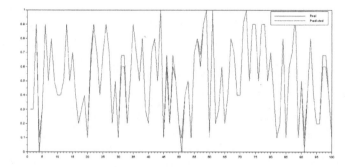

Fig. 9. MSNN performance with NTN $= 25$, $\lambda = 0.16$, ms $= 0.8$, error $= 0.0141984$

5   Conclusions

Based on the results obtained, one can conclude that the MSNN can be trained to learn the behavior of a dynamic system by a user and performance depends on the user's ability to train The MSNN has the advantage of online learning, "an easy implementation to achieve and besides it is easy to control".

Acknowledgments. We thanks to Centro de Investigación e Innovación de Desarrollo de Ingeniería y Tecnología of Facultad de Ingeniería Mecánica y Eléctrica from Universidad Autónoma de Nuevo León and Consejo Nacional de Ciencia y Tecnología for the facilities and support given for developing this work.

Appendix: Pseudocodes

1 Run State Pseudo Code

Algorithm 1: Run state pseudo code implemented in the embedded system

---

```
RunFunctionMSNN(X,W,AC,ms);
for n ← 1 to NTN do
    S = 0;
    for i ← 1 to NTI do
        S = S + (x(i) − W(n, i)²;
    end
    //fa = activation function;
    SN(n) = fa(sqrt(S), alpha);
end
Maximum Value and Position in SN;
if MaxValue > Maximum Sensibility Value then
    for o ← 1 to NTO do
        y(o) = AC(pos, o) ∗ SN(pos);
    end
else
    for o ← 1 to NTO do
        s1 = 0;
        s2 = 0;
        for n ← 1 to CN do
            s1 = SN(n) ∗ AC(n, o) + s1;
            s2 = SN(n) + s2;
        end
        y(o) = s1/s2;
    end
end
Output Value of the MSNN = y;
```

---

2 Learn State Pseudo Code Implemented in the Embedded System

Algorithm 2: Learn state pseudo code implemented in the embedded system

---

LearningFunctionMSNN(X,Ye,W,AC,ms,Lambda,U);

Maximum Value and Position in SN;;

if *Maximum Value* $\geq$ *ms* **then**

> **for** $pr \leftarrow 1$ **to** NTI **do**
> > $W(Position, pr) \leftarrow (W(Position, pr) + X(pr))/2;$
>
> **end**
> **for** $o \leftarrow 1$ **to** NTO **do**
> > $AC(Position, o) \Leftarrow (AC(Position, o) + yo(o))/2;;$
>
> **end**

else

> **if** $(CN + 1) >$ *Maximum value of neurons* **then**
> > //avaliable to use minimum Value and Position of the U;
> > **for** $pr \leftarrow 1$ **to** NTI **do**
> > > $(Position, pr) \Leftarrow X(pr);$
> >
> > **end**
> > **for** $o \leftarrow 1$ **to** NTO **do**
> > > $AC(Position, o) = yo(o);$
> >
> > **end**
>
> **else**
> > New neuron $\leftarrow$ Number of neurons actualy used $+1;$
> > **for** $pr \leftarrow 1$ **to** NTI **do**
> > > $W(NewNeuron, pr) \leftarrow X(pr);$
> >
> > **end**
> > **for** $o \leftarrow 1$ **to** NTO **do**
> > > $AC(NewNeuron, o) = yo(o);$
> >
> > **end**
>
> **end**

end

References

1. Aguilera-Ruiz, M., Torres-Trevino, L.M., Linan, J.A.R.: Control by online learning using a maximum sensibility neural network. In: 13th Mexican International Conference on Artificial Intelligence, MICAI 2014, pp. 118–120, November 2014
2. Cabrera-Gaona, D., Trevino, L., Rodriguez-Linan, A.: Control by learning in a temperature system using a maximum sensibility neural network. In: 12th Mexican International Conference on Artificial Intelligence, MICAI 2013, pp. 109–113, November 2013
3. Escamilla, I., Torres, L., Perez, P., Zambrano, P.: A comparison between back propagation and the maximum sensibility neural network to surface roughness prediction in machining of titanium (Ti 6Al 4V) alloy. In: Gelbukh, A., Morales, E.F. (eds.) MICAI 2008. LNCS (LNAI), vol. 5317, pp. 1009–1019. Springer, Heidelberg (2008)

4. Haykin, S.: Neural Networks and Learning Machines (3rd Edn.). Pearson Education, Upper Saddle River (2008)
5. Sanmiguel, G., Gonzalez, L., Torres-Trevino, L., Guerra, C.: On-line learning in an embedded maximum sensibility neural network. In: 11th Mexican International Conference on Artificial Intelligence MICAI 2012, pp. 75–79, October 2012
6. Waegeman, T., Wyffels, F., Schrauwen, B.: Feedback control by online learning an inverse model. IEEE Trans. Neural Netw. Learn. Syst. **23**(10), 1637–1648 (2012)

Chaotic Cases in a Two-Neuron Discrete Neural Network

Jorge Cervantes-Ojeda[(⊠)] and María Gómez-Fuentes

Universidad Autónoma Metropolitana – Cuajimalpa, Mexico City, Mexico
{jcervantes,mcgomez}@correo.cua.uam.mx

Abstract. We explore different cases of chaotic behavior in a two-neuron Discrete Time Recurrent Neural Network and found, until now, three cases where chaos is present in different forms. We describe how these cases of chaos are produced in a qualitative way.

Keywords: Chaos in neural networks · Discrete-time recurrent neural network dynamics · Deterministic chaos

1 Introduction

In a chaotic system, small variations in the initial conditions produce very different trajectories and irregular behavior, making it impossible in practice to predict its future state. In a Discrete Time Recurrent Neural Network (DTRNN) one can have all kinds of periodic behaviors and chaos. Knowing exactly when and why the system presents chaos is useful because, then, it is possible to select the parameter values which lead to a desired functional behavior [10] or avoid undesired ones too. Learning algorithms could make use of this to become more efficient, for instance. It is also important in the more general framework of neuroscience. For instance, Freeman [7] stated that chaos plays an in important role in the human's learning process and memory.

The sufficient and necessary conditions leading to chaos, in a DTRNN, are not established yet. If we find all possible cases where there is chaos in a DTRNN, then we will be able to draw conclusions that establish the necessary and sufficient conditions for its existence. But finding these cases is not an easy task since the parameter space in a DTRNN is huge. Instead, we wish to find some qualitative principles that could make us understand what produces chaos and what does not.

The study of the dynamic behavior of small DTRNNs (two or three neurons) is much more feasible than the analysis of more complex networks and also it can be assumed that the properties they have are also present in more complex networks [10, 11]. We report here three cases where chaos is present in different forms in a two-neuron DTRNN. We analyze the causes for chaos in a qualitative way and show how they are similar and different.

The rest of this paper is organized as follows: Sect. 2 summarizes previous related work; Sect. 3 describes the empirical methods used; Sect. 4 provides the found cases of chaos and their descriptions and in Sect. 5 we state our conclusions.

G. Sidorov and S.N. Galicia-Haro (Eds.): MICAI 2015, Part I, LNAI 9413, pp. 316–326, 2015.
DOI: 10.1007/978-3-319-27060-9_26

2 Background

Many researchers have been working in the establishment of the necessary and sufficient conditions for chaos with partial results until now. Marotto's theorem [9] says that
there is chaos in a multidimensional system when there are snap-back repellers. In [6] it
is mentioned that Shiraiwa and Kurata [12] found that, in addition to the snap-back
repellers, chaos can be present also with the existence of saddle points. However, these
findings set only sufficient conditions for chaos.

In order to simulate the neurons of the brain, Aihara et al. [2] designed the chaotic
neuron, in which the next state depends on the current state and also on some previous
states. A neural network composed of chaotic neurons can generate a chaotic response
by setting the appropriate parameters. The usefulness of chaotic neural networks has
been demonstrated in clustering [13] and in associative networks [1]. Adachi & Aihara
[1] found that the memory searching process in an associative network is improved
with a chaotic neural network.

Since Wang [14] proved analytically the existence of chaos in a two-neuron
recurrent network, some research was devoted to the study of chaos in small neural
networks. Cessac et al. [3] observed that when the weights are small in a DTRNN, the
system tends to have a single stable point of period-1, and that chaos occurs when the
weights are large. Chen & Aihara [6] stated the conditions under which a bounded
fixed point in a DTRNN evolves into a snap-back repeller generating chaotic behavior.

Potapov & Ali [10] showed that robust chaos is possible for small changes in the
interconnection weights of a DTRNN. They establish sufficient, but not necessary
robustness conditions, for a family of connection weight matrices.

Passeman [10] studied *chaotic neuromodules* which consist of two or three neurons
with feedback, in discrete time. He analyzed some sections of the input's and weights'
space, in order to display areas where non-trivial attractors co-exist.

3 Metodology

We configured a recurrent neural network in the following manner: the output of
neuron 1 (x_1), is connected to neuron 1 with a weight a, and also to the input of neuron
2 with a weight c; the output of neuron 2 (x_2), is connected to neuron 2 with a weight d,
and also to the input of neuron 2 with a weight b; u_1 and u_2 are the external inputs of
each neuron respectively. The evolution equation is then

$$\begin{bmatrix} x_1(t+1) \\ x_2(t+1) \end{bmatrix} = \begin{bmatrix} \tanh(ax_1(t) + bx_2(t) + u_1) \\ \tanh(cx_1(t) + dx_2(t) + u_2) \end{bmatrix} \tag{1}$$

where $x_1(t)$, $x_2(t)$ represent the output state of each neuron at time t.

The use of tanh() as the activation function has the advantage that whenever $\vec{u} =$
$(0,0)$ the state $\vec{x} = (0,0)$ is always a fixed point. This fact allows studying the effects

that changes in the connection weights have on the system dynamics of this point, without having to solve the fixed point equation for every set of weight values. And, more importantly, allows us to study such effects independently of the effects from changing the external inputs. In the following we will use always $\vec{u} = (0,0)$.

Using Eq. (1) we performed extensive simulations in search of representative chaotic cases with interesting properties. We used different tools to analyze them in detail:

(a) Bifurcation curves in the search space.
(b) Phase diagrams.
(c) Distance plots between different trajectories as a function of time and as a function of current state.
(d) Lyapunov exponents plots.

4   Cases of Chaos in a Two-Neuron DTRNN

4.1   Chaos Close to a Heteroclinic Bifurcation

When the weights are configured in such a way that a limit cycle emerges, and one weight is slowly varying in a continuous way, it is possible that this limit cycle reaches two saddle points at the same time. The produced bifurcation in this case, is called *heteroclinic*. It is known that there is chaos close to heteroclinic bifurcations [8].

The diagram in Fig. 1 shows bifurcations in the weights space (a, d) for the particular case: $bc = -0.56$, with $b = 0.1$ and $c = -5.6$. Note that b and c values are *unbalanced*. This means that their values are very different in absolute value. The point $(a,d) = (1.535757, 0.5)$ is marked with a big black cross.

Colored curves in Fig. 1 represent bifurcations of the fixed point at the origin [4]: the curve in red is a saddle bifurcation, the blue one is a period-doubling bifurcation and the green one is the Neimark-Sacker bifurcation. The curves in dotted lines represent the global bifurcations [5].

The two small curves in black in Fig. 1 point the place where the heteroclinic bifurcation is present. In order to have a heteroclinic bifurcation, it is necessary that b and c values are sufficiently unbalanced (with $bc < 0$), this is that either $|b| << |c|$ or $|b| >> |c|$. Chaos emerges when the point (a, d) is sufficiently close to these curves but only on the side where there are limit-cycles. In this case we mean below the black curve on the right and above the black curve on the left side.

The period-1 phase diagram of Fig. 2 (a) (corresponding to the weights stated above) is an example of a limit-cycle close to two saddle points. The red and blue lines are the nullclines of x_1 and x_2 respectively and the crossings between them are fixed points. Figure 2 (b) shows a zommed detail of the upper left corner in the limit cycle for Fig. 2 (a) and (c) shows the same but for another case where there is no chaos but instead it presents a quasiperiodic case, which is clearly very regular. The difference is

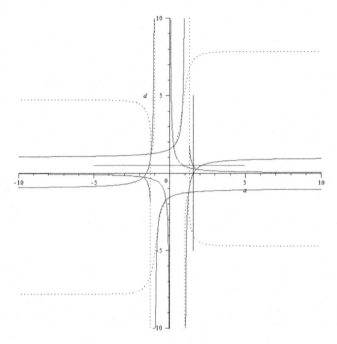

Fig. 1. Bifurcations in the weights space (a, d) for: $bc = -0.56$, with $b = 0.1$ and $c = -5.6$.

that, for the latter case, whenever the state is further ahead in the limit cycle, the next state is also ahead. This is not true in the chaotic case.

Although Fig. 2 (a) does not show an apparent chaotic behavior, we know there is some kind of chaos. See Fig. 3 where we show the measure of the distances δ_{small}, δ_{next} and δ_{opp} as a function of time (left) and δ_{small} as a function of current state $(x_1, x_2) = (x, y)$ (right). These distances are defined as follows: All distances use the current state of a reference trajectory T_r that starts at $(x_1(0), x_2(0))$.

- δ_{small} is the distance between the current states of T_r and another trajectory that starts at $(x_1(0), x_2(0) + \varepsilon)$, being $\varepsilon = 10^{-5}$ a *small* real number (green dots);
- δ_{next} is the distance between the current states of T_r and another trajectory that starts at $(x_1(1), x_2(1))$, which is the *next* state of the starting state of T_r (grey dots);
- δ_{opp} is the distance between the current states of T_r and another trajectory that starts at the *next state* of $(-x_1(0), -x_2(0))$, the latter being the *opposite* state of the starting state of T_r (blue dots).

As you can see, these distances do not show any structure, neither as a function of time nor state. This suggests there is chaotic behavior because the distances can be very low as well as very high unpredictably. This is clearer in the plot to the right hand side because, there, one can see that δ_{small} for one particular state can have very different values. These plots prove there is sensitivity to initial conditions.

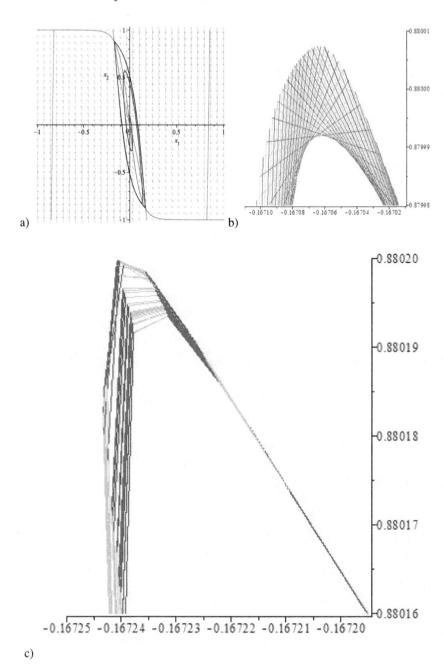

a)

b)

c)

Fig. 2. (a) Period-1 phase diagram of the case: $(a, d) = (1.535757, 0.5)$; $bc = -0.56$, with $b = 0.1$ and $c = -5.6$. (b) Detail of the corner of a quasiperiodic case. (c) Detail of the corner of the same chaotic case.

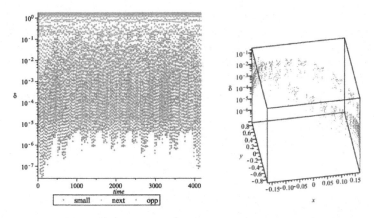

Fig. 3. Distance δ as a function of time (left) and as a function of current state $(x_1, x_2) = (x,y)$ (right)

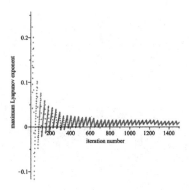

Fig. 4. Evolution of the maximum Lyapunov exponent.

Figure 4 shows the evolution of the calculation of the maximum Lyapunov exponent through one trajectory in this case. It is clear that it tends to a limit that is positive, meaning chaos. Chaotic behavior is in this case present, apparently, only in dimension 1. This means that trajectories converge to a limit cycle line but the step sizes over it are chaotic. But, as we see in Fig. 2, the visited states are not aligned but they occupy a wider space. This why this kind of chaos is difficult to spot, because the system state seems to simply flow over a limit cycle. The cause of this chaotic behavior could be the sharp turn that the state takes when close to the saddle points.

4.2   Saddle Chaos Plus Period Doubling: αC + β

In this case we use the letters: α to denote the effect of a saddle bifurcation that produces two separate period-1 fixed point attractors from another one; C to denote the presence of a modification that produces chaos; and β to denote the effect of a period doubling bifurcation that produces two period-2 fixed point attractors from another one. Thus, the expression αC + β means that we have two period-1 attractors transformed into chaotic attractors plus a separate coexisting pair of period-2 attractors.

Figure 5 shows an example of this case with $a = -1.34$, $b = 0.1$, $c = -81.1$, $d = 7$. Note that $bc = -8.11$ and that b and c are very highly unbalanced. In the top, one can see the period-2 phase diagram with two chaotic attractors and also two period-2

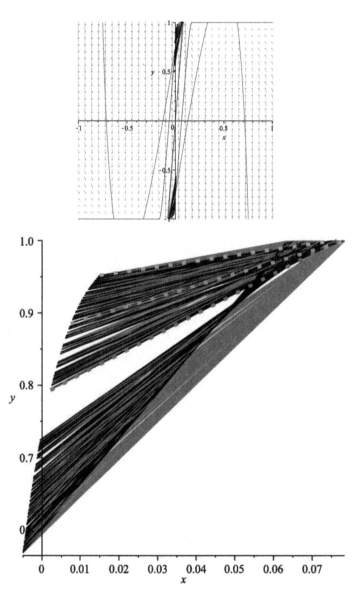

Fig. 5. Period-2 phase diagram: $a = -1.34$, $b = 0.1$, $c = -81.1$, $d = 7$ (top), zoom of one of the attractors (bottom)

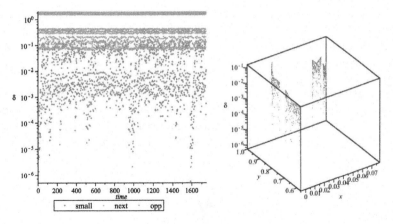

Fig. 6. Distance δ as a function of time (left) and as a function of current state $(x_1, x_2) = (x,y)$ (right)

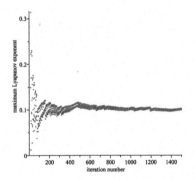

Fig. 7. Evolution of the maximum Lyapunov exponent.

attractors. In the bottom we can see a zoomed version of one of the chaotic attractors. This attractor can be described as a bunch of lines that visits 4 sites periodically, i.e., 4 period-4 strange attractors: 2 close to the vertical axis and 2 further to the right and above. In the transit from the higher one of those in the left to the right most of the other two, one can see a kind of horseshoe map. To see this, note that the yellow and red dotted lines cross each other.

In Fig. 6 one can see similar behavior as in Fig. 3 suggesting chaos. In the right hand side plot, it is clear that for each possible state the distance to the other trajectory can have different values, which means there is sensitivity to initial conditions.

The evolution of the maximum Lyapunov exponent through one trajectory is shown in Fig. 7. We can see that it tends to stabilize in a positive value.

4.3   Limit Cycle with Chaos: *I*α*C*

Here we explore the case *iα*C. We use *i* to denote a rotational behavior; α to denote that this rotational behavior does not converge to a fixed point; C to denote chaotic behavior. Thus this case presents a limit cycle that is modified to present also chaotic behavior. We want to show that a limit cycle does not need to get close to a heteroclinic (or homoclinic) bifurcation in order to present chaotic behavior. We have set the weights to $a = -0.1$, $b = 0.1$, $c = -81.1$, $d = 7$. Here we also have b and c very unbalanced with $bc = -8.11 \ll -1$.

The behavior of the system is shown in Figs. 8 and 9. A kind of horseshoe map is visible in Fig. 8 (bottom), in fact there are two horseshoes: one in the top left and one in the bottom right. See for instance the bottom right where the lines coming from the top form a curve at the bottom, then, the lines come from this curve to the left. This mixes

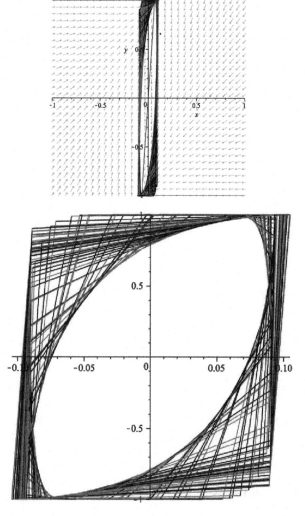

Fig. 8. Period-2 phase diagram: $a = -0.1$, $b = 0.1$, $c = -81.1$, $d = 7$ (top), zoom of one of the attractors (bottom)

the lines in a way that those that were in the middle of the bunch of lines above are now in an extreme of the bunch at the bottom, and those that were in one of the extremes are now somewhere in the middle. Then, the bunch of lines gets squeezed. So a horseshoe map has been created.

Figure 9 shows that this case is also clearly dependent on initial conditions and thus that it has some form of chaos.

From many experiments we did, we can conjecture that chaos is produced due to the strength of the unbalanced relation between b and c. This produces strong and sharp turns in the limit cycle as is the case also of Sect. 4.1.

The evolution of the maximum Lyapunov exponent for this case is shown in Fig. 10. The positive limit shows that there is chaos as in the previous case.

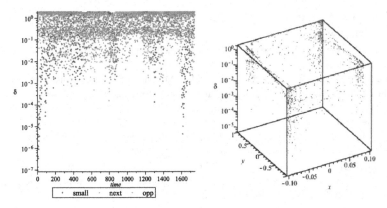

Fig. 9. Distance δ as a function of time (left) and as a function of current state $(x_1, x_2) = (x, y)$ (right)

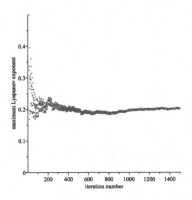

Fig. 10. Evolution of the maximum Lyapunov exponent.

5 Conclusions

We have shown that, in a two-neuron DTRNN, chaos can be caused by the existence of different forms of horseshoe maps placed in the chaotic attractors. The cases studied here are all of this type. It seems that a necessary condition for chaos is that the interconnection weights between the two neurons must have a product below zero and their magnitudes must be very unbalanced. More work still needs to be done in order to discover all possible cases of chaos in a DTRNN over the full 4-dimensional weights space, and show what exactly produces it in a qualitative and quantitative way.

References

1. Adachi, M., Aihara, K.: Associative dynamics in a chaotic neural network. Neural Netw. **10**(1), 83–98 (1997)
2. Aihara, K., Takabe, T., Toyoda, M.: Chaotic neural networks. Phys. Lett. A **144**(6/7), 333–340 (1990)
3. Cessac, B., Doyon, B., Quoy, M., Samuelides, M.: Mean-field equations, bifurcation map and route to chaos in discrete time neural networks. Physica D **74**(1), 24–44 (1994)
4. Cervantes-Ojeda, J., del Carmen Gómez-Fuentes, M.: On the connection weight space structure of a two-neuron discrete neural network: bifurcations of the fixed point at the origin. In: Gelbukh, A., Espinoza, F.C., Galicia-Haro, S.N. (eds.) MICAI 2014, Part II. LNCS, vol. 8857, pp. 85–94. Springer, Heidelberg (2014)
5. Cervantes-Ojeda J., Gomez-Fuentes M.C., Bernal-Jaquez R.: Empirical analysis of bifurcations in the weights space of a two-neuron DTRNN with balanced mutual influence between neurons. NeurocComput. (2015, submitted)
6. Chen, L., Aihara, K.: Chaos and asymptotical stability in discrete-time neural networks. Physica D **104**(3), 286–325 (1997)
7. Freeman, W.J.: The physiology of perception. Sci. Am. **264**(2), 78–85 (1991)
8. Kustnetsov, Y.: Elements of Applied Bifurcation Theory. Applied Mathematical Science, vol. 112, 2nd edn. Springer, New York (1998)
9. Marotto, F.R.: Snap-back repellers imply chaos in R^n. J. Math. Anal. Appl. **63**, 199–223 (1978)
10. Pasemann, F.: Complex dynamics and the structure of small neural networks. Netw. Comput. Neural Syst. **13**(2), 195–216 (2002)
11. Tiňo, P., Horne, B.G., Giles, C.L.: Attractive periodic sets in discrete-time recurrent networks (with emphasis on fixed-point stability and bifurcations in two-neuron networks). Neural Comput. **13**(6), 1379–1414 (2001)
12. Shiraiwa, K., Kurata, M.: A generalization of a theorem of Marotto. Proc. Jpn. Acad. **55**, 286–289 (1980)
13. Wakame M., Osana Y.: Chaotic neural network with time delay term. In: International Joint Conference on Neural Networks 2007, IJCNN 2007. pp. 880–885. IEEE, August 2007
14. Wang, X.: Period-doublings to chaos in a simple neural network: an analytical proof. Complex Syst. **5**(4), 425–44 (1991)

Dynamic Systems Identification and Control by Means of Complex-Valued Recurrent Neural Networks

Ieroham Baruch$^{(\boxtimes)}$, Victor Arellano Quintana,
and Edmundo Pérez Reynaud

Department of Automatic Control, CINVESTAV-IPN,
Ave. IPN no 2508, A.P. 14-470, 07360 Mexico D.F, Mexico
{baruch,varellano,eperez}@ctrl.cinvestav.mx

Abstract. The present article gives an extension of the real-valued recurrent neural network topology and its Back-Propagation (BP) learning to the complex-valued one. The BP learning is achieved by the use of diagrammatic rules to obtain the adjoint recurrent neural network topology aimed to propagate the output learning error through it so to learn the neural network weights. Then, this BP learning methodology is applied to the Recurrent Complex-Valued Neural Network (RCVNN) BP-learning using two type RCVNN topologies considering two different kinds of activation functions. After that, the second system identification scheme is incorporated in a total direct complex value control scheme of nonlinear oscillatory plants, introducing also an I-term. The total control scheme contained tree RCVNNs. Furthermore, comparative simulation results of one degree of freedom flexible-joint robot model illustrating system identification and control are obtained. The obtained comparative simulation results confirmed the good quality of the proposed control methodology.

Keywords: Direct adaptive neural control · Diagrammatic rules · Complex-valued Back-propagation learning · Recurrent complex-valued neural network topology · System identification of nonlinear oscillatory plants

1 Introduction

The rapid growth of available computational resources has led to the developments of a wide number of Neural Networks (NN) based modeling, identification, prediction and control applications [1–3]. Some other applications of neural and fuzzy-neural networks have been done for oscillatory chaotic systems, [4, 5]. The main NN property, namely the ability to approximate complex nonlinear relationships without prior knowledge of model structure, makes them a very attractive alternative to the classical modeling and control techniques [6–8]. Among several possible network architectures the ones most widely used are the Feed-Forward NN (FFNN) and Recurrent NN (RNN) [6]. In the last decade there has been a rise in applications using Recurrent Complex-Valued NNs (RCVNN) [9–14]. Most of them deal with oscillatory systems which, by their physical nature, are convenient to be treated in the complex domain, such as electromagnetic waves, light waves, image processing, electric power systems,

© Springer International Publishing Switzerland 2015
G. Sidorov and S.N. Galicia-Haro (Eds.): MICAI 2015, Part I, LNAI 9413, pp. 327–337, 2015.
DOI: 10.1007/978-3-319-27060-9_27

evaporator systems and mechanical systems [9–11]. In [12], the authors derived a Complex Value BP (CVBP) algorithm used for pattern classification. However, the learning algorithm has some problems because the activation functions presented singularity points in their domains. Some other works [13, 14] propose different activation functions that avoid singularity points. To simplify the BP learning for the RCVNN, the present work proposes the use of diagrammatic rules (see [16]) to construct an adjoint network and propagate the complex output error through it in order to obtain the weight adjustment, with two different RCVNN topologies considered, each with different activation functions avoiding singularities.

The BP learning technique, based on gradient-descent optimization technique [6], is used for nonlinear oscillatory plant identification and oscillation suppression by means of direct integral term adaptive neural control using RCVNN. Lastly, some comparative simulation results of RCVNN identification and control of flexible-joint robot are given and discussed, furthermore a validation stage is presented in order to confirm the good quality of the proposed learning algorithm.

2 Topology and BP Learning of Recurrent Complex-Valued NN

The general RCVNN topology in consideration is an extension of the real-valued Recurrent Neural Network topology, presented in [8], to the complex-valued case. The RCVNN topology has complex inputs, outputs, and state vectors, and complex A, B, C weight matrices. It is defined as follows:

$$X(k+1) = AX(k) + BU(k) \tag{1}$$

$$A = \text{diag}(A_i), \quad |A_i| < 1, \quad i = 1, \ldots, N \tag{2}$$

$$E(k) = Y_P(k) - Y(k) \tag{3}$$

$$Z(k) = G[X(k)] \tag{4}$$

$$V(k) = CZ(k) \tag{5}$$

$$Y(k) = S[V(k)] \tag{6}$$

The vectors and matrices dimensions of the RCVNN topology are given as follows: $A \in \mathbb{C}^{n \times n}$ is the feedback weight matrix, $B \in \mathbb{C}^{n \times m}$ is the input weight matrix, $C \in \mathbb{C}^{p \times n}$ is the output weight matrix, $X \in \mathbb{C}^n$ is the internal state vector, $Z \in \mathbb{C}^n$ is the hidden state vector, $U \in \mathbb{C}^m$ is the network input, $Y \in \mathbb{C}^p$ is the network output and $G[\cdot]$, $S[\cdot]$ are complex-valued vector activation functions. The inequality in (2) is a stability preserving condition, imposed on the diagonal blocks of the matrix A. This condition is imposed also to all the weights of the matrices B, C.

We consider two particular RCVNN with different activation functions. In the same way as in the real-valued case, [8], we apply complex-valued diagrammatic rules so to derive an adjoint network for each case.

The performance index to be minimized is given by:

$$\zeta(k) = \frac{1}{2}\sum_j \left[E_j(k) \cdot E_j^*(k) \right], \quad \zeta = \frac{1}{N_e}\sum_k \zeta(k) \tag{7}$$

The function $\zeta(k)$ is a mapping of the form $f : \mathbb{C} \to \mathbb{R}$, which is non-analytic in the sense that it does not have derivative and also it does not satisfy the Cauchy-Riemann equations. This complicates the use of the gradient descendent algorithm, because we have to use the so-called Wirtinger's calculus. Using diagrammatic rules (see [16]) it is possible to avoid this particular problem.

The instantaneous Means Squared Error (MSE) $\zeta(k)$ is used in real-time applications, while the total MSE ζ is used for one epoch N_e in off-line applications. The general RVRNN real-time BP learning algorithm with momentum term is given by the following equation:

$$W(k+1) = W(k) + \eta \cdot \Delta W(k) + \alpha \cdot \Delta W(k-1),$$
$$|W(k)| < W_0 \tag{8}$$

Where: W is a general weight matrix (A, B, C); ΔW is the change in W, η is a diagonal constant matrix of learning, α is a diagonal constant momentum term matrix and W_0 is a restricted region for the weight matrix W.

2.1 Topology and BP Learning of RCVNN with First Type Activation Function

The first type activation function is defined as follows:

$$f(z) = tanh(z), \quad z \in \mathbb{C} \setminus \left\{ z : z = 0 \pm \frac{2n-1}{2}\pi i, \quad \forall n \in \mathbb{N} \right\} \tag{9}$$

This activation function has singularities in some points of the complex domain and because of this, we avoided them. The topology of RCVNN using this activation function is given in Fig. 1.

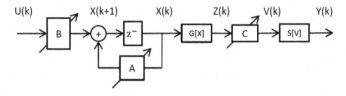

Fig. 1. Topology of the first type RCVNN

Applying the diagrammatic rules proposed in [16] to the RCVNN topology, we obtain the adjoint RCVNN model, given on Fig. 2. The adjoint RCVNN is used for the backward propagation of the output error signals of the BP algorithm.

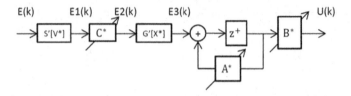

Fig. 2. Adjoint topology of the first type RCVNN

The BP learning algorithm can be defined in the complex domain with the same significance of the participating variables [12, 14]. Using the adjoint RCVNN topology we derive the following weight update algorithm:

$$E_1(k) = S'[Y(k)] \cdot E(k) \tag{10}$$

$$\Delta C(k) = E_1(k) \cdot Z^*(k) \tag{11}$$

$$E_2(k) = C^*(k) \cdot E_1(k) \tag{12}$$

$$E_3(k) = G'[Z^*(k)] \cdot E_2(k) \tag{13}$$

$$\Delta A(k) = E_3(k) \cdot X^*(k) \tag{14}$$

$$\Delta B(k) = E_3(k) \cdot U^*(k) \tag{15}$$

Where: $G'[\cdot]$, $S'[\cdot]$ are the derivatives for the activation functions $G[\cdot]$, $S[\cdot]$ and $(*)$ is the transpose and complex conjugate operation. The application of the diagrammatic rules and the obtained adjoint RCVNN topology simplified the learning algorithm, with respect to the classical gradient descent algorithm [12, 14].

2.2   Topology and BP Learning of RCVNN with Second Type Activation Function

The second type activation function ([11, 14]) does not have any singularity points and it is defined by the following equation:

$$f(z) = \tanh[\text{Re}(z)] + i \cdot \tanh[\text{Im}(z)] \tag{16}$$

In this case, the RCVNN topology is given by the following equations:

$$X(k+1) = AX(k) + BU(k) \tag{17}$$

$$Z(k) = G[X_{\text{Re}}(k)] + i \cdot G[X_{Im}(k)] \tag{18}$$

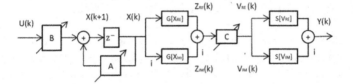

Fig. 3. Topology of the second type RCVNN

$$V(k) = C_{\text{Re}} Z_{\text{Re}}(k) + i \cdot C_{\text{Im}} Z_{\text{Im}}(k) \tag{19}$$

$$Y(k) = S[V_{\text{Re}}(k)] + i \cdot S[V_{\text{Im}}(k)] \tag{20}$$

Where the (Re) and (Im) subscripts are the real and imaginary part respectively. The topology of the RCVNN for this case is described by Fig. 3.

The vectors and matrices of the RCVNN topology are defined in the same way as in the previous topology. The complex state feedback matrix A is defined as block-diagonal with the same restriction as (2). Applying the complex-valued dia-

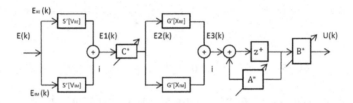

Fig. 4. Adjoint topology of the second type RCVNN

grammatic rules we could obtain the adjoint RCVNN, given on Fig. 4.

Using the adjoint RCVNN topology we can derive the following weight update algorithm:

$$E_1(k) = S'[Y_{\text{Re}}(k)] \cdot E_{\text{Re}}(k) + i \cdot S'[Y_{\text{Im}}(k)] \cdot E_{Im}(k) \tag{21}$$

$$\Delta C(k) = E_1(k) \cdot Z^*(k) \tag{22}$$

$$E_2(k) = C^*(k) \cdot E_1(k) \tag{23}$$

$$E_3(k) = G'[Z_{\text{Re}}^*(k)] \cdot E_{2,\text{Re}}(k) + i \cdot G'[Z_{\text{Im}}^*(k)] \cdot E_{2,Im}(k) \tag{24}$$

$$\Delta A(k) = E_3(k) \cdot X^*(k) \tag{25}$$

$$\Delta B(k) = E_3(k) \cdot U^*(k) \tag{26}$$

The stability and convergence of the above given BP learning algorithms could be proven extending the Theorem of stability given in [8, 15] for the real-valued case to the Complex value case.

3 Identification and Control of Nonlinear Plants

The application of the given models of RCVNN for the identification of nonlinear oscillatory plants is illustrated by Fig. 5. The input signal of the plant is the same as the input signal of the RCVNN model. Here the desired complex target vector is the output of the plant and the identification objective is to adjust the complex weight parameters of the RCVNN in a way that the RCVNN output follows the plant output with minimum MSE. The RCVNN training is then validated by a generalization step, where an unknown input signal is used and a MSE is computed with fixed RCVNN weights.

The input plant signals used for system identification and generalization are chosen as a sum of sine functions with different frequency and amplitude. The input signal of RCVNN model and the output signal of the plant are discretized in other to perform the complex BP algorithm of learning and the RCVNN model generalization (see Fig. 5).

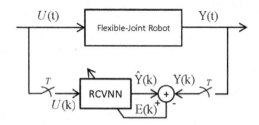

Fig. 5. Block-diagram of RCVNN plant identification

The block diagram of the neural control system is given on Fig. 6.

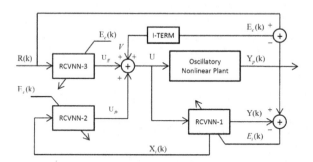

Fig. 6. Block-diagram of the direct adaptive neural control system with I-term and state feedback

It has a RCVNN-1 identifier estimating parameters and states of the nonlinear oscillatory plant; a RCVNN-2 feedback controller which uses the estimated states for feedback control; and a RCVNN-3 feed-forward controller which uses the system reference to create an inverse model of the closed-loop system. The control input of the plant also has an I-term feedback in order to eliminate the steady state error from the output of the plant. The I-term of the error is given by the following equation:

$$V(k+1) = V(k) + T_0 \cdot k_i \cdot E_C(k) \tag{27}$$

Where: V is the integral action control signal, T_0 is the sampling time, k_i is the integral gain and E_C is the control error, defined by the following equation:

$$E_C(k) = R(k) - Y_P(k) \tag{28}$$

R is the reference signal for the plant. The control input of the plant is a sum of the mentioned three components (see Fig. 6) as follows:

$$U(k) = U_{ff}(k) + U_{fb}(k) + V(k) \tag{29}$$

Where: U is the total control input for the plant, U_{ff} is the feed-forward control term and U_{fb} is the feedback control term.

The model, the output and the input of the plant are given in continuous time. In order to use a recurrent neural network for control, the output signal of the plant and the system reference signal are discretized with a sampling time T_0.

4   Simulation Results

4.1   Description of the Nonlinear Oscillatory Plant Model

The plant under neural identification and control is an idealized nonlinear model of a flexible-joint robot manipulator, illustrated in Fig. 7. The flexibility of the robot joint is caused by a harmonic drive, which is a type of robot gear mechanism with high torque transmission, low backlash and compact size.

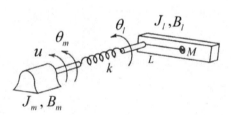

Fig. 7. An idealized joint model representing robot joint flexibility

The first robot joint consists of an actuator connected to a load through a torsional spring representing the joint flexibility. We take the motor torque as the plant input. The equations of motion of the flexible-joint robot are given as follows.

$$
\begin{aligned}
J_l\ddot{\theta}_l + B_l\dot{\theta}_l + Mgl\sin\theta_l + k(\theta_l - \theta_m) &= 0 \\
J_m\ddot{\theta}_m + B_m\dot{\theta}_m - k(\theta_l - \theta_m) &= u
\end{aligned}
\tag{30}
$$

Where: J_l, J_m, are load and motor inertias, B_l, B_m are load and motor damping constants, u is the input torque applied to the motor shaft, M and L are the mass of the link and the length between the shaft and the center of mass of the link, and k. represents the torsional stiffness constant of the harmonic drive gear. The plant is described by two second order differential equations, representing a system with two degrees of freedom but only one input which makes the system sub-actuated.

4.2   Simulation Results of System Identification

The RCVNN used has three neurons in the hidden layer, one input and one output neurons. The RCVNN dimensions are $n = 3$, $m = 1$, $p = 1$, with a sampling time of $T_0 = 0.01$. The numerical values of the plant parameters used in the plant model are: $J_l = 1$, $J_m = 3.003$, $B_l = 1$, $B_m = 3.003$, $M = 0.5$, $g = 9.81$, $l = 0.5$, $k = 100$. The input plant signals used for system identification $u_L(t)$ and generalization $u_G(t)$ are given by:

$$u_L(t) = \sin(0.1t) + 0.5sin(0.04t) \tag{31}$$

$$u_G(t) = 0.5\sin(0.1t) + 0.8sin(0.033t) \tag{32}$$

Simulation Results of Plant Identification and State Estimation. The graphical results of plant identification for the first case of RCVNN with the first activation function are given on Fig. 8(a) where the output of the plant is compared with the output of the RCVNN. The graphical results of RCVNN generalization are given on Fig. 8(b), where the NN weights are fixed and the input signal is changed. The output of the plant is compared with the output of the RCVNN exhibiting a good generalization. The final results of the RVCNN learning and generalization steps are both given on Table 1 for 1000, 2000, and 3000 steps. The validation results show a constant MSE decreasing, exhibiting a good RCVNN convergence and generalization.

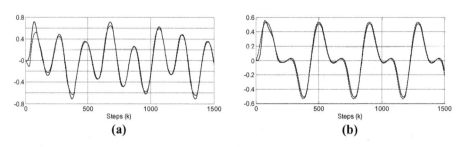

Fig. 8. Simulation results of BP (a) learning and (b) generalization for the first case of activation function; RCVNN output (dotted line); plant output (continue line)

In the same way, the graphical results of plant identification for the second case of RCVNN with second activation function are given on Fig. 9(a) for the learning step and (b) for the generalization step. The final MSEs of RCVNN convergence during system identification is also given on Table 1. The validation results showed a constant MSE decreasing, exhibiting a good performance in the RCVNN generalization.

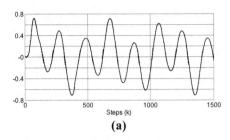 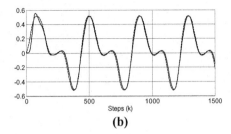

Steps (k)
(a)

Steps (k)
(b)

Fig. 9. Simulation results of BP (a) learning and (b) generalization for the second case of activation function; RCVNN output (dotted line); plant output (continue line)

Comparative Final MSE Simulation Results of Nonlinear Oscillatory Plant Identification and Generalization. The final MSE values obtained during identification and generalization experiments with both RCVNNs (see Table 1) show that the RCVNN with second type activation function outperformed the RCVNN with first type one because the first type possess singular points that affects the BP learning, while the second type does not possess such singular points. In the generalization stage the results are still showing a good performance of the RCVNN.

Table 1. Final MSE of learning and generalization during system identification

Learning		
N. of steps	1st type activation function	2nd type activation function
1000	0.0264	0.0045
2000	0.0178	0.0029
3000	0.0097	0.0028
Generalization		
N. of steps	1st type activation function	2nd type activation function
1000	0.00	0.00
2000	0.00	0.00
3000	0.0014	0.0025

4.3   Simulation Results of Direct Adaptive System Control

The control system is made by three RCVNN using second type activation functions and one output error I-term feedback. The controlled plant is one degree of freedom robot joint possessing nonlinearity and oscillations. In fact the plant is an oscillatory system given by two second order differential equations, representing two degrees of freedom but only one input which makes the system sub-actuated. The response of direct I-term adaptive neural control of the plant is given on Fig. 10(a). While the response for the same plant, applying the same control without I-term is shown in Fig. 10(b). We observe that the I-term control component eliminates the steady-state error of the system.

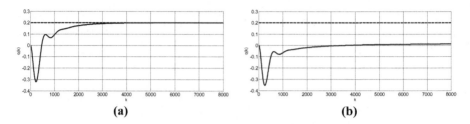

Fig. 10. Simulation results of RCVNN BP direct adaptive neural control (a) with I-term and (b) without I-term; closed loop system output (continuous line); system reference (dashed line)

The final MSE of control after 8000 iterations of RCVNN learning is 0.0105 for the control scheme with the I-term, while the final MSE for the control scheme without the I-term is 0.0519. We observe a better performance of the adaptive control when the I-term is included.

5   Conclusions

In the present work we used diagrammatic rules for the complex case and applied them to obtain the BP training algorithm for each RCVNN learning. We studied two different RCVNN topologies with two different activation functions. The obtained comparative simulation results for system identification and generalization of a nonlinear oscillatory plant using both topologies confirm the quality of the BP learning algorithm. The comparison of the results for RCVNNs with both types of activation functions yields better results for the RCVNN with second case of activation function. The scheme of RCVNN identification and state estimation has been used for direct adaptive feedback/feedforward neural control scheme with I-term where also a good performance of the network has been obtained, having a better performance when the I-term is included.

Acknowledgments. The authors Victor M. Arellano Quintana and Edmundo P. Reynaud would like to thank CONACyT, Mexico, for the student grant received during their studies at DCA, CINVESTAV-IPN, Mexico City, Mexico.

References

1. Amer, R.A., Morsy, G.A., Yassin, H.A.: SCG stability enhancement using STATCOM based-ANN controller. WSEAS Trans. Syst. Control **6**(9), 325–338 (2011)
2. Zhang, Y., Hongsheng, S.: Turbo-generator vibration fault diagnosis based on PSO-BP neural networks. WSEAS Trans. Syst. Control **5**(1), 37–47 (2010)
3. Zemouri, R., Gouriveau, R., Patic, P.C.: Combining a recurrent neural network and a PID controller for prognostic purpose: away to improve the accuracy of predictions. WSEAS Trans. Syst. Control **5**(5), 353–371 (2010)

4. Lin, D., Wang, X., Nian, F., Zhang, Y.: Dynamic fuzzy neural networks modeling and adaptive back-stepping tracking control of uncertain chaotic systems. Neurocomputing **73** (11–18), 2873–2881 (2010)
5. Zhang, H., Wang, X., Lin, X., Liu, C.: Stability and synchronization for discrete-time complex-valued neural networks with time varying delays. PLOS ONE **9**(4), 6 (2014). e93838.pdf
6. Haykin, S.: Neural Networks: A Comprehensive Foundations. Macmillan College, New York (1994)
7. Narendra, K.S., Parthasarasi, K.: Identifications and control of dynamic systems using neural networks. IEEE Trans. Neural Netw. **1**(1), 4–27 (1990)
8. Baruch, I.S., Mariaca-Gaspar, C.R.: A Levenberg-Marquardt learning applied for recurrent neural identification and control of a wastewater treatment bioprocess. Int. J. Intell. Syst. **24**, 1094–1114 (2009). ISSN 0884-8173
9. Hirose, A.: Complex-Valued Neural Networks, vol. 400, 2nd edn. Springer, Berlin (2012)
10. Hirose, A.: Motion controls using complex-valued neural networks with feedback loops. In: Proceedings of IEEE International Conference on Neural Networks, vol. 1, pp. 156–161, San Francisco, CA (1993)
11. Minin, A., Chistyakov, Y., Kholodova, E., Zimmermann, H.G., Knoll, A.: Complex-valued open recurrent neural network for power transformer modeling. Int. J. Appl. Math. Inform. **6**(1), 41–48 (2012)
12. Leung, H., Haykin, S.: The complex back-propagation algorithm. IEEE Trans. Signal Process. **39**(9), 2101–2104 (1991)
13. Woo, C., Hong, D.S.: Adaptive equalization using the complex back-propagation algorithm. In: Proceedings of IEEE International Conference on Neural Networks, vol. 4, pp. 2136–2141, Washington, DC (1996)
14. Miklos, N., Salik, B.: Neural networks with complex activations and connection weights. Complex Syst. **8**, 115–126 (1994)
15. Nava, F., Baruch, I., Poznyak, A., Nenkova, B.: Stability proofs of advanced recurrent neural networks topology and learning. C. R. (Proc. Bul. Acad. Sci.) **57**(1), 27–32 (2004)
16. Wan, E., Beaufays, F.: Diagrammatic method for deriving and relating temporal neural networks algorithms. Neural Comput. **8**, 182–201 (1996)

Segmentation of Carbon Nanotube Images Through an Artificial Neural Network

María Celeste Ramírez Trujillo[1]([⊠]), Teresa E. Alarcón[1],
Oscar S. Dalmau[2], and Adalberto Zamudio Ojeda[1]

[1] Universidad de Guadalajara, Jalisco, Mexico
mcramirez@gdl.cinvestav.mx, teresa.alarcon@profesores.valles.udg.mx,
nanozam@gmail.com
[2] Centro de Investigación en Matemáticas, Guanajuato, Mexico
dalmau@cimat.mx

Abstract. The segmentation of nanotube is an important task for Nanotechnology. The performance of segmentation stage determines the accuracy of the measurement process of nanotube when assessing the quality of nanomaterials. In this work we propose two algorithms for segmenting carbon nanotube images. The first one uses a matched filter bank in the preprocessing step and a neural network for segmenting images from Scanning Electron Microscopy. The second algorithm includes the Perona-Malik filter for enhancing the nanotube information. The segmentation phase is composed by the relaxed Otsu's threshold and an artificial neural network. This algorithm is applied on images from Transmission Electron Microscopy. After the segmentation, for both algorithms, a preprocessing based on mathematical morphology is carried out. The performance of the proposed algorithms is numerically evaluated by using real image databases. Overall accuracy of 92.74 % and 73.99 % were obtained for the first and second algorithm respectively.

Keywords: Segmentation · Artificial neural network · Filter bank · Thresholding

1 Introduction

Carbon nanotubes (CNT) are tubular structures with nanometric dimensions which are studied by nanoscientists and nanotechnologists. The dimensions of the nanotube, in particular the diameter, determine its electrical, mechanical and thermal properties. Depending on their properties, nanotubes are used in different fields of industry, electronics and biology [20]. Nanoscience and Nanotechnology have been favored with the use of computers. Specialists in these fields use the computer for automatic or semiautomatic detection of the nanotube structures in digital images. Afterward the detected nanotubes are measured for characterization purposes [7].

There are several approaches for segmenting images using Digital Image Processing: thresholding [1] and clustering techniques [5], histogram methods

© Springer International Publishing Switzerland 2015
G. Sidorov and S.N. Galicia-Haro (Eds.): MICAI 2015, Part I, LNAI 9413, pp. 338–350, 2015.
DOI: 10.1007/978-3-319-27060-9_28

[19], edge based segmentation [14], region growing techniques [15], and probabilistic approaches [8] among others [10]. Segmentation of tubular structures as nanotubes is a very difficult and time consuming task. In [3] the authors present a segmentation algorithm of the human karyotyping based on thresholding, edge linking and the laplacian operator. A similar problem is addressed in [18] through a Multidirectional Block Ranking algorithm. The segmentation of retinal vessel also engages the detection of tubular structures, this problem is addressed in [6] by combining a Matched filter bank with a cellular automata.

In this work we provide nanotube segmentation algorithms for images obtained from Scanning Electron Microscopy (SEM) and from Transmission Electron Microscopy (TEM). The main problems, in both types of images are: the nanotube overlaps, poor illuminations, and different artifacts that make it very difficult to segment the image. For TEM images the complexity increases due to the presence of the grid during the synthesis step, the noticeable similarity between nanotube and background zones and holes that could appear inside nanotubes. Therefore, the elaborated proposal includes an algorithm for segmenting SEM images and an algorithm for segmenting TEM images. Both algorithms consider three steps: preprocessing, segmentation and postprocessing. In the preprocessing step, we enhance the nanotube information by filtering the image. For SEM images we use a bank of matched filters [6,12] and for TEM images, the Perona-Malik approach [17]. The segmentation of SEM images uses a neural network trained with samples of intensity levels of nanotube and background regions. The segmentation of TEM images is achieved by means of two phases: firstly an automatic Otsu's threshold [16] is computed and then is relaxed. This phase results in three classes: CNT, background and uncertainty zone. In the second phase a neural network is trained taking into consideration the homogeneity, the energy, the correlation and the intensity levels of pixels falling in CNT and background classes. The homogeneity, energy and correlation are computed from coocurrence matrix [11]. During the generalization stage the neural network classifies the pixels in uncertainty zone. The complexity of TEM images leads to design a specific neural network for each TEM image to be analyzed. After the segmentation of both kinds of images follows a preprocessing step through morphological operators. The segmentation results are compared with manually-segmented images by an expert. The overall accuracy for SEM images was 92.74 %. When we considered a whole TEM image the overall accuracy was 73.99 %, in the case of analyzing a region of interest indicated by an expert the overall accuracy reaches the value of 84.07 %.

The structure of this manuscript is the following. Section 2 describes the images under study and two algorithms for segmenting CNT, one algorithm for each type of image. Section 3 explains and discusses the experimental work and finally, in Sect. 4 we present the conclusions.

2   Segmentation Algorithm

2.1   Study Images

The structure of a carbon nanotube is like a sheet of graphite rolled upon itself. There are different techniques for capturing images of carbon nanotubes. In this research the images under study are acquired using two techniques: Scanning Electron Microscopy (SEM) and Transmission Electron Microscopy (TEM)[1]. Figure 1 shows examples of SEM and TEM images.

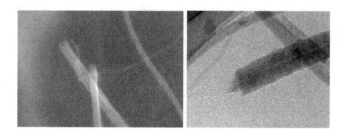

Fig. 1. Left: SEM carbon nanotube image. Right: TEM carbon nanotube image

In SEM images, pixels associated with nanotube information present a higher gray level, however, the intensity level distribution inside nanotube is not uniform. Furthermore, changes in brightness in the background cause confusion between nanotube and background. The overlaps of nanotubes on the edges cause a decreasing intensity and shadow areas. The lack of sharpness in the images makes difficult to find the exact delimitation between the background and the nanotube. Therefore, the edge information seems to be not useful for segmenting this type of images. On the other hand, TEM images also present some problematics that make them very hard to segment. They may contain elements other than carbon, for example, iron spots. Nanowires or nanoparticles can be found inside the tubes. In TEM images one can observe cavities with a trapezoid shape. In most cases, the intensity of cavities is very similar to the background of the image. The grid used for nanotube synthesis sometimes appears in the image, with a gray distribution similar to the nanotube. Certain TEM images may have an artifact in the background, similar to the expansion of water waves. All these mentioned facts lead to changes in luminosity and deformation of nanontube edges, what makes a very difficult segmentation process. The above explanation justifies the elaboration of two algorithms: one for the segmentation of SEM images and the other one for TEM images.

---

[1] The images used in this project were provided by Research and Development of Nanomaterials, SA CV RENIECYT 17567 (National Registry of Scientific and Technological Institutions and Enterprises CONACYT), through MsC. Daniel Ramirez Gonzalez and funded by the PROMEP/103.5/11/6834 project.

2.2   Segmentation Algorithm for SEM Images

For SEM images we follow a semiautomatic segmentation approach. However, the previous idea is not applied directly on the original image. In our case, we take advantage of the geometry of the structure to be segmented, in particular, nanotubes are elongated structures. Hence, we propose the following segmentation steps for SEM images:

1. **Preprocesing.** In this step we transform the original image in order to enhance the nanotube information. For increasing the contrast between nanotube and non-nanotube (background) we propose to apply an appropriate filter bank. In this work we use a matched filter bank, see Refs. [4,6,12] for details. The filter bank is composed by a set of kernels with Gaussian profiles. First, a main kernel is built with cross section, or profile, based on a Gaussian function. The remaining kernels are obtained from the previous kernel by means of rotations and scale changes. The filter bank allows us to enhance the nanotube information and remove illuminance variations in the background of the image.

2. **Feature extraction.** As feature vector we simply use the maximum response of the Matched Filter Bank of pixels belonging to the regions of interest, i.e., nanotubes regions and background regions, because the maximum response provides a good contrast between nanotubes and non-nanotubes regions. Figure 2 depicts an example of this part of the algorithm, in which a user selects the corresponding training set. Although we could be tempted to use a more sophisticated feature vector in order to get a good segmentation result, as we will see in the experiment section, the use of other local features does not guarantee a better result.

3. **Segmentation.** For the segmentation process, a multilayer perceptron (MLP) neural network was selected. Table 1 shows the configuration of the artificial neural network. The neural network was trained using the data set obtained in the previous step.

4. **Postprocessing.** Due to the problematics of SEM images the MLP could obtain nanotubes which are not well-defined, mainly with holes, or it could appear some granularity. These artifacts should be removed in order to obtain

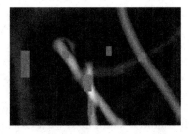

Fig. 2. Extraction of regions of interest. In red: samples of nanotube zones, in blue: samples of background regions (Color figure online)

Table 1. Selected configuration for the multilayer perceptron. SEM images.

Number of layers	*1 hidden layer with 20 neurons*
Activation function in the hidden layer	*logistic sigmoid*
Activation function in the output layer	*Lineal*
Training algorithm	*Levenberg-Marquardt* [2,9,13]
Maximum number of iterations	*100*
Error validation function	*mse*
Gradient value	10^{-4}

a good characterization of nanotubes. Therefore, in general, a post processing is required. All implemented operations are summarized below:

(a) *Removing holes and granularity.* For removing holes and granularities we simply use morphological operators of *closing* and *opening* with a structural element (SE) of type diamond, clearly the size of SE depends on the maximum size of hole needed to fill, in our case the parameters are obtained experimentally. Of course, a more pragmatic alternative could be to fill or remove 'small holes', for example, regions with area less than 1 % with respect to the total size of the processed image, and again, the parameters can be experimentally calculated or trained.

(b) *Edge smoothing.* Finally, with the goal of obtaining nanotube with smooth edges, a median filter is applied on the image obtained in the previous step.

2.3 Segmentation Algorithm for TEM Images

In the case of TEM images we present an automatic segmentation alternative. Although the idea is similar to the previous algorithm, we adapt it for TEM images because, as explained above, they have different characteristics. For example, we change the *preprocessing* step because the application of the Matched Filter bank does not produce good results.

1. **Preprocessing.** The general idea is to increase the contrast between nanotube and non-nanotube information, to remove noise and preserve the edge of nanotubes. For the previous reasons, we use the Perona-Malik [17] filter. The application of Perona-Malik algorithm allows us, at the same time, to enhance the information of nanotubes in TEM images, to preserve the nanotube borders and attenuate noise.

2. **Segmentation.** Now we can find pixels that belong to nanotubes and background by means of Otsu's method [16]. Then, we can binarize the image by using the automatic threshold U computed with Otsu's. However, this simple idea does not yield good segmentation results. Instead, the threshold U, is relaxed by a certain value (θ), that leads to two new thresholds, $U_1 = U - \theta$

and $U_2 = U + \theta$. Equation (1) explains how the two new thresholds are used on the segmentation process:

$$F(g(r)) = \begin{cases} background & \text{if } g(r) < U_1 \\ nanotube & \text{if } g(r) > U_2 \\ uncertaintyarea & \text{otherwise} \end{cases} \qquad (1)$$

where $g(r)$ represents the gray level of the pixel r in the image. Pixels with intensities greater than U_2 have high confidence to belong to the nanotube region and are classified as nanotube, and pixels with intensities less than U_1 have high confidence to belong to the background and are classified as non-nanotube. For classifying pixels with intensities in $[U_1, U_2]$, i.e., pixels with low confidence, we use a neural network. The training set is obtained by considering pixels with high confidence to belong to a class, as background or nanotube. As feature vector we use the homogeneity, energy, contrast and correlation which are computed based on the coocurrence matrix, and also, the intensity levels of the image. Table 2 describes the artificial neural network used for segmenting the uncertainty region. It is important to note, that in the case of TEM images, the neural network is trained and applied for each particular image, due to the complexity of this type of images.

Table 2. Selected configuration for the multilayer perceptron. TEM images.

Number of layers	*1 hidden layer with 20 neurons*
Activation function in the hidden layer	*hyperbolic tangent sigmoid*
Activation function in the output layer	*Lineal*
Training algorithm	*Levenberg-Marquardt* [2,9,13]
Maximum number of iterations	*100*
Error validation function	*mse*
Gradient value	10^{-4}

3. **Postprocessing.** Similar to SEM images, after applying the segmentation step, one can obtain an image with holes or with some granularity. In order to remove these artifacts we apply the same postprocessing used for SEM images, i.e., *removing holes and granularity* and *edge smoothing*.

3   Experiments and Discussion

In this section we discuss about different experiments using SEM and TEM images. The performance of the proposed algorithms is numerically evaluated by using real image databases. Based on these databases, which are manually segmented by an expert, we compute the overall accuracy measure in order to evaluate the efficiency of the proposal.

3.1   Segmentation of SEM Images

For the experimental work we use 14 SEM images of size 640 × 430 pixels. First row of Fig. 3 depicts examples of theses images. Second row of Fig. 3 shows the results after applying the filter bank. Note that, the nanotube information have been significantly improved, even for the case with poor illumination, and the smooth illuminance variation in the background has also been removed.

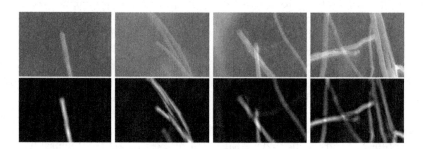

Fig. 3. Examples of SEM images. First row: (from left to right) real SEM images with different levels of complexity: easy, intermediate and difficult levels. Second row: corresponding preprocessed images after applying the Matched Filter Bank.

In order to train the multilayer neural network, we perform experiments with different feature vectors. First, we select patches that belong to nanotubes and non-nanotubes regions. In particular, the patches were taken from the image illustrated in the second row and third column in Fig. 3, see also Fig. 2. We carry out 5 experiments: one per each feature vector. The feature vectors are taken over pixels belonging to regions containing nanotubes and background. The explored features are: intensity levels of the image (Experiment I), vector composed by the local mean, variance and entropy (Experiment II), vector whose components include the intensity level and the local mean, variance and entropy (Experiment III), vector composed by the homogeneity, energy, contrast and correlation which are calculated from the co-occurrence matrix (Experiment IV), vector whose components include the intensity level and the homogeneity, energy, contrast and correlation calculated from the co-occurrence matrix (Experiment V).

In order to assess the neural network we use the remaining 13 images. First row of Fig. 4 shows the result after applying the neural network with different feature vectors. Second row of Fig. 4 shows the corresponding result after the postprocessing step. Observe the significant improvement of the postprocessing step for each executed experiment. The holes and discontinuities are removed and the body of nanotubes is recovered.

For numerically evaluating the performance of the proposed algorithm, see Sect. 2.2, we consider manually-segmented images by an expert. The third column of Table 3 shows a summary of the average of the overall accuracy computed over the 13 testing images. The evaluation considers the results of segmentation for the training and generalization phase after the postprocessing step. From the

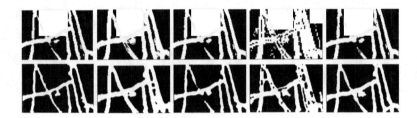

Fig. 4. Final result of the segmentation algorithm for SEM images. First row represents the outputs of the artificial neural network for the Experiments I, II, III, IV and V. Second row represents the results of the postprocessing step corresponding to the output of the artificial neural net (first row).

Table 3. SEM images: Average of the Overall accuracy for the five executed experiments.

Experiment	Training (%)	Generalization (%)
Experiment I	**98.39**	**92.74**
Experiment II	95.58	89.92
Experiment III	97.15	92.42
Experiment IV	89.80	84.65
Experiment V	97.55	92.25

results in Table 3 we conclude that the neural network trained with the feature vector given by the intensity levels (Experiment I) leads to the best result.

3.2 Segmentation of TEM Images. Experiments

For the experimental work we use 41 TEM images, Fig. 5 shows examples of these images. All of them are manually segmented by an expert. As we can see, the images have different level of complexity: easy level when there is only one nanotube; intermediate when there are two o more nanotubes; difficult level when there are overlaps between nanotubes, noise and the grid used is visible; very difficult level when they have the same problems as in images of difficult level and the nanotubes appear with interior holes. An example of the Preprocessing step is shown in Fig. 6.

Due to the complexity of the images, the neural network is applied per each image, i.e., the neural neural network is trained using pixels in the image with high confidence to belong to nanotube or background. Then the neural network is applied to pixels with low confidence to belong to the classes. For the previous reasons, the segmentation process for TEM images is more time consuming than for SEM images. In particular, the training process considers the 20 % of pixels falling in zones with high reliability (background and nanotube class according to expression (1). In the generalization step the built networks classify pixels in uncertainty zones, see Eq. (1).

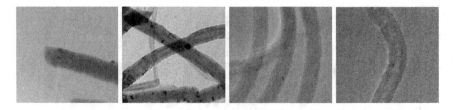

Fig. 5. Example of used TEM images. From left to right: images with easy, intermediate, difficult and very difficult levels

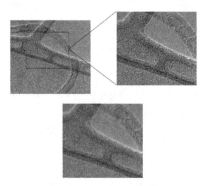

Fig. 6. Example of preprocessing step. The zoomed region contains the holes in the interior part of the nanotube and the background is very noisy (first row). The image is smoothed and the edges are preserved (second row)

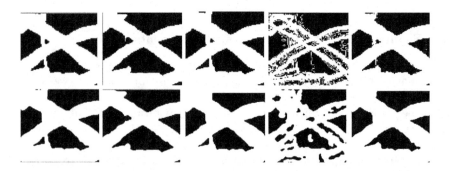

Fig. 7. Final result of the segmentation algorithm for TEM images. First row represents the outputs of the artificial neural network for the Experiments I, II, III, IV and V. Second row represents the results of the postprocessing step corresponding to the output of the artificial neural net (first row).

Similar to the experiments for SEM images, Subsect. 3.1, we perform 5 experiments by using different feature vectors. Figure 7 shows an example of the result for the segmentation process and postprocessing for each experiment. Note that, the postprocessing step allows us to eliminate small holes and to smooth edges.

Table 4. TEM images: Average of the Overall accuracy for the five executed experiments.

Experiment	Training (%)	Generalization (%)
Experiment I	85.74	70.32
Experiment II	85.43	60.65
Experiment III	**85.97**	69.38
Experiment IV	77.71	48.71
Experiment V	82.72	**73.99**

In order to assess the performance of the proposed algorithm, see Subsect. 2.3, we consider the 41 manually-segmented images by an expert. Table 4 gives a quantitative comparison of the average of the overall accuracy computed over these images. The evaluation includes the results of segmentation for the training and generalization phase and after the postprocessing step. According to the values in Table 4, we conclude that the feature vector of Experiment V, i.e., the feature vector that includes the intensity levels, the contrast, correlation, homogeneity and energy; yields the best results. Note that, the highest accuracy value is equal 73.99 %, which is less than the highest accuracy for SEM images (92.74 %).

On the other hand, we note that the segmentation algorithm mainly misclassifies zones belonging to the background, which affects the overall accuracy. Some preliminary results show that if we increase the nanotube information in the learning process, the overall accuracy could also increase. For experiments in which the nanotechnologist indicates regions of interest, and then applies the whole algorithm, using the feature vector of Experiment V, one obtains an accuracy of 84.07 %. This suggest that the algorithm can be used interactively, i.e., the expert selects a region of interest and then applies the segmentation algorithm. Figure 8 illustrates an example of the previous experiment.

Finally, we note that most errors of this algorithm occur in images with poor illumination, with very granular texture, when the distribution of intensity levels of nanotube and background are very similar, or when the nanotube has interior

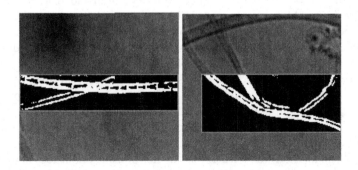

Fig. 8. Examples of segmented images using a region of interest given by an expert.

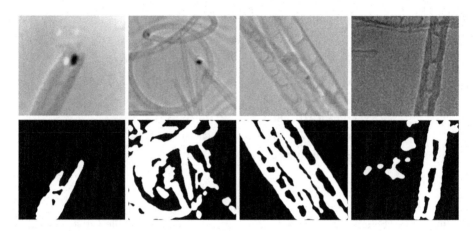

Fig. 9. Examples of segmentation results with errors due to the complexity of the image.

holes. Figure 9 depicts some examples of these images and the corresponding segmentation. According to the experimental work, we recommend a value of the relaxation parameter θ in the interval $[1, 2]$ for very noisy images, for less noisy images θ can take values in the interval $[3, 7]$. When there are noticeable variations of intensity levels within classes, θ can take values in the interval $[15, 50]$.

4   Conclusions

We proposed two algorithms for segmentation of carbon nanotube images: one for images obtained from Scanning Electron Microscopy and the other for segmenting images from Transmission Electron Microscopy. Both algorithms consider three steps: preprocessing, segmentation and postprocessing. The preprocessing step allowed to increase the contrast between nanotube and background using appropriate filters. The segmentation stage is based on a neural network approach. For TEM images a threshold technique is included with the goal of detecting regions of high confidence to belong to nanotube or background classes, which are considered as training data for the neural network. Due to the complexity of carbon nanotube images a postprocessing step was required with the aim of removing artifacts, such that holes inside nanotubes and granularities. The performance of both algorithms was evaluated using real image databases, which were manually segmented by an expert. According to the experimental work the segmentation of SEM images obtained an excellent accuracy. On the other hand, the accuracy of the algorithm for TEM images was good, although, it can be improved if an expert selects regions of interest in the image. The performance of the method was sensitive to the holes inside nanotubes and artifacts like the grid used in the synthesis for TEM images.

Acknowledgments. This research was partially supported by the Project PROMEP/ 103.5/11/6834.

References

1. Batenburg, K.J., Sijbers, J.: Adaptive thresholding of tomograms by projection distance minimization. Pattern Recogn. **42**(10), 2297–2305 (2009)
2. Bates, D.M., Watts, D.G.: Nonlinear regression: iterative estimation and linear approximations. Wiley Online Library (1988)
3. Chaku, P., Shah, P., Bakshi, S.: A digital image processing algorithm for automation of human karyotyping. Int. J. Comput. Sci. Commun. (IJCSC) **5**(1), 54–56 (2014)
4. Chaudhuri, S., Chatterjee, S., Katz, N., Nelson, M., Goldbaum, M.: Detection of blood vessels in retinal images using two-dimensional matched filters. EEE Trans. Med. Imaging **8**(3), 263–269 (1989)
5. Chuang, K.S., Tzeng, H.L., Chen, S., Wu, J., Chen, T.J.: Fuzzy c-means clustering with spatial information for image segmentation. Comput. Med. Imaging Graph. **30**, 9–15 (2006)
6. Dalmau, O., Alarcon, T.: MFCA: matched filters with cellular automata for retinal vessel detection. In: Batyrshin, I., Sidorov, G. (eds.) MICAI 2011, Part I. LNCS, vol. 7094, pp. 504–514. Springer, Heidelberg (2011)
7. Gao, Y., Li, Z., Lin, Z., Zhu, L., Tannenbaum, A., Bouix, S., Wong, C.: Automated dispersion and orientation analysis for carbon nanotube reinforced polymer composites. Nanotechnol. **23**(43), 435706 (2012)
8. Geman, S., Geman, D.: Stochastic relaxation, gibbs distributions and bayesian restoration of images. IEEE Trans. Pattern Anal. Mach. Intell. **6**(6), 721–741 (2004)
9. Gill, P.R., Murray, W., Wright, M.H.: The Levenberg-Marquardt Method. Academic Press, Practical Optimization, London (1981)
10. Gonzalez, R., Woods, R.: Digital image processing. Pearson/Prentice Hall, Upper Saddle River (2008). http://books.google.com.mx/books?id=8uGOnjRGEzoC
11. Haralick, R.M., Shanmugam, K., Dinstein, I.: Textural features for image classification. IEEE Trans. Syst. Man Cybern. **3**(6), 610–621 (1973)
12. de Jesús Guerrero, J., Dalmau, O., Alarcón, T.E., Zamudio, A.: Frequency filter bank for enhancing carbon nanotube images. In: Gelbukh, A., Espinoza, F.C., Galicia-Haro, S.N. (eds.) MICAI 2014, Part I. LNCS, vol. 8856, pp. 316–326. Springer, Heidelberg (2014)
13. Levenberg, K.: A method for the solution of certain problems in least squares. Quart. Appl. Math. **2**, 164–168 (1944)
14. Lindeberg, T., Li, M.X.: Segmentation and classification of edges using minimum description length approximation and complementary junction cues. Comput. Vis. Image Underst. **67**, 88–98 (1997)
15. Nock, R., Nielsen, F.: Statistical region merging. IEEE Trans. Pattern Anal. Mach. Intell. **26**, 1452–1458 (2004)
16. Otsu, N.: A threshold selection method from gray-level histogram. IEEE Trans. Syst. Man Cybern. **SMC–9**(1), 62–66 (1979)
17. Perona, P., Malik, J.: Scale-space and edge detection using anisotropic diffusion. IEEE Trans. Pattern Anal. Mach. Intell. **12**(7), 629–639 (1990)
18. Rajaraman, S., Vaidyanathan, G., Chokkalingam, A.: Segmentation and removal of interphase cells from chromosome images using multidirectional block ranking. Int. J. Bio-sci. Bio-Technol. **5**(3), 79–91 (2013)

19. Shapiro, L.G., Stockman, G.C.: Computer Vision. Prentice-Hall, Upper Saddle River (2001)
20. Torres, A.D.: Procesamiento digital de imgenes. Perfiles Educativos, pp. 1–15, abril-junio 1996

Evolutionary Algorithms

Finding the Optimal Sample Based on Shannon's Entropy and Genetic Algorithms

Edwin Aldana-Bobadilla[1,2(✉)] and Carlos Alfaro-Pérez[1,2]

[1] Facultad de Ingeniería UNAM, Ciudad Universitaria, México D.F, Mexico
edwynjavier@yahoo.es, carlos.alfaro26@gmail.com
[2] Facultad de Estudios Superiores-UNAM, Naucalpan
Estado de México, Mexico

Abstract. A common task in data analysis is to find the appropriate data sample whose properties allow us to infer the parameters of the data population. The most frequently dilemma related to sampling is how to determine the optimal *size* of the sample. To solve it, there are typical methods based on asymptotical results from the Central Limit Theorem. However, the effectiveness of such methods is bounded by several considerations as the sampling strategy (simple, stratified, cluster-based, etc.), the size of the population or even the dimensionality of the space of the data. In order to avoid such constraints, we propose a method based on a measure of information of the data in terms of Shannon's Entropy. Our idea is to find the optimal sample of size N whose information is as similar as possible to the information of the population, subject to several constraints. Finding such sample represents a hard optimization problem whose feasible space disallows the use of traditional optimization techniques. To solve it, we resort to Genetic Algorithms. We test our method with synthetic datasets; the results show that our method is suitable. For completeness, we used a dataset from a real problem; the results confirm the effectiveness of our proposal and allow us to visualize different applications.

Keywords: Sampling data · Genetic algorithms · Shannon's entropy · Feature selection

1 Introduction

The goal of sampling is to choose a representative subset S from a set called population denoted by P. One way in which S may be obtained is by a random process where each element in P has an equal probability of being selected (simple sampling). When this process allows us to choose an element from P more than once, it is called sampling with replacement [1] otherwise it is called sampling without replacement [2]. Alternative ways to obtain S are: systematic sampling [3], stratified sampling [4] and cluster sampling [5]. Regardless of the *sampling strategy*, an important concern is how to determine the cardinality or size of S. Usually this value is determined resorting to asymptotical results from the Central Limit Theorem (CLT) [6]. Assuming a sample S_i of size N drawn from P with mean μ_{S_i}, let $\bar{X}$ be a set of means μ_{S_i} of the form:

© Springer International Publishing Switzerland 2015
G. Sidorov and S.N. Galicia-Haro (Eds.): MICAI 2015, Part I, LNAI 9413, pp. 353–363, 2015.
DOI: 10.1007/978-3-319-27060-9_29

$$\bar{X} = \{\mu_{S_1}, \mu_{S_2}, \ldots, \mu_{S_M}\} \tag{1}$$

From CLT, it is said that there is a relationship between the mean of $\bar{X}$ denoted as $\mu_{\bar{X}}$ and the mean of the population P denoted as μ which is given by:

$$\mu_{\bar{X}} \cong \mu \tag{2}$$

Likewise, it is said that there is a relationship between the deviation of $\bar{X}$ denoted as $\sigma_{\bar{X}}$, and the standard deviation of the population σ which is given by:

$$\sigma_{\bar{X}} \cong \frac{\sigma}{\sqrt{N}} \tag{3}$$

Since $\sigma_{\bar{X}}$ represents a dispersion measure of the samples S_i (usually called standard error), its value must be as small as possible. There is an optimal value of N that allows satisfying such condition. We illustrate this fact in Fig. 1, with a synthetic dataset in $\mathbb{R}$ of size 6000. Every point is the standard error obtained with different values of N. We can see that the value of N that minimizes the standard error is the closest to the population size. Obviously, for practical purposes, such value is unsuitable. An error value must be assumed to choose a value of N less than the cardinality of P.

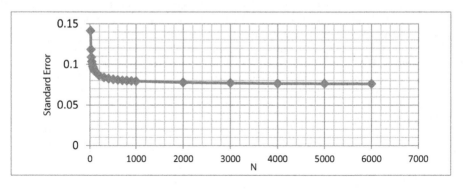

Fig. 1. Standard error in function of the sample size

From (3) and based on such error, the size of a sample is given by:

$$N \cong \frac{\sigma^2}{\sigma_{\bar{X}}^2} \tag{4}$$

From (4), typically the value of $\sigma_{\bar{X}}$ is defined in a discretionary way. From our example (see Fig. 1), if we assume that $\sigma_{\bar{X}} = 0.05$, the value of N will be greater than the size or cardinality of P. It means that not always given a value of $\sigma_{\bar{X}}$ the value of N is appropriate. We are facing an optimization problem which involves to find the breakeven point between N and $\sigma_{\bar{X}}$. An important consideration in the above discussion is that the asymptotical relationships in (2) and (3) assume that the samples are obtained by a simple random sampling; usually more complex *sampling strategies* are not taken into account. Another consideration is that these asymptotical relationships do not consider random variables in a multidimensional space. We propose a method that allows us to find the optimal sample S' from a population P without the above considerations. The idea is to find a sample of size N whose information is as similar as possible to the information of the population and the value of N is minimal. In order to measure the information, we resort to Shannon's Entropy [7]. The size of the search space is given by:

$$\sum_{N=1}^{|P|} \binom{|P|}{N} = \sum_{N=1}^{|P|} \frac{|P|!}{N!(|P| - N)!} \tag{5}$$

where $\binom{|P|}{N}$ is the number of ways of picking N elements from P. Since this search space is huge, it is necessary to resort to a method that allows us to explore it efficiently. Among the many methods that have arisen, we mention tabu search [8], simulated annealing [9], ant colony optimization [10], particle swarm optimization [11] and evolutionary computation [12]. Furthermore, among the many variations of evolutionary computation, we find evolutionary strategies [13], evolutionary programming [14], genetic programming [15] and genetic algorithms (GAs) [16]. All of these methods are used to find approximate solutions for complex optimization problems. It was proven that an elitist GA always converges to the global optimum [17]. Such a convergence, however, is not bounded in time, and the selection of the GA variation with the best dynamic behavior is very convenient. In this regard, we rely on the conclusions of previous analyses [18, 19], which showed that a breed of GA, called the eclectic genetic algorithm (EGA), achieves the best relative performance.

Having determined the measure of information and chosen the appropriate method to explore the wide search space, in the following section, we present the details of our proposal. The rest of this work has been organized as follows: In Sect. 2 we show the background to guide the discussion about our proposal. We show how to measure the information of the data based on Shannon's Entropy and how to extend such measure to data in multidimensional space. In Sect. 3, we show in detail our proposal. In Sect. 4, we show the experimental methodology and its results. Finally, we present the conclusions and infer several applications.

2 Preliminaries

2.1 Measuring the Expected Information Value

The so-called entropy [20] appeals to an evaluation of the information content of a random variable Y with possible values $\{y_1, y_2, \ldots, y_n\}$. From a statistical viewpoint, the information of the event $(Y = y_i)$ is inversely proportional to its likelihood. This information is denoted by $I(y_i)$, which can be expressed as:

$$I(y_i) = \log\left(\frac{1}{p(y_i)}\right) = -\log(p(y_i)) \tag{6}$$

From information theory [21], the entropy of Y is the expected value of I. It is given by:

$$H(Y) = -\sum_{i=1}^{n} p(y_i) \log(p(y_i)) \tag{7}$$

Typically, the *log* function may be taken to be *log₂*, and then, the entropy is expressed in bits; otherwise, as *ln*, in which case the entropy is in nats. We will use log_2 for the computations in this paper. We can visualize P and S as random variables, thus their entropies can be calculated from (7). We want to choose a sample S of **SIZE** N (in what follows denoted as S_N) from P such that:

$$\frac{|H(S_N) - H(P)|}{H(P)} \leq \varepsilon \tag{8}$$

Where ε is a parameter that represents the maximum permissible error between the information of P and S. To calculate the entropy, an important issue is how to determine the probability $p(y_i)$. Since usually the probability distribution function (PDF) of Y is unknown, we approximate such PDF through a method based on quantiles. Such method can be extended to multidimensional random variables ($Y \in \mathbb{R}^n, n \geq 2$). In what follows, we expand the discussion about this.

2.2   Fitting Distribution of Y

We can divide the space of Y into a set of intervals usually called quantiles [22]. The PDF of Y is approximated by the proportion of the elements that lies in each quantile. This is illustrated in Fig. 2.

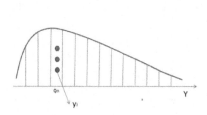
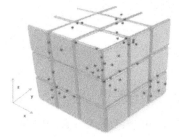

Fig. 2. A possible division of the space of Y in a one-dimensional space

Fig. 3. A possible division of the space of Y in a 3-dimensional space

The above idea may be extended to a multidimensional space, in which case, a quantile is a multidimensional partition of the space of Y as is shown in Fig. 3 ("hyper-quantile"). In both cases the probability $p(y_i)$ is the density of the quantile to which $p(y_i)$ belongs in terms of data contained in it. To determine the number of quantiles in which the space of Y must be divided, typically, Sturges' rule [23] is used. There are other alternative rules which attempt to improve the performance of Sturges's without a normality assumption as Doane's formula [24] and the Rice rule [25]. We prefer the Rice rule, which is to *set the number of intervals to twice the cube root of the number of observations.* In the case of 1000 observations, the Rice rule yields 20 intervals instead of the 11 recommended by Sturges' rule.

Having defined the way to measure the information of P and S_N, in the following section, we present important details to find the optimal S_N.

3 Proposal

3.1 Defining the Objective Function

We want to find the minimal value of N that allows us to obtain a sample S_N from P, whose entropy is as close as possible to entropy of P. Finding such sample is an optimization problem of the form:

$$Minimize : f(N) = \frac{N}{|P|}$$

$$subject\ to :$$

$$\frac{|H(S_N) - H(P)|}{H(P)} \leq \varepsilon \tag{9}$$

$$N \in [2, |P|)$$

The value of the objective function tends to 1 when the value of N is close to $|P|$. Otherwise this value tends to decrease as the value of N is away from $|P|$. As mentioned, ε is a parameter that represents the maximum permissible error between the information of P and S. The problem in (9) is a constrained optimization problem. To solve it, we use EGA with a constraint handling strategy which is described in Subsect. 3.3.

3.2 Encoding the Problem

EGA proposes M candidate values of N which allow us to obtain M samples S_N. The fitness value of these candidates is determined by the objective function. Additionally each candidate must satisfy the constraints defined in (9). The fitness of those candidates that does not satisfy such constraints is punished through a penalty function (see Subsect. 3.3). Each candidate is encoded as a binary string of length 32. EGA generates a population of candidates (binary strings) and evaluates them in accordance with their **integer** representation and the objective function (9). Evolution takes place after the repeated application of the genetic operators [18, 19]. *It is important to remark that our*

method is independent of the sampling strategy to select the elements from P. We can
choose any strategy and use it throughout of the evolutionary process of EGA.

3.3   Constraints Handling Strategy

To solve a constrained optimization problem, the most common way is resorting to a
penalty function [26]. In this approach, the objective function in (9) can be transformed
as follows:

$$F(N) = \begin{cases} f(N) & \text{if } N \text{ is a feasible solution} \\ f(N) + penalty(N) & \text{otherwise} \end{cases} \quad (10)$$

There are many variations of penalty functions. Based on the results of a comprehensive analysis reported in [27], we use the method that exhibited the best performance, where the objective function $f(N)$ is transformed as follows:

$$F(N) = \begin{cases} \left[K - \sum_{i=1}^{s} \frac{K}{p} \right] & s \neq p \\ f(N) & otherwise \end{cases} \quad (11)$$

where K is a large constant $[O(10^9)]$, p is the number of constraints and s is the number
of these which have been satisfied.

3.4   Getting the Optimal Sample

When the evolutionary process of EGA is finished, the population will have the best
candidate whose genome (the value of N) allows us to find the optimal sample S_N.
Given a population[1] P (dataset), such process involves the following:

1. Generate a random set C with candidate solutions in accordance to the problem
   encoding.
2. For each candidate or individual in C, decode its genome in order to obtain a value
   of N and a sample S_N from P.
3. Determine the fitness value of each individual based on objective function (9).
4. Determine the feasibility of each individual in C and apply the penalty function (if
   necessary).
5. Sort C in ascending order, based on the fitness values.
6. Apply genetic operators of EGA (see [18, 19]).
7. Repeated 2-4 until convergence criteria are met (usually the number of generations).
8. Select the top candidate from C; decode it in order to obtain a value of N.
9. Obtain a sample S_N from P. This is the optimal sample which satisfies:
   $\frac{|H(S_N) - H(P)|}{H(P)} \leq \varepsilon$

---

[1] To avoid ambiguities, the word *population* and the term P refer to the dataset to be sampled rather
than the set of candidate solutions of EGA. Instead, this last set is denoted as C.

As mentioned, we can choose *any sampling strategy* to obtain S_N throughout of the evolutionary process. The value of ε must be given a priori, we set $\varepsilon = 0.01$, which represents an error of 1 % between the entropies of the sample and the population.

3.5   Setting Additional Parameters

The EGA was executed with the following parameter values: $Pc = 0.90$, $Pm = 0.009$, $|C| = 70$, $G = 300$. It is based on a mentioned study [18], which showed that from a statistical view point, EGA converges to the optimal solution around such values when the problems are demanding (those with a non-convex feasible space).

4   Results

We wanted to show some **preliminary results** as evidence of the effectiveness of our method. Subsequently, we defined a performance measure relative to the ratio between the size of S_N and P. We executed systematically a set of experiments (with synthetic datasets) which allowed us to find the behavior of such ratio from the statistical view point. Finally, we show the effectiveness of our method with a real problem.

4.1   Preliminary Results

We executed preliminary experiments whose results allow us to show that our method is promissory. The datasets in such experiments included:

- A dataset of 10000 elements in a one-dimensional space drawn from a gaussian distribution (see Fig. 4).
- A dataset of 10000 elements in a bi-dimensional space drawn from a gaussian distribution (see Fig. 5).
- A dataset of 10000 elements in bi-dimensional space that represent a sinusoidal function (see Fig. 6).

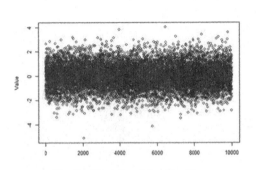

Fig. 4. Gaussian dataset in $\mathbb{R}$

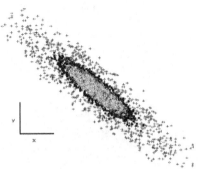

Fig. 5. Gaussian dataset in $\mathbb{R}^2$

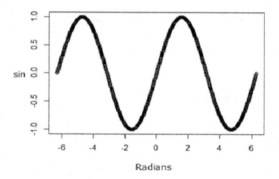

Fig. 6. Sinusoidal dataset

Our hypothesis is that our method will find the optimal sample (one with the minimal value of N) from these datasets, retaining their properties (e.g. probability distribution or spatial arrangement). In Figs. 7, 8, 9, 10, 11 and 12 we can see that the samples retain several properties of the population. Additional properties are shown in Table 1. As extended work, we will show that in general, the properties of the PDF (e.g. unimodality, skweness, kurtosis, etc.) are similar to those of the dataset. In this regard the reader can find an interesting work in [28].

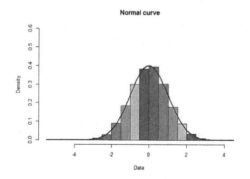

Fig. 7. Density of the dataset in $\mathbb{R}$

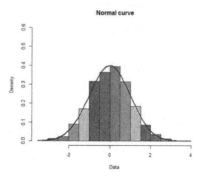

Fig. 8. Density of the sample in $\mathbb{R}$

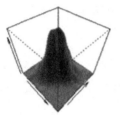

Fig. 9. Density of the dataset in $\mathbb{R}^2$

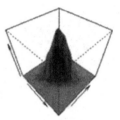

Fig. 10. Density of the sample in $\mathbb{R}^2$

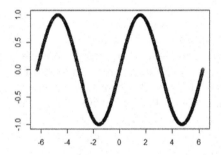

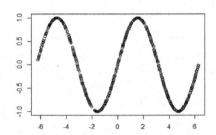

Fig. 11. Spatial arrangement of the sinusoidal dataset

Fig. 12. Spatial arrangement of the sinusoidal sample

Table 1. Additionaly properties of the datasets and the samples

	Dataset 1		Dataset 2		Dataset 3	
	Population	Sample	Population	Sample	Population	Sample
Size	10000	1860	10000	1512	10000	768
Entropy	3.0534	3.0527	3.9261	3.9937	3.7281	3.7194

4.2   Measuring the Performance

To measure the performance of our method, we resort to the *space saving metric* (SS) from compression data which is given by:

$$SS = 1 - \frac{N}{|P|} \tag{12}$$

A large value of SS (closer to 1) implies better performance. We calculated such metric with a wide set of experiments (about 5000) which included random datasets of size 1000, 5000, 10000 and 100000. The results are shown in Table 2. For completeness, we determine the confidence interval of the results with a *p*-value of 0.05.

Table 2. Summary of results obtained with differents datasets (gaussian a non-gaussian)

SS	0.7895
Standard deviation	0.3181
Lower limit	0.7806
Upper limit	0.7983
Confidence level	95 %

The experiments shows that in average the sampling process allows us to reduce the size of the dataset in more than 70 %. In this sense our method can be considered a lossy compression method.

4.3   Real World Dataset

We tested our method with a dataset whose elements represent information of the handwritten digit recognition problem. The problem is to separate the highly confusible digits '4' and '9'. Such dataset was obtained from UCI repository [29]. This dataset has 6000 instances (elements) with 5000 attributes. We applied our method in order to *reduce the number of such attributes*. For each instance, we executed our method to obtain the most informative attributes (those whose entropy is close to entropy of all attributes of the instance). Based on the above, 6000 experiments were executed. These experiments allow us to find the relative frequency of each attribute. We chose those with frequency greater than 0.15. Such decision allows us to reduce the number of attributes to 890. To test that such reduction retains the properties of the original data, we applied a Multi-layer Perceptron Network (MLPN) with the reduced dataset. The labeling set obtained by MLPN was compared with the labeling set of the original dataset. The proportion of identical elements (labels) between these sets was 97.68 %.

5   Conclusions

A new sampling method based on the entropy has been defined in order to find a sample of minimal size from a dataset (population). Finding the optimal sample involves an optimization problem that requires an efficient method to explore the huge feasible space. We use EGA as the best alternative. A first approach allows us to determine that our. method is able to find a sample from a dataset that retains the original properties related to the probability distribution or spatial arrangement. Based on these results a wide set of experiments on synthetic datasets was executed. On average the method achieved a value of SS of 0.78. It means that we can reduce the size of a dataset in more than 70 % and obtain the optimal samples that retain the information of the original datasets with an error of 1 % (given by the value of ε). Based on the above, we can tackle many applications that require lossy compression data. We showed that our method can be applied to those problems related to feature selection, where removing redundant attributes is compulsory.

References

1. Mukhopadhyay, P.: Theory and Methods of Survey Sampling. PHI Learning Pvt. Ltd., New Delhi (2009)
2. Sukhatme, P.V.: Sampling Theory of Surveys with Applications. Iowa State University Press, Ames (1957)
3. Israel, G.D.: Sampling the evidence of extension program impact. University of Florida Cooperative Extension Service, Institute of Food and Agriculture Sciences, EDIS (1992)
4. Cochran, W.G.: Sampling Techniques. Wiley, New York (2007)
5. Särndal, C.-E., Swensson, B., Wretman, J.: Model Assisted Survey Sampling. Springer, New York (2003)

6. Barany, I., Vu, V.: Central limit theorems for Gaussian polytopes. Ann. Probab. **34**, 1593–1621 (2007)
7. Shannon, C.E.: A mathematical theory of communication. ACM SIGMOBILE Mob. Comput. Commun. Rev. **5**(1), 3–55 (2001)
8. Glover, F.: Tabu search-part I. ORSA J. Comput. **1**(3), 190–206 (1989)
9. Kirkpatrick, S., Gelatt, C.D., Vecchi, M.P.: Optimization by simulated annealing. Science **220**(4598), 671–680 (1983)
10. Dorigo, M., Birattari, M.: Ant colony optimization. In: Sammut, C., Webb, G.I. (eds.) Encyclopedia of Machine Learning, pp. 36–39. Springer, New York (2010)
11. Kennedy, J.: Particle Swarm Optimization. Encyclopedia of Machine Learning, pp. 760–766. Springer, New York (2010)
12. Spears, W.M., et al.: An overview of evolutionary computation. In: Brazdil, P.B. (ed.) ECML 1993. LNCS, vol. 667, pp. 442–459. Springer, Heidelberg (1993)
13. Geritz, S.A.H., Mesze, G., Metz, J.A.J.: Evolutionarily singular strategies and the adaptive growth and branching of the evolutionary tree. Evol. Ecol. **12**(1), 35–57 (1998)
14. Kim, J.-H., Myung, H.: Evolutionary programming techniques for constrained optimization problems. IEEE Trans. Evol. Comput. **1**(2), 129–140 (1997)
15. Koza, J.R., Bennett III, F.H., Stiffelman, O.: Genetic programming as a Darwinian invention machine. In: Langdon, W.B., Fogarty, T.C., Nordin, P., Poli, R. (eds.) EuroGP 1999. LNCS, vol. 1598, pp. 93–108. Springer, Heidelberg (1999)
16. Goldberg, D.E., Holland, J.H.: Genetic algorithms and machine learning. Mach. Learn. **3**(2), 95–99 (1988)
17. Rudolph, G.: Convergence analysis of canonical genetic algorithms. IEEE Trans. Neural Netw. **5**(1), 96–101 (1994)
18. Kuri-Morales, A., Aldana-Bobadilla, E.: The best genetic algorithm I. In: Castro, F., Gelbukh, A., González, M. (eds.) MICAI 2013, Part II. LNCS, vol. 8266, pp. 1–15. Springer, Heidelberg (2013)
19. Morales, A.K., Quezada, C.V.: A universal eclectic genetic algorithm for constrained optimization. Proceedings of the 6th European Congress on Intelligent Techniques and Soft Computing, vol. 1 (1998)
20. Shannon, C.E.: A note on the concept of entropy. Bell Syst. Tech. J. **27**, 379–423 (1948)
21. Shannon, C.E., Weaver, W.: The mathematical theory of information (1949)
22. Hyndman, R.J., Fan, Y.: Sample quantiles in statistical packages. Am. Stat. **50**(4), 361–365 (1996)
23. Hyndman, R.J.: The problem with Sturges' rule for constructing histograms. Monash University (1995)
24. Doane, D.P.: Aesthetic frequency classifications. Am. Stat. **30**(4), 181–183 (1976)
25. Soo, N.H., Halim, Y.: Feature selection methodology in quality data mining (2004)
26. White, D.J., Anandalingam, G.: A penalty function approach for solving bi-level linear programs. J. Glob. Optim. **3**(4), 397–419 (1993)
27. Kuri-Morales, Á.F., Gutiérrez-García, J.O.: Penalty function methods for constrained optimization with genetic algorithms: a statistical analysis. In: Coello Coello, C.A., de Albornoz, Á., Sucar, L., Battistutti, O.C. (eds.) MICAI 2002. LNCS (LNAI), vol. 2313, pp. 108–117. Springer, Heidelberg (2002)
28. Kuri-Morales, A., Rodríguez-Erazo, F.: A search space reduction methodology for data mining in large databases. Eng. Appl. Artif. Intell. **22**(1), 57–65 (2009)
29. Lichman, M.: UCI Machine Learning Repository. http://archive.ics.uci.edu/ml/datasets/Gisette. University of California, School of Information and Computer Science, Irvine (2013)

Geometric Differential Evolution in MOEA/D: A Preliminary Study

Saúl Zapotecas-Martínez[1]([✉]), Bilel Derbel[2,3], Arnaud Liefooghe[2,3], Hernán E. Aguirre[1], and Kiyoshi Tanaka[1]

[1] Faculty of Engineering, Shinshu University, 4-17-1 Wakasato, Nagano 380-8553, Japan
{zapotecas,ahernan,ktanaka}@shinshu-u.ac.jp
[2] Université Lille, CNRS, Centrale Lille, UMR 9189 - CRIStAL - Centre de Recherche en Informatique Signal et Automatique de Lille, 59000 Lille, France
{bilel.derbel,arnaud.liefooghe}@univ-lille1.fr
[3] Inria Lille - Nord Europe, 59650 Villeneuve d'Ascq, France

Abstract. The multi-objective evolutionary algorithm based on decomposition (MOEA/D) is an aggregation-based algorithm which has became successful for solving multi-objective optimization problems (MOPs). So far, for the continuous domain, the most successful variants of MOEA/D are based on differential evolution (DE) operators. However, no investigations on the application of DE-like operators within MOEA/D exist in the context of combinatorial optimization. This is precisely the focus of the work reported in this paper. More particularly, we study the incorporation of geometric differential evolution (gDE), the discrete generalization of DE, into the MOEA/D framework. We conduct preliminary experiments in order to study the effectiveness of gDE when coupled with MOEA/D. Our results indicate that the proposed approach is able to outperform the standard version of MOEA/D, when solving a combinatorial optimization problem having between two and four objective functions.

1 Introduction

Multi-objective optimization problems (MOPs) appear in several application fields, e.g. logistics, planning, green-IT, clouds, etc. They are used to model a situation where one wants to optimize several objective functions. Such objectives are generally in conflicting, i.e., optimizing one leads inevitably to deteriorate the others. As such, it is unlikely to find a solution which is able to optimize all target objectives. Hence, solving a MOP consists in finding an entire set of solutions showing different compromises between the objectives. This set can then be provided to the final decision maker who is responsible for choosing one solution in the computed set.

More formally, a multi-objective optimization problem can be defined by a set of $M \geq 2$ objective functions $\boldsymbol{F} = (f_1, f_2, \ldots, f_M)^{\mathsf{T}}$, and a set X of feasible solutions in the *decision space*, where X is a discrete set in the combinatorial case. Let $Z = \boldsymbol{F}(X) \subseteq \mathbb{R}^M$ be the set of feasible outcome vectors in the *objective space*. To each solution $\boldsymbol{x} \in X$ is then assigned exactly one objective vector

© Springer International Publishing Switzerland 2015
G. Sidorov and S.N. Galicia-Haro (Eds.): MICAI 2015, Part I, LNAI 9413, pp. 364–376, 2015.
DOI: 10.1007/978-3-319-27060-9_30

$z \in Z$, on the basis of the vector function $F : X \to Z$ with $z = F(x)$. Without loss of generality, in a maximization context, an objective vector $z \in Z$ is dominated by an objective $z' \in Z$, denoted by $z \prec z'$, iff $\forall m \in \{1, 2, \ldots, M\}$, $z_m \leq z'_m$ and $\exists m \in \{1, 2, \ldots, M\}$ such that $z_m < z'_m$. By extension, a solution $x \in X$ is dominated by a solution $x' \in X$, denoted by $x \prec x'$, iff $F(x) \prec F(x')$. A solution $x^* \in X$ is termed *Pareto optimal* if there does not exist any other solution $x \in X$ such that $x^* \prec x$. The set of all Pareto optimal solutions is called the *Pareto set* i.e., solutions for which there exist no other solutions providing better trade-off in all objectives. Its mapping in the objective space is called the *Pareto front*. One of the most challenging task in multi-objective optimization is to identify a minimal complete Pareto set, i.e., one Pareto optimal solution for each point from the Pareto front. This task is usually intractable for several optimization problems and one seeks instead a good *Pareto front approximation*.

Different approaches and techniques exist in order to tackle MOPs. In this work, we are interested in evolutionary multi-objective optimization (EMO) methods which have been shown to be well-applicable for a broad range of MOPs while being particularly accurate in finding high quality approximations [2,4]. There exist several EMO algorithms relying on different concepts and having seemingly different properties. Besides the popular class of Pareto-dominance based algorithms, e.g. **NSGA-II** [7] and **SPEA2** [22], we can report a recent and growing interest in the so-called *aggregation-based* algorithms, and especially the **MOEA/D** (multi-objective evolutionary algorithm based on decomposition) framework [21]. MOEA/D decomposes a MOP into a number of single-objective optimization subproblems; each single-objective optimization problem is defined by a scalarizing function using a different weight vector.

The original idea of MOEA/D is to define a neighborhood relation between subproblems and to solve each problem using standard evolutionary operators (crossover, mutation) as in the single-objective setting, but cooperatively based on the solutions computed at the neighboring subproblems. Each time a subproblem is considered, some parents are selected among neighbors in order to generate a new offspring which could replace the solutions of neighboring subproblems if an improvement is observed.

In this paper, we are specifically interested in the incorporation of alternative evolutionary operators into the MOEA/D framework for combinatorial optimization problems. In fact, for continuous problems, the most successful variants of MOEA/D so far are based on differential evolution (DE) [18] operators. However, no investigations on the application of DE within MOEA/D exist in the context of combinatorial optimization. Accordingly, the contribution of this paper comes into two flavors. First, we propose to incorporate the so-called geometric differential evolution (**gDE**) [16], the discrete generalization of DE, which provides an alternative instantiation of the MOEA/D framework. Secondly, we conduct a comprehensive study on the accuracy of the so-obtained multi-objective algorithm and the impact of its parameters. As test problem, we consider the well-known Knapsack problem having two, three and four objective functions.

The rest of this paper is organized as follows. In Sect. 2, we recall the main algorithmic components of the MOEA/D framework. We also describe the geometric Differential Evolution operator that we shall incorporate into MOEA/D. In Sect. 3, we describe the experimental setup we consider in order to conduct our analysis, and we draw a comprehensive picture of our experimental findings. In Sect. 4, we conclude the paper and discuss some open questions and future research directions.

2   MOEA/D-gDE: Description of the Algorithmic Components

2.1   Multi-objective Evolutionary Algorithm Based on Decomposition

Contrary to existing Pareto-based EMO algorithms, such as NSGA-II [7] or SPEA2 [22], which explicitly use the Pareto dominance relation in their selection mechanism, decomposition-based EMO algorithms [9], see e.g. MSOPS [10] or MOEA/D [21], rather seek a good-performing solution in multiple regions of the Pareto front by *decomposing* the original multi-objective problem into a number of *scalarized* single-objective sub-problems, which can be solved independently as in MSOPS [10], or in a dependent way as in MOEA/D [21] (which is the focus of this paper). Many different scalarizing functions have been proposed in the literature. Among these methods, perhaps the two most widely used are the *Tchebycheff* and the *Weighted Sum* approaches. However, the approaches based on boundary intersection have certain advantages over those based on either Tchebycheff or the Weighted Sum, see [3,21]. In the following, we briefly describe a method based, precisely, on the boundary intersection approach, which is referred to in this work. Note however, that other scalarizing approaches could also be coupled to this work, see for example those presented in [8,14,19].

Penalty Boundary Intersection. The Penalty Boundary Intersection (PBI) approach proposed by Zhang and Li [21], uses a weighted vector $\boldsymbol{\lambda}$ and a penalty value θ for minimizing both the distance to the reference vector d_1 and the direction error to the weighted vector d_2 from the solution $\boldsymbol{F}(\boldsymbol{x})$. Therefore, assuming maximization, the optimization problem can be stated as[1]:

$$\text{minimize:} \quad g(\boldsymbol{x}|\boldsymbol{\lambda}, \boldsymbol{z}^\star) = d_1 + \theta d_2 \tag{1}$$

where,

$$d_1 = \frac{||(\boldsymbol{z}^\star - \boldsymbol{F}(\boldsymbol{x}))^\mathsf{T}\boldsymbol{\lambda}||}{||\boldsymbol{\lambda}||} \quad \text{and} \quad d_2 = \left|\left|(\boldsymbol{F}(\boldsymbol{x}) - \boldsymbol{z}^\star) + d_1\frac{\boldsymbol{\lambda}}{||\boldsymbol{\lambda}||}\right|\right|$$

such that: $\boldsymbol{x} \in X$, $\boldsymbol{\lambda} = (\lambda_1, \ldots, \lambda_M)^\mathsf{T}$ is a weighting coefficient vector with $\lambda_i \geqslant 0$ and $\sum_i^M \lambda_i = 1$; $\boldsymbol{z}^\star = (z_1^\star, \ldots, z_M^\star)^\mathsf{T}$ is the reference point, i.e., $\forall i, \forall \boldsymbol{x}, z_i^\star > f_i(\boldsymbol{x})$,

---

[1] Note, however, that in the minimization case $d_1 = \frac{||(\boldsymbol{F}(\boldsymbol{x})-\boldsymbol{z}^\star)^\mathsf{T}\boldsymbol{\lambda}||}{||\boldsymbol{\lambda}||}$, $d_2 = ||(\boldsymbol{F}(\boldsymbol{x})-\boldsymbol{z}^\star) - d_1\frac{\boldsymbol{\lambda}}{||\boldsymbol{\lambda}||}||$ and the reference point is such that $\forall i \in \{1, \ldots, M\}, \forall \boldsymbol{x} \in X, z^\star < f_i(\boldsymbol{x})$.

Algorithm 1. General overview of MOEA/D

Input: $\{\lambda^1, \ldots, \lambda^\mu\}$: weight vectors w.r.t sub-problems;
g: a scalarizing function;
$\mathcal{B}(i)$: the neighbors of sub-problem $i \in \{1, \ldots, \mu\}$;
$P = \{p^1, \ldots, p^\mu\}$: the initial population.

1 **while** STOPPING CONDITION **do**
2   **for** $i \in \{1, \ldots, \mu\}$ **do**
3         $k, \ell \leftarrow rand(\mathcal{B}(i))$;
4         $o \leftarrow crossover\_mutation(p^k, p^\ell)$;
5   **if** o *is infeasible* **then**
6            $o' \leftarrow repair(o)$
7   **else**
8            $o' = o$
9   **shuffle**$(\mathcal{B}(i))$;
10   **for** $j \in \mathcal{B}(i)$ **do**
11   **if** $g(o'|\lambda^j, z^\star)$ *better than* $g(p^j|\lambda^j, z^\star)$ **then** $p^j \leftarrow o'$;

---

for all $i \in \{1, \ldots, M\}$. Since $z^\star$ is unknown, MOEA/D states each component $z_i^\star$ by the maximum value for each objective f_i found during the search process.

Let g be a scalarizing function and let $\{\lambda^1, \ldots, \lambda^\mu)$ be a set of μ uniformly distributed weighting coefficient vectors, corresponding to μ sub-problems to be optimized. For each sub-problem $i \in \{1, \ldots, \mu\}$, the goal is to approximate the solution x with the best scalarizing function value $g(x|\lambda^i, z^\star)$. For that purpose, MOEA/D maintains a population $P = (p^1, \ldots, p^\mu)$, each individual corresponding to a good-quality solution for one sub-problem.

For each sub-problem $i \in \{1, \ldots, \mu\}$, a set of neighbors $\mathcal{B}(i)$ is defined with the T closest weighting coefficient vectors (in terms of Euclidean distance). To evolve the population, the subproblems are optimized iteratively. At a given iteration corresponding to one sub-problem i, two solutions are selected at random from $\mathcal{B}(i)$ (line 3, Algorithm 1), and an offspring solution o is created by means of variation operators (mutation and crossover, line 4 in Algorithm 1). A problem-specific repair or improvement heuristic is potentially applied on solution o to produce o' (line 6, Algorithm 1). Then, for every sub-problem $j \in \mathcal{B}(i)$, if o' improves over j's current solution p^j then o' replaces it.

The algorithm continues looping over sub-problems, optimizing them one after the other, until a stopping condition is satisfied. For a more detailed description of MOEA/D, the interested readers are referred to [21].

2.2 Geometric Differential Evolution

As depicted in the previous algorithm, MOEA/D requires the use of some crossover and mutation operators. For continuous problems, and in its very initial variant, MOEA/D was first coupled with the so-called simulated binary crossover

(SBX) [5] and parameter-based mutation (PBM) [6]. Later, it was proven that incorporating the so-called Differential Evolution (DE) [18] into MOEA/D is much more efficient in order to deal with difficult continuous benchmarks having complicated Pareto sets (the well-known **MOEA/D-DE** [12]). DE, is in fact, widely established in the continuous optimization community as one of the most efficient variation operators for single-objective problems as well as for multi-objective problems. One can find different DE-like variants and several studies about their performance and their accuracy when applied to continuous multi-objective optimization problems, see for instance the well-known **PDE** [1] and **GDE3** [11] algorithms. In this paper, however, we consider combinatorial problems and one may wonder whether there exist an adaptation of DE for discrete problems. For single-objective combinatorial optimization problem, such a variant, called geometric DE, was recently proposed in [15,16]. This evolutionary operator can be seen as a generalization of the DE for any metric space (Euclidean, Hamming, etc.). To understand the differential mutation operator referred to in this work, the following concepts are introduced.

Convex Combination. The notion of convex combination (CX) in metric spaces was introduced in [15]. The convex combination $C = CX((A, W_A), (B, W_B))$ of two points A and B with weights W_A and W_B (positive and summing up to one) in a metric space endowed with distance function d returns the set of points C such that $d(A, C)/d(A, B) = W_B$ and $d(B, C)/d(A, B) = W_A$ (the weights of the points A and B are inversely proportional to their distances to C). In fact, as it was pointed out in [15], when specified to Euclidean spaces, this notion of convex combination coincides exactly with the traditional notion of convex combination of real vectors.

Extension Ray. The weighted extension ray (ER) is defined as the inverse operation of the weighted convex combination, as follows. The weighted extension ray $ER((A, w_{ab}), (B, w_{bc}))$ of the points A (origin) and B (through) and weights w_{ab} and w_{bc} returns those points C such that their convex combination with A with weights w_{bc} and $w_{ab}, CX((A, w_{ab}), (C, w_{bc}))$, returns the point B. The set of points returned by the weighted extension ray ER can be characterized in terms of distances to the input points of ER, see [16]. This characterization may be useful to construct procedures to implement the weighted extension ray for specific spaces.

Differential Mutation Operator. The differential mutation operator $U = DM(X1, X2, X3)$ with scale factor $F \geq 0$ can now be defined for any metric space following the construction of U presented in [15] as follows:

1. Compute $W = \frac{1}{1+F}$
2. Get E as the convex combination $CX(X1, X3)$ with weights $(1 - W, W)$
3. Get U as the extension ray $ER(X2, E)$ with weights $(W, 1 - W)$

After applying differential mutation (DM), the DE algorithm applies discrete recombination to U and $X(i)$ with probability parameter Cr generating V. This operator can be thought as a weighted geometric crossover and readily generalized as follows: $V = CX(U, X(i))$ with weights $(Cr, 1 - Cr)$ [15].

Having the previous description, we can see that incorporating gDE into MOEA/D can be done as follows. For each single weight vector $\boldsymbol{\lambda}^i$ (the inner loop in Algorithm 1), select in a random way, three different indices r_1, r_2 and r_3 such that $r_1 \neq r_2 \neq r_3 \neq i$ from the corresponding neighborhood $\mathcal{B}(i)$. The selected indices state the solutions (associated to their corresponding subproblems) which are used in the geometric recombination, that is $X1 = p^{r_1}, X2 = p^{r_2}$ and $X3 = p^{r_3}$. Then, the convex combination $E = CX(X1, X3)$ and the extension ray $U = ER(X2, E)$ operators with their respective weights $(1 - W, W)$ and $(W, 1 - W)$ are carried out. Finally, the offspring solution $\boldsymbol{o}$ is created by using discrete recombination between U and the current solution p^i, that is $\boldsymbol{o} = CX(U, p^i)$ with weights $(Cr, 1 - Cr)$. This offspring solution is considered for replacement in the same manner than the previously described MOEA/D.

3   Experimental Study

3.1   The Multi-objective Knapsack Problem: A Case Study

In order to test the performance of the proposed MOEA/D-gDE, the knapsack problem, one of the most studied NP-hard problems from combinatorial optimization, is adopted in a multi-objective optimization context. Given a collection of n items and a set of M knapsacks, the $0 - 1$ multi-objective knapsack problem seeks a subset of items subject to capacity constraints based on a *weight function* vector $w : \{0, 1\}^n \to \mathbb{N}^M$, while maximizing a *profit function* vector $p : \{0, 1\}^n \to \mathbb{N}^M$. More formally, it can be stated as:

$$\begin{aligned} \text{maximize} \quad & f_i(\boldsymbol{x}) = \sum_{j=1}^n p_{ij} \cdot x_j && i \in \{1, 2, \ldots, M\} \\ \text{s.t.} \quad & \sum_{j=1}^n w_{ij} \cdot x_j \leqslant c_i && i \in \{1, 2, \ldots, M\} \\ & x_j \in \{0, 1\} && j \in \{1, \ldots, n\} \end{aligned}$$

where $p_{ij} \in \mathbb{N}$ is the profit of item j on knapsack i, $w_{ij} \in \mathbb{N}$ is the weight of item j on knapsack i, and $c_i \in \mathbb{N}$ is the capacity of knapsack i. We consider the conventional instances proposed in [23], with random uncorrelated profit and weight integer values from $[10, 100]$, and where capacity is set to half of the total weight of a knapsack. A random problem instance of 500 items is investigated for each objective space dimension throughout the paper. Notice that different repair mechanism exist for knapsack. In this paper, we use a standard procedure to handle constraints as proposed in [23].

3.2   Experimental Setup

The performance of MOEA/D-gDE is evaluated by using different parameter settings. Since the scalar factor F in gDE states the value of $W \in (0, 1]$, i.e. $W = \frac{1}{1+F}$, and W is the unique parameter employed in both the convex combination CX and the extension ray ER, we set directly the value of W instead of F. In Table 1, we summarize the different parameters considered in our analysis.

Table 1. Parameter setting.

pop size	μ	200 (resp. 210, 200) for $M = 2$ (resp. 3, 4)
neighborhood size	T	20
PBI	θ	5
crossover/mutation rate		1.0
gDE	Cr	$\{0.1, 0.2, 0.3, \cdots, 0.9, 1.0\}$
	W	$\{0.1, 0.2, 0.3, \cdots, 0.9, 1.0\}$
stopping condition		5,000 generations

Notice that we essentially vary the values of Cr and W in order to study their impact on gDE when plugged into MOEA/D.

As a baseline we consider the conventional version of MOEA/D as initially described in [21]. Notice that the conventional MOEA/D employs the well-established one-point crossover with probability 1. For all algorithms, we apply the flip bit mutation with probability $1/n$ and it takes place after performing their corresponding crossover, where n denotes the number of decision variables (in this work, we consider $n = 500$ items for all the instances). The neighborhood size is the same for all the algorithms and it is set to 20. In order to generate the weight vectors corresponding to the different subproblems, we adopt the simplex-lattice design [17] (the same strategy used in the original MOEA/D [21]), i.e., the settings of μ and $\{\boldsymbol{\lambda}^1, \ldots, \boldsymbol{\lambda}^{\mu}\}$ are controlled by a parameter H. More precisely, $\boldsymbol{\lambda}^1, \ldots, \boldsymbol{\lambda}^{\mu}$ are all the weight vectors in which each individual weight takes a value from $\left\{ \frac{0}{H}, \frac{1}{H}, \ldots, \frac{H}{H} \right\}$. Therefore, the number of such vectors is given by $\mu = C_{H+M-1}^{M-1}$, where M is the number of objective functions. In our comparative study, the set of weights was defined with $H = 99$ (resp. 19 and 9) for two objectives (resp. three and four objectives). It is worth noticing that when the number of objectives increases, the use of the simplex-lattice design becomes impractical. Nonetheless, other strategies can be considered, see for instance the one presented in [20].

3.3   Experimental Analysis

Overall Impact of Parameters. In Fig. 1, we analyze the overall performance of MOEA/D-gDE as a function of the two control parameters Cr and W. More precisely, we report the average normalized hypervolume indicator [24] (to be maximized) obtained over the 30 executed runs. Different interesting observations can be seen. First, both parameters Cr and W have a deep impact on the performance of the algorithm. In particular, the impact of W appears to be more critical with low values being overall better. We also notice that for the small values of W, parameter Cr has a relatively marginal effect, whereas this impact is more pronounced for the lower values of W. For $M = 2$, that is for the bi-objective knapsack problem, we notice that the best configuration of MOEA/D-gDE is obtained with parameter values of $W = 0.6$ and $Cr = 0.1$.

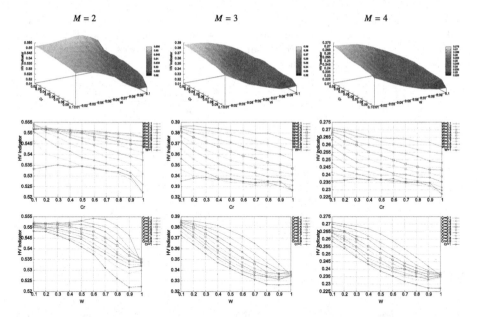

Fig. 1. Hypervolume Indicator as a function of W and Cr for the knapsack problem with respectively 2, 3 and 4 objectives. Larger hypervolume indicates better performances.

Interestingly, the situation is seemingly different for $M = 2$ and $M = 3$ for which the best configuration is obtained with $W = 0.1$ and $Cr = 0.1$. Note however that, since $W = \frac{1}{1+F}$, the smaller the value of W, the greater the value of F.

Comparison with Conventional MOEA/D. In Table 2, we compare the performance of MOEA/D-gDE and MOEA/D. We recall that the only difference is that MOEA/D is using the standard one-point crossover. Due to space restriction, we only report results for $Cr = 0.1$ (for which MOEA/D-gDE performs better) while varying parameter W (which was observed to have a more critical effect on the performance). We remark that MOEA/D-gDE is able to outperform MOEA/D and the difference is statistically significant for a large number of values of parameter W. One can notice that the results of Table 2 confirm the fact that lower values of W are more beneficial for the search process. On the other hand, we notice that when the number of objectives grows, the values of W where MOEA/D-gDE is able to outperform MOEA/D are less numerous, which we attribute to the difficulty of optimizing many-objective problems, i.e., MOEA/D-gDE is relatively less robust to the range of W values when solving difficult problems with a large number of objectives.

EAF Analysis. In order to have a more clear information about the relative performance of MOEA/D-gDE as a function of parameter W, we use the empirical attainment functions (EAFs) [13] dedicated to bi-objective problems; and

Table 2. Hypervolume and standard deviation ($\times 10^{-2}$). Cr is fixed to 0.1 for MOEA/D-gDE. Symbol + (resp. − and =) indicates that the performance of MOEA/D-gDE is essentially better than (resp. worst, same) than MOEA/D according to a Wilcox unpaired statistical test with confidence level 0.05.

			$M = 2$		$M = 3$		$M = 4$	
		MOEA/D	$54.78_{(0.24)}$		$37.77_{(0.34)}$		$26.18_{(0.56)}$	
MOEA/D-gDE	W	0.1	$55.17_{(0.23)}$	+	$38.64_{(0.20)}$	+	$27.12_{(0.48)}$	+
		0.2	$55.16_{(0.22)}$	+	$38.59_{(0.28)}$	+	$26.99_{(0.49)}$	+
		0.3	$55.18_{(0.24)}$	+	$38.41_{(0.14)}$	+	$26.85_{(0.43)}$	+
		0.4	$55.24_{(0.24)}$	+	$38.17_{(0.16)}$	+	$26.7_{(0.33)}$	+
		0.5	$55.32_{(0.25)}$	+	$37.71_{(0.19)}$	−	$26.36_{(0.31)}$	=
		0.6	$55.42_{(0.35)}$	+	$37.20_{(0.12)}$	−	$25.91_{(0.22)}$	−
		0.7	$55.38_{(0.29)}$	+	$36.51_{(0.19)}$	−	$25.35_{(0.28)}$	−
		0.8	$55.07_{(0.18)}$	+	$35.62_{(0.19)}$	−	$24.8_{(0.34)}$	−
		0.9	$54.63_{(0.26)}$	−	$34.59_{(0.29)}$	−	$24.19_{(0.35)}$	−
		1	$53.32_{(0.24)}$	−	$33.52_{(0.42)}$	−	$23.59_{(0.27)}$	−

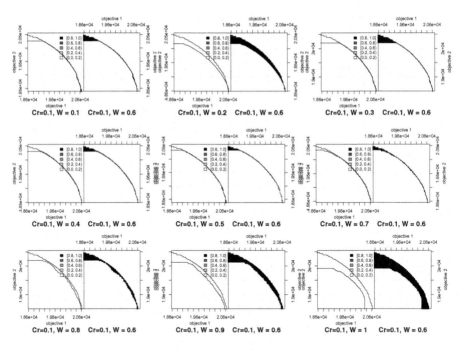

Fig. 2. EAF differences ($M = 2$) for MOEA/D-gDE with Cr = 0.1 and W = 0.6 (Right subfigures) compared to MOEA/D-gDE with Cr = 0.1 and W $\neq$ 0.6 (left subfigures).

we compare the sets of solutions obtained by MOEA/D-gDE when configured with the best value of W, i.e., $W = 0.6$, and MOEA/D-gDE when configured with the other values considered in our experiments. The EAF provides the probability, estimated from several runs, that an arbitrary objective vector is dominated by, or equivalent to, a solution obtained by a single run of the algorithm. The difference between the EAFs for two different algorithms enables to identify the regions of the objective space where one algorithm performs better than another. The magnitude of the difference in favor of one algorithm is plotted within a gray-colored graduation as illustrated in Fig. 2. We can clearly see that for large W values, the algorithm produces solutions that are very likely dominated almost everywhere by solutions produced with the best configuration. For low W values, the difference in performance is less pronounced and the best configuration (W=0.6) is essentially able to find better solution at the extreme parts of the Pareto front.

Anytime Behavior. Up to now, we only considered the relative performance of the different algorithm configurations at the end of their executions. In the following we shall consider the performance as a function of the running time or equivalently the number of generations. In fact, a desirable and important behavior of an algorithm is to be able to output the best possible results at

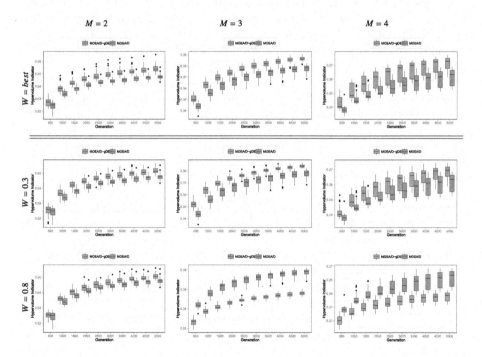

Fig. 3. Runtime behavior of MOEA/D-gDE compared to baseline MOEA/D. Hypervolume indicator is considered. Top figures are with respect to the best setting of parameters obtained for MOEA/D-gDE, i.e., $Cr = 0.1$ and $W = 0.6$ for $M = 2$ and $Cr = 0.1$ and $W = 1$ for $M = 3$ and $M = 4$. Other figures are with respect to respectively a relatively low W-value (0.3) and a relatively high W-value (0.8) and $Cr = 0.1$.

any time of its execution and not only after a large fixed amount of functions evaluations which can then bias our judgment for the relative performance of an algorithm. For this purpose, we depict in Fig. 3, the hypervolume obtained by MOEA/D-gDE and MOEA/D as a function of the number of generations. We recall that a generation refer to the full execution of the main loop of the algorithm where the solution of every sub-problem is evolved exactly once, i.e., one generation is equivalent to μ fitness function evaluations (all objectives count one) where μ is the population size. From Fig. 3, it is clear that the previous discussion about the relative performance of MOEA/D-gDE holds at any time of the algorithm execution. In fact, we can see that the best W value extracted from the last generation ($W = 0.6$) remains also very efficient compared to MOEA/D at any generation of the algorithm. We can also clearly see that lower values of W are more beneficial for the search process, which is to contrast to the higher values independently of the considered generation.

4   Conclusions and Future Works

In this paper, we conducted the first experimental study on the performance of a generalized form of differential evolution, i.e., geometric differential evolution (gDE), for solving multi-objective combinatorial optimization problems. We considered extending the widely used MOEA/D framework to incorporate gDE and to analyze its behavior as a function of its control parameters. Our experimental results indicate that gDE is a well performing evolutionary operator that can be successfully applied in the context of multi-objective optimization. This constitutes a first and promising step toward the application of gDE for solving a large panel of multi-objective combinatorial optimization problems. In fact, several open issues are left open and several research challenges have to be addressed in order to better assess the accuracy of gDE. Some interesting research paths are sketched in the following:

- Other optimization problems with different properties (e.g., convexity, objective correlation, fitness landscape difficulty, etc.) have to be considered in order to better understand the behavior of gDE and its ruling parameters.
- Other DE variants can be adapted to the combinatorial case by taking inspiration from the basic gDE used in this paper. In fact, the community has proposed different design strategies for DE in the case of continuous problems. Generalizing those variants in the combinatorial case is a challenging issue which is in our opinion a very promising research path. One particularly interesting question would be to study self-adaptive strategies mixing different gDE designs.
- We considered the incorporation of gDE within the standard variant of MOEA/D. It is worth-mentioning that other more advanced variants of MOEA/D exist in the literature and could benefit much from the incorporation of gDE to solve difficult multi-objective combinatorial problems. A systematic study on the application of gDE within those variants is one

open research issue that deserves more investigations and design efforts. Moreover, gDE does not depend on the MOEA/D framework. Although we believe that MOEA/D provides much flexibility when considering gDE-like operators, other algorithmic frameworks could also be potential candidates with an eventually improved performance and hence should be considered in future work.

References

1. Abbass, H.A., Sarker, R., Newton, C.: PDE: a Pareto-frontier differential evolution approach for multi-objective optimization problems. In: CEC 2001, vol. 2, pp. 971–978. IEEE Service Center, Piscataway, May 2001
2. Coello Coello, C.A., Lamont, G.B., Van Veldhuizen, D.A.: Evolutionary Algorithms for Solving Multi-Objective Problems, 2nd edn. Springer, New York (2007). ISBN 978-0-387-33254-3
3. Das, I., Dennis, J.E.: Normal-boundary intersection: a new method for generating Pareto optimal points in multicriteria optimization problems. SIAM J. Optim. **8**(3), 631–657 (1998)
4. Deb, K.: Multi-Objective Optimization using Evolutionary Algorithms. John Wiley & Sons, Chichester (2001)
5. Deb, K., Agrawal, R.B.: Simulated binary crossover for continuous search space. Complex Syst. **9**(2), 115–148 (1995)
6. Deb, K., Agrawal, R.B.: A Niched-Penalty approach for constraint handling in genetic algorithms. Artificial Neural Networks and Genetic Algorithms, pp. 235–243. Springer, Vienna (1999)
7. Deb, K., Pratap, A., Agarwal, S., Meyarivan, T.: A fast and elitist multiobjective genetic algorithm: NSGA-II. IEEE TEVC **6**(2), 182–197 (2002)
8. Ehrgott, M.: Multicriteria Optimization, 2nd edn. Springer, Berlin (2005)
9. Giagkiozis, I., Purshouse, R.C., Fleming, P.J.: Generalized decomposition. In: Purshouse, R.C., Fleming, P.J., Fonseca, C.M., Greco, S., Shaw, J. (eds.) EMO 2013. LNCS, vol. 7811, pp. 428–442. Springer, Heidelberg (2013)
10. Hughes, E.: Multiple single objective Pareto sampling. In: IEEE 2003 Congress on Evolutionary Computation (CEC 2003), vol. 4, pp. 2678–2684, December 2003
11. Kukkonen, S., Lampinen, J.: GDE3: the third evolution step of generalized differential evolution. In: IEEE Congress on Evolutionary Computation, vol. 1, pp. 443–450, September 2005
12. Li, H., Zhang, Q.: Multiobjective optimization problems with complicated Pareto sets, MOEA/D and NSGA-II. IEEE Trans. Evol. Comput. **13**(2), 284–302 (2009)
13. López-Ibáñez, M., Paquete, L., Stützle, T.: Exploratory analysis of stochastic local search algorithms in biobjective optimization. In: Bartz-Beielstein, T., Chiarandini, M., Paquete, L., Preuss, M. (eds.) Experimental Methods for the Analysis of Optimization Algorithms, chap. 9, pp. 209–222. Springer, Heidelberg (2010)
14. Miettinen, K.: Nonlinear Multiobjective Optimization. Kluwer Academic Publishers, Boston (1999)
15. Moraglio, A., Togelius, J.: Geometric differential evolution. In: GECCO 2009, pp. 1705–1712. ACM (2009)
16. Moraglio, A., Togelius, J., Silva, S.: Geometric differential evolution for combinatorial and programs spaces. Evol. Comput. **21**(4), 591–624 (2013)

17. Scheffé, H.: Experiments with mixtures. J. Roy. Stat. Soc.: Ser. B (Methodol.) **20**(2), 344–360 (1958)
18. Storn, R.M., Price, K.V.: Differential Evolution - a simple and efficient adaptive scheme for global optimization over continuous spaces. Technical report TR-95-012, ICSI, Berkeley, March 1995
19. Vincke, P.: Multicriteria Decision-Aid. John Wiley & Sons, New York (1992)
20. Zapotecas-Martínez, S., Aguirre, H.E., Tanaka, K., Coello Coello, C.A.: On the Low-Dyscrepancy sequences and their use in MOEA/D for high-dimensional objective spaces. In: 2015 IEEE Congress on Evolutionary Computation (CEC 2015), pp. 2835–2842. IEEE Press, Sendai, May 2015
21. Zhang, Q., Li, H.: MOEA/D: a multiobjective evolutionary algorithm based on decomposition. IEEE TEVC **11**(6), 712–731 (2007)
22. Zitzler, E., Laumanns, M., Thiele, L.: SPEA2: Improving the strength Pareto evolutionary algorithm. In: Giannakoglou, K., Tsahalis, D., Periaux, J., Papailou, P., Fogarty, T. (eds.) EUROGEN 2001, Evolutionary Methods for Design, Optimization and Control with Applications to Industrial Problems, Athens, Greece (2001)
23. Zitzler, E., Thiele, L.: Multiobjective evolutionary algorithms: a comparative case study and the strength Pareto approach. IEEE TEVC **3**(4), 257–271 (1999)
24. Zitzler, E., Thiele, L., Laumanns, M., Fonseca, C.M., Grunert da Fonseca, V.: Performance assessment of multiobjective optimizers: an analysis and review. IEEE TEC **7**(2), 117–132 (2003)

Energy Efficient Routing Based on NSGA-II for Context Parameters Aware Sensor Networks

Angela Rodríguez[1]([⊠]), Armando Ordoñez[1], and Hugo Ordoñez[2]

[1] Foundation University of Popayán, Popayán, Colombia
{angela.rodriguez,armando.ordonez}@docente.fup.edu.co
[2] University of San Buenaventura, Cali, Colombia
haordonez@usbcali.edu.co

Abstract. A wireless sensor network collects crucial data for decision making in several domains even under extreme deployment conditions. In this scenario, network availability is usually affected by diverse environment variables. The present approach adapts an evolutionary multi-objective technique in order to get network structures that let to perform data routing efficient in energy consumption. The resulting algorithm, MOR4WSN, comes up from a new solution encoding done to the NSGA-II as well as adapting user-preferences handling even if preference context parameters to optimize are contradictory. MOR4WSN allows optimizing data gathering paths, which contributes to increase network longevity. Experimental evaluation shows that network lifecycle is increased when MOR4WSN is used, compared to other routing mechanisms.

Keywords: Evolutionary optimization techniques · Sensor networks · Multi-objective algorithms

1 Introduction

Internet of things (IoT) is based on the pervasive presence of elements such as sensors and actuators which interact with each other in order to reach a common goal [1]. Among this wide set of elements, wireless sensor networks (WSNs) play an important role as they allow to collect information from the context which is useful for decision making [1]. Nowadays one of the main challenges of WSN is energy saving [2], given the fact that sensors have limited energy sources which usually cannot be recharged once networks are deployed in large scale and difficult access areas. In a WSN the major energy consumption is produced during data transmission phase due to the use of radiofrequency modules [3, 4]. In this sense, the higher the transmission distance, the higher energy expense. Consequently, battery saving can be achieved by reduction of data transmission by optimization of information gathering paths, i.e. optimization of WSN routing topology. Regarding topology optimization, diverse factors must be considered such as: distance between sender and receiver sensors, packets length, etc.; therefore this optimization may be seen as a multi objective optimization problem.

© Springer International Publishing Switzerland 2015
G. Sidorov and S.N. Galicia-Haro (Eds.): MICAI 2015, Part I, LNAI 9413, pp. 377–388, 2015.
DOI: 10.1007/978-3-319-27060-9_31

Some approaches [3–7] used bio inspired techniques for routing optimization in hierarchical WSNs; however, these works don't consider multi objective optimization. The authors in [8] used a multi-objective evolutionary optimization algorithm called NSGA-II to select the optimal active nodes set of a WSN in a target coverage area by maximizing the coverage range using a relative small quantity of sensor nodes in order to conserve system energy; as the work done in [8] aims to putting some sensors into low-power sleep mode, they didn't consider the optimization of the radiofrequency module of the active ones, which is meant to be the most energy consuming module even more when the communication distance between sensors is appreciable. In the work documented in [9], the recent MOAA (Multi-Objective Alliance Algorithm) was applied for the optimization of WSN in order to maximize their coverage and lifetime. Comparisons of results were done with NSGA-II and SPEA2 algorithms, however the discussion is more focused on the mathematical issues (such as Pareto front values), than on terms of WSN energy node's conservation. Another Pareto-based optimization algorithm (called FLEX) was developed by the authors of [10], when looking for an optimal positioning of wireless sensor nodes. The metrics used for the multi-objective function were three: coverage, connectivity and energy cost. The work in [10] doesn't specify how a unique solution was chosen from the Pareto set.

MOR4WSN [11] is a hierarchical WSN routing mechanism based on the NSGA-II [12] that uses objective functions for creating a set of optimal WSN routes [13] and subsequently uses a binary index for refining the search [14]. In this paper, the WSN routing tree topology representation according to genetic algorithm elements is presented, the drawback with the common random initial population of the NSGA-II is described as well as its associated solution: a model for the network initial deployment and a technique for generating the initial population allowing only valid chromosomes for large area contexts. Also, a method for selecting a unique optimized network structure from the N (N is the network size) solutions calculated by NSGA-II is presented. Finally the power saving algorithm, MOR4WSN, is emerged which preserves valid chromosomes during its evolution. The experimental tests of MOR4WSN show promising results in terms of network longevity.

The rest of this paper is organized as follows: Sect. 2 presents a background of the proposal; Sect. 3 shows the multi-objective problem statement; Sect. 4 presents the algorithm design for initial population adapting, Sect. 5 presents how the binary index was implemented, Sect. 6 shows experimental evaluation of MOR4WSN regarding its lifetime, and Sect. 7 details conclusions and future work.

2   Background

2.1   WSN Concepts

WSNs are composed of sensors known as *source nodes* whose function is to gather information from environment and to communicate with other nodes through wireless technologies in order to send data to a central point known as *base station* where information analysis can be performed. As WSN lacks of physical infrastructure, it can adopt different topologies according to its needs. A common topology for high scale network deployments is tree based or hierarchical. Figure 1 shows a directed acyclic graph representing a WSN rooted with the *base station* while the rest of the nodes are data sources and the directed edges indicate its next hop node for data transmission. WSN routing is concerned as the path to carry out data transmission from source to destination [15], and network longevity is the time period counted from WSN start-up until the moment in which one node or a percentage of nodes is unable of sending data to base station.

Fig. 1. WSN with hierarchical topology.

2.2   Multi- Objective Genetic Algorithms (MOGA)

In contrast to simple (mono-objective) genetic algorithms [13, 16], multi-objective genetic algorithms (MOGA) aim to find solutions that require optimization of several objectives at the same time, which may be opposed to each other. Most of the existing multi-objective evolutionary algorithms have a computational complexity of $O(mN^3)$ [12], where m is the number of objectives and N is the population size. In order to get a lower complexity, NSGA II (*Fast Elitist Non Dominated Sorting Genetic Algorithm*) reduces search spaces by applying two concepts: *elitism* and *diversity preservation*. With this modification, NSGA II reduces complexity to $O(mN^2)$ [11, 17]. However, NSGA II gives not a unique solution but a set of them, which are all optimized solutions having all objectives into account; this concept is called Pareto dominance and will be treated in Sect. 4.

2.3   WSN Modelling in Genetic Algorithms

The basic information unit in a genetic algorithm is the chromosome (or *individual*) that consist of a set of gens. Gens at chromosomes keep data and value through indices and alleles that represent any possible problem solution as shown in Fig. 2. All chromosomes along generations have equal quantity of gens. In MOR4WSN hierarchical WSNs are modelled in chromosomes as treated in [5–7]. Let N be the total of source nodes in a WSN (see Fig. 3a), each node is labelled with an integer from 0 to N-1; *base station* is always marked as N. Chromosome in Fig. 3b represents such routing scheme; the index corresponds to the identifier of a source node and the allele indicates the next-hop node of such index. i.e. in Fig. 3b the gen value in index 0 is 2 indicating that node 0 selects node 2 to transmit its data, node 2 transmits to node 5, the value in 5 is 6 indicating that the next node is the *base station*; therefore the full gathering path from node 0 is expressed as the path $0 \rightarrow 2 \rightarrow 5 \rightarrow 6$. In MOR4WSN one important condition of chromosomes to be a valid routing solution, is that the next-hop node of a source node has to be within its communication range (*neighbor nodes*), what is known during WSN deployment.

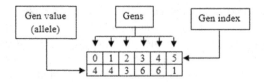

Fig. 2. Chromosome with 6 gens.

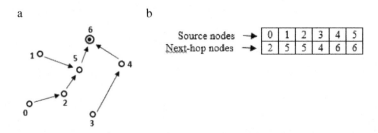

Fig. 3. (a) Directed routing tree in a WSN; (b) chromosome representing the directed tree.

2.4   Pareto Set Solutions

When using an evolutionary multi-objective approach like MOR4WSN, selecting the more adequate solution is not an easy task because solution is not one but a set of them known as the Pareto set, having the same size of the population (N = 100, 200 …). Pareto dominance is illustrated in Fig. 4, here a solution *a* 'dominates' *b* provided that: *a* is not worse than *b* in all objectives, and *a* is strictly better than *b* in at least one objective. That way, the solution set that are not dominated by any other else conform the Non Dominated Front also known as Pareto non dominated solutions. In Fig. 8 these non-dominated solutions are represented with the points marked as 3 and 5.

To select an *a posteriori* multicriteria solution in the Pareto set, some methods (outranking methods) perform peer comparison in order to establish if there exists preference, indifference or they are incomparable. However, these methods require the decision maker to establish some weights [18].

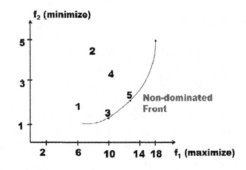

Fig. 4. Pareto front and dominance [17].

3   Problem Statement

The nodes in a hierarchical network (as the one in Fig. 3a) receiving and retransmitting lots of incoming data from other network nodes, will drain their batteries more quickly than those nodes performing few retransmissions. That way, a monitoring WSN with tree structure is long-lived as in its number of leaf nodes and its depth are decreased [15]. That's called network *load balancing*. Load balancing is used to balance the energy consumption between all network nodes by performing a fair distribution of sent, processed and received data packets. Figure 5 shows that reducing simultaneously the value of both parameters *leaf nodes* and *depth* in a routing tree is contradictory situation. That's why a MOGA is an adequate metaheuristic for the routing problem.

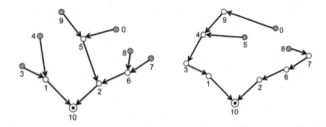

Fig. 5. Routing trees in a WSN

4   Initial Population in MORWSN

As mentioned earlier, in a genetic algorithm the initial population is usually randomly generated; it means that the alleles of chromosomes being part of the initial population can take any value between 0 and N. Specifically, known NSGA-II implementations [19] let the user to set min and max limits for each index of chromosome and from the range [*min, max*] the corresponding allele value is randomly chosen. i.e. if for index 0, the min and max values are fixed as 3 and 5 respectively, the allele at position 0 of the chromosome can only take the values 3, 4 or 5. Range limits of each index are inserted just once during the algorithm execution and those values are applied for all chromosomes in initial population.

As depicted in Fig. 3, in MOR4WSN an allele value identifies the next-hop node of the source node identified with its index number. In this sense, the process described in the foregoing paragraph allows an index (source node) of a chromosome of the initial population to take an allele value (next-hop node) that not necessarily is part of its neighbor's nodes list. In MOR4WSN is strongly necessary that and index node value and its corresponding allele node value are neighbor nodes in order the chromosomes to be valid solutions for the routing scheme.

As an example, Figs. 6 and 7 show a 10-source node WSN deployment chart. Neighboring nodes, understood as those which covering ranges are overlapped, are shown in Fig. 6. Overlapped covering ranges means possibility of communication between the pair of nodes; in graph terms this is represented by an edge as shown in

Fig. 7. One cannot assure that neighboring nodes has consecutive identifier numbers, what implies that the way as allele values are chosen in generic NSGA-II must be adapted to MOR4WSN conditions, what is explained at once.

At the level of initial population, next points to solve in MOR4WSN are identified: (i) in a chromosome each allele must be a neighbor node of its corresponding index, (ii) Each tree (represented as a chromosome) must be rooted with the base station, (iii) Avoid cycle formation in the WSN topology (represented as a chromosome).

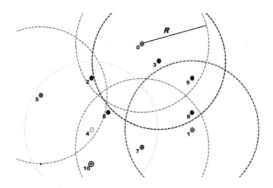

Fig. 6. Covering range of source nodes. R = covering range radius.

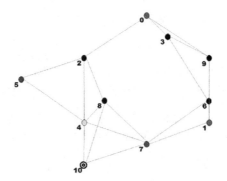

Fig. 7. WSN as a graph.

4.1   Neighbor's Matrix

Covering range radius and location of each sensor node at the deployment area are beforehand known values; carrying out some straightforward calculus one can assign neighboring nodes over the whole network.

In this sense, MOR4WSN uses a neighbor's matrix M. Matrix associated to WSN in Fig. 7 is shown in Fig. 8 where its size is $(N + 1) \times V$; V is the maximum quantity of neighbors that a source node has. In M, the first column lists the identifiers of all nodes of the WSN and the rows shows the identifiers of its corresponding neighbor's nodes.

Now, *min* and *max* limit numbers needed by NSGA-II to generate a random allele value, have another meaning in MOR4WSN; they indicate how many neighbors' nodes has a source node (an index at chromosome). That way, *min* will always be 0, while *max* is the quantity of neighbors. The random chosen value in [*min, max*] is not anymore the allele value, but the position column at *M*. In Fig. 9 one can see a chromosome formed from *M* conditions; i.e. for index i = 2 MOR4WSN generates a random value between 0 and 3 because according to *M* the node 2 has 4 neighbors in total (identified as 0, 4, 5, and 9). The random value between 0 and 3 will led place to a coordinate (*i, max*) giving an exact element position at *M* having the allele value for index 2. For example, if the random value is 1, then the allele value at i = 2 will be 4 (the next-hop node).

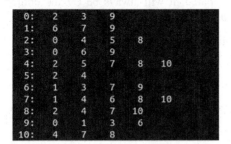

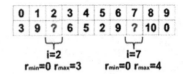

Fig. 8. Neighbors node's matrix *M*; the last one (*BS*) for information purposes.

Fig. 9. Randomly generated chromosome.

4.2 Valid Chromosomes Generating

Once guaranteed that next-hop nodes will be always neighbors of their respective source nodes, one have to face the other points of adapting the algorithm in order to have real valid solutions in the initial population: avoid cycling graphs, avoid not connected graphs or isolated nodes.

To solve it, Algorithm 1 was developed; here, base station is referred as *BS*.

inTree ← {*BS*}
pending ← {0, 1, 2, ..., *N* − 1}

While (*pendings* ≠ 0) *do*
    r ← *random*(*inTree*)
    Q ← *neighbors*(*r*) ∩ *pendings*
If (*Q* ≠ ∅) *then*
inTree ← *inTree* − {*r*}
    Continue
h ← *random* (*Q*)
allele (*h*) = *r*
inTree = inTree + {*h*}
pendings = pendings − {*h*}
End − *while*

Algorithm 1. Initial population adapting in MOR4WSN.

5   Selecting in Pareto Set Using a Binary Index

In MOR4WSN a criteria for selecting just one solution from the Pareto set, is avoiding outliers which often are present in non-dominated set because they are not dominated by another solution in just one objective; that way, solutions at Pareto set are peer compared using a binary index that represents each routing tree. Using such index outlier solutions are avoided to be selected as a final routing structure. Using the binary index, each tree of the Pareto Front is compared with an outlier structure and MOR4WSN selects the tree having the least similitude with such outlier. This scenario is illustrated in Fig. 10. Comparative process is as follows: let $G1$ and $G2$ be the labeled graphs (representing routing trees) to be compared, it will always be $G1$ the outlier solution while $G2$ is a non-dominated not outlier solution like in Fig. 10. So, Fig. 11 are the corresponding chromosomes: $G1 \rightarrow C1$ y $G2 \rightarrow C2$.

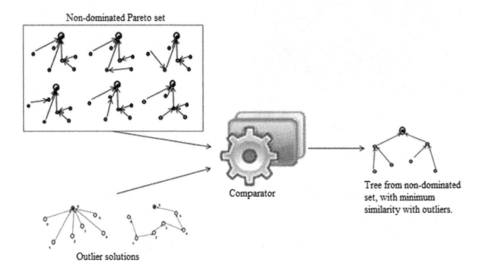

Non-dominated Pareto set

Comparator

Tree from non-dominated set, with minimum similarity with outliers.

Outlier solutions

Fig. 10.   Graph comparison

Starting from $C1$ and $C2$, matrix S is created as shown in Fig. 11 which size is $N \times 3$. S is created as follows:

$$S = \left\{ x_{ij}/x_{io} = C1, x_{i1} = C2, x_{i3} = 0 \; si \; x_{i0} = x_{i1} \; o \; x_{i3} = 1 \; si \; x_{i0} \neq x_{i1} \right\},$$

where $i = 0,1,\dots,N$ y $J = 0, 1, 2$

The column S_{i3} underlined in red in Fig. 11, is a binary vector formed from coincidences of the elements in each row of S. Let i be the row under consideration, if the elements $(i, 0)$ and $(i, 1)$ of S match exactly, the element at i-th position of S_{i3} is 1, otherwise its value is 0. Matrix S is the index of our algorithm; each graph has associated its own index given that S orders the necessary information to define similarity between graphs $G1$ and $G2$.

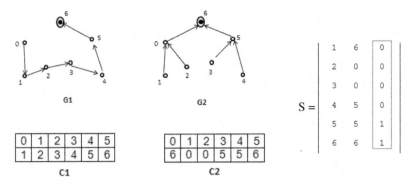

Fig. 11. Index comparison process

Then, from the elements of column $j = 3$ of each graph index, a similitude relation is established as follows:

Let $t = \{x_{i3}/x_{i3} \in S\}$ where $i = 0, 1, \ldots N$

$z = \sum_{k=1}^{N-1} (t_k)$, for each $t = 1$

and $p = (z/N) * 100\%$.

For the example in Fig. 10 we have: N = 6, t = {0, 0, 0, 0, 1, 1}, z = 2, p = 33.33 %.

The above means that similitude level between G1 and G2 is of 33.33 %, value taken as selection criteria in Pareto set elements since it determines a similitude percentage. As a decision maker, MOR4WSN selects finally an only tree: the one having the smaller p value between the $(N - 2) * 2\,p$ calculated values.

6 Evaluation

Evaluation compares WSN lifecycle (in terms of sensing and gathering rounds) using MOR4WSN as routing scheme with other routing technique for hierarchical topologies Tree Routing (TR, which is used by ZigBee). Table 1 lists simulation parameters values; homogeneous networks are assumed, that means all nodes having the same initial energy level and its covering range being the same. Results of comparative tests are shown in Figs. 12 and 13 where one can realize that inclusion of multi objective

Table 1. Simulation parameters

Parameter	Value	Unity/observation
Population size	N	N = number of nodes
Generations	2N	
Crossing probability	0.5	——
Mutation probability	0.5	——
Initial node energy	1000	Unities of energy timer
Packet size	128	Bytes
Covering range of nodes	2 %	Percent of total deployment area
Minimal energy threshold	10 %	Percent of initial energy

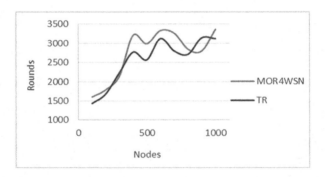

Fig. 12. WSN life cycle until the first node dies.

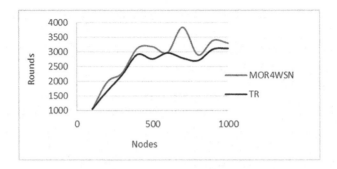

Fig. 13. WSN life cycle until 10 % of nodes die.

alternative for selecting tree topology increases network longevity even up to 23 %. In both evaluated cases, albeit fluctuations in curves showing the number of rounds, MOR4WSN exceeds in 85 % of measures the longevity of the standard Tree Routing whose only criteria for selecting paths is the number of hops from source node to base station [15]. Equally, Figs. 11 and 12 shows that advantages in life cycle of MOR4WSN are independent of the number of nodes in the network.

7   Conclusions

Generation of valid individual of the initial population can be seen as a key treatment in MOR4WSN since all thenceforth generations depends on the initial population whose composition is changed through the operators of selection, crossover and mutation also previously adapted for MOR4WSN [11, 13, 14].

Although multiple works [3–7] focused on designing the fitness function according to hierarchical network performance needs in order to reduce its energy consumption, no one of them referenced any adaptation to genetic algorithm operators or initial population, not even considered using a multi-objective approach.

This paper presents the initial population adapting in MOR4WSN for preserving energy efficient routing trees in hierarchical WSN based on NSGA-II. Besides, MOR4WSN uses a binary index column matrix that helps to select the best optimized solution from the Pareto set, avoiding the normal randomly selection. MOR4WSN finds routing structures where valid trees along generations are guaranteed in spite the application of NSGA-II therefore optimized solutions in Pareto front are also valid routing trees, where a unique solution is chosen by using a binary index as exposed in [14].

As seen on results from Figs. 12 and 13, using an evolutionary meta-heuristic allows to make a topology network that advantages WSN lifetime by choosing transmission paths according to network conditions.

Adaptation of NSGA-II allows to conclude that other genetic operators (crossover, mutation) must also be tuned carefully to WSN conditions. As future work, it is envisaged to test MOR4WSN in IoT networks with different devices and features.

Acknowledgements. The authors acknowledge to GIT group of the University of Cauca in Colombia for the academic support to this work as well as to the I3A institute of the University of Castile-La Mancha in Spain. Financial support is acknowledged to University of Cauca and to the Administrative Department of Science Technology and Innovation of Colombia – Colciencias.

References

1. Atzori, L., Antonio, I., Morabito, G.: The internet of things: a survey. Comput. Netw. **54** (15), 2787–2805 (2010)
2. Giusto, D., Iera, A., Morabito, G., Atzori, L. (eds.): The Internet of Things. Springer, Berlin (2010). ISBN: 978-1-4419-1673-0
3. Bari, A., Wazed, S., Jaekel, A., Bandyopadhyay, S.: A genetic algorithm based approach for energy efficient routing in two-tiered sensor networks. Ad Hoc Netw. **7**(4), 665–676 (2009)
4. Chakraborty, A., Kumar, S.: Kanti M (2011) A genetic algorithm inspired routing protocol for wireless sensor networks. Int. J. Comput. Intell. Theor. Pract. **6**(1), 1–8 (2011)
5. Gupta, S.K., Kuila, P., Jana, P.K.: GAR: an energy efficient GA-based routing for wireless sensor networks. In: Hota, C., Srimani, P.K. (eds.) ICDCIT 2013. LNCS, vol. 7753, pp. 267–277. Springer, Heidelberg (2013)
6. Islam, O., Hussain, S., Zhang, H.: Genetic Algorithm for Data Aggregation Trees in Wireless Sensor Networks. IET Digital Library, London (2007)
7. Apetroaei, I., Oprea, I.A., Proca, B.E., Gheorghe, L.: Genetic algorithms applied in routing protocols for wireless sensor networks. In: 2011 10th Roedunet International Conference (RoEduNet), pp. 1–6. IEEE (2011)
8. Jia, J., et al.: Coverage optimization based on improved NSGA-II in wireless sensor network. In: IEEE International Conference on Integration Technology, 2007. ICIT 2007, pp. 614–618. IEEE (2007)
9. Lattarulo, V., Parks, G.T., Parks, G.T.: Application of the MOAA for the optimization of wireless sensor networks. EVOLVE-A Bridge Between Probability, Set Oriented Numerics, and Evolutionary Computation V, pp. 231–245. Springer International Publishing, Berlin (2014)
10. Chaudhry, S.B., et al.: Pareto-based evolutionary computational approach for wireless sensor placement. Eng. Appl. Artif. Intell. **24**(3), 409–425 (2011)

11. Rodríguez, A.M., Corrales, J.C.: Adaptación de una Metaheurística Evolutiva para Generar Árboles Enrutadores en una Red de Sensores Inalámbricos del Contexto de la Agricultura de Precisión. Revista Ingenierías Universidad de Medellín, N° 30 (2016, approved - publication awaited)

12. Deb, K., Agrawal, S., Pratap, A.: A fast elitist non-dominated sorting genetic algorithm for multi-objective optimization: NSGA-II. In: Schoenauer, M., Deb, K., Rudolph, G., Yao, X., Lutton, E., Merelo, J.J., Schwefel, H.-P. (eds.) PPSN VI. LNCS, vol. 1917, pp. 849–858. Springer, Heidelberg (2000)

13. Rodriguez, A., Ordóñez, A., Falcarin, P.: Energy optimization in wireless sensor networks based on genetic algorithms. In: SAI Intelligent Systems Conference 2015 (IntelliSys 2015), London

14. Rodriguez, A., Armando O., Ordonez, H.: Energy consumption optimization for sensor networks in the IoT. In: 2015 IEEE Colombian Conference on Communications and Computing (COLCOM). IEEE (2015)

15. Ortiz, T., Manuel, A.: Técnicas de enrutamiento inteligente para redes de sensores inalámbricos. Phd Thesis, University of Castille La Mancha, Albacete – Spain (2011)

16. León Javier, A.: Diseño e implementación en hardware de un algoritmo bioinspirado. Master Thesis, Instituto Politécnico Nacional, México (2009)

17. Deb, K., Pratap, A., Agarwal, S., Meyarivan, T.: A fast and elitist multiobjective genetic algorithm: NSGA-II. IEEE Trans. Evol. Comput. 6(2), 182–197 (2002)

18. Cabezas, I., Trujillo, M.: A method for reducing the cardinality of the Pareto front. In: Alvarez, L., Mejail, M., Gomez, L., Jacobo, J. (eds.) CIARP 2012. LNCS, vol. 7441, pp. 829–836. Springer, Heidelberg (2012)

19. NSGA-II C source code. http://www.egr.msu.edu/ ~ kdeb/codes.shtml. Accessed June 2015

On Analysis and Performance Improvement of Evolutionary Algorithms Based on its Complex Network Structure
A Summary Overview

Ivan Zelinka[✉]

Department of Computer Science,
Faculty of Electrical Engineering and Computer Science,
VSB-Technical University of Ostrava, 17. listopadu 2172/15,
708 00 Ostrava-Poruba, Czech Republic
ivan.zelinka@vsb.cz
http://navy.cs.vsb.cz

Abstract. In this participation there is sketched and explained mutual intersection between complex networks and evolutionary computation including summarization of our previous results. It is sketched how dynamics of evolutionary algorithm can be converted into a complex network and based on its properties like degree centrality etc. can be improved performance of used evolutionary algorithm. Results presented here are currently numerical demonstration rather than theoretical mathematical proofs. Paper discusses results from differential evolution, self-organizing migrating algorithm, genetic algorithms and artificial bee colony. We open question whether evolutionary algorithms really create complex network structures and whether this knowledge can be successfully used like feedback for control of evolutionary dynamics and its improvement in order to increase the performance of evolutionary algorithms.

Keywords: Evolution · Algorithm · Complex networks · Performance · Dynamics

1 Introduction

In this paper there is summarized synthesis of two partially different areas of research: complex networks, evolutionary computation. Ideas, results and methodologies reported and mentioned here are based on our previous results and experiments. We report here our latest results as well as propositions on further research that is in process in our group[1]. In order to understand what is the main idea, lets briefly discuss an overview of the two main areas: complex networks and dynamics of the evolutionary algorithms.

---

[1] http://navy.cs.vsb.cz/.

© Springer International Publishing Switzerland 2015
G. Sidorov and S.N. Galicia-Haro (Eds.): MICAI 2015, Part I, LNAI 9413, pp. 389–400, 2015.
DOI: 10.1007/978-3-319-27060-9_32

Large-scale networks, exhibiting complex patterns of interaction amongst vertices exist in both nature and in man-made systems (i.e., communication networks, genetic pathways, ecological or economical networks, social networks, networks of various scientific collaboration, Internet, World Wide Web, power grid etc.). The structure of complex networks thus can be observed in many systems. The word complex networks [1–6] comes from the fact that they exhibit substantial and non-trivial topological features, with patterns of connection between vertices that are neither purely regular nor purely random. Such features include a heavy tail in the degree distribution, a high clustering coefficient, hierarchical structure, amongst other features. In the case of directed networks, these features also include reciprocity, triad significance profile and other features. Amongst many studies, two well-known and much studied classes of complex networks are the scale-free networks and small-world networks (see examples in Fig. 1), whose discovery and definition are vitally important in the scope of this research. Specific structural features can be observed in both classes i.e. so called power-law degree distributions for the scale-free networks and short path lengths with high clustering for the small world networks. Research in the field of complex networks has joined together researchers from many areas, which were outside of this interdisciplinary research in the past like mathematics, physics, biology, chemistry computer science, epidemiology etc. For more recent details discussing research on complex networks and its various applications it is recommended to read for example [3–6].

Evolutionary computation is a sub-discipline of computer science belonging to the bio-inspired computing area. Since the end of the second world war, the main ideas of evolutionary computation have been published [17] and widely introduced to the scientific community [18]. Hence, the golden era of evolutionary techniques began, when Genetic Algorithms (GA) by Holland [18], Evolutionary Strategies (ES), by Schwefel [19] and Rechenberg [20] and Evolutionary Programming (EP) by Fogel [21] had been introduced. All these designs were favored by the forthcoming of more powerful and more easily programmable computers, so that for the first time interesting problems could be tackled and evolutionary computation started to compete with and became a high quality alternative to other optimization methods.

As a representative example of evolutionary algorithms we can mention for example Genetic algorithm (GA) [18, 26], Evolutionary strategies (ES) [20] and Schwefel [19], Ant Colony Optimization (ACO), [27], Particle Swarm (PS) or SOMA (Self-Organizing Migrating Algorithm) [28], Memetic Algorithms (MA) [29–32]. Differential Evolution (DE) [25] or the latest Firefly [34] (FF), CoCoo algorithm [33] (CC) or Bat algorithm (BA) [35] amongst the others. In this paper, we would like to summarize few results of our continuing research on mutual intersection of complex networks, evolutionary algorithms dynamics.

The main question (already sketched in our research papers as for example in [36–41]) is whether it is possible to visualize and simulate underlying dynamics of evolutionary process like complex network [1, 2, 10]. Reason for this is that today various techniques for analysis and control of complex networks exist and if complex network structure is hidden behind EA dynamics, then we believe, that existing control techniques could be used to improve dynamics of evolutionary algorithms (EAs).

We demonstrated that dynamics of evolutionary algorithms, that are based on Darwin theory of evolution and Mendel theory of genetic heritage [7] (or also on swarm principles), can be also visualized as complex networks, as in Fig. 2, [1,2,11]. Vertices in such a network are individuals of population and edges "capture" its interactions in offspring creation, i.e. evolutionary dynamics can be understood as a growth (dynamics) of the network [12,13]. It can be analyzed by classical tools for complex networks (e.g. Fig. 2, as we did for genetic algorithms [22], differential evolution [37] and SOMA algorithm [39]).

The main idea of our research is to show in this article that the dynamics of evolutionary algorithms, in general, shows properties of complex networks and evolutionary dynamics can be analyzed and visualized like a complex networks. We open and answer question whether evolutionary algorithms really create complex network structures and whether this knowledge can be successfully used like feedback for control of evolutionary dynamics and its improvement in order to increase the performance of evolutionary algorithms.

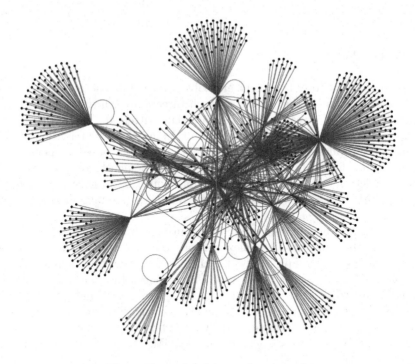

Fig. 1. Example of a complex network.

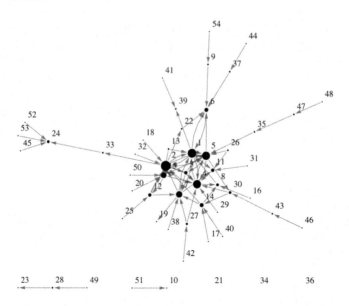

Fig. 2. Degree centrality of genetic algorithm as complex network in 50th generation, [22].

2   Motivation

Different problems solved by EAs are solved with different performance and results quality. One of theoretical research directions is how to improve EAs performance. Lot of research papers have been written and discuss this topic. The new approach reported here is based on EAs individuals interactions and its recording as a complex network. Evolutionary algorithms, based on its canonical central dogma (following darwinian ideas) clearly demonstrate intensive interaction amongst individual in the population, which is, in general, one of the important attributes of complex networks (intensive interaction amongst the vertices).

The main aim of our research reported in this paper, is to sketch how to convert EAs dynamics into complex network then interpret tools of complex networks analysis on complex networks that are given by evolutionary dynamics. Reason for this is that today various techniques for analysis and control of complex networks exist. If complex network structure is hidden behind EA dynamics, then we believe, that for example above mentioned control techniques could be used to improve dynamics of EAs. The first steps (i.e. conversion of the EA dynamics to the complex network and to CML system) have been done in the [10,12,23] and in [36–41].

3   Experiment Design

3.1   Conversion

Based on above mentioned principles and algorithms, we believe that there is no universal approach, but rather a personal one, based on the knowledge of algorithm principle. Lets take as an example DE, e.g. DERand1Bin in which each individual is selected in each generation to be a parent. Thus in DE, we have recorded only those individuals-parents, that have been replaced by better offspring (like vertex with added connections). In the DE class of algorithms we have omitted the philosophy that a bad parent is replaced by a better offspring, but accepted philosophical interpretation, that individual (worse parent) is moving to the better position (better offspring in original DE philosophy). Thus no vertex (individual) has to be either destroyed or replaced in the philosophical point of view. If, for example, DERand1Bin has a parent replaced by offspring, then it was considered as an activation (new additional links, edges) of vertex-worse parent from three another vertices (randomly selected individuals, see [10,12,23,25]). In fact, such general approach can be used also in another algorithms. If interaction amongst N individuals leads to the improvement of another arbitrary one, say M_{th}, then it is equivalent to the situation that N vertices give incoming edges to the M_{th} vertex. And vice versa. Edges can be weighted by integer numbers ($+1$ = successive support of the M_{th} vertex, -1 = nonsuccessive support) or simply by differences in fitness before interaction and after interaction. Again, this very general idea has to be adopted for each used algorithm. As reported in [36–39], we have tried this conversion for SOMA, DE, PSO, ABC (Artificial Bee Colony) and GA. Few selected results from ABC and DE are reported at the end of chapter. Complex networks can be then visualized as for example in Fig. 3 [9] or Fig. 4. From both figures it is visible that different algorithm dynamics produce different complex networks structure. Another visualizations can be found in [36–39].

3.2   Test Problems

The test function applied in [10] was selected from the test bed of 17 well known test function like Schwefels, Rastrigin's, Rana's function amongst the others. Evolution was searching for global extreme in 50 dimensions, i.e. individual has 50 parameters. Test functions have been selected due to their various complexity and mainly for the fact that these functions are widely used by researchers working with evolutionary algorithms. Another reason was that speed of convergence and thus evolutionary dynamics itself is different on that function, compared to simple test functions. Results are reported in more details in [36–39].

4   Results

As reported in [10] test function (to reveal its complex networks dynamics) with constant level of test function dimensionality (i.e. individual length). All

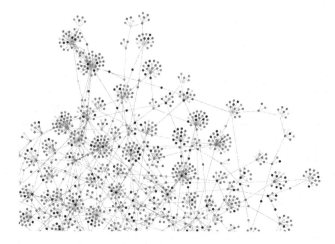

Fig. 3. Example of a network based on PSO. Network structure capture time development of PSO in certain time window.

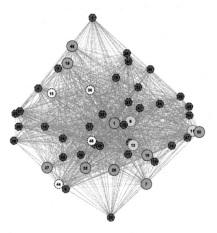

Fig. 4. Example of a network based on SOMA.

data have been processed graphically. Visual emergence of complex network structure behind evolutionary dynamics depends on many factors. However some special versions of used algorithms did not show complex network structure despite the fact that the number of generations was quite large, see [10, 12, 23]. The main tools of *Mathematica* software were used on basic analysis and are proposed here. Visualized and analyzed graphs have multiple edges that can be understand like weight of single edge. Attributes of proposed analysis are represented by subgraph colors and vertices size in graphs. Our proposed interpretation, based on terms and command from Wolfram *Mathematica* used for all of our experiments is reported in [15, 16]. Here we report shortly 2 selected case studies.

4.1   Case Study 1 - Artificial Bee Colony

Proposed approach has been tested on Artificial Bee Colony algorithm (ABC) and presented in [36,38]. The main idea was to test ABC on scheduling problems as well as on continuous test problems. The complex network analysis was used for adaptive control of the population. The structure of the algorithm was as follows: firstly, the weighted adjacency matrix was created throughout the algorithm iterations, for some fixed number of iterations, a fraction of the total expected number of iterations before algorithm termination. The complex network recorded this way is then analyzed, and this information was subsequently used to identify the nodes (solutions) that dont play a significant role in the population dynamics. In this algorithm, such nodes are replaced by the new randomly generated ones, although different schemas of the replacements generation could also be used.

The measures used to identify the nodes that do not contribute significantly to the population improvement were chosen to be the three types of vertex centrality, the weighted degree centrality (strength), closeness and betweenness centrality, as described in [36,38]. The vertices representing solutions were ranked according to these measures, and the fixed ratio of the solutions corresponding to the lowest ranking nodes was removed and regenerated. The adjacency matrix was then reset. The entire procedure of network recording and the nodes ranking and replacement is repeated until the algorithm terminates. This concept is illustrated in Figs. 5, 6 and 7.

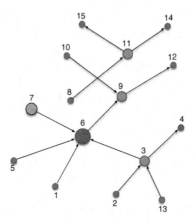

Fig. 5. The network with labelled nodes (individuals) ranked by centrality. The larger centrality nodes are marked in bigger size and different colors. The smallest blue nodes have the lowest centrality, the largest red node has the highest centrality value (Color figure online).

ABC was used in other 2 (so in total in 3) variants. The 2nd variant (called in [38] Adaptive ABC 2) is based on use of three fully separated sub-populations,

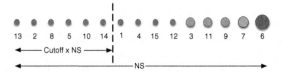

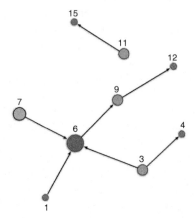

Fig. 6. The nodes (individuals) sorted according to their centrality score in ascending order. The first Cutoff NS nodes will be removed.

Fig. 7. The network after the low centrality nodes (individuals) removal. The most important nodes are preserved.

each with their own network (or better sub-network, if whole EAs dynamics is taken like network itself). Each of them was evaluated using different centrality measure type. After the less influential nodes are pruned and the networks reset, the tournament selection of size two is performed to select every next-generation solution of every sub-population, choosing the better of two solutions randomly selected from all three sub-populations. In this way the information sharing between sub-populations is ensured.

Third version, named Adaptive ABC 3 was created in order to explore the influence of distinct centralities on the speed of convergence. It takes the centrality measure to be used for network analysis and nodes evaluation as a parameter. The algorithm is fully described in [38].

Based on results reported in above referenced papers, it can be stated that concept proposed here was successful and has improved ABC performance significantly [38].

4.2   Case Study 2 - Differential Evolution

In this case of [37, 40, 41] is discussed use of the weighted clustering coefficient [4, 5] in order to improve DE performance. One of the main goals of weighted clustering coefficient use on DE is to find the way how to select the parents in the mutation step to improve DE convergence rate. In the variant DE/best/1/bin, the best individual is the individual with the smallest (in minimizing problems) or greatest (in maximizing problems) fitness value. As it was described in former research, DE/best/1/bin does not reach the best results in the non-separable and multimodal functions. This fact led us to search for another criterion of the best individual selection. From the rules that we have presented, we know that the edges between nodes representing the individuals are created only if the individuals represented by these nodes contributed to the population improvement. The nodes representing the individuals becoming the parents will have the greater out-degree (the number of out-going edges will be greater) more often and the weights of the edges leading from these nodes will be higher. Such parents have the genomes of high quality and it is important to spread these genomes. The weighted clustering coefficient is one of the most appropriate candidate to be chosen as the criterion of parents selection in the mutation step from two reasons:

1. It enables to capture spreading of the genomes from the node to another node (individual).
2. Unlike the local clustering coefficient the weights of the edges are took into consideration.

When the adjacency matrix A_G for the generation G is created, the weighted clustering coefficient of each node is computed. Then, for each individual the probability of selection is computed according to the following equation:

$$p_i = \frac{\widetilde{C}_{i,Z}}{\sum_{j=1}^{NP} \widetilde{C}_{j,Z}}, \tag{1}$$

where p_i denotes the probability of the i-th individual selection and $\widetilde{C}_{i,Z}$ is the weighted clustering coefficient of the node representing the i-th individual. Individual represented by the node with the higher weighted clustering coefficient has the higher probability to be selected as the parent in the mutation step. As reported in [40,41], this approach has improved DE's performance significantly. Similar research is reported in [37].

5   Conclusion

In this paper we refer possible interpretation [16] and use of selected well known tools and terminology from complex networks analysis [1–6] to the evolutionary algorithms dynamics converted to the complex network structures as firstly reported in [14]. This paper is only overview of our previous research presented in above mentioned papers and latest research reported in [22,40,41], where we proposed all necessary steps joining evolutionary dynamics, complex networks and so called CML systems [7,8].

Based on many research papers more or less mentioned here it is clear that for EAs applications as well as in EAs dynamics itself lot of open research questions can be raised. It is clear that EAs are nothing else than a kind of discrete dynamical systems exhibiting complex structures and dynamics that can be studied by means of various tools of mathematics as classical statistics or/an by tools of complex networks and chaotic systems [1–26]. It is clear that there is a lot of interesting questions like (for example) *what is the impact of specific dynamic regimes in EAs dynamics on its performance? What are limitations of EAs performance when complex network methodology proposed here is used?* or more practical questions joined with EAs performance.

The volume of this paper is too small to mention and explain all the possible interpretations and tools. This is only a mid-step in our research presented in [10, 12, 23, 36–39], where we proposed all necessary steps joining evolutionary dynamics, complex networks and CML systems.

Acknowledgment. The following grants are acknowledged for the financial support provided for this research: Grant Agency of the Czech Republic - GACR P103/15/06700S and SP2015/142.

References

1. Dorogovtsev, S.N., Mendes, J.F.F.: Evolution of networks. Adv. Phys. **51**, 1079–1187 (2002)
2. Boccaletti, S., et al.: Complex networks: structure and dynamics. Phys. Rep. **424**, 175–308 (2006)
3. Meyn, S.: Control Techniques for Complex Networks. Cambridge University Press, Cambridge (2007)
4. Steen, M.: Graph Theory and Complex Networks: An Introduction, Maarten van Steen (2010). ISBN: 978-9081540612
5. Chen, G., Wang, X., Li, X.: Fundamentals of Complex Networks: Models, Structures and Dynamics. Wiley, New York (2015)
6. Barrat, A., Barthlemy, M., Vespignani, A.: Dynamical Processes on Complex Networks. Cambridge University Press, Cambridge (2008)
7. Zelinka, I., Celikovsky, S., Richter, H., Chen, G. (eds.): Evolutionary Algorithms and Chaotic Systems. SCI, vol. 267. Springer, Heidelberg (2010)
8. Schuster, H.G.: Handbook of Chaos Control. Wiley-VCH, New York (1999)
9. Pluhacek, M., Janostik, J., Senkerik, R., Zelinka, I., Davendra, D.: PSO as complex network - capturing the inner dynamics, an initial study. In: Proceedings of Nostradamus 2015: International Conference on Prediction, Modeling and Analysis of Complex Systems, AECIA, France. AISC. Springer (2015) (accepted, in print)
10. Zelinka, I., Davendra, D., Chadli, M., Senkerik, R., Dao, T.T., Skanderova, L.: Evolutionary dynamics and complex networks. In: Zelinka, I., Snasel, V., Ajith, A. (eds.) Handbook of Optimization. Springer, Heidelberg (2012)
11. Zelinka, I., Snasel, V., Ajith, A. (eds.): Handbook of Optimization. Springer, Heidelberg (2012)
12. Zelinka, I., Davendra, D., Senkerik, R., Jasek, R.: Do evolutionary algorithm dynamics create complex network structures? Complex Syst. **20**(2), 127–140 (2011). ISSN: 0891-2513

13. Zelinka, I.: Mutual relations of evolutionary dynamics, deterministic chaos and complexity. In: Tutorial at IEEE Congress on Evolutionary Computation, Mexico (2013)
14. Zelinka, I.: On close relations of evolutionary dynamics, chaos and complexity. In: Keynote at International Workshop on Chaos-Fractals Theories and Applications, Dalian, China (2012)
15. Zelinka, I.: Controlling complexity. In: AIP Conference Proceedings, vol. 1479, no. 1, pp. 654–657 (2012)
16. Zelinka, I., Skanderova, L., Saloun, P., Senkerik, R., Pluhacek, M.: Hidden complexity of evolutionary dynamics - analysis. In: Sanayei, A., Zelinka, I., Rossler, O.E. (eds.) ISCS 2013, vol. 8. Springer, Heidelberg (2014)
17. Turing, A.: Intelligent machinery, unpublished report for National Physical Laboratory. In: Michie, D. (ed.) Machine Intelligence, vol. 7 (1969), Turing, A.M. (ed.): The Collected Works, vol. 3, Ince D. North-Holland, Amsterdam (1992)
18. Holland, J.: Adaptation in Natural and Artificial Systems. University of Michigan Press, Ann Arbor (1975)
19. Schwefel, H.: Numerische Optimierung von Computer-Modellen, Ph.D. thesis (1974). Reprinted by Birkhauser (1977)
20. Rechenberg, I.: Evolutionsstrategie - Optimierung technischer Systeme nach Prinzipien der biologischen Evolution, Ph.D. thesis (1971). Printed in Fromman-Holzboog (1973)
21. Fogel, D.B.: Unearthinga fossil from the history of evolutionary computation. Fundamenta Informaticae 35(1–4), 116 (1998)
22. Zelinka, I., Davendra, D., Lampinen, J., Senkerik, R., Pluhacek, M.: Dynamics, evolutionary algorithms, its hidden complex network structures. In: IEEE Congress on Evolutionary Computation, WCCI 2014, 6–11 July 2014, Beijing, pp. 3246–3251 (2014). doi:10.1109/CEC.2014.6900441
23. Zelinka, I., Davendra, D., Snasel, V., Jasek, R., Senkerik, R., Oplatkova, Z.: Preliminary investigation on relations between complex networks and evolutionary algorithms dynamics. In: CISIM, Poland (2010)
24. Bornholdt, S., Schuster, H.G. (eds.): Handbook of Graphs and Networks: From the Genome to the Internet. Wiley-VCH, New York (2003)
25. Price, K.: An introduction to differential evolution. In: Corne, D., Dorigo, M., Glover, F. (eds.) New Ideas in Optimization, pp. 79–108. McGraw-Hill, London (1999)
26. Goldberg, D.: Genetic Algorithms in Search, Optimization, and Machine Learning. Addison-Wesley Publishing Company Inc., Boston (1989). ISBN: 0201157675
27. Dorigo, M., Sttzle, T.: Ant Colony Optimization. MIT Press, Cambridge (2004). ISBN: 978-0262042192
28. Zelinka, I.: SOMA - self organizing migrating algorithm. In: Onwubolu, G.C., Babu, B.V. (eds.) New Optimization Techniques in Engineering, pp. 167–218. Springer, New York (2008). ISBN: 3-540-20167X
29. Goh, C., Ong, Y., Tan, K. (eds.): Multi-Objective Memetic Algorithms. SCI. Springer, New York (2009). ISBN: 978-3-540-88050-9
30. Schonberger, J.: Operational Freight Carrier Planning: Optimization Models and Advanced Memetic Algorithms. Springer, Heidelberg (2005). ISBN: 978-3-540-25318-1
31. Onwubolu, G., Babu, B.: New Optimization Techniques in Engineering. Springer, New York (2004). ISBN: 3-540-20167X
32. Hart, W., Krasnogor, N., Smith, J.: Recent Advances in Memetic Algorithms, vol. 166. Springer, Heidelberg (2005). ISBN: 978-3-540-22904-9

33. Yang, X.-S., Deb, S.: Cuckoo search via Lvy flights. In: World Congress on Nature and Biologically Inspired Computing (NaBIC 2009), pp. 210–214. IEEE Publications, December 2009

34. Yang, X.-S.: Firefly algorithms for multimodal optimization. In: Watanabe, O., Zeugmann, T. (eds.) SAGA 2009. LNCS, vol. 5792, pp. 169–178. Springer, Heidelberg (2009)

35. Yang, X.S.: A new metaheuristic bat-inspired algorithm. In: Gonzalez, J.R., Pelta, D.A., Cruz, C., Terrazas, G., Krasnogor, N. (eds.) NISCO 2010. SCI, vol. 284, pp. 65–74. Springer, Heidelberg (2010)

36. Metlicka, M., Davendra, D.: Chaos-driven discrete artificial bee colony. In: IEEE Congress on Evolutionary Computation, pp. 2947–2954 (2014)

37. Davendra, D., Zelinka, I., Metlicka, M., Senkerik, R., Pluhacek, M.: Complex network analysis of differential evolution algorithm applied to flowshop with no-wait problem. In: IEEE Symposium on Differential Evolution, 9–12 December, Orlando, FL, USA, pp. 65–72 (2014)

38. Davendra, D., Metlicka, M.: Ensemble centralities based adaptive artificial bee algorithm. In: IEEE Congress on Evolutionary Computation (2015)

39. Zelinka, I.: Evolutionary algorithms as a complex dynamical systems. In: Tutorial at IEEE Congress on Evolutionary Computation, Sendai (2015)

40. Zelinka, I.: On mutual relations amongst evolutionary algorithm dynamics, its hidden complex network structures.: an overview and recent advances. In: Meghanathan, N. (ed.) Advanced Methods for Complex Network Analysis. IGI (2015)

41. Skanderova, L., Zelinka, I.: Differential evolution dynamic analysis by the complex networks. In: Meghanathan, N. (ed.) Advanced Methods for Complex Network Analysis. IGI (2015)

Scheduling Projects by a Hybrid Evolutionary Algorithm with Self-Adaptive Processes

Virginia Yannibelli[1,2(✉)] and Analía Amandi[1,2]

[1] ISISTAN Research Institute, UNCPBA University, Campus Universitario,
Paraje Arroyo Seco, 7000 Tandil, Argentina
{vyannibe,amandi}@exa.unicen.edu.ar
[2] CONICET, National Council of Scientific and Technological Research,
Buenos Aires, Argentina

Abstract. In this paper, we present a hybrid evolutionary algorithm with self-adaptive processes to solve a known project scheduling problem. This problem takes into consideration an optimization objective priority for project managers: to maximize the effectiveness of the sets of human resources assigned to the project activities. The hybrid evolutionary algorithm integrates self-adaptive processes with the aim of enhancing the evolutionary search. The behavior of these processes is self-adaptive according to the state of the evolutionary search. The performance of the hybrid evolutionary algorithm is evaluated on six different instance sets and then is compared with that of the best algorithm previously proposed in the literature for the addressed problem. The obtained results show that the hybrid evolutionary algorithm considerably outperforms the previous algorithm.

Keywords: Project scheduling · Human resource assignment · Multi-skilled resources · Hybrid evolutionary algorithms · Evolutionary algorithms · Simulated annealing algorithms

1 Introduction

Project scheduling is a really central, complex and costly task in most organizations and companies. This task means defining start times and human resource assignments feasible for the activities of a given project, in such a way that a given optimization objective is achieved. In addition, defining human resource assignments for project activities implies considering the available knowledge about the effectiveness of the human resources with regard to project activities. This is because the results as well as the development of any project activity depend on the effectiveness of the human resource assignment defined for it [1, 2].

Based on the above-mentioned, a wide variety of project scheduling problems have been presented and addressed in the literature. Nonetheless, only few of these project scheduling problems consider that human resources usually have very different levels of effectiveness [3–6, 10], a really essential aspect in the context of real project scheduling problems. These project scheduling problems differ significantly in the assumptions considered regarding the effectiveness of human resources.

© Springer International Publishing Switzerland 2015
G. Sidorov and S.N. Galicia-Haro (Eds.): MICAI 2015, Part I, LNAI 9413, pp. 401–412, 2015.
DOI: 10.1007/978-3-319-27060-9_33

In the project scheduling problem formally described in [6], it is supposed that the effectiveness level of a human resource depends on different factors inherent to its work context (i.e., the project activity to which the resource is assigned, the skill to which the resource is assigned within the project activity, the set of human resources assigned to the project activity, and the attributes of the resource). This assumption about the effectiveness of human resources is really valuable. This is mainly because, in the context of real project scheduling problems, human resources have different levels of effectiveness with regards to different work contexts, and therefore, the effectiveness level of a human resource is usually considered in relation to its work context [1, 2]. To the best of our knowledge, the influence of the factors inherent to the work context on the effectiveness levels of human resources is not taken into account in other project scheduling problems described in the literature. Therefore, the project scheduling problem described in [6] supposes valuable and also novel assumptions regarding the effectiveness levels of human resources in the context of project scheduling problems.

In this paper, we present a hybrid evolutionary algorithm with self-adaptive processes to solve the project scheduling problem described in [6]. It is necessary to mention that this problem takes into account an optimization objective priority for project managers: to maximize the effectiveness levels of the sets of human resources assigned to the project activities. This algorithm integrates self-adaptive processes which adapt their behavior in accordance with the state of the evolutionary search. The integration of self-adaptive processes has the aim of enhancing the evolutionary search, in both exploration and exploitation [18–20].

We present this hybrid evolutionary algorithm mainly due to the next reasons. The addressed project scheduling problem is a special case of the RCPSP (Resource Constrained Project Scheduling Problem) [9], and therefore, is an NP-Hard problem. In this respect, hybrid evolutionary algorithms that integrate self-adaptive processes have been shown to be much more effective than hybrid evolutionary algorithms with non-adaptive processes in the resolution of a wide variety of NP-Hard problems [18–20]. Thus, we consider that the hybrid evolutionary algorithm presented could outperform the best algorithm previously presented in the literature for the addressed problem. We refer to the hybrid evolutionary algorithm presented in [8].

The remainder of the paper is organized as follows. In Sect. 2, we present a description of the addressed problem. In Sect. 3, we present the hybrid evolutionary algorithm. In Sect. 4, we present the computational experiments developed in order to evaluate the performance of the hybrid evolutionary algorithm and also an analysis of the obtained results. In Sect. 5, we review reported project scheduling problems in which the effectiveness of human resources is considered. Finally, in Sect. 6 we present the conclusions of the present work.

2   Problem Description

In this paper, we address the project scheduling problem formally presented in [6]. We give a description of this project scheduling problem below.

Consider that a project contains a set A of N activities, $A = \{1, ..., N\}$, which have to be scheduled (i.e., the starting time and the human resources of each activity have to be defined). The duration, precedence relations and resource requirements of each activity are known.

The duration of each activity j is notated as d_j. Moreover, it is considered that pre-emption of activities is not allowed (i.e., the d_j periods of time must be consecutive).

Among some project activities, there are precedence relations. The precedence relations establish that each activity j cannot start until all its immediate predecessors, given by the set P_j, have completely finished.

Project activities require human resources – employees – skilled in different knowledge areas. Specifically, each activity requires one or several skills as well as a given number of employees for each skill.

It is considered that organizations and companies have a qualified workforce to develop their projects. This workforce is made up of a number of employees, and each employee masters one or several skills.

Considering a given project, set SK represents the K skills required to develop the project, $SK = \{1,\ldots, K\}$, and set AR_k represents the available employees with skill k. Then, the term $r_{j,k}$ represents the number of employees with skill k required for activity j of the project. The values of the terms $r_{j,k}$ are known for each project activity.

It is considered that an employee cannot take over more than one skill within a given activity. In addition, an employee cannot be assigned more than one activity at the same time.

Based on the previous assumptions, an employee can be assigned different activities but not at the same time, can take over different skills required for an activity but not simultaneously, and can belong to different possible sets of employees for each activity.

As a result, it is possible to define different work contexts for each available employee. It is considered that the work context of an employee r, denoted as $C_{r,j,k,g}$, is made up of four main components. The first component refers to the activity j which r is assigned (i.e., the complexity of j, its domain, etc.). The second component refers to the skill k which r is assigned within activity j (i.e., the tasks associated to k within j). The third component is the set of employees g that has been assigned j and that includes r (i.e., r must work in collaboration with the other employees assigned to j). The fourth component refers to the attributes of r (i.e., his or her experience level in relation to different tasks and domains, the kind of labor relation between r and the other employees of g, his or her educational level in relation to different knowledge areas, his or her level with respect to different skills, etc.). It is considered that the attributes of r could be quantified from available information about r (e.g., curriculum vitae of r, results of evaluations made to r, information about the participation of r in already executed projects, etc.).

The four components described above are considered the main factors that determine the effectiveness level of an employee. For this reason, it is assumed that the effectiveness of an employee depends on all the components of his or her work context. Then, for each employee, it is possible to consider different effectiveness levels in relation to different work contexts.

The effectiveness level of an employee r, in relation to a possible context $C_{r,j,k,g}$ for r, is notated as $e_{rCr,j,k,g}$. The term $e_{rCr,j,k,g}$ represents how well r can handle, within activity j, the tasks associated to skill k, considering that r must work in collaboration with the other employees of set g. The mentioned term $e_{rCrj,k,g}$ takes a real value over the range $[0, 1]$. The values of the terms $e_{rCrj,k,g}$ inherent to each employee available for the project are known. It is considered that these values could be obtained from available information about the participation of the employees in already executed projects.

The problem of scheduling a project entails defining feasible start times (i.e., the precedence relations between the activities must not be violated) and feasible human resource assignments (i.e., the human resource requirements must be met) for project activities in such a way that the optimization objective is reached. In this sense, a priority objective is considered for project managers at the early stage of the project schedule design. The objective is that the most effective set of employees be assigned each project activity. This objective is modeled by Formulas (1) and (2).

Formula (1) maximizes the effectiveness of the sets of employees assigned to the N activities of a given project. In this formula, set S contains all the feasible schedules for the project in question. The term $e(s)$ represents the effectiveness level of the sets of employees assigned to project activities by schedule s. Then, $R(j,s)$ is the set of employees assigned to activity j by schedule s, and the term $e_{R(j,s)}$ represents the effectiveness level corresponding to $R(j,s)$.

Formula (2) estimates the effectiveness level of the set of employees $R(j,s)$. This effectiveness level is estimated calculating the mean effectiveness level of the employees belonging to $R(j,s)$.

For a more detailed discussion of Formulas (1) and (2), we refer to [6].

$$\max_{\forall s \in S} \left(e(s) = \sum_{j=1}^{N} e_{R(j,s)} \right) \tag{1}$$

$$e_{R(j,s)} = \frac{\sum_{r=1}^{|R(j,s)|} e_{rCr,j,k(r,j,s),R(j,s)}}{|R(j,s)|} \tag{2}$$

3   Hybrid Evolutionary Algorithm with Self-Adaptive Processes

In order to solve the addressed problem, we present a hybrid evolutionary algorithm with self-adaptive processes. This algorithm integrates self-adaptive processes which adapt their behavior in accordance with the state of the evolutionary search. The integration of self-adaptive processes has the aim of enhancing the evolutionary search, in both exploitation and exploration [18–20].

The main behavior of the hybrid evolutionary algorithm is shown in Fig. 1 and is described below.

Taking into account a given project to be scheduled, the algorithm creates a random initial population of solutions. In this population, each solution encodes a feasible

```
BEGIN
    CREATE initial population;
    EVALUATE each solution of the population;
    REPEAT UNTIL ( number of iterations is reached ) DO
        SELECT parents;
        RECOMBINE pairs of parents to produce offspring;
        MUTATE the resulting offspring;
        EVALUATE new solutions;
        CREATE new population;
        IMPROVE solutions via Simulated Annealing;
    OD
    PROVIDE best solution;
END
```

Fig. 1. Main behavior of the hybrid evolutionary algorithm

project schedule. Then, the algorithm decodes and evaluates each solution of the population by a fitness function. Specifically, the schedule related to each solution is built and then evaluated with respect of the optimization objective of the problem. As was detailed in Sect. 2, the optimization objective implies maximizing the effectiveness of the sets of employees assigned to the project activities. In relation to this objective, the fitness function evaluates the employee assignments of each solution based on knowledge of the effectiveness of the employees considered in the solution.

After each solution of the population is evaluated, a parent selection process is utilized to determine which solutions of the population will integrate the mating pool. The solutions with the highest fitness values will have more chance of being selected. Once the mating pool is complete, the solutions in the mating pool are organized in pairs. After that, a crossover process is applied to each pair of solutions with a self-adaptive probability AP_c to generate new feasible ones. After that, a mutation process is applied to each solution obtained by the crossover process, with a self-adaptive probability AP_m. After that, a survival selection process is applied in order to determine which solutions from the solutions in the population and the solutions generated from the mating pool will integrate the new population. Finally, a self-adaptive simulated annealing algorithm is applied to the solutions of the new population. The above-described process is repeated until a predefined number of iterations is reached.

3.1 Representation of Solutions

We used the representation described in [6] in order to encode the solutions. By this representation, each solution is encoded by two lists with as many positions as activities in the project.

The first list is a traditional activity list. This list is a feasible precedence list of the activities in the project (i.e., each activity j can appear on this list in any position higher than the positions of all its predecessors). The activity list defines the order in which activities shall be added to the schedule.

The second list is an assigned resources list. This list details the employees assigned to each activity of the project (i.e., position j on this list details the employees of every skill k assigned to activity j).

In order to decode the schedule related to the representation, we used the serial schedule generation process described in [6]. By this process, each activity j is scheduled at the earliest possible time.

3.2   Fitness Function

To evaluate the encoded solutions, we used a fitness function specially designed. Given an encoded solution, this function decodes the schedule s related to the solution by the serial schedule generation process mentioned in Sect. 3.1. After that, the fitness function calculates the value of the term $e(s)$ corresponding to s (Formulas (1) and (2)). This value defines the fitness level of the solution. The term $e(s)$ takes a real value on $[0,\ldots, N]$.

In order to calculate the value of term $e(s)$, the fitness function utilizes the values of the terms $e_{rCr,j,k,g}$ inherent to s (Formula 2). In this respect, the values of the terms $e_{rCr,j,k,g}$ inherent to each available employee r are known, as was detailed in Sect. 2.

3.3   Parent Selection and Survival Selection

To develop the parent selection, we used the process named roulette wheel selection [18]. In this process, a selection probability is defined for each solution of the current population. The selection probability of each solution is proportional to its fitness value. Thus, the solutions with the best fitness values have more probability of being selected for the mating pool.

To develop the survival selection, we utilized the process named fitness-based steady-state selection [18]. By this process, the worst λ solutions of the current population are replaced by the best λ solutions generated from the mating pool. This process preserves the best solutions reached by the hybrid evolutionary algorithm [18].

3.4   Self-Adaptive Crossover and Self-Adaptive Mutation

In respect of the crossover process and the mutation process, we utilized self-adaptive processes feasible for the representation of the solutions.

The crossover process is composed by a crossover process feasible for activity lists and a crossover process feasible for assigned resources lists. In respect of the crossover for activity lists, we applied a process named two-point crossover [21]. For assigned resources lists, we applied a process named uniform crossover [18].

The mutation process is composed by a mutation process feasible for activity lists and a mutation process feasible for assigned resources lists. In relation to the mutation for activity lists, we applied a process named adjacent pairwise interchange [21]. For assigned resources lists, we applied a process named random resetting [18].

In order to apply the crossover process and the mutation process, we considered self-adaptive probabilities AP_c and AP_m, respectively. Specifically, we considered the known self-adaptive probabilities AP_c and AP_m described in [11]. These probabilities are defined by Formulas (3) and (4). In these formulas, f_{max} is the maximal fitness of the population, f_{avg} is the average fitness of the population, and $(f_{max} - f_{avg})$ is a measure of the state of the evolutionary search. In Formula (3), f' is the higher fitness of the two solutions to be crossed, and AP_{cLA} and AP_{cUA} are predefined values for the crossover probability, considering $0 \leq AP_{cLA}, AP_{cUA} \leq 1$. In Formula (4), f'' is the fitness of the solution to be mutated, and AP_{mLA} and AP_{mUA} are predefined values for the mutation probability, considering $0 \leq AP_{mLA}, AP_{mUA} \leq 1$.

Probabilities AP_c and AP_m are adaptive according to the state of the evolutionary search. Specifically, when the evolutionary search starts to converge, AP_c and AP_m are increased in order to encourage the exploration of new regions of the search space and therefore to avoid the premature convergence of the evolutionary search. In contrast, when the evolutionary search is scattered in the search space, AP_c and AP_m are reduced in order to encourage the exploitation of known regions of the search space.

$$AP_c = \begin{cases} \frac{AP_{cUA}(f_{max}-f')}{(f_{max}-f_{avg})} & f' \geq f_{avg} \\ AP_{cLA} & f' < f_{avg} \end{cases} \tag{3}$$

$$AP_m = \begin{cases} \frac{AP_{mUA}(f_{max}-f'')}{(f_{max}-f_{avg})} & f'' \geq f_{avg} \\ AP_{mLA} & f'' < f_{avg} \end{cases} \tag{4}$$

3.5   Self-Adaptive Simulated Annealing Algorithm

We applied a self-adaptive simulated annealing algorithm to the solutions of the population obtained by the survival selection process, except to the solution with the highest fitness value of this population which is preserved. The applied self-adaptive simulated annealing algorithm is a variation of the simulated annealing algorithm presented in [8].

The main behavior of the self-adaptive simulated annealing algorithm is described as follows. Given an encoded solution s, the algorithm generates a new encoded solution s' from the solution s by using a move process, and then decides if the solution s must be replaced or not by the new solution s'. If the fitness value of the new solution s' is better than that of the solution s, the algorithm replaces to the solution s by the solution s'. In contrast, if the fitness value of the new solution s' is worse than or equal to that of the solution s, the algorithm replaces to the solution s by the solution s' based on an acceptance probability which is $exp(-delta / T_c)$. In this probability, term T_c is the current value of the temperature parameter and $delta$ is the difference between the fitness values of the solutions s and s'. Thus, the acceptance probability is proportional to the current value of the temperature parameter.

The above-described process is repeated until a predetermined number of iterations is reached. It is necessary to mention that, at the end of each iteration, the value of the temperature parameter is reduced by a predefined cooling factor.

In relation to the initial value T_i of the temperature parameter, we defined the value T_i based on the evolutionary search state reached after the survival selection process, considering that such state is measured by calculating the term $(f_{max} - f_{avg})$ on the population obtained by the survival selection process. Specifically, we calculated the value T_i by using the next formula: $T_i = 1 / (f_{max} - f_{avg})$. By this formula, when the evolutionary search is scattered in the search space, the value T_i is low, and thus the acceptance probability of the algorithm is also low. As consequence of this, the algorithm promotes the exploitation of known regions of the search space. When the evolutionary search starts to converge, the value T_i increases, and thus the acceptance probability of the algorithm also increases. As consequence of this, the algorithm promotes the exploration of new regions of the search space. Based on the mentioned, the algorithm is self-adaptive to promote either the exploitation or exploration of the search space, according to the state of the evolutionary search.

Move Process. The self-adaptive simulated annealing algorithm utilizes a move process to produce a new encoded solution from a given encoded solution. In this respect, we applied a move process feasible for the representation of the solutions. The move process is composed by a move process feasible for activity lists and a move process feasible for assigned resources lists. In respect of the move process for activity lists, we applied a move process named simple shift [21]. For assigned resources lists, we applied a move process which is considered as a variation of the process named random resetting [18].

4   Computational Experiments

4.1   Instance Sets

We used the six instance sets introduced in [7] in order to evaluate the performance of the hybrid evolutionary algorithm. Each one of these six instance sets contains 40 instances. Each instance contains a number of activities to be scheduled as well as a number of available employees for these activities. The main characteristics of these six instance sets are presented in Table 1. For a more detailed description of these six instance sets, we refer to [7].

It is necessary to mention that each instance of these six instance sets has a known optimal solution with a fitness level equal to N. Note that N is the number of activities to be scheduled in the instance. These known optimal solutions of the instances are considered as references to evaluate the performance of the algorithm.

4.2   Main Results

We evaluated the performance of the hybrid evolutionary algorithm on each of the six instance sets. Specifically, we run the algorithm a predetermined number t of times (i.e.,

Table 1. Main characteristics of the instance sets

Instance set	Number of activities per instance	Number of possible sets of employees per activity
j30_5	30	1 to 5
j30_10	30	1 to 10
j60_5	60	1 to 5
j60_10	60	1 to 10
j120_5	120	1 to 5
j120_10	120	1 to 10

$t = 30$ times) on each instance of the six instance sets. In order to develop these runs, we set the algorithm parameters as follows: population size = 90; number of generations = 300; crossover process: $AP_{cLA} = 0.9$ and $AP_{cUA} = 0.6$; mutation process: $AP_{mLA} = 0.1$ and $AP_{mUA} = 0.05$; survival selection process: $\lambda = 45$; simulated annealing algorithm: number of iterations = 25 and cooling factor = 0.9. It is necessary to mention that we set the algorithm parameters with these values based on exhaustive preliminary experiments. By these preliminary experiments, we considered many different settings for the algorithm parameters, and then we selected the best of these settings for the algorithm parameters.

We analyzed the results obtained by the hybrid evolutionary algorithm for each of the six instance sets. Specifically, for each instance set, we analyzed the average percentage deviation from the optimal value (Av. Dev. (%)) as well as the percentage of instances for which the optimal value is reached at least once among the t runs developed (Opt. (%)).

For j30_5, j30_10, j60_5 and j60_10, the algorithm obtained an Av. Dev (%) equal to 0 % and an Opt. (%) equal to 100 %. These results indicate that the algorithm reached an optimal solution in each run developed on each instance of these sets.

For j120_5 and j120_10, the algorithm obtained Av. Dev (%) values equal to 0.1 % and 0.36 %, respectively. Because the optimal solutions of the instances of both sets have a fitness level equal to 120, these results indicate that the average fitness level of the solutions obtained by the algorithm for j120_5 and j120_10 is 119.88 and 119.57, respectively. Therefore, the algorithm obtained very near-optimal solutions for the instances of both sets.

Moreover, for j120_5 and j120_10, the algorithm obtained an Opt. (%) value equal to 100 %. These results indicate that, for each instance of these two sets, the algorithm reached an optimal solution at least once among the t runs developed on the instance.

4.3   Comparison

In this section, we compare the performance of the hybrid evolutionary algorithm with that of the best algorithm previously presented in the literature for solving the addressed problem. We refer to the hybrid evolutionary algorithm presented in [8].

For simplicity, we will refer to the hybrid evolutionary algorithm presented in [8] as algorithm H. Like the hybrid evolutionary algorithm presented here, the algorithm

H integrates an adaptive simulated annealing algorithm into the framework of an evolutionary algorithm. Unlike the hybrid evolutionary algorithm presented here, the algorithm H uses non-adaptive crossover and mutation processes. These processes do not consider the state of the evolutionary search.

In [8], the algorithm H has been evaluated on the six instance sets presented in Table 1 and has obtained the following results. For j30_5, j30_10, j60_5 and j60_10, the algorithm H obtained an Av. Dev (%) equal to 0 % and an Opt. (%) equal to 100 %. For j120_5 and j120_10, the algorithm H obtained Av. Dev (%) values equal to 0.64 % and 0.8 %, respectively. Moreover, for j120_5 and j120_10, the algorithm obtained an Opt. (%) value equal to 100 %.

Comparing the results obtained by the algorithm H and the hybrid evolutionary algorithm presented here, we can mention the following points. Both algorithms have obtained an optimal effectiveness level for j30_5, j30_10, j60_5 and j60_10 (i.e., the less complex instance sets). However, the effectiveness level obtained by the hybrid evolutionary algorithm for j120_5 and j120_10 (i.e., the more complex instance sets) is significantly higher than that obtained by the algorithm H. Therefore, the hybrid evolutionary algorithm outperforms the algorithm H on the more complex instance sets. This is mainly because of the following reasons.

The hybrid evolutionary algorithm integrates self-adaptive crossover and mutation processes. These processes adapt their behaviour according to the state of the evolutionary search, in order to promote either the exploitation or exploration of the search space and thus enhance the evolutionary search. In contrast with the hybrid evolutionary algorithm, the algorithm H utilizes non-adaptive crossover and mutation processes. These processes do not consider the state of the evolutionary search and thus do not have the possibility of enhancing the evolutionary search.

5   Related Works

A wide variety of reported project scheduling problems consider the effectiveness of human resources. Nonetheless, these project scheduling problems differ significantly in the assumptions considered regarding the effectiveness of human resources. In this respect, only few of these project scheduling problems consider that human resources usually have very different levels of effectiveness [3–6, 10], a really essential aspect in the context of real project scheduling problems. In this section, we review the assumptions considered about the effectiveness of human resources in reported project scheduling problems.

In the multi-skill project scheduling problems reported in [12–17], each project activity requires a given number of skills and a given number of human resources for each required skill. Each available human resource masters one or several skills, and all the human resources that master a given skill have the same effectiveness level in relation to such skill.

In the multi-skill project scheduling problem reported in [3], hierarchical levels of skills are considered. Given a skill, for each human resource that masters the skill, an effectiveness level is defined in relation to the skill. Thus, the human resources that master a given skill have different levels of effectiveness in relation to the skill. Then, each project activity requires one or several skills, a minimum effectiveness level for each skill, and a number of human resources for each pair skill-level. This problem assumes that all sets of human resources that can be assigned to a given activity have the same effectiveness on the development of the activity. Specifically, with respect to effectiveness, such sets are merely treated as unary resources with homogeneous levels of effectiveness.

In the multi-skill project scheduling problems reported in [4, 5], most activities require only one human resource with a particular skill, and each available human resource masters different skills. The human resources that master a given skill have different levels of effectiveness with respect of such skill. Then, the effectiveness of a human resource in a given activity is defined by considering only the effectiveness level of the human resource in relation to the skill required for the activity.

In contrast to the problems above-mentioned, in the project scheduling problem reported in [6], it is supposed that the effectiveness level of a human resource depends on different factors inherent to its work context. Therefore, for each human resource, it is possible to define different effectiveness levels with respect to different work contexts. This assumption about the effectiveness levels of human resources is really valuable. This is mainly because, in the context of real project scheduling problems, human resources have different levels of effectiveness with regards to different work contexts, and therefore, the effectiveness level of a human resource is usually considered in relation to its work context [1, 2]. Based on the above-mentioned, the project scheduling problem reported in [6] supposes valuable assumptions about the effectiveness levels of human resources in the context of project scheduling problems.

6   Conclusions

In this paper, we addressed the project scheduling problem described in [6]. This problem considers really valuable assumptions about the effectiveness of human resources. Moreover, this problem considers an optimization objective priority for project managers: maximizing the effectiveness levels of the sets of human resources assigned to the project activities.

We presented a hybrid evolutionary algorithm with self-adaptive processes for solving the addressed problem. This algorithm integrates self-adaptive processes which adapt their behavior in accordance with the state of the evolutionary search. The integration of self-adaptive processes has the aim of enhancing the evolutionary search, in both exploration and exploitation.

We evaluated the performance of the hybrid evolutionary algorithm on different instance sets. Then, we compared the performance of the hybrid evolutionary algorithm with that of the best algorithm previously reported in the literature for solving the addressed problem. Based on the obtained results, we may state that the hybrid evolutionary algorithm considerably outperforms the previous algorithm.

In future works, we will evaluate the integration of other self-adaptive process into the framework of the evolutionary algorithm. In particular, we will evaluate other self-adaptive local search and optimization techniques, other self-adaptive crossover processes, as well as other self-adaptive mutation processes.

References

1. Heerkens, G.R.: Project Management. McGraw-Hill, New York (2002)
2. Wysocki, R.K.: Effective Project Management, 3rd edn. Wiley, Hoboken (2003)
3. Bellenguez, O., Néron, E.: Lower bounds for the multi-skill project scheduling problem with hierarchical levels of skills. In: Burke, E.K., Trick, M.A. (eds.) PATAT 2004. LNCS, vol. 3616, pp. 229–243. Springer, Heidelberg (2005)
4. Hanne, T., Nickel, S.: A multiobjective evolutionary algorithm for scheduling and inspection planning in software development projects. Eur. J. Oper. Res. **167**, 663–678 (2005)
5. Gutjahr, W.J., Katzensteiner, S., Reiter, P., Stummer, Ch., Denk, M.: Competence-driven project portfolio selection, scheduling and staff assignment. Central Eur. J. Oper. Res. **16**(3), 281–306 (2008)
6. Yannibelli, V., Amandi, A.: A knowledge-based evolutionary assistant to software development project scheduling. Expert Syst. Appl. **38**(7), 8403–8413 (2011)
7. Yannibelli, V., Amandi, A.: A memetic approach to project scheduling that maximizes the effectiveness of the human resources assigned to project activities. In: Corchado, E., Snášel, V., Abraham, A., Woźniak, M., Graña, M., Cho, S.-B. (eds.) HAIS 2012, Part I. LNCS, vol. 7208, pp. 159–173. Springer, Heidelberg (2012)
8. Yannibelli, V., Amandi, A.: A diversity-adaptive hybrid evolutionary algorithm to solve a project scheduling problem. In: Corchado, E., Lozano, J.A., Quintián, H., Yin, H. (eds.) IDEAL 2014. LNCS, vol. 8669, pp. 412–423. Springer, Heidelberg (2014)
9. Blazewicz, J., Lenstra, J., Rinnooy Kan, A.: Scheduling subject to resource constraints: classification and complexity. Discrete Appl. Math. **5**, 11–24 (1983)
10. Yannibelli, V., Amandi, A.: Project scheduling: a multi-objective evolutionary algorithm that optimizes the effectiveness of human resources and the project makespan. Eng. Optim. **45**(1), 45–65 (2013)
11. Srinivas, M., Patnaik, L.M.: Adaptive probabilities of crossover and mutation in genetic algorithms. IEEE Trans. Syst. Man Cybern. **24**(4), 656–667 (1994)
12. Bellenguez, O., Néron, E.: A branch-and-bound method for solving multi-skill project scheduling problem. RAIRO – Oper. Res. **41**(2), 155–170 (2007)
13. Drezet, L.E., Billaut, J.C.: A project scheduling problem with labour constraints and time-dependent activities requirements. Int. J. Prod. Econ. **112**, 217–225 (2008)
14. Li, H., Womer, K.: Scheduling projects with multi-skilled personnel by a hybrid MILP/CP benders decomposition algorithm. J. Sched. **12**, 281–298 (2009)
15. Valls, V., Pérez, A., Quintanilla, S.: Skilled workforce scheduling in service centers. Eur. J. Oper. Res. **193**(3), 791–804 (2009)
16. Aickelin, U., Burke, E., Li, J.: An evolutionary squeaky wheel optimization approach to personnel scheduling. IEEE Trans. Evol. Comput. **13**(2), 433–443 (2009)
17. Heimerl, C., Kolisch, R.: Scheduling and staffing multiple projects with a multi-skilled workforce. OR Spectrum **32**(4), 343–368 (2010)
18. Eiben, A.E., Smith, J.E.: Introduction to Evolutionary Computing, 2nd edn. Springer, Berlin (2015)
19. Rodriguez, F.J., García-Martínez, C., Lozano, M.: Hybrid metaheuristics based on evolutionary algorithms and simulated annealing: taxonomy, comparison, and synergy test. IEEE Trans. Evol. Comput. **16**(6), 787–800 (2012)
20. Talbi, E.: Hybrid metaheuristics. SCI, vol. 434. Springer, Berlin (2013)
21. Kolisch, R., Hartmann, S.: Experimental investigation of heuristics for resource-constrained project scheduling: an update. Eur. J. Oper. Res. **174**, 23–37 (2006)

E-HIPS: An Extention of the Framework HIPS for Stagger of Distributed Process in Production Systems Based on Multiagent Systems and Memetic Algorithms

Arnoldo Uber Junior[✉], Paulo José de Freitas Filho,
and Ricardo Azambuja Silveira

Postgraduate Program in Computer Science – PPGCC,
Federal University of Santa Catarina – UFSC, Florianópolis, Brazil
arnoldo.u.jr@gmail.com,
{freitas.filho,ricardo.silveira}@ufsc.br

Abstract. This work proposes a new framework for implementing control systems for distributed scheduling. The framework E-HIPS (Extended Hybrid Intelligent Process Scheduler) aims to scale processes in production systems as an extension to the framework HIPS, proposed by the authors in previous work. The original proposal presented a methodology and a set of tools that use the theory of agents and the heuristic search technique Genetic Algorithms (GA) for the implementation of computer systems that have the purpose of managing the scheduling of production processes in the industry. This article proposes an extension to the framework HIPS, by substitution of GA on Memetic Algorithms (MA). The article is an analysis of the problem, under the computational viewpoint, a retrospective of the original proposal, and a new description of the framework with these changes. Aiming to evaluate the framework and its extension, an implementation was made of a control application for scheduling flow to a section of a yarn dyeing industry raw materials for clothing. And a comparison of the results with actual production data obtained from the ERP industry where the system was applied.

Keywords: Multiagent systems (MAS) · Stagger of process · Job shop schedule problem (JSSP) · Genetic algorithms · Memetic algorithms

1 Introduction

The demand for real-time information becomes reality every moment and production systems require a continuous flow of information agile. This way can improve the manufacturing processes, to meet the wide variety of settings that make up their products, which flexibly, reduces costs, improves quality and delivering on time, and the amount requested.

The study of techniques for process scheduling refers to the creation of the first operating systems (OS) with the algorithms without preemption process schedulers (FCFS - first come first run, SJF - first with less time), And algorithms with preemption

© Springer International Publishing Switzerland 2015
G. Sidorov and S.N. Galicia-Haro (Eds.): MICAI 2015, Part I, LNAI 9413, pp. 413–430, 2015.
DOI: 10.1007/978-3-319-27060-9_34

(Round-Robin, Priority, SRTF - first the process missing less time, multilevel queues). The use of schedulers also reaches other areas besides OS, and involves problems in that there are a set of tasks to be performed and performing a number of units, and end the execution time of the tasks is directly affected by execution sequence adopted.

Scheduling is the allocation of resources over time to perform a set of tasks. Schedulers are devices that assign tasks to their respective resources, determining the chronological sequence and satisfying the rules for assignment [9, 22, 32].

These types of problems are found in areas such as sequencing projects, Job Shop Scheduling Problem (JSSP), production planning and others. Because it is a problem that tends to be NP - Full and enable broad application, the problem of process scheduling in production systems has been studied in this work, resulting in the framework proposed in this paper.

The tools that allow the use of these techniques, independently or together, forming new hybrid technologies allow satisfactory solution of complex problems from other perspectives, making what was once unthinkable in real solutions [9, 11, 14].

The framework HIPS (Hybrid Intelligent Process Scheduler) are presented by [28, 29], to perform distributed scheduling processes, applied to industrial production systems, based on the theory of agents and the heuristic search technique Genetic Algorithms. This paper presents an extension of the framework HIPS, which proposes the use of Memetic Algorithms.

This new proposal is presented using another class of local search algorithm called evolutionary Memetic Algorithms which is partly based on genetic algorithm but also takes into account both the biological evolution, cultural evolution, in other words, each individual help in the search process without a generation elapses.

The paper is organized into sections. In the next section an analysis is made of the problem of process scheduling scenario in industrial production and its complexity, from the point of view of computational treatment. In the following section, a brief review is made of the theoretical framework used in the development of the proposal, involving Multiagent Systems, genetic algorithms and Memetic Algorithms. The following is the Framework HIPS in its original proposal and its proposed new extension. Finally, it is shown an implementation of the framework in an actual production environment, the results obtained in a comparative assessment and final conclusions.

2 Problem

The planning of a production system is commonly done in three levels: the long, medium and short term [27]. Long-term planning seeks to mount a Production Plan or Strategic Planning Production that meets the needs determined by the sales forecast long-term, and also the production capacity needed to meet it. This level of long-term planning is called strategic because it is directly related to and will be directly affected because of the strategy that the company will adopt the use of its financial resources and infrastructure. The medium-term takes into account the production plan and therefore already have definitions of needs, thus creating the Master Production Plan (MPP). The MPP aims to operationalize the production, using the best tactic for the production system, planning efficiently the capacity utilization (plant), which seeks to meet the needs of the production plan. This level is called tactical planning, considering different ways of using the production system to accomplish their goals. In the short term, the production system will run through the Production Scheduling, which the production plan defined and operationalized through the PMP the best tactic. Thus, the production schedule is the operational level [27].

The Production Scheduling taken by PPC (Planning and Production Control) defines short-term and based on the MPP, as and when making raw material, and all other items necessary for the production of the final product.

At this level of planning are defined production orders and also staggering, with the goal of maximizing the use of productive resources. In the short term it is also made for monitoring and control of production, through the analysis of data obtained at checkpoints in production is possible to determine whether the production schedule is correct and according to plan. Having problems in the production system, the PCP can define corrective measures in order to meet planned. One of these measures is to make the operation of production scheduling. Therefore, the production scheduling is to make the production schedule, adding new orders to the production system, and also, by decision of the PPC to identify a problem caused by a given event in production.

In summary, the activity scale production in the textile sector is held by the Planning, Programming and Production Control (PPPC). To achieve this, analyzes strategic, tactical and operational in the company, seeking to define the strategic planning and master production. After these settings, the activity of production scheduling is performed, thus generating production orders to be staggered [22, 27].

This research focuses on the production scheduling activity, so the steps mentioned earlier production scheduling, and later, part of the activities performed by the ERP system will not be described in detail, with specific literature on the subject [22, 27, 31].

Most production scheduling problems studied applies context known as Job Shop Schedule Problem (JSSP). The traditional JSSP is characterized by enabling different flows of orders between the machines and different numbers of order operations, which are processed only once on each machine or device [22]. JSSP problems consist of a finite set of processes P_i, i = 1, 2, ... m, to be processed in a finite set of machines M_x, x = 1, 2, ... n. Each of the processes is processed on a machine, obeying the rules of precedence and capacity, generating a sequence of operations on each machine. The objective of the problem is to reduce the total process time, optimizing the deadlines, delays [10].

A typical type JSSP is one in which the materials moving on the production line of a factory with routes depending on the type of work to be performed. Already, on the other hand, a flow shop type environment characterized by the fact that the materials and parts to move routes set at the factory. The actual production situations fall between these two types, or as a combination of both [22, 32].

The problem JSSP is a combinatorial problem, which become NP – complete in certain situations (implicit or explicit enumeration of all possible alternatives to ensure the optimal solution). Thus, algorithms are computationally feasible when applied to real problems small, with limited objectives. For problems of similar size to those found in the real environment, it is customary to sacrifice to obtain an optimal solution by heuristic methods, which result in a suboptimal solution with reasonable computational time [10, 22]. The solution proposed in this paper considers a problem of composite features job shop and flow shop which will be quoted in this just like JSSP.

Scheduling problems have been extensively studied in the last decades. Many researches have been done in different areas to modeling and algorithms for JSSP Problem. The reason for this popularity comes from the fact that the problem of organizing the execution of a set of tasks by a group of finite resources is present in almost any kind of productive activity and can be easily described, but their mathematical complexity is extremely challenging. It is known that the problem JSS is a combinatorial problem becomes NP-Hard in certain situations, especially when there are explicit or implicit enumeration of all possible alternatives to ensure the optimal solution [9, 20, 22].

The optimization approaches, which are included in dynamic programming and branch-and-bound, performing a partial enumeration of the possible solutions, but the number of possibilities grows exponentially as the problem variables increase [14, 23]. Thus, only optimization algorithms are computationally feasible when applied to real problems, with limited objectives [32]. For problems of similar size to those found in real production environment, customarily sacrifice to obtain the optimal solution by heuristic methods, which result in a satisfactory solution with acceptable computational time, for example: sequence rules, branch-and-bound, Lagrangian relaxation, bottleneck [30], dynamic programming and decision trees [17], neural networks [23] and others local search and meta-heuristics.

The meta-heuristics for the JSS problem, are usually applied individually, such as Tabu Search [19], GA [12, 20, 25], Ant Colony [7], Simulated Annealing and local searches [33]. But there are cases where the combination of various techniques can generate better results [3], according to studies by [19, 20, 28].

2.1 Scenario Production

A hypothetical scenario was developed for the production representation of the problem and follows the model shown in Fig. 1 below. The model shown in Fig. 1 represents the dyeing yarn [1] having a production stream consisting of seven distinct phases (numbered 2 through 8 in the model) where transformation process material in all of them, but not necessarily in sequence. The model also gives the Planning, Programming and Production Control (PPPC) with the number one and ending inventory of product, with the number nine, which depending on the sector to be scaled, it may be the stock of finished product or a stock broker another sector, starting a new model [28].

Enterprise Resource Planning are software systems that integrate applications in finance, production, logistics, sales, marketing, human resources and other areas of a company. This integration is performed through a database shared by all applications [31].

Each production phase has a different set of processes having specific features for performing each step in the production of the product. A stock broker may possibly occur in the process, because of the production resources available do not meet the demand or upon the occurrence of problems during process execution. Once the

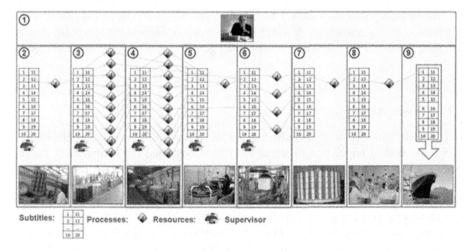

Fig. 1. Production scenario [28]

process performed in each production resource, the product resulting intermediate feed stock another intermediate that will supply the productive resources of the next stage, which may or may not be further presented.

Depending on the size of this intermediate stock, the number of alternatives to select the next process to run and also the sequence that will be executed, control flow optimally can become an operation that requires considerable time supervising the production. This is multiplied a considerable number of times, if we consider that the local choice in a certain stage, cause a change in sequencing all subsequent stages, may cause advance or late deliveries of products at the end of the stream.

Sequencing of a phase or particular resource by imposing other commonly generates a loss of local efficiency, making the objectives are achieved at the expense of overall system efficiency.

Characterized so therefore the need for a tool that enables communication between the phases of production, seeking to strike a balance between local efficiency of each phase and the overall efficiency of the sector, through communication, cooperation and self-organization of resources. This is the problem that it intends to address through modeling and development of a system, called TNT (TiNTuraria, portuguese translation of dyeing) framework implemented using the E-HIPS presented in the remaining sections.

3   Theoretical Reference

The development of the framework HIPS based on the Theory of Multi-Agent Systems [5, 6, 24] and heuristic search technique Genetic Algorithms. The extension proposed in this paper seeks to improve the results obtained by extending this framework, using for this the Memetic Algorithms. The following is a brief summary of the theoretical framework used in this work, in order to contextualize the reader to the presentation of the proposed model.

The chosen platform is known for JADE (Java Agent Development Framework) [2], which is a framework for developing agent-based applications in accordance with the specifications FIPA (Foundation for Intelligent Physical Agents) for multi-agent systems [13].

3.1 Genetic Algorithms and Memetic

GA not deterministic and probabilistic technique to search for the solution of complex problems. With a population of initial problem solvers and the definition of certain parameters can be found several different solutions each execution cycle. The algorithm works by keeping a population of these structures, called individuals or chromosomes that behave similar to the model of evolution in nature [15, 23]. The so called genetic operators are applied to these structures, where each cycle, each individual receives an evaluation, or passes through the objective function, which classifies the quality and resolution of the problem. Analogous to the natural process, genetic operators are applied to simulate the survival of the fittest individual.

The MA is a new class of evolutionary algorithm, partly based on GA. However, while the GA was inspired to try to mimic the biological evolution, the MA tries to imitate the cultural evolution [18, 26]. In MA each individual can come to make a significant contribution to the search process, but while in the GA genes are passed down through generations, memes (unit of cultural information) can be transmitted from one individual to another without a generation elapse. This mechanism allows you to have a higher evolution than only using crossover and mutation.

Figure 2 is a flowchart comparing MA and GA. Notice the similarity between the two flows, however, it is important to check for new processes of local search in the flow of MA, held shortly after the startup of the population, then the mutation. The processes of local search performed by MA are performed independently for each individual.

It should be clear that both GA and MA did not seek the optimal solution to the problem, but a satisfactory solution in accordance with a function or processing time established. During processing will be found local maxima and minima, coming or not the global maximum.

Using memetic algorithms to solve complex problems, the computational point of view, is widely explored in the literature. Some research in the area were made using MA applying the JSSP problem, such as [34] proposed a clonal selection extending memetic algorithms; reference [16] uses MA to improve the utilization of a Flow Shop problem; reference [4] proposed an improvement in the activity of selection of parents to produce a new generation. Thus, it is natural to extend the framework with the use of HIPS MA, in view of the significant gains identified in the research cited.

GA and MA are not deterministic and probabilistic techniques, namely with the same initial population and parameters, different solutions can be found for each application. It should be clear that the use of GA and MA seek an optimal solution to the problem, and this is a satisfactory solution according to a function or set processing time. During processing will be found local maxima and minima, coming or not the

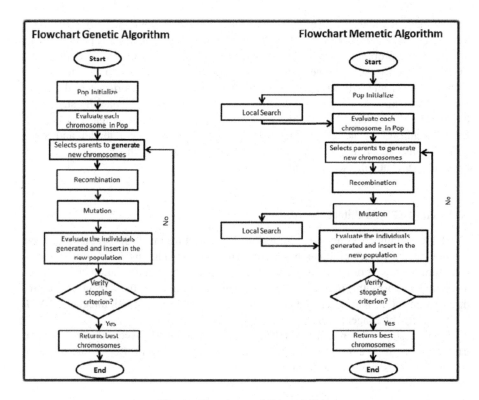

Fig. 2. Flowcharts of GA and MA

global maximum, but the method itself does not guarantee obtaining the optimal solution. However, for complex problems that require real-time solution or rapid responses such as JSSP of these solutions appear quite adequate.

The combined use of two techniques: Multiagent Systems and Genetic Algorithms (or memetic) has the advantage of using manipulation capabilities knowledge bases, autonomous, distributed and cooperative resolution of problems, typical of multi-agent systems, with the non-determinism of these algorithms.

4 Framework Hips and Extension

The framework HIPS proposed by [28] and presented in [29], allows modeling of process scheduling problems in production scenarios that meet the specifications of the type of problems JSSP and also execute and monitor the system through a multi-agent environment associated with the application developed from it.

The HIPS framework has three stages: modeling, development and execution. The modeling stage is done in HIPS Architect tool, which identifies the operations, resources, methods and rules for scheduling optimization. The second stage, the development of agents use a structure of agents provided by the framework HIPS. This basic structure, called JHIPS, assists in the implementation of agents and business rules specific to the problem. It also able to use the model developed in HIPS Architect and the base frame for the implementation of multi-agent system. This step also defines the roles of agents and scheduling. One of the roles of greater importance is the agent phase, which aims to define the operations to be scheduled and make the staggering through metaheuristic GA. The third step, which is the execution is made in the tool HIPS Architect. Agents are implemented as multi-agent system model and starts executing its life cycle. Thus, the interaction of agents with each other and the environment, generates the schedule of production.

4.1   The HIPS Architect

The HIPS Architect is the tool responsible for modeling the JSSP problem, and the creation of the model production scenario you want to administer. It allows you to configure the layout of production and define the parameters optimization and its form. Thus, it composes the multiagent environment necessary for the execution of production control. In Hips Architect can then run the scenario designed, integrated JADE platform, in which agents run.

Figure 3 shows the interface of HIPS Architect, configuring Agent Phase. No detail can be observed parameters [28] for the MA used by this agent. Recall that for comparison are the same ones used by GA originally.

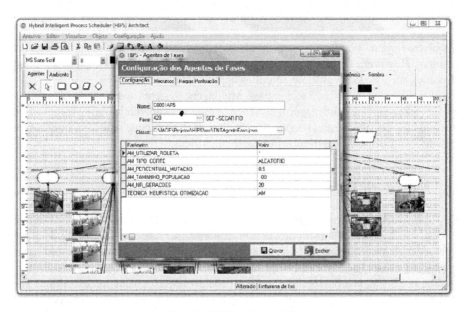

Fig. 3. HIPS architect [28]

4.2   JHIPS Package

The package implements JHIPS the basic classes needed to represent the production scenario modeled on Hips Architect, structuring and loading the settings configured in the model.

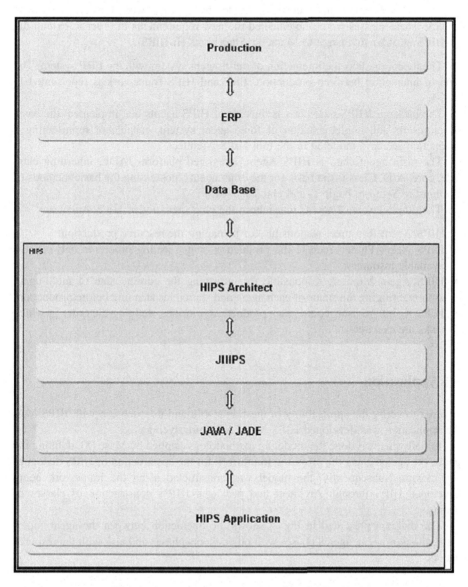

Fig. 4. Interaction Production × ERP × HIPS [28]

Packages JHIPS are Java classes implemented from the JADE framework and are divided into three groups:

- JHIPS Ontology: are the classes that make up the ontology of multi-agent system;
- JHIPS Base: agents are based HIPS, and have the basic structures for the implementation of multi-agent system to represent a production scenario modeled in HIPS Architect;
- JHIPS Tools: are ancillary classes provided by the framework for data access and GA. These classes were implemented the new requirements in order to extend the HIPS in order to change to Memetic Algorithms (E-HIPS).

The model predicts the interaction of multi-agent system with the ERP system. The type of interaction between production, ERP and HIPS framework is represented in Fig. 4.

The package JHIPS base class is thus set of HIPS agents that implement the basic structures for the implementation of multi-agent system, capable of representing a production scenario modeled in the tool HIPS Architect.

The main agent class is HIPS Agent, integrated platform JADE, inheriting class jade. core. AID. Class is the basis for the other agents, possessing the basic methods of configuring Setup to begin () and end Takedown ().

The other classes of agents that inherit the characteristics of HIPS Agent are:

- HIPS Agent Resource: responsible for managing the resource production;
- HIPS Agent Phase: manage the production stage, scaling processes between the available resources;
- HIPS Agent Monitor: responsible for informing the current state of multi-agent system, bringing the status of each agent and started his standing before production;
- HIPS Agent Advisor: coordinates production priorities, defining the order in which tasks are executed.

5   Application

In order to verify the applicability of the framework and its extension with HIPS MA, the application was developed HIPS MA TNT (yarn dyeing).

Initially this was done the modeling methodology applied by Mase [8], defining the goals, the agents using the proposed framework for the construction of HIPS dialogues and classes. Subsequently, the model was constructed using the framework being developed HIPS through Architect and packages JHIPS construction of classes of agents.

The diagram presented in Fig. 5 shows the interaction between the agent supervisor, monitor agent, agents phases with other agents phases and also with the resource agents.

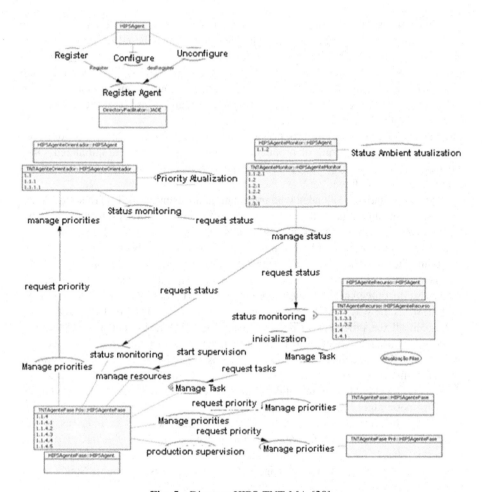

Fig. 5. Diagram HIPS TNT MA [28]

5.1 Life Cycle

The life cycle defined for the application HIPS MA TNT starts with the instantiation Advisor Agents (TNTAdvisorAgents) and Monitor Agents (TNTMonitorAgents). Subsequently, are started Phase Agents (TNT Phase Agents) for each of the phases making up the stage of production and, finally, the instantiation Resource Agents (TNTResourceAgent).

The TNTAdvisorAgents initialize seeking production priorities, which were defined as priorities Agent Advisor and also the policies for the delivery dates of the requests for production, in order to determine the priority of applications. The update of the priorities of production is done at intervals of a minute, through its own behavior Agent Advisor. The TNTAdvisorAgent also has two other behaviors, which are: to inform your agent status and return TNTMonitorAgent production priorities Phase Agents TNTPhaseAgent.

The agent responsible for informing the user what the status of each agent in the production scenario is TNTMonitorAgent. Their behavior is based on monitoring the production scenario, searching for new registered agents in JADE platform, through constant consultation with the directory service platform (DF). Also monitor agent assignment, ask the agents phases, information about resources and guidance, as well as the current status of each, presenting the user through an interface, the information for each registered agent in platform.

Agents Phase oversee the production phase defined for them in HIPS Architect. Come to exercise monitoring of production resources when they are initialized. Once you receive the request for early TNTResourcesAgent agents, they start to get the processes to be scheduled.

After being started and loaded with information, the agents seek TNTResourceAgent their respective Agent Phase, through the settings in HIPS Architect, informing him that the resource production that are managing and what is the number of processes in its queue fixed. Once initialized before his Agent Phase, agents TNTResourceAgent now have to monitor the behavior of their respective resource production through integration with the database of the ERP system. By realizing the expiration of any of the processes, agents TNTResourceAgent ask the agent Phase the next order to be added to your queue fixed, it works the way first-in, first-out, in other words, First In, First Out (FIFO).

Loaded all the processes to be scheduled, the TNTPhaseAgent performs scaling procedure. The agent checks the parameters determined for the production scenario through the HIPS Architect, which in turn are used by the optimization algorithm to determine the most appropriate scaling. It was originally used in the application HIPS TNT, Genetic Algorithm, but the extended version, this agent was changed to the use of memetic algorithm (MA).

The optimization is performed by the MA TNTPhaseAgent at intervals of one minute. Each execution of the optimization procedure updates the list of pending production, checks for new features, check the fixed list of each feature, query priorities Agent Advisor and Agents Phase neighbors, in other words, all agents Stage, which orders to be scheduled later processes have to be scheduled.

These same criteria were used in the first version of the system that used the GA and are used also for the new version that uses MA. Through this consultation, it is possible, at each new moment, determine production priorities of the sector and also of each production phase later, seeking to optimize the schedule periodically. To calculate the score sequencing, i.e. the fitness AM is also considered weights defined in HIPS Architect when configuring agent phase to each scoring rules.

The agents also have the type TNTPhaseAgent behaviors return the status to TNTMonitorAgent, returning production orders sequenced agent TNTResourceAgent and return to the other agents Stage your priority production also calculated through the discretion of the delivery date.

Running this production scenario, by applying HIPS MA TNT can be visualized in Fig. 6, which were also used, some features of the JADE platform for viewing the agents and servants of the dialogue being exchanged at that moment.

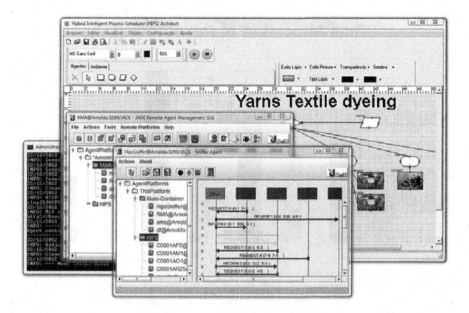

Fig. 6. HIPS TNT MA executing

6   Results Obtained

To carry out a comparative study with the objective of evaluating the results obtained from the implemented system, we used information from the real production sector yarn dyeing, which contains all the productive resources of this sector and pending orders production, from the system ERP and treated with HIPS MA TNT (implementing the process of optimizing the production flow that sector). The results obtained were compared with the results obtained in [28].

The analysis performed in this study is to examine the current situation of the process scheduling in a production stage, the object of the study, carried out by specialists in charge of the management of the production process, termed ordinary scaling, and compare them with the situation obtained, on the same production phase, with resources being staggered by applying HIPS MA TNT over a period of time.

The phase chosen for this study was the fifth stage of the production scenario shown in Fig. 1, in other words, the phase of the drying wire after the dyeing operation. In real production scenario, this phase has six productive resources, but the application was modeled with four features just because two were under maintenance. The period chosen for analysis was a week, or seven days after a Monday.

The execution starts with seventy-four production orders waiting to be scheduled at this stage. Among its features, however, three orders in each feature obey a scaling existing, according to the parameters defined in HIPS Architect. Only at the end of the day, agents TNTResourceAgent requested new orders to the agents TNTPhaseAgent.

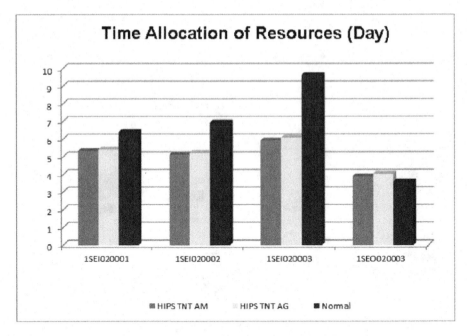

Fig. 7. Charts of time allocation of resources

A comparative analysis was made between the three schedules made as to the time allocation of each resource in order to indicate which allocated in the best way, the production resources available.

Determining the distribution of resources to the production processes, scaling HIPS MA TNT got a better use of time, avoiding stops for process equipment configuration. This difference in scaling relation to normal and scaling generated by the application HIPS TNT GA can be seen in Fig. 7, which shows the comparative graph. In red are shown the results obtained regarding time allocation (amount of time used in relation to the time available) by scaling normal obtained from the data recorded in the ERP system that controls the production line used in the research sector. In yellow shows the results obtained by the system originally developed from the first version of the implemented system using the model based on Genetic Algorithms. In green shows the results obtained by the new system developed from the version of the system implemented using the model E-HIPS, based on memetic algorithms. Each data set refers to a resource on the production line.

As can be seen in three of the four available resources, scheduling HIPS TNT GA took less time where the resource allocated more time compared to scaling usually done, this is justified by better distribution processes. The application HIPS MA TNT could better results than those obtained by experts and, in addition, in all cases exceeded, the results obtained by the application based on GA.

Another analysis takes into account the total time used by schedules, in other words, the sum of the times of all the resources of these two scales. In the graph of Fig. 8, can be observed sums of the times of all the features of each and the staggering

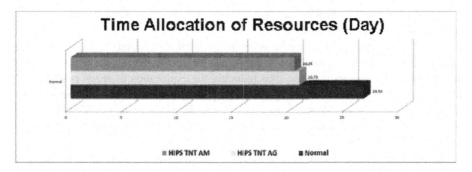

Fig. 8. Charts of time allocation of total resources

number of days spent by scheduling more regular. Each color of the displayed graph represents the results of each of the allocation modes as in the previous figure.

As can be observed in this comparison, the improvement obtained by use of MA becomes even more evident considering that the gain GA using shown above in staggered relation to normal but becomes even greater with the use of BF.

Directly comparing the scaling normal and HIPS TNT GA, we have HIPS TNT GA scaling a saving of time of 5.8 days, which represents a gain of 27.98 % compared to the usual scheduling. The gain between applications HIPS TNT GA and MA was 0.5 days, which represents 2.36 % compared to HIPS and 31 % TNT GA in relation to the standard scheduling.

Whereas, according to the data used in the experiment obtained from the ERP system, the seventy-four orders production were moving 12,943.97 kg of yarn, in practical terms, scaling using the TNT HIPS GA and MA could have been dried 3621.72, 4012.63 kg and more KG respectively, therein.

Through these comparisons, you can check the amount of time used by scheduling more regular and better distribution of cases between the resources available, carried out by applying HIPS TNT GA and MA, respectively. Thus, the possibility of staggering almost in real time, with heuristic optimization techniques and multi-agent system can provide high productivity gains in the production process.

It is worth noting, too, that scaling standard has remained unchanged since the beginning of the process, in other words, what is planned at the beginning of the period of analysis is considered valid until the end of the production cycle. Interventions undertaken by the supervision phase, or production management could assist in obtaining the best values of efficiency scaling normal but decision making should occur for this situation and actions should be performed in the ERP system. However this process is not online and the production scenario is constantly changing.

7 Conclusion

Using memetic algorithms for agents allowed phase gains in choosing a satisfactory place, avoiding the analysis of the entire set of possibilities to sequence the pending cases. Another important advantage of MA is the processing time, making it possible to return a sequencing satisfactory, not requiring a large amount of time as needed agents stage. Both inherited traits of GA.

Another situation was observed that due to the local search, and the processing time relation, the execution of local search can consume considerable time, lowering thus the generation of new individuals, thus reducing the exploration of space possibilities. In this regard, a simulation may be performed by increasing the number of generations GA and compared with the initial number of generations of the meme. Thus it can be checked whether convergence due to local search can be overcome by a higher repetition of the original algorithm GA.

In comparison, the use of MA obtained a significant result in relation to the GA, and [4, 16, 34]. The real gain from the use of MA depends largely on the processing time and the quality of local search heuristics employed, otherwise can aggravate the situation where the search is exploring a local maximum, depending on the genetic operators to evolve. In relation to those mentioned yet, the proposed solution is dynamic, i.e. intermittently generates solutions to the problem of scaling. Moreover, it allows if necessary, the distribution of processing by instantiating agents in multiple locations.

Improvements can still be made in the framework HIPS, such as the inclusion of techniques of negotiation between the agents and advisor for phase change priorities, using their own strategies for dealing or stemmed from game theory, such as games of incomplete information, such as auctions. Besides the change in the interaction of the agents can be added more search options, an option to GA and MA, such as those cited by [21]: Simulated Annealing, Ant Colony e Tabu Search. Having more search options, can be modeled behavior of agents in phase that allows the choice of method to be employed, including using more than one [11].

References

1. Araújo, M., De Melo E Castro, E.M.: Manual de Engenharia Têxtil, vol. 1. Fundação Calouste Gulbenkian, Lisboa (1986)
2. Bellifemine, F., Caire, G., Greewood, D.: Developing Multiagent Systems with JADE, 300 p. Wiley, New York (2007)
3. Bittencourt, G.: Inteligência artificial: ferramentas e teorias, 3edn, p. 371. Editora da UFSC, Florianópolis (2006)
4. Boudia, M., Prins, C.A.: Memetic algorithm with dynamic population management for an integrated production–distribution problem. Eur. J. Oper. Res. **195**, 703–715 (2009)
5. Brenner, W., Zarnekow, R., Wittig, H.: Intelligent Software Agents: Foundations and Applications. Springer, Berlin (1998)
6. Bradshaw, J.M. (ed.): Software Agents. MIT Press, Cambridge (1997)
7. Carvalho, E.M., Ramos, G.S.: Otimização por colônia de formigas. Departamento de Informática, Universidade Federal do Paraná, Curitiba (2007)
8. DeLoach, S.A., Wood, M.: Developing multiagent Systems with agentTool. In: Castelfranchi, C., Lespérance, Y. (eds.) ATAL 2000. LNCS (LNAI), vol. 1986, pp. 46–60. Springer, Heidelberg (2001)

9. Dissaux, P., Marc, O., Rubini, S., Fotsing, C., Gaudel, V., et al.: The SMART project: multi-agent scheduling simulation of real-time architectures. In: Embedded Real Time Software and Systems, Toulouse, France, February 2014

10. Geyik, F., Cedimoglu, I.H.: The strategies and parameters of tabu search for job-shop scheduling. J. Intell. Manuf. **15**, 439–448 (2004)

11. Gutièrrez, T.N., Ciarletta, L., Chevrier, V.: Multi-agent simulation based control of complex systems. In: AAMAS, pp. 1517–1518 (2014)

12. Gonçalves, J.F., Mendes, M.J.J., Resende, M.G.C.: A hybrid genetic algorithm for the job shop scheduling problem. Eur. J. Oper. Res. **167**, 77–95 (2005). ISSN 0377-2217

13. JADE: Java agent development framework. http://jade.tilab.com. Accessed June 2015

14. Hüning, C., Wilmans, J., et al.: MARS- a next-gen multi-agent simulation framework. http://mars-group.org/. Accessed June 2015

15. Linden, R.: Algoritmos Genéticos: uma importante ferramenta da Inteligência Computacional, 372 p. Brasport, Rio de Janeiro (2006)

16. Liu, B., Wang, L., Jin, Y.: An effective PSO-based memetic algorithm for flow shop scheduling. IEEE Trans. Syst. Man Cybern. B Cybern. **37**(1), 18–27 (2007)

17. Morton, T., Pentico, D.W.: Heuristic Scheduling Systems: With Applications to Production Systems and Project Management, p. 720. Wiley, EUA, New York (1993)

18. Moscato, J.P.: On evolution, search, optimization, GAs and martial arts: toward memetic algorithms. Ph.D. dissertation, California Institute of Technology, Pasadena, USA (1989)

19. Müller, G.I., Gomez, A.T.: Utilização da busca tabu para a geração de um modelo aplicado ao job-shop scheduling problem considerando um sistema de manufatura flexível, p. 10. Universidade do Vale do Rio dos Sinos, São Leopoldo (2006)

20. Oliveira, R.L., Walter, C.: Escalonamento de um job-shop: um algoritmo com regras heurísticas. UFRGS (2000)

21. Petrowski, A., Dréo, J., Taillard, E., Siarry, P.: Metaheuristics for Hard Optimization: Simulated Annealing, Tabu Search, Evolutionary and Genetic Algorithms, Ant Colonies,… - Methods and Case Studies. Springer, Berlin (2006)

22. Pinedo, M.L.: Planning and Scheduling in Manufacturing and Services. Springer, New York (2009)

23. Russell, S., Norvig, P.: Inteligência artificial: tradução, 2 edn, 1040 p. Editora Campus, Rio de Janeiro (2004)

24. Sacile, R., Paolucci, M.: Agent-Based Manufacturing and Control Systems. CRC Press LLC, Flórida (2005)

25. Soares, M.M., et al.: Otimização do planejamento mestre da produção através de algoritmos genéticos. In: XXII ENEPGEP - Encontro Nacional de Engenharia de Produção, Curitiba (2002)

26. Tavakkoli-Moghaddama, R., Safaei, N., Sassani, F.: A memetic algorithm for the flexible flow line scheduling problem with processor blocking. Comput. Oper. Res. **36**, 402–414 (2009)

27. Tubino, D.F.: Planejamento e controle da produção: teoria e prática, p. 196. Editora Ática, São Paulo (2007)

28. Junior, A.U., Silveira, R.A.: Using multiagent systems and genetic algorithms to deal with problems of staggering. In: Demazeau, Y., Pavón, J., Corchado, J.M., Bajo, Javier (eds.) 7th International Conference on Practical Applications of Agents and Multi-Agent Systems (PAAMS 2009). AISC, vol. 55, pp. 567–575. Springer, Heidelberg (2009)

29. Junior, A.U., Silveira, R.A.: HIPS: Um Framework para Escalonamento Distribuído de Processos em Sistemas de Produção Utilizando Sistemas Multiagente. Avances en sistemas e informatica **7**, 7–15 (2010)

30. Varela, M.L.R.: Uma contribuição para o escalonamento da produção baseado em métodos globalmente distribuídos, p. 224. Tese. Universidade do Minho, Braga. Programa de Pós-Graduação em Produção e Sistemas (2007)
31. Vollmann, T.E., et al.: Sistemas de planejamento & controle da produção para o gerenciamento da cadeia de suprimentos, 5 edn, p. 648. Bookman, Porto Alegre (2006)
32. Xhafa, F., Abraham, A.: Metaheuristics for scheduling in Industrial and Manufacturing Applications. Studies in Computational Intelligence, vol. 128. Springer, Heidelberg (2008)
33. Yamada, T., Nakano, R.: Job Shop Scheduling by Simulated Annealing Combined with Deterministic Local Search, pp. 237–248. Kluwer Academic Publishers, Boston (1996)
34. Yang, J.-H., Liang, S., Heow, P.L., Yun, Q., Liang, Y.: Clonal selection based memetic algorithm for job shop scheduling problems. J. Bionic Eng. 5, 111–119 (2008)

Fuzzy Logic

A New Bat Algorithm Augmentation Using Fuzzy Logic for Dynamical Parameter Adaptation

Jonathan Pérez[✉], Fevrier Valdez, and Oscar Castillo

Tijuana Institute of Technology, Tijuana, BC, Mexico
tecjonathan@gmail.com

Abstract. We describe in this paper a new approach to enhance the bat algorithm using a fuzzy system to dynamically adapt its parameters. The original method is compared with the proposed method and also compared with genetic algorithms, providing a more complete analysis of the effectiveness of the bat algorithm. Simulation results on a set of benchmark mathematical functions show that the fuzzy bat algorithm outperforms the traditional bat algorithm and genetic algorithms.

Keywords: Bat algorithm · Mathematical functions · Fuzzy system

1 Introduction

This paper focuses on the study of the Bat Algorithm, which has proven to be one of the best to face problems of nonlinear global optimization.

The bat algorithm is a metaheuristic optimization method proposed by Yang in 2010 and this algorithm is based on the behavior of micro bats echolocation pulses with different emissions and sound.

The bat algorithm has the characteristic of being one of the best methods to solve problems of nonlinear global optimization. In this paper, the use of the bat algorithm with a fuzzy system is presented in order to dynamically configure some parameters in the algorithm to obtain improvement in performance against other metaheuristic algorithms in optimization problems. To validate our proposed approach a set of mathematical functions was used.

From a Literature survey, we found the following Bat Algorithm variants: a fuzzy logic bat algorithm (FLBA) was presented in [2] as a variant by introducing fuzzy logic into Bat Algorithm, a Multi-objective bat algorithm (MOBA) was presented in [8] as an extended Bat Algorithm to deal with multi-objective optimization, which has demonstrated its effectiveness for solving a few design benchmarks in engineering, a K-means bat algorithm (KMBA) in [3] presented a combination of K-Means and bat algorithm for efficient clustering, Chaotic bat algorithm (CBA) [4] presented a chaotic bat algorithm using Levy flights and chaotic maps to carry out parameter estimation in dynamic biological systems.

This paper is organized as follows in Sect. 2 describes the original bat algorithm, Sect. 3 describes the benchmark mathematical functions, in Sect. 4 we describe the

© Springer International Publishing Switzerland 2015
G. Sidorov and S.N. Galicia-Haro (Eds.): MICAI 2015, Part I, LNAI 9413, pp. 433–442, 2015.
DOI: 10.1007/978-3-319-27060-9_35

results between genetic algorithm and bat algorithm, in Sect. 5 we describe a statistical test, in Sęct. 6 we describe the proposed method and results, and in Sect. 7 we describe the conclusions.

2 Bat Algorithm

This section describes the basic concepts of the Bat Algorithm. If we idealize some of the echolocation characteristics of microbats, we can develop various bat-inspired algorithms or bat algorithms. For simplicity, we now use the following approximate or idealized rules [7]:

1. All bats use echolocation to sense distance, and they also know the difference between food/prey and background barriers in some magical way.
2. Bats fly randomly with velocity v_i at position x_i which a fixed frequency f_{min}, varying wavelength λ and loudness A_0 to search for prey. They can automatically adjust the wavelength (or frequency) of their emitted pulses and adjust the rate of pulse emission r ϵ [0, 1], depending on the proximity of their target.
3. Although loudness can vary in many ways, we assume that the loudness varies from a large (positive) A_0 to a minimum constant value A_{min}.

For simplicity, the frequency $f \epsilon$ [0, f_{max}], the new solutions x_i^t and velocity v_i^t at a specific time step t are represented by a random vector drawn from a uniform distribution [1].

2.1 Pseudo Code for the Bat Algorithm

The basic steps of the bat algorithm, can be summarized as the pseudo code shown in Fig. 1.

Initialize the bat population $x_i(i=1, 2,..., n)$ and v_i
Initialize frequency f_i, pulse rates r_i and the loudness A_i
While *(t<Max numbers of iterations)*
   Generate new solutions by adjusting frequency
   and updating velocities and locations/solutions [equations (1) to (3)]
   if(rand>r_i)
      Select a solution among the best solutions
      Generate a local solution around the selected best solution
   end if
   Generate a new solutions by flying randomly
   if *(rand <A_i& $f(x_i) < f(x_*)$)*
      Accept the new solutions
      Increase r_i and reduce A_i
   end if
   Rank the bats and find the current best x_*
end while

Fig. 1. Pseudo code of the bat algorithm

2.2 Movements in the Bat Algorithm

Each bat is associated with a velocity v_i^t and location x_i^t, at iteration t, in a dimensional search or solution space. Among all the bats, there exist a current best solution x_*. Therefore, the above three rules can be translated into the updating equations for x_i^t and velocities v_i^t:

$$f_i = f_{min} + (f_{max} - f_{min})\beta, \tag{1}$$

$$v_i^t = v_i^{t-1} + (x_i^{t-1} - x_*)f_i, \tag{2}$$

$$x_i^t = x_i^{t-1} + v_i^t, \tag{3}$$

Where $\beta \in [0, 1]$ is a random vector selected from a uniform distribution [6].

As mentioned earlier, we can either use wavelengths or frequencies for implementation, and we will use $f_{min} = 0$ and $f_{max} = 1$, depending on the domain size of the problem of interest. Initially, each bat is randomly assigned a frequency which is drawn uniformly from $[f_{min} - f_{max}]$. The loudness and pulse emission rates essentially provide a mechanism for automatic control and auto zooming into the region with promising solutions [9].

2.3 Loudness and Pulse Rates

In order to provide an effective mechanism to control the exploration and exploitation and switch to the exploitation stage when necessary, we have to vary the loudness A_i and the rate r_i of pulse emission during the iterations. Since the loudness usually decreases once a bat has found its prey, while the rate of pulse emission increases, the loudness can be chosen as any value of convenience, between A_{min} and A_{max}, assuming $A_{min} = 0$ means that a bat has just found the prey and temporarily stop emitting any sound, where α and γ are constants. In essence, here α is similar to the cooling factor of a cooling schedule in simulated annealing. For any $0 < \alpha < 1$ and $\gamma > 0$, with these assumptions, we have [1]

$$A_i^{t+1} = \alpha A_i^t, \quad r_i^{t+1} = r_i^0[1 - \exp(-\gamma^t)], \tag{4}$$

3 Benchmark Mathematical Functions

This section lists a number of the benchmark mathematical functions used to evaluate the performance of the optimization algorithms. The mathematical functions are defined below:

- **Sphere**

$$f_1(x) = \sum_{j=1}^{n_x} x_j^2 \tag{8}$$

where $x_j \in [-100, 100]$ and $f^*(x) = 0.0$

- **Rosenbrock**

$$f_2(x) = \sum_{j=1}^{n_z/2} [100(x_{2j} - x_{2j-1}^2)^2 + (1 - x_{2j-1})^2]$$ (9)

where $x_j \in [-2.048, 2.048]$ and $f^*(x) = 0.0$

- **Rastrigin**

$$f_3(x) = \sum_{j=1}^{n_x} (x_j^2 - 10\cos(2\pi x_j) + 10)$$ (10)

where $x_j \in [-5.12, 5.12]$ and $f^*(x) = 0.0$

- **Ackley**

$$f_4(x) = -20e^{-0.2\sqrt{\frac{1}{n_x}\sum_{j=1}^{n_x} x_j^2 - \frac{1}{n_x}\sum_{j=1}^{n_x} \cos(2\pi x_j)}} + 20 + e$$ (11)

where $x_j \in [-30, 30]$ and $f^*(x) = 0.0$

- **Zakharov**

$$f_5(x) = \sum_{i=1}^{n} x_i^2 + (\sum_{i=1}^{n} 0.5ix_i)^2 + (\sum_{i=1}^{n} 0.5ix_i)^4$$ (12)

where $x_i \in [-5, 10]$ and $f^*(x) = 0.0$

The mathematical functions were integrated directly into the code of the bat algorithm and genetic algorithm.

4   Results Between GA and the Bat Algorithm

In this section the Bat algorithm is compared against the genetic algorithm. In each of the algorithms, 5 Benchmark math functions were used separately for a dimension of 10 variables, and 30 tests were made for each function with different parameters in the algorithms. The parameters in the Bat algorithm are as follows: Population size 2 to 40 Bats, Loudness 0.5 to 1, Pulse frequency 0.5 to 1, Frequency min 0 to 2, Frequency max.: 0 to 2. The parameters for the genetic algorithm are shown: Number of Individuals 4 to 40, StochasticSelection, Remainder, Uniform, Roulette, Scattered Crossover, Single Point, Two Point, Heuristic, Arithmetic, Mutation Gaussian, and Uniform.

Once the modification in the bat algorithm is performed, tests were made with benchmark mathematical functions to analyze its effectiveness. Also the original method is compared with the proposed method and with genetic algorithms, providing a more complete analysis of the effectiveness of bat algorithm. Simulation results with the fuzzy bat algorithm outperform the traditional bat algorithm and genetic algorithms.

The results of the tests are shown below in Table 1.

Table 1. The comparison between the bat algorithm and genetic algorithm

Population	Function	Bat algorithm	Genetic algorithm
		Mean	Mean
2/4	F1	0.366906	0.50145
	F2	0.200877	0.56189
	F3	0.610017	0.53238
	F4	0.006825	0.34634
	F5	0.404631	0.44289
5	F1	0.235177	0.29767
	F2	0.097149	0.47668
	F3	0.613184	0.48465
	F4	0.098505	0.55591
	F5	0.371813	0.36849
10	F1	0.000286	0.61649
	F2	1.133775	0.21288
	F3	0.530195	0.59146
	F4	0.396806	0.30968
	F5	0.000277	0.47577
20	F1	1.77E-05	0.25064
	F2	0.02374	0.15163
	F3	0.153645	0.41605
	F4	0.198577	0.21732
	F5	0.000221	0.44479
30	F1	0.00031	0.52185
	F2	0.628592	0.05068
	F3	0.576684	0.40294
	F4	0.991825	0.0131
	F5	1.73E-05	1.51853
40	F1	5.39E-05	0.55895
	F2	0.178972	0.24298
	F3	0.303122	0.30482
	F4	0.098321	0.22942
	F5	0.000116	1.30143

5   Statistical Test of the Bat Algorithm and Genetic Algorithm

The statistical test was performed as follows: the comparison is made between the bat algorithm and the genetic algorithm with the experiments corresponding to the results of tests performed for each algorithm. In this case each algorithm is applied separately to the benchmark mathematical functions. The experiments are with six functions for algorithms and 30 experiments were performed for each function for a total 180 experiments for method.

The statistical test used for the comparison is the z-test, whose parameters are set out in Table 2.

Table 2. Parameters for the statistical test

Parameter	Value
Level significance	95 %
Alfa	5 %
H_a	$\mu_1 < \mu_2$
H_0	$\mu_1 \geq \mu_2$
Critical value	1.96

The alternative hypothesis states that the average performance of the bat algorithm is lower than the average of the results of the genetic algorithm, and therefore the null hypothesis tells us that the average bat algorithm is greater than or equal to the average of the algorithm genetic, with a reject region for all values less than -1.96. The equation of the statistical test is the following:

$$Z = \frac{(\overline{X_1} - \overline{X_2}) - (\mu_1 - \mu_2)}{\sigma_{\overline{X_1} - \overline{X_2}}} \tag{14}$$

The data of the values of the mean, standard deviation are found in Table 3.

Table 3. Statistical data of the comparison of the algorithms

Algorithm	Number sample	Mean	Standard deviation	Level significance α
Genetic	30	0.446659	0.306969	0.05
Bat	30	0.274021	0.303970	

With a significance level of 95 % and a value of $Z = -2.1888$, we can affirm that the alternative hypothesis is accepted that the average mentioning of the bat algorithm is below the average of the genetic algorithm.

6   Proposed Method

The Bat Algorithm has the characteristic of being one of the best to face problems of nonlinear global optimization. In this paper the enhancement of the bat algorithm using a fuzzy system is presented with the objective of dynamically setting some of the parameters in the algorithm. The goal is improving the performance of the algorithm against other metaheuristics in optimization problems by testing through the use of benchmark mathematical functions. In the area of fuzzy logic for adapting parameters in metaheuristics we can find as similar work: Dynamic Fuzzy Logic Parameter Tuning for ACO and its Application in TSP Problems [5].

Usually in the bat algorithm, the modification of the parameters is done by trial and error, modifying the parameters, which are wavelength λ, loudness (volume) A_0, low frequency and high frequency. In the present work an implementation of a fuzzy system, which can be responsible for setting any of these parameters dynamically in order to improve the performance of the algorithm achieving greater effectiveness is presented. Once the modification in the bat algorithm is performed, tests were made with benchmark mathematical functions to analyze its effectiveness. At the end, the original method is compared with the proposed method and also compared with the genetic algorithm, providing a more complete analysis of the effectiveness of the bat algorithm. Simulation results with the fuzzy bat algorithm outperform the traditional bat algorithm and genetic algorithms. The general approach of the proposed bat algorithm method can be seen in Fig. 2.

The proposed fuzzy system is of Mamdani type because it is more common in this type of fuzzy control and the defuzzification method was the centroid. The membership functions are of triangular form in the inputs and Gaussian for the outputs. For the input1 variable (Iterations) the membership functions are of triangular form and shown in Fig. 3. The output1 variable (Loudness) the membership functions are of Gaussian form shown in Fig. 4. The output2 variable (Pulse) the membership functions are of Gaussian as shown in Fig. 5 and the Mamdani fuzzy system has 9 rules is a show in Fig. 6.

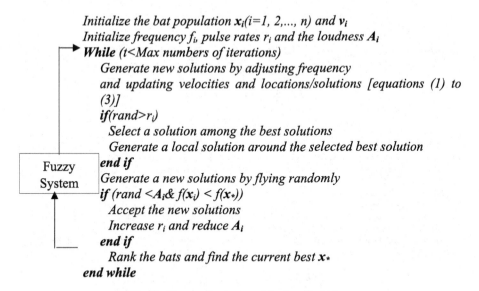

Fig. 2. Proposed scheme of the bat algorithm.

To test the proposed approach, we use the benchmark mathematical functions. In Table 4 we show for function 1 for the fuzzy bat algorithm the results of our proposed approach, where we obtain on average better results when compared with the original method.

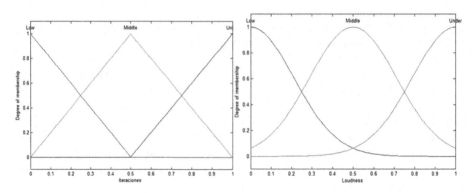

Fig. 3. Variable input 1   **Fig. 4.** Variable output 1

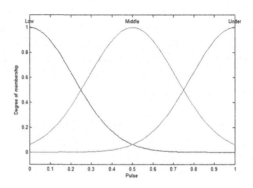

Fig. 5. Variable output 2

```
1. If (Iteraciones is Low) then (Loudness is Low)(Pulse is Low) (1)
2. If (Iteraciones is Low) then (Loudness is Middle)(Pulse is Middle) (1)
3. If (Iteraciones is Low) then (Loudness is Under)(Pulse is Under) (1)
4. If (Iteraciones is Middle) then (Loudness is Low)(Pulse is Low) (1)
5. If (Iteraciones is Middle) then (Loudness is Middle)(Pulse is Middle) (1)
6. If (Iteraciones is Middle) then (Loudness is Under)(Pulse is Under) (1)
7. If (Iteraciones is Under) then (Loudness is Low)(Pulse is Low) (1)
8. If (Iteraciones is Under) then (Loudness is Middle)(Pulse is Middle) (1)
9. If (Iteraciones is Under) then (Loudness is Under)(Pulse is Under) (1)
```

Fig. 6. Rules of the fuzzy system

In Table 5 we show the function 2 for the fuzzy bat algorithm, the results show that our proposed approach obtains on average better results when compared with the original method.

Table 4. Average results from the experiments with function 1

Numbers bats	Best	Worst	Mean
2	9.33E-06	0.372297	0.124107
5	2.36E-06	0.702742	0.197137
10	1.86E-06	0.000481	0.000250
20	1.51E-09	0.947046	0.450914
30	2.98E-09	1.024096	0.512048
40	3.00E-10	0.810889	0.445072

Table 5. Average results from the experiments with function 2

Numbers bats	Best	Worst	Mean
2	0.003374	1.596956	0.867861
5	0.025269	1.332906	0.491555
10	0.031700	2.449012	1.091745
20	0.102419	1.509615	0.949192
30	0.152072	1.897880	1.249411
40	0.000328	1.559541	0.883111

7 Conclusions

In this paper we have presented a fuzzy logic approach for parameter adaptation in the bat algorithm. In Sects. 4 and 6 of the paper the analysis of the comparative study of the Bat Algorithm and the proposed fuzzy modification of the Bat Algorithm, we find that there are promising results, but we plan to continue improving the algorithm. Based on these results we can say that using fuzzy logic for parameter adaptation is a good choice for metaheuristics, in particular for the bat algorithm. The application of the bat algorithm to various problems has been a very wide field, where the revised items its effectiveness is demonstrated in various applications, their use can be mentioned in the processing digital pictures, search for optimal values, neural networks, and many applications.

References

1. Goel, N., Gupta, D., Goel, S.: Performance of firefly and bat algorithm for unconstrained optimization problems. Department of Computer Science Maharaja Surajmal Institute of Technology GGSIP University C-4, Janakpuri, New Delhi, India (2013)
2. Khan, K., Sahai, A.: A Comparison of BA, GA, PSO, BP and LM for training feed forward neural networks in e-learning context. Department of A chaotic Levy flight bat algorithm for parameter estimation in nonlinear dynamic Computing and Information Technology, University of the West Indies, St. Augustine, Trinidad And Tobago (2012)
3. Komarasamy, G., Wahi, A.: An optimized K-means clustering technique using bat algorithm. Int. J. Interact. Multimedia. Art Intell. **1**(7), 26–32 (2012)

4. Lin, J.H., Chou, C.W., Yang, X., Tasi, H.L.: A chaotic levy flight bat algorithm for parameter estimation in nonlinear dynamic biological systems. J. Comput. Inf. Technol. **2**(2), 56–63 (2015)
5. Neyoy, H., Castillo, O., Soria, J.: Dynamic fuzzy logic parameter tuning for ACO and its application in TSP problems. In: Castillo, O., Melin, P., Kacprzyk, J. (eds.) Recent Advances on Hybrid Intelligent Systems. SCI, vol. 451, pp. 259–272. Springer, Heidelberg (2013)
6. Rodrigues, D., Pereira, L., Nakamura, R., Costa, K., Yang, X., Souza, A., Papa, J.P.: A wrapper approach for feature selection based on bat algorithm and optimum-path forest. Department of Computing, Universidade Estadual Paulista, Bauru, Brazil (2013)
7. Yang, X.: A new metaheuristic bat-inspired algorithm. Department of Engineering, University of Cambridge, Trumpington Street, Cambridge CB2 1PZ, UK (2010)
8. Yang, X.: Bat algorithm for multi-objective optimization. Int. J. Bio-Inspired Comput. **3**(5), 267–274 (2011)
9. Yang, X.: Bat algorithm: literature review and applications. School of Science and Technology, Middlesex University, The Burroughs, London NW4 4BT, United Kingdom (2013)

An Embedded Fuzzy Self-tuning PID Controller for a Temperature Control System of Peltier Cells

Aldebaran A. Alonso-Carreón, Miguel Platas, and Luis Torres-Treviño[✉]

DIE FIME, Universidad Autónoma de Nuevo León,
San Nicolás de los Garza, Mexico
luis.torres.ciidit@gmail.com

Abstract. The aim of the present work is to describe the performance of a fuzzy agent that is implemented in an embedded system to make an on-line tuning of a embedded PID controller. The fuzzy agent inputs are steady-state error, overshooting and settling time, with this input the fuzzy agent is able to automatically adjust the PID parameter in order to have a better performance. The Peltier cells are used to control the temperature of a small chamber.

Keywords: On-line tuning · Fuzzy agent · Self-tuning PID controller

1 Introduction

1.1 Fuzzy Logic Systems

Fuzzy logic has recently emerged as an important tool for controlling complex systems and industrial processes. this is because fuzzy logic allows us to find intermediate values in order to rate conventional statements as true or false, so we can design applications for machines to respond with more intelligence to the imprecision and conditions of the outside world, thereby imitate human behavior. Creating a machine with fuzzy logic is the same as creating an expert system, where the behavior of the machine will be solely based on expert knowledge or the person who provides their empirical knowledge to operate it. Expert knowledge is empirical knowledge of how to control the phenomenon, without knowing any model of the system to be controlled.

1.2 PID Control Systems

Based on Classic Control Theory, the PID controller is a closed-loop feedback controller that calculates an error value as the sum of the difference between a measured process variable and a desired setpoint, the history of that difference and how that difference has change through time. The objective of this controller is to minimize error. This definition for PID in the continuous domains is described as:

$$u(t) = K_p e(t) + K_i \int_0^t e(\tau)\, d\tau + K_d \frac{d}{dt} e(t) \tag{1}$$

G. Sidorov and S.N. Galicia-Haro (Eds.): MICAI 2015, Part I, LNAI 9413, pp. 443–451, 2015.
DOI: 10.1007/978-3-319-27060-9_36

In the PID formula the K_p is the proportional gain, the K_i is the integral gain and the K_d is the derivative gain, the controller operates on the measured reference error $e(t)$. By tuning the three parameters (K_p K_i K_d) in the PID controller algorithm, the controller can provide control action designed for specific process requirements. The response of the controller can be described in terms of the responsiveness of the controller to an error, the degree to which the controller overshoots the setpoint, and the degree of system oscillation. Nowadays, there is an existing problem generalized with the tuning of PID control systems, which generally are set through the expert experience, which means, that the gains are set in an heuristic way [1].

1.3   Fuzzy Logic in PID Control Systems

In terms of Control, fuzzy systems can be applied as controller or tuning system. A controller based on fuzzy logic (FLC), gather information on how to control a process. With this information set of rules can be expressed in the logical structure (if A and B then C), which dictate how the controller should react to changes in the controlled variable. A tuning system based on fuzzy logic in nature an FLC in which the process to control is the controller [4].

Using constant values in the PID tuning parameters, gives a satisfactory performance indices for first order linear systems, however it is not the case for the higher order systems subject to load disturbances or noise. In this sense, this opens the possibility of improving the performance of the classic PID controller using the dynamic adjustment of the tuning parameters. Since there is no standardized method for tuning parameters to ensure good performance in general method. This dynamic adjustment can be made by Intelligent PID control that arise at the historic moment. The most common intelligent PID control methods are Fuzzy PID control, Neural Network PID control, genetic algorithm PID control and hybrid PID control [1]. Fuzzy tuning of PID control is the outcome combination of the fuzzy theory, the fuzzy technology and PID control algorithm.

The diagram for a Fuzzy Tuning PID is illustrated below [3] (Fig. 1).

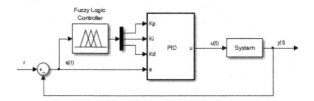

Fig. 1. Basic diagram for a fuzzy self-tuning PID.

The fuzzy tuning system to perform the establishment of the parameters, we have to settle rules in the fuzzy control chart which will connect the three parameters of the PID and the three properties of the steady-state, in the precisely moment in which the control parameters are established [1].

2   System Description

The fuzzy tuning system and the PID controller was implemented in a microcontroller (MCU), in order to have a full embedded system. We use the Arduino Due a microcontroller board that is based on the Atmel SAM3X8E ARM Cortex-M3 CPU (Fig. 2).

The aim of the PID controller is to regulate the temperature of the Peltier cells according to the value of a potentiometer (setpoint), this is accomplish by using a PWM output as the controller output. The feedback of the temperature is made by a temperature sensor (LM35). Basically the whole system can be illustrate as:

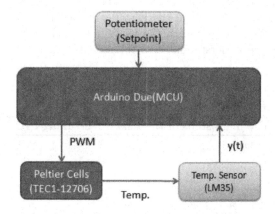

Fig. 2. Description of the implemented system.

As we know the MCU operates in the discrete domain, so in order to implement the PID we have to use the discrete formula for The PID

$$u(n) = K_p e(n) + K_i T s \sum_{n=1}^{N} e(n) + \frac{K_d}{Ts} \Delta e(n) \qquad (2)$$

$$\Delta e(n) = e(n) - e(n-1) \qquad (3)$$

Where $e(t)$ is the error, $u(t)$ is the control signal and T_s is the sampled period.

For the tuning problem we apply the fuzzy agents, which are the ones that manipulates K_p, K_i and K_d, by manipulating this parameters, the system provides different responses curves, so we measure steady-state properties, the properties that we considered are the overshoot, the settle time and the steady state error, we use these properties as qualifiers that evaluate the performance of the system response and therefore the input of the the fuzzy agents.

Each Fuzzy Agent use a set of fuzzy rules in order to make the modification of the PID controller's gains. We use the Takagi-Sugeno-Kahn (TSK) model as structure for the rule set, following the standard procedure of fuzzy controller's design, which consist of fuzzification, control rule base establishments, inference engine, and defuzzifier [1].

1. **Fuzzifier:** a normalized input (value mapped between 0 and 1) is classified in fuzzy values, which can be read in a linguistic way as very low, low, medium, high, very high. The membership value is computed according to the value of the input.
2. **Knowledge base:** where the rules that decide the behavior of the system are stored as a IF-THEN rules, this rules are generally provided by experts.
3. **Inference engine:** the output is calculated but it has a fuzzy value, according to the membership values from the Fuzzifier based on the knowledge base.
4. **Defuzzifier:** the stage in which the fuzzy output changes into a numerical values that can be understandable to the mechanism.

The Fuzzy self-tuning PID controller was design with the following the steps:

Algorithm 1. The main steps of the Fuzzy Self-tuning PID controller

---

Initialize the System;
repeat
    repeat
       | PID controller;
    until *until the system reaches the steady state*;
    Steady State properties are computed;
    Fuzzification;
    Inference Engine;
    Defuzzification;
until *requirements are met*;

Combining these fuzzy agents and the PID controller, creates an intelligent tuning system that search for the optimal combination of PID parameter's.

3 Implementation

We use Arduino DUE because it is based on a microcontroller that fits on our needs. Since the Arduino Due board runs at 3.3V, we condition the system.

The proposed system for the application of the PID controller are Peltier cells that are connected to the development board Arduino DUE (MCU) through an Darlington NPN transistor (TIP122), in order to have a feedback of the temperature of the Peltier cells we use the LM35 a temperature sensor a potentiometer is used as setpoint.

Table 1. Computational environment configuration

Microcontroller	AT91SAM3X8E
Operating voltage	3.3 V
Digital I/O pins	54 (12 PWM output)
Analog input pins	12
Flash memory	512 KB
SRAM	96 KB
Clock speed	84 MHz

When the system starts, the parameters of the PID controller is set as $K_p = 0.1$, $K_i = 0.1$ and $K_d = 0.1$. The fuzzy system is in charge of minimizing the errors based on the response of the PID, when the system reach the steady state, we measure the overshoot, steady state error and the settle time, these variables are normalize so we use them as input of the fuzzy system, The TKS model was designed for only one output and we need to modify three gains. So we use 3 complete system in order to calculate the gains value. Each fuzzy system has 3 inputs, 1 output and 5 fuzzy sets which are Very Low (1), Low (2), Medium (3), High (4), Very High (5). Using a fuzzy rule set [1], each gain has 125 different rules, as an example, a part of Fuzzy Rules for K_d is shown below (Table 2).

Table 2. Part of the Fuzzy Rules for K_d behaviour

OS	ESS	ST	O
1	4	4	5
2	2	1	5
3	1	1	3
4	5	3	2
5	5	5	4

Where OS is the overshoot, ESS is steady-state error, ST is the settle time and O is the output and the optimal value is Medium for all the inputs. The rules of Table 1 can be describe as follows:

If OS is 1 AND if ESS is 4 AND if ST is 4 THEN O is 5.
If OS is 2 AND if ESS is 2 AND if ST is 1 THEN O is 5.
If OS is 3 AND if ESS is 1 AND if ST is 1 THEN O is 3.
If OS is 4 AND if ESS is 5 AND if ST is 3 THEN O is 2.
If OS is 5 AND if ESS is 5 AND if ST is 5 THEN O is 4.

The output of the defuzzifier controls the change of the PID controller's gains, this output is normalized, so the gains are computed as.

$$K_x = K_x + \beta \Delta K_x \qquad (4)$$

Where K_x represent any gain, and β is a factor that describes how K_x changes ($\beta_{Kp} = 10$, $\beta_{Ki} = \beta_{Kd} = 0.1$), ΔK_x represent the defuzzifier output and $-1 \leq \Delta K_x \leq 1$.

4   Results

For this test, the setpoint is set to 41.5°C, the system starts at room temperature (30°C), so we wait until the system reaches a steady state, the sample time (T_s) is 100 ms. The performance of the system through iteration is shown in Table 3, the table shows how the steady state properties and the value of the gains are change through each iteration.

Table 3. Fuzzy self-tuning PID behavior through iterations

Iteration	K_p	K_i	K_d	OS	ESS	ST
1	0.10	0.10	0.10	0.78	0.66	0.99
2	8.79	0.11	-0.09	0.87	0.69	0.99
4	17.88	-0.05	0.10	0.64	0.79	0.83
6	19.97	0.30	0.30	0.85	0.70	0.99
8	20.06	0.20	0.20	0.63	0.33	0.99
12	21.95	-0.01	0.11	0.55	0.36	0.80
16	24.62	-0.07	0.20	0.49	0.30	0.75
20	29.54	-0.19	0.40	0.52	0.43	0.67

Where the optimum vale for the properties of the steady state are 0.5. The complete description of the behavior of the system in each iteration exposed in the table is shown below (Figs. 3, 4, 5, 6, 7, 8, 9 and 10).

As we can see the evolution of the behavior of the system depends on the criteria used in the fuzzy rules, in this case we expect to see low values (three in the fuzzy set) of steady-state error, overshoot and settling time.

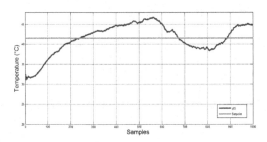

Fig. 3. System behavior with $k_p = 0.1$ $K_i = 0.10$ $K_d = 0.1$

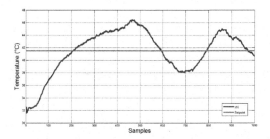

Fig. 4. System behavior with $k_p = 8.79$ $K_i = 0.11$ $K_d = -0.09$

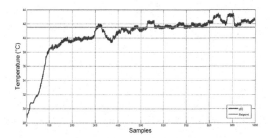

Fig. 5. System behavior with $k_p = 17.88$ $K_i = -0.05$ $K_d = 0.10$

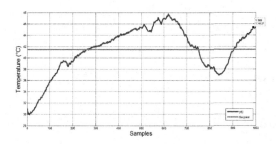

Fig. 6. System behavior with $k_p = 19.79$ $K_i = 0.30$ $K_d = 0.30$

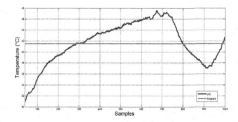

Fig. 7. System behavior with $k_p = 20.06$ $K_i = 0.20$ $K_d = 0.20$

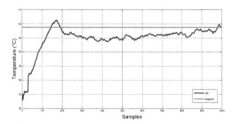

Fig. 8. System behavior with $k_p = 21.95$ $K_i = -0.01$ $K_d = 0.11$

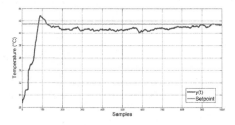

Fig. 9. System behavior with $k_p = 21.95$ $K_i = -0.07$ $K_d = 0.20$

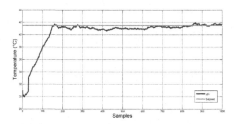

Fig. 10. System behavior with $k_p = 29.54$ $K_i = -0.19$ $K_d = 0.40$

5   Conclusion

Since the Peltier cells has non-linear behavior we use PID controller but there is
no standardized method for tuning parameters that ensure good performance,
this justifies the implementation of the Fuzzy Self-tuning PID controller. The
result of the experiment showed that for each iteration the performances of the
system response improves. Finally we can conclude that the Fuzzy Self-tuning
PID controller is a good option to solve complex objects control problems of
uncertainly, non-linearity, and time variances [1–4].

References

1. Alvarado-Yañez, L.A., Torres-Treviño, L.M., Rodríguez-Liñán, A.: An embedded fuzzy agent for online tuning of a PID controller for position control of a DC motor. In: Castro, F., Gelbukh, A., González, M. (eds.) MICAI 2013, Part II. LNCS, vol. 8266, pp. 225–232. Springer, Heidelberg (2013)
2. Cabrera-Gaona, D., Trevino, L., Rodriguez-Linan, A.: Control by learning in a temperature system using a maximum sensibility neural network. In: 12th Mexican International Conference on Artificial Intelligence (MICAI), pp. 109–113, November 2013
3. Yang, Z., Ye, Y., Lu, Q.: Design of self-tuning fuzzy PID controller on PWM $dc - dc$ converter. In: Xing, S., Chen, S., Wei, Z., Xia, J. (eds.) Unifying Electrical Engineering and Electronics Engineering. Lecture Notes in Electrical Engineering, vol. 238, pp. 685–691. Springer, New York (2014)
4. Zhang, R., Song, L., Yang, J., Hoffman, T.: DC motor speed control system simulation based on fuzzy self-tuning PID. In: Cao, B., Li, T.-F., Zhang, C.-Y. (eds.) Fuzzy Information and Engineering Volume 2. AISC, vol. 62, pp. 967–975. Springer, Heidelberg (2009)

Fuzzy Chemical Reaction Algorithm

David de la O[(✉)], Oscar Castillo, Leslie Astudillo, and José Soria

Division of Graduate Studies, Tijuana Institute of Technology, Tijuana, Mexico
ddsh@live.com, ocastillo@tectijuana.mx,
leslie.astudillo@suntroncorp.com

Abstract. In this paper, a Fuzzy Chemical Reaction Algorithm (FCRA) is proposed. In order to overcome the problems of the basic Chemical Reaction Algorithm (CRA), we improve the CRA by proposing a FCRA that takes into account the diversity of the population. Comparative experimental results with benchmark functions show that our proposed method performs much better than the original algorithm in problems with many dimensions.

Keywords: Chemical algorithm · Control · Fuzzy logic · Robot

1 Introduction

In this paper we propose a method based on CRA that automatically changes parameters in adapting to the characteristics of the problem. It has been demonstrated [1–5], that the combination of several systems offers new possibilities for solutions and improvements, instead of using methods separately.

CRA is an optimization algorithm proposed by Astudillo et al. [6–10], this algorithm is based on a static population metaheuristic, which applies an abstraction of several chemical reactions as intensifiers (substitution, double substitution reactions) and other reactions as diversifying (synthesis, decomposition reactions) mechanisms.

This paper is organized into four sections as follows: Sect. 2 describes the main problem and recent research work is presented. Sections 3 and 4 describe the theory underlying the present work, in which issues such as fuzzy logic, the CRA algorithm and a little on the operation of autonomous mobile robot are discussed. Section 5 shows the results of the simulations.

2 The Chemical Optimization Paradigm

The proposed chemical reaction algorithm is a metaheuristic strategy that performs a stochastic search for optimal solutions within a defined search space. In this optimization strategy, an element (or compound) represented every solution, and the fitness or performance of the element is evaluated in accordance with the objective function.

This algorithm has the advantage of not having external parameters (kinetic/potential energies, mass conservation, thermodynamic characteristics, etc.) as occurs in other optimization algorithms; this is a very straight forward methodology that takes the characteristics of the chemical reactions (synthesis, decomposition, substitution and double-substitution) to find the optimal solution [6] (Fig. 1).

G. Sidorov and S.N. Galicia-Haro (Eds.): MICAI 2015, Part I, LNAI 9413, pp. 452–459, 2015.
DOI: 10.1007/978-3-319-27060-9_37

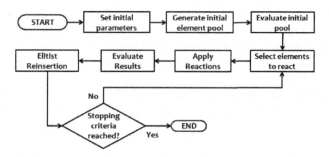

Fig. 1. General flowchart of the chemical reaction algorithm

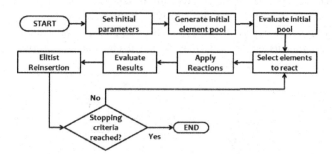

Fig. 2. Decomposition possibilities

This approach is based on a static population metaheuristic, which applies an abstraction of chemical reactions as intensifiers (substitution, double substitution reactions) and diversifying (synthesis, decomposition reactions) mechanisms. The elitist reinsertion strategy allows the permanence of the best elements and thus the average fitness of the entire element pool increases with each iteration. Figure 2 shows the flowchart of the algorithm.

The main components of this chemical reaction algorithm are described below.

The synthesis and decomposition reactions are used to diversify the resulting solutions; these procedures prove to be highly effective and rapidly lead the results to a desired value.

The single and double substitution reactions allow the algorithm to search for optimal values around a good previously found solution and they're described as follows.

The algorithm works mainly with chemical reactions with a change in at least one substance (element or possible solution), that changes its composition and property sets. Such reactions are classified into 4 types, which are described below:

2.1 Type 1: Combination Reactions

$$B + X \rightarrow BX \tag{1}$$

A combination reaction is a reaction of two reactants to produce one product. The simplest combination reactions are the reactions of two elements to form a compound. After all, if two elements are treated with each other, they can either react or not.

2.2   Type 2: Decomposition Reactions

$$BX \rightarrow B + X \qquad (2)$$

The second type of simple reaction is decomposition. This reaction is also easy to recognize. Typically, only one reactant is given. A type of energy, such as heat or electricity, may also be indicated. The reactant usually decomposes to its elements, to an element and a simpler compound, or to two simpler compounds.

Binary compounds may yield two elements or an element and a simpler compound. Ternary (three-element) compounds may yield an element and a compound or two simpler compounds (See Fig. 3).

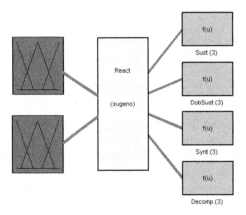

Fig. 3. Fuzzy system for parameter adaptation

2.3   Type 3: Substitution Reactions

$$X + AB \rightarrow AX + B \qquad (3)$$

Elements have varying abilities to combine. Among the most reactive metals are the alkali metals and the alkaline earth metals. On the opposite end of the scale of reactivities, among the least active metals or the most stable metals are silver and gold, prized for their lack of reactivity. Reactive means the opposite of stable, but means the same as active.

When a free element reacts with a compound of different elements, the free element will replace one of the elements in the compound if the free element is more reactive than the element it replaces. In general, a free metal will replace the metal in the compound, or a free nonmetal will replace the nonmetal in the compound. A new compound and a new free element are produced.

2.4 Type 4: Double-Substitution Reactions

Double-substitution or double-replacement reactions, also called double-decomposition reactions or metathesis reactions, involve two ionic compounds, most often in aqueous solution [4].

In this type of reaction, the cations simply swap anions. The reaction proceeds if a solid or a covalent compound is formed from ions in solution. All gases at room temperature are covalent. Some reactions of ionic solids plus ions in solution also occur. Otherwise, no reaction takes place.

Just as with replacement reactions, double-replacement reactions may or may not proceed. They need a driving force.

In replacement reactions the driving force is reactivity; here it is insolubility or covalence.

At first sight, chemical theory and definitions may seem complex and none or few are related to optimization theory, but only the general schema will be considered here in order to focus on the control application.

The steps to consider in this optimization method are illustrated in Fig. 4 and given as follows.

- First, we need to generate an initial pool of elements/compounds.
- Once we have the initial pool, we have to evaluate it.
- Based on the previous evaluation, we will select some elements/compounds to "induce" a reaction.
- Given the result of the reaction, we will evaluate the obtained elements/compounds.
- Repeat the steps until the algorithm meets the criteria (desired result or maximum number of iterations is reached) [6].

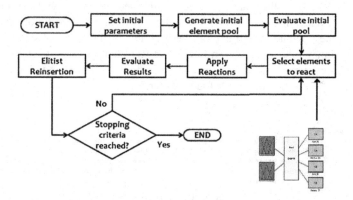

Fig. 4. CRA flowchart with fuzzy system

3   Methodology

Normally the algorithm uses fixed parameters for each of the reactions: synthesis, decomposition, substitution and double-substitution, propose the idea of adapting the parameters of the reactions, to control the ability of exploration and exploitation, these parameters will be used as output of a fuzzy system (Fig. 3) and as input the level of diversity Eq. 4 which is in the population and the percentage of iterations Eq. 5 [1].

$$Diversity(S(t)) = \frac{1}{n_s} \sum_{i=1}^{n_s} \sqrt{\sum_{j=1}^{n_x} \left(x_{ij}(t) - \bar{x}_j(t)\right)^2} \tag{4}$$

$$Iteration = \frac{Curren\, Iteration}{Maximum\, of\, Iterations} \tag{5}$$

Where *current iteration* is the number of iterations elapsed and *maximum iterations* is the number of iterations established for CRA to find the best solution. In Eq. 4, S is the population of the CRA; t is the current iteration or time, n_s is the size of the population, i is the number of the particle, n_x is the total number of dimensions, j is the number of the dimension, x_{ij} is the j dimension of the particle i, j is the j dimension of the current best particle of the population.

Figure 3 shows the adaptation of the CRA fuzzy system for adjusting the parameters of the chemical reactions, which change at every iteration, before performing the chemical reaction of the elements, then the elements are evaluated, this in order that they can adapt to every possible circumstance.

We obtain the rule set for the fuzzy system used to adapt the parameters of the CRA, using knowledge about the effects of the parameters as intensifiers (substitution, double substitution reactions) and diversifying (synthesis, decomposition reactions) mechanisms, for example: when we use a synthesis higher than decomposition reactions and substitution lower than double substitution reactions the effect is that the population will explore the space of search, and when we use a synthesis lower than decomposition reactions and substitution higher than double substitution reaction the effect is that the population will exploit the best area of the space of search found.

With the fuzzy rule set shown in Fig. 5, we want that in early iterations the CRA algorithm will explore the space of search and in final iterations the CRA will exploit the best area of the space of search found so far.

1. If (Iteration is low) and (Diversity is low) then (Sust is low)(DobSust is low)(Synt is high)(Decomp is high) (1)
2. If (Iteration is medium) and (Diversity is medium) then (Sust is medium)(DobSust is medium)(Synt is medium)(Decomp is mf2) (1)
3. If (Iteration is high) and (Diversity is high) then (Sust is high)(DobSust is high)(Synt is low)(Decomp is low) (1)
4. If (Iteration is high) and (Diversity is low) then (Sust is medium)(DobSust is medium)(Synt is low)(Decomp is low) (1)
5. If (Iteration is medium) and (Diversity is high) then (Sust is medium)(DobSust is medium)(Synt is high)(Decomp is high) (1)

Fig. 5.   Fuzzy rules set

4 Simulation Results

To validate the proposed approach we performed some tests with benchmark functions, and these functions are described below in Table 1.

Table 1. Benchmark functions.

Test Function	Definition	Search domain	f_{min}
f_1	$f(x) = \sum_{i=1}^{n} x_i^2$	[-100, 100]	0
f_2	$f(x) = \sum_{i=1}^{n} i * x_i^2$	[-100, 100]	0
f_3	$f(x) = \sum_{i=1}^{n} \left(\sum_{j=1}^{i} x_j \right)^2$	[-65, 65]	0
f_4	$f(x) = \sum_{i=1}^{n} 5i * x_i^2$	[-100, 100]	0
f_5	$f(x) = \sum_{i=1}^{n-1} \left[100(x_{i+1} - x_i^2)^2 + (1 - x_i)^2 \right]$	[-30, 30]	0
f_6	$f(x) = 10n + \sum_{i=1}^{n} \left[x_i^2 - 10\cos(2\pi x_i) \right]$	[-100, 100]	0
f_7	$f(x) = \sum_{i=1}^{n} -x_i \sin\left(\sqrt{|x_i|} \right)$	[-600, 600]	$-n \cdot 418.9829$

Testing was performed using 30 and 1500 dimensions. Table 2 shows the mean and standard deviation obtained for each function.

Table 2. Mean and standard deviation of FCRA.

Function	Dimensions	Mean	Standard deviation
F1	30	1.39E-74	5.14E-74
	1500	4.57E-84	2.35E-83
F2	30	4.83E-74	2.09E-73
	1500	9.41E-75	5.15E-74
F3	30	6.60E-21	3.62E-20
	1500	7.72E-09	4.14E-08
F4	256	7.45E-70	4.08E-69
	1500	3.75E-78	2.03E-77
F5	30	2.90E+01	1.87E-02
	1500	1.50E+03	3.84E-02
F6	30	0	0
	1500	0	0
F7	30	−1.05E+08	−3.78E+08
	1500	8.48E+07	2.31E+08

5   Comparison of Results

We made comparisons against others works and these works are briefly described below.

The first comparison is against Astudillo et al. [4], Tables 3 and 4 summarize the results presented in [4], and we add our results using the proposed approach (FCRA).

Table 3. Mean and standard deviation 30 dimensions.

Function		Mean	Standard deviation	t	P
F1	CRA	9.51E-33	3.41E-32	−0.02	0.494
	FCRA	1.39E-74	5.14E-74		
F2	CRA	6.78E-31	3.70E-30	−1	0.162
	FCRA	4.83E-74	2.09E-73		
F3	CRA	6.78E-31	3.70E-30	1	0.837
	FCRA	6.60E-21	3.62E-20		
F4	CRA	2.38E-26	1.54E-25	−0.85	0.202
	FCRA	7.45E-70	4.08E-69		
F5	CRA	2.9E+01	2.62E-02	0	0.50
	FCRA	2.90E+01	1.87 E-02		
F6	CRA	0	0		
	FCRA	0	0		
F7	CRA	−3.96E+04	4.19E+04	−6.78	0
	FCRA	−1.05E+08	8.48 E+04		

Table 4. mean and standard deviation 1500 dimensions.

Function		Mean	Standard deviation	t	P
F1	CRA	9.03E-27	2.83E-26	−1.75	0.046
	FCRA	4.57E-84	2.35E-83		
F2	CRA	1.14E-25	3.78E-25	−1.65	0.055
	FCRA	9.41E-75	5.15E-74		
F3	CRA	1.31E-25	6.52E-25	1.02	0.842
	FCRA	7.72E-09	4.14E-08		
F4	CRA	3.86E-24	1.99E-23	−1.06	0.148
	FCRA	3.75E-78	2.03E-77		
F5	CRA	1.50E+03	1.04E-02	0	0.50
	FCRA	1.50E+03	3.84E-02		
F6	CRA	0	0		
	FCRA	0	0		
F7	CRA	−4.05E+05	6.82E+05	−8.95	0
	FCRA	−3.78E+08	2.31E+08		

6   Conclusion

This paper proposed a fuzzy system for the CRA algorithm. The CRA is a new optimization algorithm for optimization problem inspired by the nature of chemical reactions. We improve this algorithm by using a fuzzy system in the adaptation of parameters of the chemical reactions. So our proposed FCRA method is better than CRA. The comparative experiments show that our proposed method is more efficient and robust in problem with many dimensions.

Acknowledgements. The authors would like to thank CONACYT and Tijuana Institute of Technology for the facilities and resources granted for the development of this research.

References

1. Olivas, F., Valdez, F., Castillo, O.: An interval type-2 fuzzy logic system for dynamic parameter adaptation in particle swarm optimization. In: 2014 IEEE Conference on Norbert Wiener in the 21st Century (21CW), pp. 1–6, 24–26 June 2014
2. Castillo, O., Neyoy, H., Soria, J., Melin, P., Valdez, F.: A new approach for dynamic fuzzy logic parameter tuning in ant colony optimization and its application in fuzzy control of a mobile robot. Appl. Soft. Comput. **28**, 150–159 (2015)
3. Soto, J., Melin, P., Castillo, O.: Time series prediction using ensembles of ANFIS models with genetic optimization of interval type-2 and type-1 fuzzy integrators. Int. J. Hybrid Intell. Syst. **11**(3), 211–226 (2014)
4. Amezcua, J., Melin, P.: Optimization of modular neural networks with the LVQ algorithm for classification of arrhythmias using particle swarm optimization. In: Recent Advances on Hybrid Approaches for Designing Intelligent Systems, pp. 307–314 (2014)
5. Melin, P., Soto, J., Castillo, O., Soria, J.: A new approach for time series prediction using ensembles of ANFIS models. Expert Syst. Appl. **39**(3), 3494–3506 (2012)
6. Valdez, F., Melin, P., Castillo, O.: A survey on nature-inspired optimization algorithms with fuzzy logic for dynamic parameter adaptation. Expert Syst. Appl. **41**(14), 6459–6466 (2014)
7. Astudillo, L., Melin, P., Castillo, O.: Nature optimization applied to design a type-2 fuzzy controller for an autonomous mobile robot. In: 2012 Fourth World Congress on Nature and Biologically Inspired Computing (NaBIC) (2012)
8. Melin, P., Astudillo, L., Castillo, O., Valdez, F., Garcia, M.: Optimal design of type-2 and type-1 fuzzy tracking controllers for autonomous mobile robots under perturbed torques using a new chemical optimization paradigm. Expert Syst. Appl. **40**(8), 3185–3195 (2013)
9. Astudillo, L., Melin, P., Castillo, O.: Introduction to an optimization algorithm based on the chemical reactions. Inf. Sci. **291**, 85–95 (2015)
10. Sanchez, C., Melin, P., Astudillo, L.: Chemical optimization method for modular neural networks applied in emotion classification. In: Castillo, O., Melin, P., Kacprzyk, J. (eds.) Recent Advances on Hybrid Approaches for Designing Intelligent Systems, vol. 547, pp. 381–390. Springer, Berlin, Heidelberg (2014)

A Fuzzy Bee Colony Optimization Algorithm Using an Interval Type-2 Fuzzy Logic System for Trajectory Control of a Mobile Robot

Leticia Amador-Angulo[(✉)] and Oscar Castillo

Division of Graduate Studies, Tijuana Institute of Technology, Tijuana, Mexico
`leticia.amadorangulo@yahoo.com.mx`,
`ocastillo@tectijuana.mx`

Abstract. A new fuzzy Bee Colony Optimization (FBCO) algorithm with dynamic adaptation in the alpha and beta parameters using an Interval Type-2 Fuzzy Logic System is presented in this paper. The Bee Colony Optimization meta-heuristic belongs to the class of Nature-Inspired Algorithms. The objective of the work is based on the use of Interval Type-2 Fuzzy Logic to find the best Beta and Alpha parameter values in BCO. We use BCO specifically for tuning membership functions of the fuzzy controller for stability of the trajectories in a mobile robot. We implemented the IAE and MSE metrics as performance metrics of control. We added perturbations in the model with the pulse generator so that the Interval Type-2 Fuzzy Logic System is better analyzed under uncertainty and to verify that the FBCO shows better results than the traditional BCO.

Keywords: Bee · Colony optimization algorithm · Interval Type-2 Fuzzy Logic System · Dynamic adaptation · Mobile robots

1 Introduction

In recent years, many works have been developed on control and system stabilization. However, all these control design methods require the exact mathematical model of the physical systems which may not be available in practice. On the other hand, fuzzy logic control has been successfully applied for solving many nonlinear control problems [1, 2, 5]. Fuzzy Logic or multi-valued logic is based on fuzzy set theory proposed in [17–19], which helps us in modeling knowledge, through the use of if-then rules. In Type-2 fuzzy systems, the membership functions can now return a range of values, which vary depending on the uncertainty involved in not only the inputs, but also in the same membership functions [10, 12, 19].

BCO has recently received many improvements and applications. The BCO algorithm mimics the food foraging behavior of swarms of honey bees [9]. Honey bees use several mechanisms, like the waggle dance to optimally locate food sources and search new ones. It is a very simple, robust and population based stochastic optimization algorithm [15].

Mobile robots have attracted considerable interest in the robotics and control research community; because they have non-holonomic properties caused by non-integrable

© Springer International Publishing Switzerland 2015
G. Sidorov and S.N. Galicia-Haro (Eds.): MICAI 2015, Part I, LNAI 9413, pp. 460–471, 2015.
DOI: 10.1007/978-3-319-27060-9_38

differential constrains [10]. The main contribution of the paper is the proposed fuzzy BCO approach using Interval Type-2 Fuzzy Logic System to provide efficient control of mobile robots.

This paper starts with related works in Sect. 2. Section 3 describes the Theoretical basis. Section 4 describes the problem statement. Section 5 describes the Bee Colony Optimization algorithm. Section 6 describes the proposed method. Section 7 describes the experimental results, Sect. 8 describes a comparison of results, and finally Sect. 9 presents the conclusion and future works of this research.

2 Related Works

Many intelligent optimization techniques, such as Ant Colony Optimization [8, 13], and Particle Swarm Optimization [11], Differential Evolution [13] have been proposed to tune Fuzzy Controllers. However, the BCO algorithm is a new technique to solve complex problems and can also be used for tuning fuzzy controllers.

The problem of controlling the trajectory of the amobile robot, such as in [7, 10], with different meta-heuristics algorithms. In addition, most related works are realized with the classical algorithm, in [7, 11, 13] implemented the dynamic adaptation of the parameters in bio-inspired algorithms finding good results. In [1] fixed values are recommended for the Alpha and Beta parameters in the BCO algorithm are both 1.0, and several experiments were realized to find the optimum values of these parameters. To overcome this problem, we proposed to use the dynamic adaptation parameter of the BCO with type-1 fuzzy logic and interval type-2 fuzzy logic system to find the best values of the Alpha and Beta parameters in the BCO algorithm.

3 Theoretical Basis

The main idea of fuzzy logic systems was introduced by Zadeh in 1965 [17–19], and was first applied to control theory in 1974 by Mamdani [5]. Based on these works, the fuzzy controllers have successfully been used in various applications [1, 5, 7, 8, 10, 13, 14, 16].

3.1 Interval Type-2 Fuzzy Logic Systems

If we have a type-1 membership function, and we are blurring it to the left and to the right, then, for a specific value x', the membership function (u'), takes on different values, which are not all weighted the same, so we can assign an amplitude distribution to all of those points. Doing this for all $x \in X$, we create a three-dimensional membership function – a type-2 membership function – that characterizes an interval type-2 fuzzy set [6, 14]. Figure 1 shows the Interval Type-2 membership function.

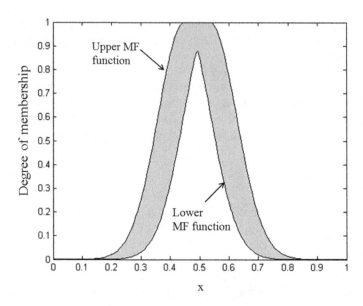

Fig. 1. Interval Type-2 membership function.

A Type-2 fuzzy set, $\tilde{A}$, is characterized by Eq. (1).

$$\tilde{A} = \{(x, u), u\tilde{A}(x, u))|\forall x \in X, \forall u \in Jx \subseteq [0, 1]\} \tag{1}$$

Where $0 \le u\tilde{A}(x, u) \le 1$

The footprint Uncertainty affects decisions in a number of different ways. The concept of information is fully connected to the concept of uncertainty. The most fundamental part of this connection is that the uncertainty involved in any solution of a problem is the result of poor information, which may be incomplete, imprecise, fragmentary, not fully reliable, vague, contradictory, or deficient in some way or another [1, 2].

4 Problem Statement

4.1 General Description of the Problem

The model that is used is of a unicycle mobile robot [10, 16], consisting of two driving wheels located on the same axis and a front free wheel. Figure 2 shows a graphical description of the robot model.

The robot model assumes that the motion of the free wheel can be ignored in its dynamics, as shown in Eqs. (2) and (3).

$$M(q)\dot{v} + C(q, \dot{q})v + Dv = \tau + P(t) \tag{2}$$

Where,

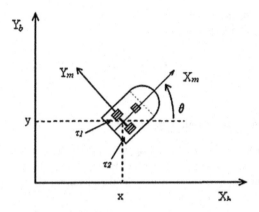

Fig. 2. Mobile robot model.

$q = (x, y, \theta)^T$ is the vector of the configuration coordinates,

$\upsilon = (v, w)^T$ is the vector of velocities,

$\tau = (\tau_1, \tau_2)$ is the vector of torques applied to the wheels of the robot where τ_1 and τ_2 denote the torques of the right and left wheel,

$P \in R^2$ is the uniformly bounded disturbance vector,

$M(q) \in R^{2 \times 2}$ is the positive-definite inertia matrix,

$C(q, \dot{q})\vartheta$ is the vector of centripetal and Coriolis forces, and

$D \in R^{2 \times 2}$ is a diagonal positive-definite damping matrix.

The kinematic system is represented by Eq. (3).

$$
\dot{q} = \underbrace{\begin{bmatrix} \cos\theta & 0 \\ \sin\theta & 0 \\ 0 & 1 \end{bmatrix}}_{J(q)} \underbrace{\begin{bmatrix} v \\ w \end{bmatrix}}_{\upsilon} \tag{3}
$$

Where,

(x, y) is the position in the X − Y (world) reference frame,

θ is the angle between the heading direction and the x-axis,

v and w are the linear and angular velocities.

Furthermore, Eq. (4) shows the non-holonomic constraint, which this system has, which corresponds to a no-slip wheel condition preventing the robot from moving sideways.

$$
\dot{y}\cos\theta - \dot{x}\sin\theta = 0 \tag{4}
$$

The system fails to meet Brockett's necessary condition for feedback stabilization, which implies that no continuous static state-feedback controller exists that can stabilize the closed-loop system around the equilibrium point. The control objective is to design a fuzzy logic controller of τ that ensures:

$$\lim_{\tau \to \infty} \|qd(t) - q(t)\| = 0 \tag{5}$$

4.2 Design of the Fuzzy Logic Controller

The main problem to study is controlling the stability of the trajectory in a mobile robot. The mobile robot was modeled with a Mandani Fuzzy Controller [16]. The linear (ϑ_d) and the angular (w_d) velocity errors are taken as input variables and the right (τ_1) and left (τ_2) torques as the outputs.

The Fuzzy Controller has two inputs and two outputs. The membership functions used in the input are of trapezoidal form for the Negative (N) and Positive (P) and triangular for the Zero (Z) linguistics terms. The first input is called ev (error in linear velocity), which has three membership functions with linguistic values of N (Negative), Z (Zero) and P (Positive). The second input variable is called ew (error in angular velocity) with three membership functions with the same linguistic values. The Outputs are called T1 (Torque 1), and T2 (Torque 2), which are composed of three triangular membership functions with the following linguistic values, respectively: N (Negative), Z (Zero), P (Positive). Figures 3 and 4 show the representation of the rules and the design of the Type-1 Fuzzy Logic System, respectively.

The test criteria is a series of Performance Indices; where the MSE (Mean Square Error), and the IAE (Integral Absolute Error) were used, and are respectively shown in Eqs. (6–7).

$$MSE = \frac{1}{n} \sum_{i=1}^{n} (\overline{Y}_i - Y_i)^2 \tag{6}$$

$$\text{Minimize } IAE = \int_0^t (|\Delta P(t)| + |\Delta Q(t)|) dt \tag{7}$$

1. If (ev is N) and (ew is N) then (T1 is N)(T2 is N) (1)
2. If (ev is N) and (ew is Z) then (T1 is N)(T2 is Z) (1)
3. If (ev is N) and (ew is P) then (T1 is N)(T2 is P) (1)
4. If (ev is Z) and (ew is N) then (T1 is Z)(T2 is N) (1)
5. If (ev is Z) and (ew is Z) then (T1 is Z)(T2 is Z) (1)
6. If (ev is Z) and (ew is P) then (T1 is Z)(T2 is P) (1)
7. If (ev is P) and (ew is N) then (T1 is P)(T2 is N) (1)
8. If (ev is P) and (ew is Z) then (T1 is P)(T2 is Z) (1)
9. If (ev is P) and (ew is P) then (T1 is P)(T2 is P) (1)

Fig. 3. Rules of the Fuzzy Logic System.

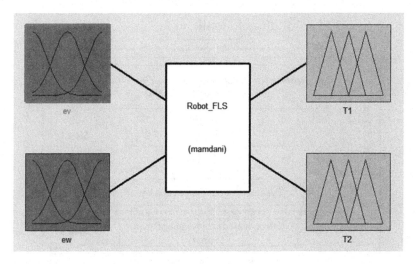

Fig. 4. Design of the Type-1 Fuzzy Logic System.

5   Bee Colony Optimization Algorithm

The BCO is inspired by the bees´ behavior in the nature. The basic idea behind the BCO is to create the multi agent system (colony of artificial bees) capabilities to successfully solve difficult combinatorial optimization problems [15]. The BCO metaheuristic [3, 4] has been introduced fairly recently by Lučić and Teodorović as a new direction in the field of Swarm Intelligence, and has not previously been applied in Interval Type-2 FLS applied to Fuzzy Controller design. The general steps are shown in the flowchart in Fig. 5.

6   Proposed Method

The dynamics of BCO are defined in Eqs. (8-11).

$$Pij, n = \frac{[\rho ij, n]^{\alpha} \cdot [\frac{1}{dij}]^{\beta}}{\sum\limits_{j \in Ai,n} [\rho ij, n]^{\alpha} \cdot [\frac{1}{dij}]^{\beta}} \tag{8}$$

$$D_i = K \cdot \frac{Pf_i}{Pf_{colony}} \tag{9}$$

$$Pf_i = \frac{1}{L_I}, L_i = \text{Tour Length} \tag{10}$$

$$Pf_{colony} = \frac{1}{N_{Bee}} \sum_{i=1}^{N_{Bee}} Pf_i \tag{11}$$

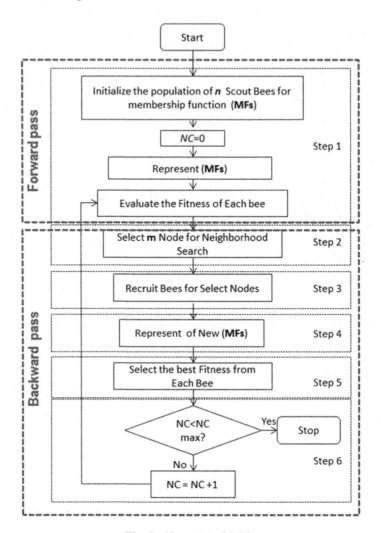

Fig. 5. Flowchart of BCO.

Equation (8) represents the probability of a bee k located on a node i selects the next node denoted by j, where β is the probability of visiting the following node. Note that the ρij is inversely proportional to the city distance. d_{ij} represents the distance of node i until node j, for this algorithm indicates the total the dance that a bee have in this moment. Finally ∝ is a binary variable that is used for to find better solutions in the algorithm.

Equation (9) represents that a waggle dance will last for certain duration, determined by a linear function, where K denotes the waggle dance scaling factor, Pf_i denotes the profitability scores of bee i as defined in Eq. (10) and Pf_{colony} denotes the bee colony's average profitability as in Eq. (11) and is updated after each bee completes its tour.

For measuring the iterations of the algorithm, it was decided to use the percentage of iterations as a variable, i.e. when we are at the initial stages of the algorithm the iterations will be considered "low", and when the iterations are completed it will be considered "high" or close to 100 %. To represent this idea we use:

$$\text{Iteration} = \frac{\text{Current Iteration}}{\textit{Maximum of Iterations}} \tag{12}$$

The diversity measure is defined by Eq. (13), which measures the degree of dispersion of the bee, i.e. when the bees are closer together, there is less diversity as well as when bees are separated then diversity is high. As the reader will realize the equation of diversity can be considered as the average of the Euclidean distances between each bee and the best bee.

$$\text{Diversity}(S(t)) = \frac{1}{n_s} \sum_{i=1}^{n_x} \sqrt{X_{ij}(t) - \bar{X}_j(t))^2} \tag{13}$$

We realized three FLSs; the design in inputs for each FLS is with two inputs called Iteration and Diversity; each input has three triangular membership functions with the linguistic value of Low, Medium and High. The output changed depending on the type of the FLS implemented; i.e. the first is FBCO1 has dynamic adjustment the value of alpha and value of beta is 2, the second is FBCO2 with dynamic value of the beta and value of alpha is 0.01. Finally, the third is FBCO3 with dynamic adjustment in alpha and beta. The outputs have five triangular membership functions granulated as; Low, Medium Low, Medium, Medium High and High for alpha and beta. The design and the rules of the fuzzy system are shown in Figs. 6 and 7, respectively.

In BCO the value of alpha indicates the exploitation; and beta represents the exploration. With the same methodology, we can design the Interval Type-2 Fuzzy Logic Systemand both are Mamdani style.

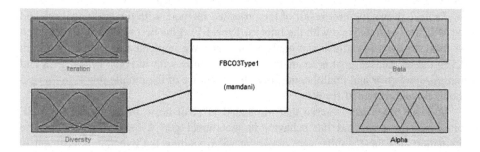

Fig. 6. Type-1 Fuzzy Logic System.

1. If (Iteration is Low) and (Diversity is Low) then (Beta is High)(Alpha is Low) (1)
2. If (Iteration is Low) and (Diversity is Medium) then (Beta is MediumHigh)(Alpha is Medium) (1)
3. If (Iteration is Low) and (Diversity is High) then (Beta is MediumHigh)(Alpha is MediumLow) (1)
4. If (Iteration is Medium) and (Diversity is Low) then (Beta is MediumHigh)(Alpha is MediumLow) (1)
5. If (Iteration is Medium) and (Diversity is Medium) then (Beta is Medium)(Alpha is Medium) (1)
6. If (Iteration is Medium) and (Diversity is High) then (Beta is MediumLow)(Alpha is MediumHigh) (1)
7. If (Iteration is High) and (Diversity is Low) then (Beta is Medium)(Alpha is High) (1)
8. If (Iteration is High) and (Diversity is Medium) then (Beta is MediumLow)(Alpha is MediumHigh) (1)
9. If (Iteration is High) and (Diversity is High) then (Beta is Low)(Alpha is High) (1)

Fig. 7. Rules for the Type-1 Fuzzy Logic System.

7   Experimental Results

The experimentation was performed with perturbations. We used some specific noise generators, like the Pulse Generator noise. Where the height of the Power Spectral Density of set to 0.5. The configuration of the experiments is shown in Table 1.

Table 1. Parameters for each method

Parameters	Traditional BCO	Fuzzy BCO 1	Fuzzy BCO 2	Fuzzy BCO 3
Population	50	50	50	50
Bee Follower	30	30	30	30
Iterations	20	20	20	20
Alpha	0.01	Dynamic	0.01	Dynamic
Beta	2	2	Dynamic	Dynamic

Simulation results in Table 2 show the best experiments without perturbation in the fuzzy logic controller for each bio-inspired algorithm. These results are of the best results and average of the MSE of 30 experiments for each method.

Table 2 shows the best result of the proposed method, with the traditional method the MSE was of **0.006** and with the Interval Type-1 FLS the best result was **0.004** when we used the dynamic adjustment in alpha and beta. We implemented levels of noise in 0.5 in the model, the goal is to analyze the uncertainty with Interval Type-2 FLS and minimize the error and finally controlling the trajectory of the mobile robot. In Table 3 shows the experimental results.

In Table 3 we can observe that the added level of noise in the model the MSE minimizes the error and the behavior in the model gets a better trajectory in the simulation. The best results were obtaining when visiting the dynamic adjustment in

Table 2. Simulation results without a noise level.

Simulation Error					
Type of the FLS	Index	Traditional BCO	Fuzzy BCO 1	Fuzzy BCO 2	Fuzzy BCO 3
Type-1 FLS	IAE	14.382	74.622	66.218	146.485
	MSE	**0.006**	0.048	0.017	**0.004**
Average:		4.319	3.616	3.559	2.737
Interval Type-2 FLS	IAE	Not Applicable	394.639	394.63	490.7488
	MSE		0.079	0.079	0.0207
Average:			4.328	4.328	3.6818

Table 3. Simulation results with noise level.

Simulation Error					
Type of the FLS	Index	Traditional BCO	Fuzzy BCO 1	Fuzzy BCO 2	Fuzzy BCO 3
Type-1 FLS	IAE	290.311	112.8783	374.74	221.2159
	MSE	0.11	0.0443	0.0657	0.0338
Average:		4.4039	4.5121	3.6887	4.1498
Interval Type-2 FLS	IAE	Not Applicable	347.5412	435.17	349.65
	MSE		0.0352	**0.0033**	0.005
Average:			4.3857	3.5905	3.9874

Alpha because the exploitation is very important for BCO algorithm and Interval Type-2 FLS shows that the evaluation of the uncertainty applied level of noise obtain better results.

8   Comparison of Results

The experimental results realized with levels of noise allow to observer a better trajectory in the mobile robot when, we used the Interval Type-2 FLS in the adjustment dynamic in parameters alpha and beta. The behavior in the model of the two proposed methods when we applied noise level is shown in Fig. 8.

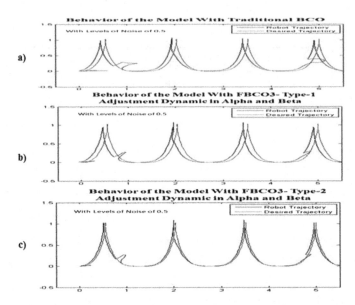

Fig. 8. (a) Behavior the Traditional BCO, (b) Behavior the FBCO3 with Type-1 FLS, and (c) Behavior the FBCO3 with Interval Type-2 FLS.

9   Conclusions

We conclude that dynamically adjusting parameters of an optimization method (in this case the Bee Colony Optimization BCO), can improve the quality of results and increase the diversity of solutions to a problem. By comparing the proposed methods and the traditional BCO, in the design of fuzzy logic systems applied to fuzzy controller it was found that in method based on the experiments that in developing this work, it was possible to develop a BCO for the optimization of FLS for controlling the trajectory in a mobile robot and we design a FBCO with adjusting in the alpha and beta parameters with Type-1 FLS and Interval Type-2 FLS. Finally, we find the optimal values in Alpha and Beta to improve the results when compared with the traditional method of BCO.

References

1. Amador-Angulo, L., Castillo, O., Pulido, M.: Comparison of fuzzy controllers for the water tank with type-1 and type-2 fuzzy logic. In: IFSA World Congress and NAFIPS Annual Meeting (IFSA/NAFIPS), pp. 1062–1067. IEEE (2013)
2. Amador-Angulo, L., Castillo, O.: Comparison of the optimal design of fuzzy controllers for the water tank using ant colony optimization. In: Castillo, O., Pedrycz, W., Kacprzyk, J. (eds.) Recent Advances on Hybrid Approaches for Designing Intelligent Systems, pp. 255–273. Springer International Publishing (2014)

3. Biesmeijer, J.C., Seeley, T.D.: The use of waggle dance information by honey bees throughout their foraging careers. Behav. Ecol. Sociobiol. **59**(1), 133–142 (2005)
4. Bonabeau, E., Dorigo, M., Theraulaz, G.: Swarm Intelligence: From Natural to Artificial Systems (No. 1). Oxford University Press, Oxford (1999)
5. Castillo, O.: Interval type-2 mamdani fuzzy systems for intelligent control. In: Trillas, E., Bonissone, P.P., Magdalena, L., Kacprzyk, J. (eds.) Combining Experimentation and Theory, pp. 163–177. Springer, Berlin (2012)
6. Castillo, O.: Type-2 Fuzzy Logic in Intelligent Control Applications, vol. 272. Springer, Heidelberg (2012)
7. Castillo, O., Neyoy, H., Soria, J., Garcia, M., Valdez, F.: Dynamic fuzzy logic parameter tuning for ACO and its application in the fuzzy logic control of an autonomous mobile robot. Int. J. Adv. Rob. Syst. **10**, 1–10 (2013)
8. Castillo, O., Martínez-Marroquín, R., Melin, P., Valdez, F., Soria, J.: Comparative study of bio-inspired algorithms applied to the optimization of type-1 and type-2 fuzzy controllers for an autonomous mobile robot. Inf. Sci. **192**, 19–38 (2012)
9. Chong, C.S., Sivakumar, A.I., Low, M.Y.H., Gay, K.L.: A bee colony optimization algorithm to job shop scheduling. In: Proceedings of the 38th Conference on Winter Simulation, pp. 1954–1961 (2006)
10. Martinez, R., Castillo, O., Aguilar, L.T.: Optimization of interval type-2 fuzzy logic controllers for a perturbed autonomous wheeled mobile robot using genetic algorithms. Inf. Sci. **179**(13), 2158–2174 (2009)
11. Melin, P., Olivas, F., Castillo, O., Valdez, F., Soria, J., Valdez, M.: Optimal design of fuzzy classification systems using PSO with dynamic parameter adaptation through fuzzy logic. Expert Syst. Appl. **40**(8), 3196–3206 (2013)
12. Mendel, J.M.: Uncertain Rule-Based Fuzzy Logic System: Introduction and New Directions. Practice Hall, New Jersey (2001)
13. Ochoa, P., Castillo, O., Soria, J.: Differential evolution with dynamic adaptation of parameters for the optimization of fuzzy controllers. In: Castillo, O., Melin, P., Pedrycz, W., Kacprzyk, J. (eds.) Recent Advances on Hybrid Approaches for Designing Intelligent Systems, pp. 275–288. Springer International Publishing (2014)
14. Sepúlveda, R., Rodriguez, A., Castillo, O.: A New Approach to Inference him in Type-2 fuzzy systems and its application to intelligent control, pp. 8–10, Tijuana, B.C. (2006)
15. Teodorović, D.: Swarm intelligence systems for transportation engineering: principles and applications. Transp. Res. Part C Emerg. Technol. **16**(6), 651–782 (2008)
16. Wang, T., Tong, S.C., Li, Y.M.: Robust adaptive fuzzy control for nonlinear system with dynamic uncertainties based on backstepping. Int. J. Innovative Comput. Inf. Control **5**(9), 2675–2688 (2009)
17. Zadeh, L.A.: The concept of a linguistic variable and its application to approximate reasoning—I. Inf. Sci. **8**(3), 199–249 (1975)
18. Zadeh, L.A.: Fuzzy sets. Inf. Control **8**(3), 338–353 (1965)
19. Zadeh, L.A.: The concept of a lingüistic variable and its application to approximate reasoning, part II. Inf. Sci. **8**, 301–357 (1975)

Time Series Prediction Using Ensembles of ANFIS Models with Particle Swarm Optimization of the Fuzzy Integrators

Jesus Soto[✉], Patricia Melin, and Oscar Castillo

Division of Graduates Studies and Research,
Tijuana Institute of Technology, Tijuana, Mexico
jesvega83@gmail.com, {pmelin, ocastillo}@tectijuana.mx

Abstract. This paper describes the Particle Swarm Optimization of the Fuzzy integrators in Ensembles of ANFIS (adaptive neuro-fuzzy inferences systems) models for the prediction time series. A chaotic system is considered in this work, which is the Mackey-Glass time series, that is generated from a model is in the form of differential equations. This benchmark time series is used to test of performance of the proposed optimization of the fuzzy integrators in ensemble architecture. We used interval type-2 and type-1 fuzzy systems to integrate the output (forecast) of each Ensemble of ANFIS models. Particle Swarm Optimization (PSO) was used for the optimization of membership function parameters of each fuzzy integrator. In the experiments we optimized Gaussian, Generalized Bell and Triangular membership functions parameters for each of the fuzzy integrators. Simulation results show the effectiveness of the proposed approach. Therefore, a comparison was made against another recent work to validate the performance of the proposed model.

Keywords: ANFIS · Ensemble learning · Fuzzy integrators · Particle swarm optimization

1 Introduction

Time series are usually analyzed to understand the past and to predict the future, enabling managers or policy makers to make properly informed decisions. Time series analysis quantifies the main features in data, such as the random variation.

These facts, combined with improved computing power, have made time series methods widely applicable in government, industry, and commerce. In most branches of science, engineering, and commerce, there are variables measured sequentially in time [1, 2]. For example, reserve banks record interest rates and exchange rates each day.

This paper reports the results of the simulations, in which the Mackey-Glass [3, 4] time series prediction using ensembles of ANFIS models with particle swarm optimization of the fuzzy integrators is achieved, where the results for each ANFIS are evaluated by the method of the root mean square error (RMSE).

The selection of the time series for the simulations was based on the fact that these time series are widely quoted in the literature by different researchers [5–8], which

© Springer International Publishing Switzerland 2015
G. Sidorov and S.N. Galicia-Haro (Eds.): MICAI 2015, Part I, LNAI 9413, pp. 472–483, 2015.
DOI: 10.1007/978-3-319-27060-9_39

allows comparing results with other approaches, such as neural networks and linear regression.

This paper is organized as follows: the next section briefly describes ensemble learning. Section 3 presents the ANFIS models architecture. Section 4 presents the Mackey-Glass time series that we used for the experiments. Section 5 presents a brief review of interval type-2 fuzzy systems. Section 6 presents the particle swarm optimization that we used to optimize the fuzzy integrators. Section 7 presents the proposed architecture for time series prediction. Section 8 presents the simulation results obtained from the experiments. The last section presents the conclusions of this work.

2 Ensemble Learning

The Ensemble consists of a learning paradigm where multiple component learners are trained for a same task, and the prediction of the component learners are combined for dealing with future instances [9]. Since an Ensemble is often more accurate than its component learners, such a paradigm has become a hot topic in recent years and has already been successfully applied to optical character recognition, face recognition, scientific image analysis, medical diagnosis and time series [10].

3 ANFIS Models

There have been proposed systems that have fully achieved the combination of fuzzy systems with neural networks, one of the most mentioned in the literature is the ANFIS (Adaptive Neuro Fuzzy Inference System) as referred to by Jang [5] (Fig. 1), which is a method for creating the rule base of a fuzzy system, using the backpropagation training algorithm from the data collection process. Its architecture is functionally equivalent to a fuzzy inference system of Takagi-Sugeno-Kang form.

The basic learning rule of ANFIS is the gradient descent backpropagation, which calculates the error rates (defined as the derivative of the squared error for each output node) recursively from the output to the input nodes.

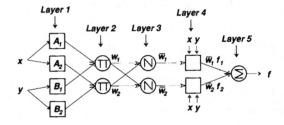

Fig. 1. ANFIS architecture.

4   Mackey-Glass Time Series

The problem of predicting future values of a time series has been a point of reference for many researchers. The aim is to use the values of the time series known at a point $x = t$ to predict the value of the series at some future point $x = t + P$. The standard method for this type of prediction is to create a mapping from D points of a Δ spaced time series, is $(x(t - (D - 1)\Delta)... x(t - \Delta), x(t))$, to a predicted future value $x(t + P)$. To allow a comparison with previous results in this work [5–8] the values $D = 4$ and $\Delta = P = 6$ were used.

The chaotic time series data that was used is defined by the Mackey-Glass [3, 4] time series, whose differential equation is given by Eq. (1):

$$x(t) = \frac{0.2x(t - \tau)}{1 - x^{10}(t - \tau)} - 0.1x(t - \tau) \tag{1}$$

For obtaining the values of the time series at each point, we can apply the Runge-Kutta method for the solution of Eq. (1). The integration step was set at 0.1, with initial condition $x(0) = 1.2$, $\tau = 17$, $x(t)$ is then obtained for $0 \le t \le 1200$, (Fig. 2) (We assume $x(t) = 0$ for $t < 0$ in the integration).

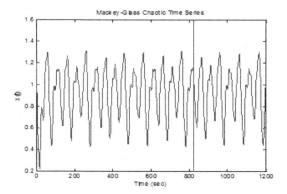

Fig. 2. The Mackey-Glass time series.

5   Interval Type-2 Fuzzy Logic Systems

Type-2 fuzzy sets are used to model uncertainty and imprecision; originally they were proposed by Zadeh [11, 12] and they are essentially "fuzzy–fuzzy" sets in which the membership degrees are type-1 fuzzy sets.

The basic structure of a type-2 fuzzy system (Fig. 3) implements a nonlinear mapping of input to output space. This mapping is achieved through a set of type-2 fuzzy if-then rules, each of which describes the local behavior of the mapping.

The uncertainty is represented by a region called footprint of uncertainty (FOU). When $\mu_{\tilde{A}}(x, u) = 1, \forall u \in l_x \subseteq [0, 1]$ we have an interval type-2 membership function.

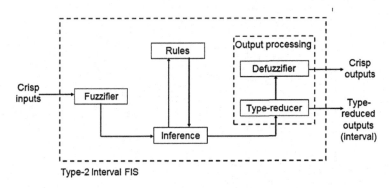

Fig. 3. Structure of the interval type-2 fuzzy logic system.

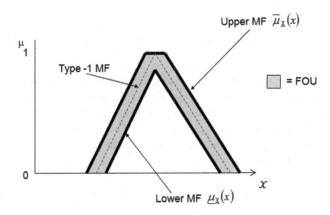

Fig. 4. Interval type-2 membership function.

The uniform shading for the FOU (Fig. 4) represents the entire interval type-2 fuzzy set and it can be described in terms of an upper membership function $\bar{\mu}_{\tilde{A}}(x)$ and a lower membership function $\underline{\mu}_{\tilde{A}}(x)$ [13].

A fuzzy logic systems (FLS) described using at least one type-2 fuzzy set is called a type-2 FLS. Type-1 FLSs are unable to directly handle rule uncertainties, because they use type-1 fuzzy sets that are certain [14]. On the other hand, type-2 FLSs are very useful in circumstances where it is difficult to determine an exact certainty value, and there are measurement uncertainties [15–17].

6   Particle Swarm Optimization (PSO)

Particle Swarm Optimization (PSO) is a metaheuristic search technique based on a population of particles (Fig. 5). The main idea of PSO comes from the social behavior of schools of fish and flocks of birds [18]. In PSO each particle moves in a D-dimensional space based on its own past experience and those of other particles.

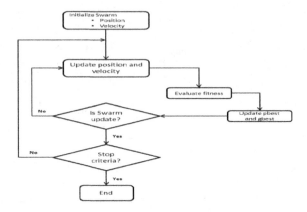

Fig. 5. Flowchart of the PSO algorithm.

Each particle has a position and a velocity represented by the vectors $x_i = (x_{i1}, x_{i2}, \ldots, x_{iD})$ and $V_i = (v_{i1}, v_{i2}, \ldots, v_{iD})$ for the i-th particle. At each iteration, particles are compared with each other to find the best particle [19, 20]. Each particle records its best position as $P_i = (p_{i1}, p_{i2}, \ldots, p_{iD})$. The best position of all particles in the swarm is called the global best, and is represented as $G = (G_1, G_2, \ldots, G_D)$. The velocity of each particle is given by Eq. (2).

$$V_{id} = wv_{id} + C_i \cdot rand_1() \cdot (pbest_{id} - x_{id}) + C_2 \cdot rand_2() \cdot (gbest - x_{id}) \qquad (2)$$

In this equation $i = 1, 2, \cdots, M, d = 1, 2, \cdots, D$, C_1 and C_2 are positive constants (known as acceleration constants), $rand_1()$ and $rand_2()$ are random numbers in [0,1], and w, introduced by Shi and Eberhart [21] is the inertia weight. The new position of the particle is determined by Eq. (3):

$$x_{id} = x_{id} + v_{id} \qquad (3)$$

7   Problem Statement and Proposed Method

The proposed general architecture combines the ensemble of ANFIS models and the use of interval type-2 and type-1 fuzzy systems as response integrators (Fig. 6) for time series prediction.

This architecture is divided into 5 sections, where the first phase represents the data base to simulate in the Ensemble of ANFIS, which in our case is the dataset of the

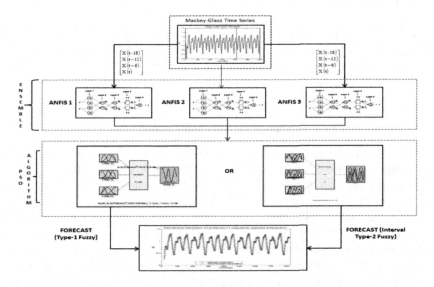

Fig. 6. Theproposed general architecture.

Mackey-Glass time series. From the Mackey-Glass time series we extracted the first 800 pairs of data points (Fig. 1), similar to [6–8].

We predict $x(t)$ from three past (delays) values of the time series, that is, $x(t-18)$, $x(t-12)$, and $x(t-6)$. Therefore the format of the training data is:

$$[x(t-18), x(t-12), x(t-6); x(t)] \tag{4}$$

Where $t = 19$ to 818 and $x(t)$ is the desired prediction of the time series.

In the second phase, training (the first 400 pairs of data are used to train the ANFIS) and validation (the second 400 pairs of data are used to validate the ANFIS models) is performed sequentially in each ANFIS model, where the number of ANFIS models to be used can be from 1 to n depending on what the user wants to test, but in our case we are dealing with a set of 3 ANFIS in the Ensemble. Therefore each ANFIS model used in the Ensemble training is formed differently, for example each of these ANFIS model uses different type of (Gaussian, triangular and Generalized Bell) MFs and different type of error goal [0.001,0.000001].

In the third phase we have to generate the results of each ANFIS used in the previous section and in the fourth phase we integrate the overall results of each ANFIS, such integration will be done by type-1 and interval type-2 fuzzy integrators of Mamdani type, but each fuzzy integrator is optimized with PSO in the membership functions. Finally the outcome or the final prediction of the Ensemble ANFIS learning is obtained.

8   Simulation Results

This section presents the results obtained through experiments on the architecture of genetic optimization of type-2 fuzzy integrators in ensembles of ANFIS models fortime series prediction, which show the performance that was obtained from each experiment to simulate the Mackey-Glass time series.

8.1   Design of the Fuzzy Inference Systems Integrators

The design of the type-1 and interval type-2 fuzzy inference systems integrators are of Mamdani type and have 3 inputs (ANFIS1, ANFIS2 and ANFIS3 predictions) and 1 output (Forecast), so each input is assigned two MFs with linguistic labels "Small and Large" and the output will be assigned 3 MFs with linguistic labels "OutANFIS1, OutANFIS2 and OutANFIS3" (Fig. 7) and have 8 rules if-then. The design of the if-then rules for the fuzzy inference system depends on the number of membership functions used in each input variable using the system (e.g. our fuzzy inference system uses 3 input variables which each entry contains two membership functions, therefore the total number of possible combinations for the fuzzy-rules is 8 (e.g. $2*2*2 = 8$)), therefore we used 8 fuzzy-rules for the experiments (Fig. 8) because the performance is better and minimized the prediction error of the Mackey-Glass time series.

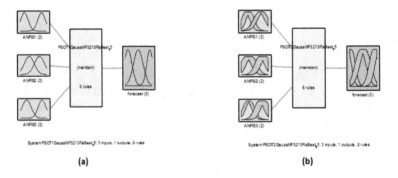

Fig. 7. Structure of the type-1 FIS (a) and interval tyep-2 FIS (b) integrators.

1. If (ANFIS1 is small) and (ANFIS2 is small) and (ANFIS3 is small) then (forecast is OutANFIS1) (1)
2. If (ANFIS1 is small) and (ANFIS2 is small) and (ANFIS3 is large) then (forecast is OutANFIS1) (1)
3. If (ANFIS1 is small) and (ANFIS2 is large) and (ANFIS3 is small) then (forecast is OutANFIS2) (1)
4. If (ANFIS1 is small) and (ANFIS2 is large) and (ANFIS3 is large) then (forecast is OutANFIS2) (1)
5. If (ANFIS1 is large) and (ANFIS2 is small) and (ANFIS3 is small) then (forecast is OutANFIS2) (1)
6. If (ANFIS1 is large) and (ANFIS2 is small) and (ANFIS3 is large) then (forecast is OutANFIS2) (1)
7. If (ANFIS1 is large) and (ANFIS2 is large) and (ANFIS3 is small) then (forecast is OutANFIS3) (1)
8. If (ANFIS1 is large) and (ANFIS2 is large) and (ANFIS3 is large) then (forecast is OutANFIS3) (1)

Fig. 8. If-then rules for the fuzzy integrators.

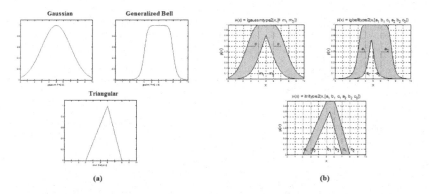

Fig. 9. Type-1 MFs (a) and interval type-2 MFs (b) for the fuzzy integrators.

In the type-1 FIS integrators we used different MFs (Gaussian, Generalized Bell, and Triangular) (Fig. 9(a)) and for the interval type-2 FIS integrators we used different MFs (igaussmtype2, igbelltype2 and itritype2) (Fig. 9(b)) [13] to observe the behavior of each of them and determine which one provides better forecast of the time series.

8.2 Design the Representation of the Particle Swarm Optimization

The PSO is used to optimize the parameters values of the MFs in each type-1 and interval type-2 fuzzy integrator. The representation in PSO is of Real-Values and the particle size will depend of the number of MFs that are used in each design of the fuzzy integrators.

The objective function is defined to minimize the prediction error as follows in Eq. (5):

$$f(t) = \sqrt{\frac{\sum_{t=1}^{n}(a_t - p_t)^2}{n}} \qquad (5)$$

Where a, corresponds to the real data of the time series, p corresponds to the output of each fuzzy integrators, t is de sequence time series, and n is the number of data points of time series.

The general representation of the particles represents the utilized membership functions. The number of parameters varies according to the kind of membership function of the type-1 fuzzy system (e.g. two parameter are needed to represent a Gaussian MF's are "sigma and mean") (Fig. 10(a)) and interval type-2 fuzzy system (e.g. three parameter are needed to represent "igaussmtype2" MF's are "sigma, mean1 and mean2") (Fig. 10(b)).

Therefore the number of parameters that each fuzzy inference system integrator has depends of the MFs type assigned to each input and output variables.

The parameters of particle swarm optimization used for optimizing the type-1 and interval type-2 fuzzy inference systems integrators are shown on Table 1.

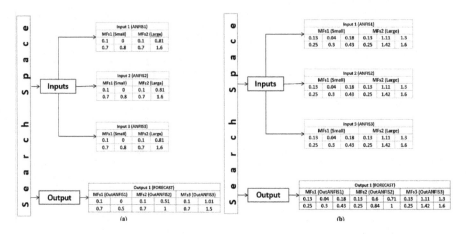

Fig. 10. Representation of the particles structure of the type-1 (a) and interval type (b) fuzzy integrators.

Table 1. Parameters of the particle swarm optimization

Parameters	Value
Particles	100
Iterations	65
Inertia Weight "ω"	Linear decrement [0.88–0]
Constriction "C"	Linear increment [0.01–0.9]
r1, r2	Random
c1	Linear decrement [2–0.5]
c2	Linear increment [0.5–2]

We performed experiments in time-series prediction, specifically for the Mackey-Glass time series in ensembles of ANFIS models using fuzzy integrators optimized with PSO.

The obtained results with the optimized type-1 fuzzy integrator (using Gaussian MFs) with particle swarm optimization are shown on Table 2. The best error is of 0.03154 and the average error is of 0.03848. The forecasts, evolution errors (for iteration), the membership functions and generated output surface were obtained for the optimized type-1 FIS integrator with PSO are shown (Fig. 11).

The obtained results with an optimized the interval type-2 fuzzy integrator (using igaussmtype2 MFs) and particle swarm optimization are shown on Table 2. The best error is of 0.01891 and the average error is of 0.01999. The forecasts, evolution errors (for iteration), the MFs and generated output surface were obtained for the optimized the interval type-2FIS integrator with PSO and are shown in Fig. 12.

In this proposal we can notice the accurate results in the prediction error of the time series Mackey-Glass. In Table 3 you can find the best results obtained by the proposed method and we also made a comparison with the proposed method by Gaxiola et al. [8].

Table 2. Resultsof the ensembles of ANFIS models using fuzzy integrators optimized with particle swarm optimization for the Mackey-Glass time series.

#	Iterations	Particles (Real)	Type-1 fuzzy integrator			Interval type-2 fuzzy integrator		
			Gaussian	Generalized bell	Triangular	igaussmtype2	igbelltype2	itritype2
1	65	100	0.03932	0.04397	0.10962	0.0194	0.02178	0.02413
2	65	100	0.04470	0.03669	0.10844	0.01971	0.02018	0.02057
3	65	100	0.03951	0.04897	0.10786	0.02051	0.02188	0.02458
4	65	100	0.03988	0.03484	0.11012	0.01942	0.02065	0.02337
5	65	100	0.03988	0.03484	0.11012	0.01942	0.02065	0.02337
6	65	100	0.03829	0.04585	0.10677	0.02062	0.02029	0.02338
7	65	100	0.03498	0.04027	0.10772	0.01947	0.0208	0.024
8	65	100	0.03667	0.05111	0.10625	0.01891	0.02081	0.02408
9	65	100	0.03154	0.04013	0.10798	0.02241	0.02021	0.0218
10	65	100	0.04003	0.04432	0.1073	0.02012	0.02007	0.02279

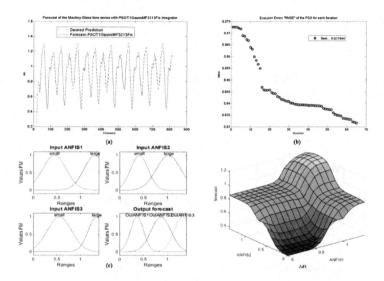

Fig. 11. The forecast time series (a), evolution error of "65 iterations" (b), inputs/output MFs (c) and surface output (d) are generated for the optimized of the type-1 FIS integrator with PSO.

Most of the results obtained by the proposed method are better than the results obtained in the work of Gaxiola et al. [8].

9   Conclusions

Time series prediction using ensembles of ANFIS models with particle swarm optimization of the fuzzy integrators was proposed. The best result with the optimized interval type-2 fuzzy inference systems (using igaussmtype2 MFs) integrator with particle swarm optimization for the Mackey-Glass time series is a prediction error of 0.01891 (as shown in Fig. 12 and Table 2). The type-1 fuzzy inference systems (using

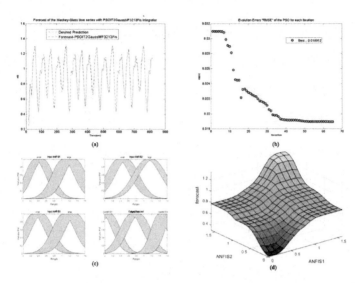

Fig. 12. The forecast time series (a), evolution error of "65 iterations" (b), inputs/output (c) and surface output (d) are generated for the optimized of the interval type-2 FIS integrator with PSO.

Table 3. Comparison of results with the method proposed by GaxiolaF. for the Mackey-Glass time series.

Method	Prediction error
Gaxiola et al. [8]	0.05061
Proposed method using Gaussian MFs	0.03154
Proposed method using G. Bell MFs	0.03484
Proposed method using igaussmtype2 MFs	0.01891
Proposed method using igbelltype2 MFs	0.02007
Proposed method using itritype2 MFs	0.02057

Gaussian MFs) were optimized with particles warm optimization obtaining a prediction error of 0.03154 (as shown in Fig. 11 and Table 2).

The proposed method presents better accuracy in almost all the experiments than the proposal by Gaxiola et al. [8] (as shown in Table 3).

These results showed efficient results in the prediction error of the time series Mackey-Glass generated by proposal method.

References

1. Brocklebank, J.C., Dickey, D.A.: SAS for Forecasting Series, pp. 6–140. SAS Institute Inc., Cary (2003)
2. Brockwell, P.D., Richard, A.D.: Introduction to Time Series and Forecasting, pp. 1–219. Springer, New York (2002)

3. Mackey, M.C., Glass, L.: Oscillation and chaos in physiological control systems. Science **197**, 287–289 (1997)
4. Mackey, M.C.: Mackey-Glass. McGill University, Canada. http://www.sholarpedia.org/-article/Mackey-Glass_equation, 5 September 2009
5. Jang, J.S.R.: ANFIS: adaptive-network-based fuzzy inference systems. IEEE Trans Syst. Man Cybern. **23**, 665–685 (1992)
6. Melin, P., Soto, J., Castillo, O., Soria, J.: A new approach for time series prediction using ensembles of ANFIS models. Expert Syst. Appl. **39**(3), 3494–3506 (2012)
7. Soto, J., Melin, P., Castillo, O.: Time series prediction using ensembles of ANFIS models with genetic optimization of interval type-2 and type-1 fuzzy integrators. Int. J. Hybrid Intell. Syst. **11**(3), 211–226 (2014)
8. Gaxiola, F., Melin, P., Valdez, F., Castillo, O.: Optimization of type-2 fuzzy weight for neural network using genetic algorithm and particle swarm optimization. In: World Congress on Nature and Biologically Inspired Computing (NaBIC), pp. 22–28, 12–14 August 2013
9. Sharkey, A.: Combining Artificial Neural Nets: Ensemble and Modular Multi-Net Systems. Springer, London (1999)
10. Sollich, P., Krogh, A.: Learning with ensembles: how over-fitting can be useful. In: Touretzky, D.S., Mozer, M.C., Hasselmo, M.E. (eds.) Advances in Neural Information Processing Systems 8, Denver, CO, pp. 190–196. MIT Press, Cambridge (1996)
11. Zadeh, L.A.: Fuzzy Logic. Computer **1**(4), 83–93 (1988)
12. Zadeh, L.A.: Fuzzy logic = computing with words. IEEE Trans. Fuzzy Syst. **4**(2), 103–111 (1996)
13. Castro, J.R., Castillo, O., Martínez, L.G.: Interval type-2 fuzzy logic toolbox. Eng. Lett. **15** (1), 89–98 (2007)
14. Castillo, O., Melin, P.: Optimization of type-2 fuzzy systems based on bio-inspired methods: A concise review. Inf. Sci. **205**(1), 1–19 (2012)
15. Mendel, J.M.: Why we need type-2 fuzzy logic systems. Article is provided courtesy of Prentice Hall, By Jerry Mendel, 11 May 2001
16. Mendel, J.M. (ed.): Uncertain Rule-based Fuzzy Logic Systems: Introduction and New Directions, pp. 25–200. Prentice Hall, Englewood Cliffs (2000)
17. Karnik, N.N., Mendel, J.M., Qilian, L.: Type-2 fuzzy logic systems. IEEE Trans. Fuzzy Syst. **7**(6), 643–658 (1999)
18. Kennedy, J., Eberhart, R.: Particle swarm optimization. IEEE International Conference on Neural Networks, Proceedings, vol. 4. pp. 1942–1948 (1995)
19. Parsopoulos, K.E., Vrahatis, M.N.: Particle Swarm Optimization Intelligence: Advances and Applications, pp. 18–40. Information Science Reference, New York (2010)
20. Shi, Y., Eberhart, R.: A modified particle swarm optimizer. In: Proceedings of the IEEE Congress on Evolutionary Computation, pp. 69–73 (1998)
21. Shi, Y., Eberhart, R.: Empirical study of particle swarm optimization. In: Proceedings of the IEEE Congress on Evolutionary Computation, pp. 1945–1950 (1999)

Machine Learning and Data Mining

Primary Clusters Selection Using Adaptive Algorithms

Shahrbanoo Ahmadi, Hamid Parvin$^{(\boxtimes)}$, and Farhad Rad

Department of Computer Engineering, Yasooj Branch,
Islamic Azad University, Yasooj, Iran
parvin@iust.ac.ir

Abstract. Data clustering means to partition the samples in similar clusters; so that each cluster's samples have maximum similarity with each other and have a maximum distance from the samples of other clusters. Due to the problem of unsupervised clustering selection of a specific algorithm for clustering a set of unknown data is involved in much risk, and we usually fail to find the best option. Because of the complexity of the issue and inefficacy of basic clustering methods, most studies have been directed toward combined clustering methods. We name output partition of a clustering algorithm as a result. Diversity of the results of an ensemble of basic clusterings is one of the most important factors that can affect the quality of the final result. The quality of those results is another factor that affects the quality of the final result. Both factors considered in recent research of combined clustering. We propose a new framework to improve the efficiency of combined clustering that is based on selection of a subset of primary clusters. Selection of a Proper subset has a crucial role in the performance of our method. The selection is done using intelligent methods. The main ideas of the proposed method for selecting a subset of the clusters are to use the clusters that are stable. This process is done by the intelligent search algorithms. To assess the clusters, stability criteria based on mutual information has been used. At last, the selected clusters are going to be aggregated by some consensus functions. Experimental results on several standard datasets show that the proposed method can effectively improve the complete ensemble method.

Keywords: Combined clustering · Cluster analysis · Mutual information · Genetic algorithm · Simulated annealing algorithm · Extended evidence accumulation clustering · Correlation matrix

1 Introduction

The main idea of information clustering, is to separate samples from each other and placing them in similar groups. This means that similar samples should be placed in a group and they should have the most differences with the samples from other groups [1, 2]. In fact, data clustering is an essential tool for finding groups with unlabeled data [3].

The next section is about the required background. The third part is about a brief review of activities in the field of combined clustering based on a subset of primary results. The proposed method for a combined clustering based on a subset of results has been described in the fourth Section. The fifth section is about interpretation of results.

© Springer International Publishing Switzerland 2015
G. Sidorov and S.N. Galicia-Haro (Eds.): MICAI 2015, Part I, LNAI 9413, pp. 487–498, 2015.
DOI: 10.1007/978-3-319-27060-9_40

The conclusion of this thesis has been collected in sixth section. Future work is going to be introduced in this section.

2 Background

In this section we are going to study the prerequisite data of this article.

2.1 Genetics Algorithm

Genetic algorithm is an approach that considers the natural evolution as a model [4]. This method is an imitation of development process using computer algorithms. The most basic principle of development is inheritance. Each generation inherits the characteristics of the previous generation and transfer it to the next generation. The characteristics transfer from one generation to the next, is done by our genes. The world which we live in is constantly changing. To survive in this dynamic system, people should be the able to fit themselves with environment. Fitness is determined that how much chances are there to survive and pass their genes to the next generation. In biological development, only winners can participate in the development process. Characteristics of all beings are coding in their genes, and during the process of inheritance, the genes transported to the Offspring.

2.2 Simulated Rolling

Simulated rolling is an optimization method that is similar to the process for metal heating and comfort cooling and this is the reason of its nomenclature [5]. At the end of the physical annealing process, the solid material is crystalline. In the optimization method, target function shows the thermodynamic process energy and optimum solution considered to be solid crystalline mode. The difference between this method and metal's heat process is that variable of basic local searching mode, searching process, will chose the best answer between the points that are in the neighborhood of the primary answer. If the best answer is not better than the original solution search process stops and the assumption is that the optimal solution is found. This method is effective for target functions that are simple and only has one point of local extreme (for minimum or maximum issues). For complex functions, for example, for minimizing problems, the optimal local point may be quietly different from general optimization and optimization model can't provide the optimal solution which is desired.

2.3 Combination of Clustering

Due to the most of basic clustering methods insist on specific features, so it works only on specific datasets. So we need the methods that can produce more optimum results, using combining the algorithm and catch their strong. In fact the main reason of combined clustering is to search better and stronger results using information combination and results of several primary clustering [3, 6]. Many studies have been done on the combination classification [7–9]. Combined clustering in this area has been considered the same as combined classification. Recent studies have shown that the clustering of data in this field can significantly benefit from the combination of several data partition. In addition, their parallel power has natural adaptation to the needs of distributed data mining. Combined clustering can has express better results in comparison with data methods in the term of, strong, novelty, stability and flexibility. In short, combined clustering has two main phases [1, 3]:

1. Produces different results from clustering, as primary results clustering based on different methods of the process, called phase variation or dispersion.
2. Combining results from different factions primary cluster for the final clustering which performed by the agreement function (combinatory algorithm).

3   Related Work

Combined clustering methods will try to produce a robust partitioning by combining different partitions which produced by basic clustering methods [3, 13, 14].

In the most recent studies, all partitions with equal weight are in the final combination, and all clusters in all partitions with equal weight are in the final combination [15]. Strehl and Ghosh [3] introduce a criterion for selecting between possible combinations based on the general quality of a cluster. For doing this they considered the stability within basic and combined partitions, and then they use a constant combined rule to have a pairwise similarity criterion on the D dimensional property area.

Azimi [16] used the concept of distribution to make combined clustering intelligent. This method dynamically select an optimum subset of results in the final composition, the simple combined clustering is done. Then this method is going to measure all the results of primary clustering and data, then tries to classified data in three levels: easy, normal and hard. In this classification, easier data collection is a data collection that the primary clustering is not such a different from obtained combined clustering. This means that a simple clustering can provide similar results about such combined clustering. This event indicates that the data set is quite a common border and a common simple method for clustering as complex and powerful combined clustering methods which are not able to isolate subjects. Then the results of all primary clustering divided into the four sub- clusters based on different factions of their carefully matched with a simple combination of clustering, each set of data categories (easy, normal and hard) are going to select one of these sub for the final result. Experimental results in [16] have also shown that the combination of primary clusters with the highest, the lowest, and the average degree of clustering will have better results in easy, hard and normal datasets. The method tries to remove the results of primary clustering. Another method that is closed to this one is Alizadeh's method [17], that all dataset sorted in the term of stability, the 33 % which are more stabled are going to be selected.

In the most of the basic algorithms, combined clustering for data sampling is going to be used. The main issue is how to evaluate clusters and clustering. In [18], authors presented a method based on resampling to investigate validation of fuzzy clustering.

In recent years, the stability of the cluster has been noticed as a cluster evaluation criterion [15, 19–21]. The initial ideas for cluster validating using resampling have been presented in [22] and have later completed in [23] and [24]. Ras and his assistants [25, 26] also, presented a method based on resampling to investigate validation of fuzzy clustering. The main element of this method that is the former completed method is the cluster stability. A stability criterion is going to measure the partitions' correlation from two independent samplings of a dataset. More stability for a cluster means that if we use clustering algorithm on samples more and more, similar results are going to be obtained [27, 28]. Also, Roth and Lange [29] presented a new algorithm for clustering that is based on the feature selecting. In this method they have used stability criterion based on data resampling, to select clustering algorithm parameters.

Some clustering validation methods have been presented based on using stability. Ben-Hur and partners [31] also provides a method for calculating the stability which based on the similarity between samples which act different in clustering. In this way, the correlation matrix obtained by using resampling. The Jaccard coefficient as a measure of stability is calculated based on the matrix. Also, Estivill-Castro and Yang [32] have presented a method for evaluating clustering partitions using Support Vector Machine (SVM). This method uses noise detection outliner data clustering to gain strength. Moller and Radke [33] use nearest neighbor resampling to validate the clustering results. This resampling method has been used in time series analysis the first time [34]. Inokuchi and partners [35] have proposed kernelized validity measure. In this method core means central function is used in support vector machine. In this method two functions have been considered: first one is total value of the fuzzy covariance in clusters, and second one is index based on Zhi-ben. In this method, two indices for evaluating the results of clustering and determining the number of clusters with non-linear boundaries have been used. Das and Sil [37] have presented a method for determining the number of clusters uses clusters validating to divide and merge them. Fern and Lin [38] have proposed a method for clustering combination that effectively subdivides the primary partitions used in the final combination. In this method, although the number of members participating in the final composition is less than a combination of clustering because of the selecting partitions with higher performance, the results will improve. The parameters considered in this study include: quality and distribution. This method tries to enter the partitions with the preliminary results into a final composition, which has the highest quality and also have the highest distribution. In this method, the measure of total normalized mutual information (for partitioning in comparison with other partitions) is used to measure the quality of a partition.

The normalized mutual information criterion (between all partitions in combination) is used to measure the distribution for the combination. Fern and Lin [38] show that their method in comparison with total combined clustering or random selection method has better performance. Law and others [19] have proposed a multi objective clustering method based on the selection of clusters generated by different algorithms for clustering, in an optimization routine. In this method, the best set of objective functions for the various sections of feature area is selected. Fred and Jain [15] have presented a mixed clustering, in which similarities between the two taught using the stability of the cluster criteria. In this method, instead of using evaluation criteria based on the final partition, partitions of fundamental algorithms in different parts of d-dimensional feature area is evaluated. In most of the above methods correlation matrix for the aggregation of primary clustering information is used. If several matrixes are present, there are various ways to produce the final correlation matrix using merge. Brossier [39] presented a method to merge multiple distance matrixes to a distance matrix. Necessary and sufficient condition for the integration process has been considered. Also Lapointe and Legendre [40] presented a method to produce random dandrogram. They have done this by associated cophenetic matrix. Each incoming $d_C(i, j)$ in the cophenetic matrix presented a level which xi and xj have met for the first time in a cluster [41]. Benfield [42] presented an algorithm to calculating distance for single connected dandrogram. This algorithm will catch a distance matrix from the entrance and minimum spanning tree is used. Distance in this algorithm is the maximum of chained connections which is going to connect any double dots of tree. In fact distances are levels from dandrogram that both of the dots are connected on that level.

3.1   Variety in Clustering

In the first stage of combined clustering, some clusters which emphasize on unique feature are going to be created. The first and simplest way to create and spread of a data set, is using different clustering algorithm. Each clustering algorithm will look at this problem with particular aspect. Thus, errors in different ways can be different. This can be cause variation in the results of basic clustering algorithms. The most important basic clustering algorithms that commonly used in combined clustering, are consist of: hierarchical algorithm [1, 10] and [43], and partitioned clustering algorithms [41, 43–45]. K-means algorithm is going to be used as basic clustering algorithm due to its simplicity and ability to fit in clusters. Another way to gain distribution is to have different results from a basic clustering method using one of these methods:

- Initialization for selected clustering algorithm [6]
- Change the selected parameters for clustering algorithm [49]
- Use the different subset of features [3, 11]
- Mapping data to another features area
- Divide main data to different subsets (resampling) [3, 46, 51]

3.2   Problems of Combined Clustering

A factor that is often used to improve the performance of combined clustering is the quality of primary results. It has been shown that the quality of the final clusters will be better if the primary results are in higher quality, as well as the required distribution [14]. Although Fern and Lin [38] have shown that simultaneous optimization of the distribution and quality in the primary results of combined clustering can significantly improve the efficiency of clustering, to compromise these two factors is a problem that is still facing many difficulties to be properly solved.

In this study, we tried to find a relatively optimized subset of the results of the primary clustering in order to be a part of the final composition and to improve the efficiency of combined clustering. For this purpose, a general framework is proposed.

3.3   Collector Function

After the preliminary results (with as much distribution as possible) are produced, these results are usually combined by using a combining function. One of the most common methods to combine the results is the correlation matrix which will be thoroughly discussed in Sects. 3–5. Extended evidence combined clustering method which is based on the correlation matrix has been introduced by Fred and Jain [6] for the first time and soon became popular. Today, other methods based on the correlation matrix have been proposed [12].

Strehl and Ghosh [3] have represented the concept of convention with the hyper-graph viewpoint. They proposed three methods based on Hyper-graph for consensus methods. They have converted data areas to a hyper-graph form in the first stage of all three consensus methods. In those hyper-graphs, clusters are known as hyper-edges and peaks are the data. Cluster-based Similarity Partitioning Algorithms can be used to separate the peaks or data points. Using minimum k cutting algorithm, k areas of this hyper-graph will be extracted. There are efficient heuristics in order to solve the problem of cutting the minimum k on a hyper-graph. Some of them have computational complexities of ($|\varepsilon|$) grade. ε represents the number of hyper-edges. Cluster-based Similarity Partitioning Algorithm (CSPA), Hyper-Graph Partitioning Algorithm (HGPA) and Meta-Clustering Algorithm (MCLA) will be discussed here.

- CSPA

In CSPA, the data points feature area is first mapped by feature area of hyper-graph correlation. Then a METIS-like minimum cutting hyper-graph algorithm is used on the recently interspaced points. As before, this method assumes that if the number of data points in a cluster in the primary partition increase, then it is more likely that those data points belong to a single cluster. CSPA is the simplest heuristic among hyper-graph-based methods. The calculation complexity is $O(kN^2M)$ in which k is the number of clusters, N is the number of points and M is the number of areas. The next two methods are of less computational complexity.

- HGPA

HGPA Algorithm assumes that peaks are the data points and clusters which have come out of the primary partition, are their hyper-edges. Now a METRIS-like minimum cutting hyper-graph algorithm is used on the hyper-graph in order to separate the peaks, the data points of the hyper-graph, into k components. The calculation complexity is $O(kNM)$ in which k is the number of clusters, N is the number of data points and M is the number of areas.

- MCLA

MCLA algorithm first separates the cluster obtained from the primary partition and then uses a mechanism based on polling in order to produce the partitions of the convention. Clustering has been performed by means of METIS. The calculation complexity is $O(k^2NM^2)$ in which the elements are as before. Refer to chapter [3] for more details on hyper-graph-based methods.

4 Framework of Proposed Procedure

The main idea of this method is to use a subset of primary clusters instead of all clusters in combined clustering. In this method, using the methods of development of distribution, B primary clustering is created. This can be done using data sampling, using different algorithms for clustering, using a subset of selected features or parameters for a clustering algorithm. K-means algorithm has been used here to generate primary results. The required distribution of primary results in K-means algorithm is obtained by random selection of primary points of the clusters' centers as well as sampling. In addition, a method for the production of the required distribution has been obtained from K-means with different K's. Then the normalized mutual information of each of the obtained clusters are calculated and put into a square matrix with all obtained clusters.

After stability was calculated for each cluster in comparison with other clusters, the next step is to choose the clusters in two subdivisions. In the first subdivision with the help of genetic algorithm a subset of the cluster is selected in a way that the selected clusters have together the greatest stability. In the second subdivision, to produce variability in the selected clusters, by means of genetic algorithm we choose those clusters which together have less stability. The suggested method for selecting clusters will be discussed in Sect. 4.2.

The next step is to combine the selected clusters and obtain the final clusters. There are different ways to combine the initial and acquire final clusters. The difference here is that in this method, of each initial clustering may exist only a number of clusters in the final convention. In this paper, the two methods suggested by Alizadeh [17] are used to combine the results of the basic clusters and to obtain the final clusters using the basic ones. These methods which can be used to generate the correlation matrix for the samples, when only a number of clusters are available, will be discussed in Sect. 4.3. After making the correlation matrix, we can obtain the final clusters using one of the hierarchical algorithms or hyper-graph-based methods.

Since combined clustering is a complicated process including several steps, its calculation is of high complexity and therefore it is a prolonged and offline process. Accordingly, there is little discussion on the computational complexity of the proposed methods in researches done in this area.

After finishing the calculation of the stability of each cluster, the next step is selection of clusters regarding their stability. A method based on evolutionary algorithms has been presented to selecting a subset of primary clusters which will be discussed in this section.

Selection of clusters is done in two phases. In phase 1, an evolutionary algorithm tries to find a subset of clusters with the most stability. This algorithm includes a bite-size chromosome with a length of the total number of produced clusters in different clustering production section. Each gene in this chromosome can take 1 or zero value. Value 1 shows that the respective cluster is among the selected clusters and value 0 in gene number m, shows that cluster number m is not among selected clusters. To assess the goodness function of this evolutionary algorithm, we calculate the difference between the stability of selected clusters' average and value 1(average of selected clusters has the maximum stability).

$$FitnessFunction = 1 - \sum_i \sum_j \frac{Similarity(C_i, C_j)}{Card.(SelectedClusters)^2} \tag{1}$$

$$, i,j \in SelectedClusters$$

Similarity (C_i, C_j) is calculated via the following equation:

$$Similarity(C_i, C_j) = NMI(P(C_i, D/C_i), P(C_j, D/C_j)) \tag{2}$$

In Eq. 2 $P(C_i, D|C_i)$ is a clustering including two clusters: C_i and $D|C_i$ (the cluster that includes all data except those of C_i). In phase 2, by means of an evolutionary algorithm a subset of the clusters is selected that has the least stability in order for the final selected clusters to be of more diversity. Here the evolutionary algorithm has one bite-size chromosome with a length of the total number of clusters. Goodness function for this algorithm is the amount of stability in selected clusters.

$$FitnessFunction = \sum_i \sum_j \frac{Similarity(C_i, C_j)}{Card.(SelectedClusters)^2} \tag{3}$$

$$, i,j \in SelectedClusters$$

It should be noted that in any case, our goal is to minimize the goodness function, therefore, whatsoever the smaller is the function, the higher will be the goodness of the set of clusters selected by chromosome. Here, the set selected by the first evolutionary algorithm is called S1 and the set selected by the second evolutionary algorithm is called S2.

5   Experiments

For a comparison between the results of the research methods at Iran University of Science and Technology, results of Table 1 have been presented with single linkage as a collecting function. As you can see in result, this method has better performance

Table 1. Comparison of the accuracy of proposed methods by the full assembly and former's

Data collection	Full Assembly	GA	SA	Alizadeh	Azimi
Wine	96.75	96.64	96.63	96.63	96.64
Breast-Cancer	97.04	95.3	95.18	95.74	95.92
BUPA	55.03	55.09	55.07	54.33	54.73
Galaxy	30.03	32.81	30.66	31.26	29.98
Glass	56.82	56.87	45.79	57.74	55.05
Half-Ring	76.39	74.5	74.5	74.47	67.69
Iris	89.6	89.33	89.33	89.33	89.33
Ionosphere	70.72	70.67	70.66	70.6	70.73
SA-Heart	63.43	63.29	63.27	63.37	56.06
Yeast	39.43	42.76	43.06	42.93	43.39
ALL	67.524	67.726	66.415	67.64	65.952

sometimes and as a whole. The reason of this work is the selected set by primary genetic algorithm is very stable and in fact it will show the simple clusters correctly. Also the second genetic algorithm will select the clusters which have most diversity and it will help the result diversity.

6 Conclusions

In this paper, a method has been proposed to improve the efficiency of combined clustering. This method is similar to previous works of Alizadeh's and Azimi's is based on the use of a subset of results. To select a subset of the initial results, we need to define the measurement criteria and in this research, NMI criterion has been used.

Experimental results on 10 datasets show the effectiveness of standard on 10 datasets in comparison with other ensemble clustering. Also results shows, although only a small amount of the preliminary results of the proposed methods are employed in the ensemble, the performance of these methods can be even improved in comparison with the complete ensemble. Edited normalized mutual information methods, in combination with ITOU (Intersection TO Union) to build the co-association matrix, indicates the most improvement in results. This improvement is tested on all 10 tested set of full ensemble method in comparison with Azimi and Alizadeh method. We can do some other works after this research such as: more searching to represent the criteria for evaluating a cluster or a partitioning of the data. If we find a criterion or a set of criteria to evaluate the clusters, without considering the clusters or data type, intelligent search methods can be employed using them. Also we can use boosting and bagging methods in production level. There are several ways in the combination of classifiers to produce diversity. By using them we can we can select more diverse classifiers. We can use these methods for ensemble clustering.

References

1. Jain, A., Murty, M.N., Flynn, P.: Data clustering: a review. ACM Comput. Surv. **31**(3), 264–323 (1999)
2. Faceli, K., Marcilio, C.P., Souto, D.: Multi-objective clustering ensemble. In: Proceedings of the Sixth International Conference on Hybrid Intelligent Systems (HIS 2006) (2006)
3. Strehl, A., Ghosh, J.: Cluster ensembles - a knowledge reuse framework for combining multiple partitions. J. Mach. Learn. Res. **3**(Dec), 583–617 (2002)
4. Melanie, M.: An Introduction to Genetic Algorithms. The MIT Press, Cambridge (1999). (A Bradford Book, Fifth printing)
5. Aarts, E.H.L., Korst, J.: Simulated Annealing and Boltzmann Machines. Wiley, Essex (1989)
6. Fred, A., Jain, A.K.: Data clustering using evidence accumulation. In: Proceedings of the 16th International Conference on Pattern Recognition, ICPR 2002, Quebec City, pp. 276–280 (2002)
7. Parvin, H., Alizadeh, H. Minaei-Bidgoli, B.: A new method for constructing classifier ensembles. Int. J. Digit. Content Technol. Appl. JDCTA (2009). ISSN 1975-9339

8. Parvin H., Alizadeh, H., Minaei-Bidgoli, B.: Using clustering for generating diversity in classifier ensemble. Int. J. Digit. Content Technol. Appl. JDCTA, **3**(1), 51–57 (2009). ISSN 1975-9339

9. Alizadeh H., Minaei-Bidgoli, B., Amirgholipour, S.K.: A new method for improving the performance of k nearest neighbor using clustering technique. Int. J. Convergence Inf. Technol. JCIT (2009). ISSN 1975-9320

10. Topchy, A., Jain, A.K., Punch, W.F.: Combining multiple weak clusterings. In: Proceedings of the 3d IEEE International Conference on Data Mining, pp. 331–338 (2003)

11. Fred, A., Lourenco, A.: Cluster ensemble methods: from single clusterings to combined solutions. In: Studies in Computational Intelligence (SCI), vol. 126, 3–30 (2008)

12. Ayad, H.G., Kamel, M.S.: Cumulative voting consensus method for partitions with a variable number of clusters. IEEE Trans. Pattern Anal. Mach. Intell. **30**(1), 160–173 (2008)

13. Fred, A.L., Jain, A.K.: Combining multiple clusterings using evidence accumulation. IEEE Trans. Pattern Anal. Mach. Intell. **27**(6), 835–850 (2005)

14. Kuncheva ,L.I., Hadjitodorov, S.: Using diversity in cluster ensembles. In Proceedings of the IEEE International Conference on Systems, Man and Cybernetics, pp. 1214–1219 (2004)

15. Fred, A., Jain, A.K.: Learning pairwise similarity for data clustering. In: Proceedings of the 18th International Conference on Pattern Recognition (ICPR 2006) (2006)

16. Azimi, J.: (1386), To study the distribution of the compound clustering, thesis, University of Science and Technology, June

17. Alizadeh H., (1387), clustering-based combination subset of the initial results, Master Thesis, Department of Computer Engineering, University of Science and Technology, March

18. Baumgartner, R., Somorjai, R., Summers, R., Richter, W., Ryner, L., Jarmasz, M.: Resampling as a cluster validation technique in fMRI. J. Magn. Reson. Imaging **11**, 228–231 (2000)

19. Law, M.H.C., Topchy, A.P., Jain, A.K.: Multiobjective data clustering. In: Proceedings of the IEEE Conference on Computer Vision and Pattern Recognition, vol. 2, pp. 424–430, Washington D.C. (2004)

20. Shamiry, O., Tishby, N.: Cluster stability for finite samples. In: 21st Annual Conference on Neural Information Processing Systems (NIPS 2007) (2007)

21. Lange, T., Braun, M.L., Roth V., Buhmann, J.M.: Stability-based model selection. In: Advances in Neural Information Processing Systems 15. MIT Press, Cambridge (2003)

22. Breckenridge, J.: Replicating cluster analysis: Method, consistency and validity. Multivar. Behav. Res. (1989)

23. Fridlyand, J., Dudoit, S.: Applications of resampling methods to estimate the number of clusters and to improve the accuracy of a clustering method. Statistics Berkeley Tech Report no. 600 (2001)

24. Levine, E., Domany, E.: Resampling method for unsupervised estimation of cluster validity. Neural Comput. **13**, 2573–2593 (2001)

25. Roth, V., Lange T., Braun, M., Buhmann, J.: A resampling approach to cluster validation. In: International Conference on Computational Statistics, COMPSTAT (2002)

26. Roth, V., Braun, M.L., Lange, T., Buhmann, J.M.: Stability-based model order selection in clustering with applications to gene expression data. In: Dorronsoro, J.R. (ed.) ICANN 2002. LNCS, vol. 2415, pp. 607–612. Springer, Heidelberg (2002)

27. Rakhlin, A., Caponnetto, A.: Stability of k-means clustering. In: Advances in Neural Information Processing Systems 19. MIT Press, Cambridge (2007)

28. Luxburg, U.V., Ben-David, S.: Towards a statistical theory of clustering. Technical report, PASCAL Workshop on Clustering, London (2005)

29. Roth, V., Lange, T.: Feature selection in clustering problems. In: Advances in Neural Information Processing Systems, NIPS 2004 (2004)
30. Lange, T., Roth, V., Braun, M.L., Buhmann, J.M.: Stability-based validation of clustering solutions. Neural Comput. 16(6), 1299–1323 (2004)
31. Ben-Hur, A., Elisseeff, A., Guyon, I.: A stability based method for discovering structure in clustered data. In: Pasific Symposium on Biocomputing, vol. 7, pp. 6–17 (2002)
32. Estivill-Castro, V., Yang, J.: Cluster Validity Using Support Vector Machines. In: Kambayashi, Y., Mohania, M., Wöß, W. (eds.) DaWaK 2003. LNCS, vol. 2737, pp. 244–256. Springer, Heidelberg (2003)
33. Moller, U., Radke, D.: A cluster validity approach based on nearest-neighbor resampling. In: Proceedings of the 18th International. Conference on Pattern Recognition (ICPR 2006) (2006)
34. Brandsma, T., Buishand, T.A.: Simulation of extreme precipitation in the Rhine basin by nearest-neighbour resampling. Hydrol. Earth Syst. Sci. 2, 195–209 (1998)
35. Inokuchi, R., Nakamura, T., Miyamoto, S.: Kernelized cluster validity measures and application to evaluation of different clustering algorithms. In: Proceedings of the IEEE International Conference on Fuzzy Systems, Canada, 16–21 July 2006
36. Xie, X.L., Beni, G.: A validity measure for fuzzy clustering. IEEE Trans. Pattern Anal. Mach. Intell. 13(4), 841–846 (1991)
37. Das, A.K., Sil, J.: Cluster validation using splitting and merging technique. In: Proceedings of International Conference on Computational Intelligence and Multimedia Applications, ICCIMA (2007)
38. Fern, X., Lin, W.: Cluster ensemble selection. In: SIAM International Conference on Data Mining (SDM 2008) (2008)
39. Brossier, G.: Piecewise hierarchical clustering. J. Classif. 7(2), 197–216 (1990)
40. Lapointe, F.J., Legendre, P.: The generation of random ultrametric matrices representing dendrograms. J. Classif. 8(2), 177–200 (1991)
41. Jain, A.K., Dubes, R.C.: Algorithms for Clustering Data. Prentice Hall, Englewood Cliffs (1988)
42. Banfield, C.F.: Ultrametric distances for a single linkage dendrogram. JSTOR: Appl. Stat. Stat. Algorithms 25(3), 313–315 (1976)
43. Duda, R.O., Hart, P.E., Stork, D.G.: Pattern Classification, 2nd edn. Wiley, New York (2001)
44. Kaufman, L., Rosseeuw, P.J.: Finding Groups in Data: An Introduction to Cluster Analysis. Wiley, New York (1990)
45. Man, Y., Gath, I.: Detection and separation of ring-shaped clusters using fuzzy clusters. IEEE Trans. Pattern Anal. Mach. Intel. 16(8), 855–861 (1994)
46. Minaei-Bidgoli, B., Topchy, A., Punch, W.F.: Ensembles of partitions via data resampling. In: Proceedings of International Conference on Information Technology, ITCC 04, Las Vegas
47. Alizadeh, H., Amirgholipour, S.K., Seyedaghaee, N.R., Minaei-Bidgoli, B.: Nearest cluster ensemble (NCE): clustering ensemble based approach for improving the performance of k-nearest neighbor algorithm. In: 11th Conference of the International Federation of Classification Societies, IFCS09, 13–18 Mar 2009
48. Mohammadi, M., Alizadeh, H., Minaei-Bidgoli, B.: Neural network ensembles using clustering ensemble and genetic algorithm. In: International Conference on Convergence and Hybrid Information Technology, ICCIT08, IEEE CS, 11–13 Nov 2008
49. Barthelemy, J.P., Leclerc, B.: The median procedure for partition. In: Cox, I.J. et al. (eds.) Partitioning Data Sets. AMS DIMACS Series in Discrete Mathematics, vol. 19, pp. 3–34 (1995)

50. Fern, X. Brodley, C.E.: Random projection for high dimensional data clustering: a cluster ensemble approach. In: Proceedings of the 20th International Conference on Machine Learning, ICML (2003)
51. Dudoit, S., Fridlyand, J.: Bagging to improve the accuracy of a clustering procedure. Bioinformatics **19**(9), 1090–1099 (2003)
52. Fischer, B., Buhmann, J.M.: Bagging for path-based clustering. IEEE Trans. Pattern Anal. Mach. Intell. 1411–1415 (2003)
53. Fred, A., Jain, A.K.: Robust data clustering. In: Proceedings of the IEEE Computer Society Conference on Computer Vision and Pattern Recognition, CVPR, vol. II, pp. 128–136 USA (2003)
54. Kuncheva, L.I., Whitaker, C.J.: Measures of diversity in classifier ensembles. Mach. Learn. (2003)
55. Newman, C.B.D.J., Hettich, S., Merz, C.: UCI repository of machine learning databases (1998). http://www.ics.uci.edu/~mlearn/MLSummary.html

A Multi-agent Ensemble of Classifiers

Jaime Calderón, Omar López-Ortega[✉], and Félix Agustín Castro-Espinoza

Área Académica de Sistemas Computacionales,
Universidad Autónoma del Estado de Hidalgo, Carretera Pachuca-Tulancingo,
km. 4.5, C. U., 42084 Pachuca, Hidalgo, Mexico
jaime@hotmail.es, lopezo@uaeh.edu.mx, fcastroe@gmail.com

Abstract. It is well-known that every classifier method or algorithm, being Multi-Layer Perceptrons, Decisions Trees or the like, are heavily dependent on data. That is to say, their performance varies significantly whether training data is balanced or not, multi-class or binary, or if classes are defined by numeric or symbolic variables. Some unwanted issues arise, for example, classifiers might be over-trained, or they could present bias or variance, all of which lead to poor performance. The classifiers performance can be analyzed by metrics such as specificity, sensitivity, F-Measure, or the area under the ROC curve. Ensembles of Classifiers are proposed as a means to improve classifications tasks. Classical approaches include Boosting, Bagging and Stacking. However, they do not present cooperation among the base classifiers to achieve a superior global performance. For example, it is desirable that individual classifiers are able to communicate each other what tuples are classified correctly and which are not so errors are not duplicated. We propose an Ensemble of Classifiers that relies on a cooperation mechanism to iteratively improve the performance of both, base classifiers and ensemble. Information Fusion is used to reach a decision. The ensemble is implemented as a Multi-Agent System (MAS), programmed on the JADE platform. The base classifiers are taken from WEKA, as well as the calculation of the performance metrics. We prove the ensemble with a real dataset that is unbalanced, multi-class, and high-dimensional, obtained from a psychoacoustics study.

Keywords: Classifiers ensemble · Multi-agent systems · Information fusion · Cooperation

1 Introduction

One of the most common data mining tasks consists in assigning a set of inputs to a given class or classes, for which it is required a statistical model representing a mapping from input data (normally described by several attributes) to the appropriate category. This model approximates the true mapping from inputs to outputs. A decision of to which category a new, unseen input belongs, can be reached [11].

© Springer International Publishing Switzerland 2015
G. Sidorov and S.N. Galicia-Haro (Eds.): MICAI 2015, Part I, LNAI 9413, pp. 499–508, 2015.
DOI: 10.1007/978-3-319-27060-9_41

Classification focuses on methods that establish a dependency within data, concentrating on the so-called target attribute [1]. Classification algorithms are intended for modeling the dependency between input attributes and the target attribute. Each object $\mathbf{x}$ is described by its attributes, which in turn define the value of the target attribute $\mathbf{Y}$. Thus, the dataset D from which the model is constructed consists of a finite set of tuples such as $D = \{(x_i, Y_i),\ i = 1 \cdots n\}$. If the target attribute Y possesses nominal values, we are dealing with a classification problem. If the target attribute is described by continuous numeric values, we face a regression problem. Along this text we employ the term *classification* referring to both tasks, and *classifier* to the algorithm that computes *classification*.

However, the usage of a single classifier might not be the best decision to complete a classification task because its performance is affected by several factors i.e. the initial parameters of the algorithm, the distribution of the training dataset, risk of overtraining, among others. This provokes that the arrival of new objects that do not match the statistical model decreases the performance of the classifier. These problems are aggravated when classifiers learn from real datasets, where the distribution of input objects might be unbalanced.

The performance of classifiers is quantified by using the confusion matrix and derived metrics such as the F-Measure and the area under the ROC curve. The F-Measure is used in multi-class problems, while the area under the ROC curve serves only for binary problems. The Weka platform implements the method proposed by Mann Whitney [15] to compute the area of the ROC curve.

It is thought that Ensembles of Classifiers (EoC) have better performance than single classifiers because they benefit from diversity. In an EoC the final conclusion is obtained by aggregating individual decisions. Information fusion is largely employed to that end. As reported in [11] the concept of EoC's has been studied at large: Stacking [4], bagging [2], boosting [5], model averaging and forecast combining are classic methods to form ensembles. A survey of Ensembles of Classifiers can be found in [17].

The main challenges regarding EoC's consist in finding a procedure to employ base classifiers and rules to combine their individual solutions. One of the essential requirements to form ensembles is that two base classifiers do not make the same mistakes on new input data. That is to say, the errors made by the individual predictors must be uncorrelated. For example, if the final solution is obtained by simple majority voting, and if it is assumed that the mistakes made by the classifiers are independent, then the ensemble will misclassify a new input object only if more than half the base classifiers make mistakes. This situation in highly unlikely in heterogeneous EoC.

Thus, the design of EoC's should include a set of base classifiers so the ensemble yields the highest possible performance [13]. To increase the efficiency of the EoC it has been suggested that each base classifier learn from a subset of the original dataset, without duplicating training subsets [7].

We explore the multi-agent paradigm to form ensembles of classifiers. We call this approach a Multi-Agent Ensemble of Classifiers (MAEoC). A software agent is a computer system that is situated in some environment and possesses a strong notion of agency (self-directed behavior). That is to say, an agent is capable of performing autonomous actions within an environment [14, 16]. A Multi-Agent System (MAS) consists of agents that respond to changes in the environment and interact with other agents by using a communication language, such as the Agent communication Language (ACL).

MAS are suitable for building dynamic ensembles of classifiers: It is feasible to develop an environment with a number of *classifier agents* where each of them performs its duties (a classification task), communicate to other agents its results (what instances where correctly and incorrectly classified), and learn from what other *classifier agents* do well. Classifier agents complement each other. To the best of the authors' knowledge, MAEoC constitute a novel approach to designing Ensembles of Classifiers.

In Sect. 2 we describe the main notions to form EoC with MAS. We test our MASEoC on a demanding classification task: To determine to which emotional tag some well-defined input parameters used to create fractal music belong. The dataset for this task is described in Sect. 3. The experimental results and comparisons with other types of ensembles is given is Sect. 4. We apply our MAEoC to assist in the creation of musical fragments. Conclusions and a roadmap leading to improvements are delineated in Sect. 5.

2   The Multi-agent Ensemble of Classifiers

The algorithm we propose to form an Ensemble of Classifiers relies on two premises: (i) the performance of base classifiers and (ii) the communication of hits (H) and failures (F) obtained by base classifiers. The steps of the algorithm are outlined next:

1. At time t = 0
   - Coordinator agent recruits m classifiers, $m > 2$, and launches m classifier agents.
   - Coordinator agent broadcasts dataset D to classifier agent$_i$, $\forall i, i \cdots m$.
   - Classifier agent$_i$ performs a ten fold cross-validation. F-Measure$_i$ is calculated.
   - Classifier agent$_i$, $\forall i, i \cdots m$, informs Coordinator Agent two subsets. Subset H_i contains objects correctly classified; subset F_i contains objects incorrectly classified.
2. At time t = 1
   - Coordinator agent forms two aggregated sets: AH and AF. $AH = \cup H_i$; $AF = \cup F_i$.
   - Coordinator agent launches classifier$_{m+1}$, based on the highest F-Measure$_i$ obtained at $t = 0$.
   - Classifier$_{m+1}$ is trained with set AF. Model M_{m+1} is added to the ensemble. F-Measure C_{m+1} is obtained by ten fold cross validation on AF.
   - Classifiers$_{1\cdots m}$ are trained with set AH. Models $M_{1\cdots m}$ are added to the ensemble. F-Measures$_{1\cdots m}$ are obtained by ten fold cross-validation on AH.

3. At time t = 2
   - Classifiers$_{1...m+1}$ are given weights according to their updated F-Measure at $t = 1$.
   - Weighted voting is used to reach a final conclusion.

To validate our EoC, we perform a classification task whose objective is to assign an input object x_{input} to one of the sixteen emotional tags of Russell's Circumplex Model of Affect [12]. Input object x_{input} possesses attributes to create fractal music as described in [9]. Target attribute Y is the emotional tag.

3   The Psychoacoustics Dataset

To test our ensemble we employ a psychoacoustic dataset, which contains the emotional responses to fractal music, as reported in [8]. It is a challenging dataset because:

- It is a multi-class dataset. There are sixteen different emotions as values of the target variable.
- It is an unbalanced dataset.
- It is a high-dimension dataset. Each object x_i is defined by fifteen attributes, on which fractal musical fragments are created.
- Each object x_i is defined by mixed attributes i.e. nominal and numeric values.
- The target attribute Y_i is an emotional tag associated to each object x_i.

Thus, $D = \{(x_i, Y_i), i = 1 \cdots n\}$ contains diverse combinations of input parameters, and the corresponding emotional tag. Input parameters refer to the chaotic system i.e. Lorenz equations, and musical parameters.

The Lorenz equations [10] are defined by variables x, y, and z, which represent the initial values of the attractor. In this case such variables represent initial notes. Variables *sigma*, r and b help determine the actual trajectory. Table 1 displays the range of values that were used to compute the Lorenz attractor (as a generator of melodic sequences).

To complete the creation of musical fragments, musical parameters are paired with the sequence yielded b the Lorenz equations. Musical parameters are: Tempos, Notes Durations, Musical Scales, Chords and Instruments.

Values for variable Tempo are in the interval (60, 220) beats per minute. Notes Durations are tied to Tempos, so they are expressed in values such as whole duration (1), half duration (1/2), a quarter (1/4), and so on. For the present study, Notes Durations lie between 1/16 and 1. Instruments are: (i) Grand Piano, Bright Acoustic and Harpsichord; (ii) Acoustic Guitar, Steel String Guitar;

Table 1. Range of Lorenz Parameters

Lorenz Parameters					
x	y	z	sigma	r	b
[0,127]			[-200, 200]		

Table 2. Sample of the psychoacoustics dataset

Instrument	Scale	Chord	TempoX	TempoY	TempoZ	DuraX	DuraY	DuraZ	x	y	z	sigma	r	b	Emotion
Piano	PGMayor	none	145	145	150	0.1	0.12	0.2	12	15	16	4	23	2	Happiness
Piano	CNMenor	major	140	165	150	0.125	0.1	0.25	23	56	16	4	23	2	Sadness
Distortion Guitar	PGMayor	none	125	135	145	0.125	0.115	0.13	23	34	67	4	8	7	Stress
Guitar Harmonics	PEMenor	none	187	180	199	0.175	0.195	0.145	63	40	77	30	57	11	Excitation
PizzicatoStrings	PCMenor	none	187	180	199	0.205	0.275	0.345	65	41	79	40	23	115	At ease
Overdriven Gtr	GAMenorr	major	255	255	255	1	1	1	80	119	90	43	14	37	Stress
String ensemble	PGMenor	major	255	255	255	0.125	0.13	0.12	67	65	68	100	100	100	Euphoria
Electric Muted Gtr	PEMenor	diminished	255	255	255	0.132	0.137	0.131	12	120	92	200	200	200	Astonishment
StringEnsemble	PGMayor	none	124	124	124	0.55	0.5	0.45	15	15	15	-10	-10	-10	Droopiness
Piano	PEMenor	minor	90	90	90	0.065	0.065	0.065	12	100	45	-3	3	-3	Satisfied
Overdriven Gtr	PGMenor	add9	80	80	80	0.125	0.125	0.125	120	12	24	-65	-65	-65	Tiredness
Piano	BMelMinor	none	60	60	60	.125	.125	.125	23	45	78	-100	-100	-100	At ease
Bright Acoustic	CMelMinor	Minor	60	60	60	.125	.125	.125	67	10	9	-100	-100	-100	At ease
Bright Acoustic	CMelMinor	Minor	60	60	60	.125	.125	.125	67	10	9	-100	-100	-100	Tiredness
Piano	GBlues	Major	220	220	220	0.125	0.125	0.125	61	9	3	-150	-150	-150	Euphoria
Cello	CBlues	Minor	140	140	140	0.125	0.125	0.125	2	2	2	150	150	150	Anger

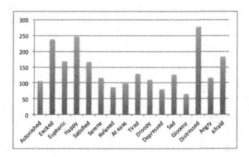

Fig. 1. Distribution of evaluations by emotional label

(iii) Electric Clean Guitar, Electric Jazz Guitar, Guitar Harmonics, Distorted Guitar, Overdriven Guitar, Electric Muted Guitar; (iv) Violin, Viola, Cello, Tremolo, Pizzicato, Orchestral Strings, String Ensembles; and Acoustic Bass, Electric Bass Finger, Electric Bass Pick, Fretless Bass, Slap Basses, Contrabass.

The Chord variable accepts the following values: Mayor chords; Minor chords; Augmented chords; Diminished Chords; Other chords, and No chords. Musical Scales are: Pentatonic Scales; Harmonic Scales; Natural Scales; Blues Scales; Melodic Scales; No scale.

Some $(x_i, Y_i) \in D$ are shown in Table 2. Altogether, dataset D contains 2312 objects at the time of performing the experiments. Figure 1 illustrates the distribution of objects by emotional label.

4   Experimental Results

The proposed algorithm is implemented on the JADE platform [3]. Classifiers and performance measures are obtained from Weka [6]. The psychoacoustics dataset is stored on a relational database implemented in the MySQL database management system. We now present the experimental results. To do so, we follow the steps of the proposed algorithm (see Sect. 2).

The Multi-Agent Ensemble of Classifiers (MAEoC) is composed of the following base classifiers C_i: (i) Naive Bayes, (ii) k-Nearest Neighbors, $k = 5$,

Table 3. Performance of the EoC vs other techniques

C_i	C_{it0}	Bagging	Boosting	Stacking Meta Ci	Oversampling	Undersampling	C_{it1}
NB	0.129	0.13	0.129	0.15	0.146	0.105	0.181
5-NN	0.201	0.201	0.201	0.167	0.305	0.154	0.277
J48	0.161	0.164	0.161	0.151	0.273	0.146	0.236
SVM	0.183	0.184	0.183	0.189	0.243	0.157	0.248
MLP	0.191	0.199	0.191	0.171	0.261	0.156	0.253
MAEoC 0.337							

(iii) Decision Tree J48, (iv) Support Vector Machine, and (v) Multi-Layer Perceptron. This ensemble ensures diversity of algorithms. The main results are summarized in Table 3.

Firstly, the F-Measure was quantified for each classifier C_i when they were trained with original dataset D. These results are presented in column C_{it0}.

A second experiment consisted in forming ensembles using bagging, boosting, and stacking on every classifier C_i.

Since dataset D is unbalanced, we modify it via Oversampling and Undersampling. Then each classifier C_i was trained with those modified datasets. The F-Measures are given in columns Oversampling and Undersampling, respectively.

We also present how the MAEoC behaves at time $t = 1$. Column C_{it1} shows the F-Measure when base classifiers C_i are trained with dataset AH. We urge reader to remember that AH is the aggregated dataset of the objects correctly classified.

Finally, the performance of the MAEoC is given.

The performance of the MAEoC can be observed in Figs. 2 and 3.

We normalized the performances based on the highest F-Measure obtained when the base classifiers were trained with original dataset D. In this experiment, that honor corresponds to k-Nearest Neighbors, $k = 5$. F-Measure = 0.201

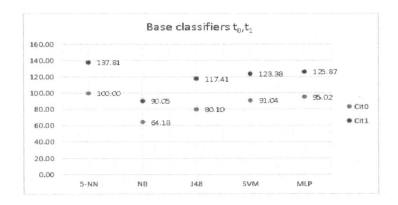

Fig. 2. Performance of classifiers at $t = 0$ and $t = 1$ (Color figure online)

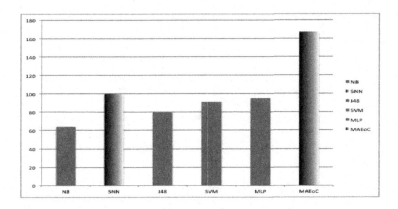

Fig. 3. Performance of base classifiers vs MAEoC

corresponds to a baseline of 100. In Fig. 2 the blue dots correspond to the normalized F-Measure obtained by the base classifiers when they were trained with the original dataset D. Thus, it can be seen that the Naive - Bayes classifier (NB) has a performance 36 % worse than 5-NN. Conversely, The red dots reflect the normalized F-Measure when the base classifiers were trained with dataset AH, that is to say, the aggregated set of correctly classified instances. Based on this data, we support our claim that communicating hits and fails is a way of reducing the influence of the data distribution in the creation of its statistical model.

Figure 3 presents a comparison of the F-Measures obtained at t = 0 and the final F-Measure obtained with the MAEoC, which improved in the order of 67 %.

4.1   Application to Computer-Assisted Creativity

The application to Computer-Assisted Creativity is presented in the following screenshots. As one of the applications of the MAEoC, we use it to help a creative subject to know what emotions will most likely be evoked by the parameters s/he enters in order to create a musical fragment. The MAEoC is used as follows. Once the MAEoC is launched, the training phase begins. This is show in Fig. 4. As stated before, dataset D contains the emotional responses to fractal music obtained in a psychoacoustics study [8]. In the let frame of the screenshot the communication among classifier agents and coordinator agent is shown.

As soon as the MAEoC is trained, the final weights are given to each classifier. This includes the classifier $m + 1$ contemplated as part of the algorithm. These results are show in Fig. 5.

When the voting weights are assigned to the classifiers, the MAEoC is ready to classify new objects. This is illustrated in Fig. 6. Variables x, y, and z are the initial values of the Lorenz attractor. Variables $sigma$, r, and b define its trajec-

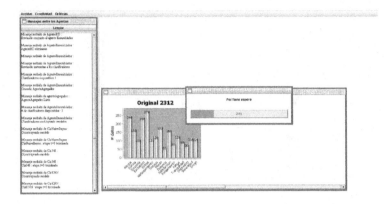

Fig. 4. Training of the MAEoC

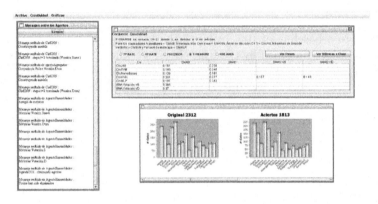

Fig. 5. Voting weights obtained by the members of the ensemble

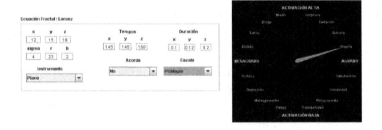

Fig. 6. Example 1. Classification of a new input object

tory. The remaining of the variables refer to the musical parameters necessary to create a musical fragment: Instrument (Instrumento) is Piano; Chord (acorde) is null; Musical Scales (Escala) is set to be G Major Pentatonic. Variables Tempo and Notes Durations defined the rhythm of the musical fragment. The MAEoC classifies this new input object X_i belongs to the class of objects that evoke *happiness* (alegría).

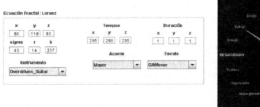
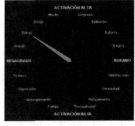

Fig. 7. Example 2. Classification of a new input object

If that were the creative subject's intention, then those input parameters would be used to render musical fragments; otherwise, the creative subject would be free to change their values. Figure 7 shows a different input object. The MAEoC determines that it belongs to the class of objects that provoke *Distress* (estres).

When the MAEoC is incorporated into a system that creates music, it guides the creative subject in her/his endeavor. The MAEoC classifies newly input values into one of the sixteen classes of the CMoA, preventing the creative subject from doing educated guesses.

5 Conclusions and Future Work

We propose a Multi-Agent Ensemble of Classifiers (MAEoC). The algorithm employed to construct and exploit such ensemble is based on the dynamic calculation of a performance measure, communication, and information fusion. We tested our proposal on a demanding classification tasks: determine the most likely emotional tag based on a number of musical and fractal parameters on which a musical fragment is created. A psychoacoustics dataset is used as training source. We also compared he MAEoC with aggregation techniques (bagging, boosting, stacking), and with data manipulation techniques (undersampling and oversampling). On our experiments the MAEoC obtained the highest F-Measure.

Future work includes development of different versions of the algorithm. For instance, we can proposed a version where objects in subset AH are weighted according to the number of classifiers that predicted them correctly. We will test the MAEoC with different datasets, taken mostly from the UCI repository. We will continue acquiring data regarding the emotional responses, and train the MAEoC with upgraded versions of the dataset.

References

1. Berthold, M.R., Borgelt, C., Hoppner, F., Klawonn, F.: Guide to Intelligent Data Analysis, 1st edn. Springer, London (2010)
2. Breiman, L.: Bagging predictors. Mach. Learning **24**, 123–140 (1996)

3. Caire, F.L.B.G., Greenwood, D.: Developing Multi-Agent Systems with JADE. Wiley, New York (2007)
4. Dzeroski, S., Zenko, B.: Is combining classifiers with stacking better than selecting the best one? Mach. Learning **54**, 255–273 (2004)
5. Freund, Y., Saphire, R.: Experiments with a new Boosting algorithm. In: Proceedings of the Thirteen International Conference on Machine Learning, pp. 148–156 (1996)
6. Holmes, G., Donkin, A., Witten, I.: Weka: a machine learning workbench. In: Proceedings of the Second Australia and New Zealand Conference on Intelligent Information Systems, Brisbane, Australia (1994)
7. Kheradpisheh, S.R., Sharifizadeh, F., Nowzari-Dalini, A., Ganjtabesh, M., Ebrahimpour, R.: Mixture of feature specified experts. Inf. Fusion **9**, 4–20 (2014)
8. Lopez-Ortega, O., Franco-Arcega, A.: Analysis of psychoacoustic responses to digital music for enhancing autonomous creative systems. Appl. Acoust. **89**, 320–332 (2015)
9. López-Ortega, O., López-Popa, S.I.: Fractals, fuzzy logic and expert systems to assist in the construction of musical pieces. Expert Syst. Appl. **39**, 11911–11923 (2012)
10. Lorenz, E.N.: Deterministic non-periodic flow. Atmos. Sci. **20**, 130–141 (1963)
11. Oza, N.C., Tumer, K.: Classifier ensembles: select real-world applications. Inf. Fusion **9**, 4–20 (2008)
12. Russell, J.A.: A circumflex model of affect. J. Pers. Soc. Psychol. **39**, 1161–1178 (1980)
13. Ruta, D., Gabrys, B.: Classifier selection for majority voting. Inf. Fusion **6**, 63–81 (2005)
14. Weiss, G.: Multiagent Systems. A Modern Approach to Distributed Artificial Intelligence, 1st edn. The MIT Press, Cambridge (1999)
15. Witten, I., Frank, E., Hall, M.: Data mining. Practical Machine Learning tools and Techniques, 3rd edn. Morgan Kaufmann, San Francisco (2011)
16. Wooldridge, M.: An Introduction to MultiAgent Systems, 2nd edn. Wiley, New York (2009)
17. Wozniak, M., Grana, M., Corchado, E.: A survey of multiple classifier systems as hybrid systems. Inf. Fusion **16**, 3–17 (2014)

A Classifier Ensemble Enriched
with Unsupervised Learning

Mehdi Hamzeh-Khani[1], Hamid Parvin[1,2(✉)], and Farhad Rad[1]

[1] Department of Computer Engineering, Yasuj Branch,
Islamic Azad University, Yasuj, Iran
`parvin@iust.ac.ir`
[2] Young Researchers and Elite Club, Nourabad Mamasani Branch,
Islamic Azad University, Nourabad, Mamasani, Iran

Abstract. A novel methodology has been suggested to automatically recognize mine in SONAR data. The suggested framework employs a possibilistic ensemble method to classify SONAR instances as mine or mine-like object. The suggested algorithm minimizes an objective function that merges background identification, multi-algorithm fusion criteria and a learning term. The optimization wants to discover backgrounds as solid clusters in subspaces of the high-dimensional feature-space via a possibilistic semi-supervised learning and feature discrimination. The proposed clustering element allocates a degree of typicality to each data instance in order to recognize and decrease the power of noise instances and outliers. After that the approach results in optimal fusion parameters for each background. The trials on artificial datasets and standard SONAR dataset show that our proposed ensemble does better than individual classifiers and unsupervised local fusion.

Keywords: Unsupervised learning · Ensemble learning · Classifier fusion

1 Introduction

Classifiers ensemble has nowadays emerged as successful methods that assume complementary information yields more accurate decisions. In other words, if the Classifiers collaborate, combined results would take advantage of the strengths of the individual Classifiers, and decrease the impact of their errors in order to improve the ultimate classification performance. A host of models have been suggested for classifier ensembles. Most of them count on the hypothesis that classifiers are not dependent to each other. This hypothesis hardly ever holds, and the opinions of several classifiers are highly likely to be dependent in reality. A fuzzy optimization to partition the feature space has been adopted for classifier ensembles [1].

In the current paper, we suggest a possibilistic local methodology that adjusts multi-classifier ensemble to diverse areas of the feature space. The suggested methodology begins by placing the training samples into a set of dissimilar groups. This stage is a difficult optimization problem that is prone to local optimum. To resolve this problem we introduce a semi-supervised learning term in the proposed objective function [2]. This grouping procedure allocates a possibilistic membership, characterizing the grade

© Springer International Publishing Switzerland 2015
G. Sidorov and S.N. Galicia-Haro (Eds.): MICAI 2015, Part I, LNAI 9413, pp. 509–517, 2015.
DOI: 10.1007/978-3-319-27060-9_42

of typicality, to each instance in order to recognize and decrease the power of noisy instances and outliers [6]. Furthermore a classifier is employed for each group. These classifiers determine the best classifiers for the related context (group). After that the weights are approximated by the combining component for each classifier. Each weight reveals the performance of the classifier in its context. Finally, for a test instance, the fusion of the individual confidence values is attained using the aggregation weights allocated with the closest context.

2 Proposed Method

Let $T = \{t_j | j = 1, \ldots N\}$ be the preferred output of N training instances. These outputs are obtained using K classifiers. Each classifier k uses its own feature set $X_k = \{x_j^k | j = 1 \ldots N\}$ and creates the confidence values $Y_k = \{y_j^k | j = 1 \ldots N\}$. The K feature sets are then concatenated to produce one global descriptor, $\chi = \bigcup_{k=1}^{K} \chi^k = \{x_j = [x_j^1, \ldots, x_j^K] | j = 1, \ldots, N]\}$. The possibilistic context extraction for local fusion algorithm has been formulated as partitioning the instances into C groups minimizing an objective function. However, this grouping approach requires the estimation of various parameters using complex optimization and is prone to local optimum. To overcome this drawback, we suggest a semi-supervised version of the algorithm in [6]. The supervision information relies on two sets of pairwise constraints. The first one is *Should-link (SL)* ones which specify the instance pairs that are expected to belong to the same cluster. The second set of constraints is the *ShouldNot-link (NL)* which specifies that the instance pairs that are expected to belong to dissimilar clusters. Let SL be the set of SL pairs of instances. If a pair (X_i, X_j) belongs to SL, then X_i and X_j are expected to be assigned to the same cluster. Similarly, let NL be the set of NL pairs. If a pair (X_i, X_j) belongs to NL, then X_i and X_j are expected to be assigned to different clusters. We reformulate the problem of discovering the C clusters as a constrained optimization problem as follows.

$$
J = \sum_{j=1}^{N} \sum_{i=1}^{C} u_{ij}^m \sum_{k=1}^{K} v_{ik}^q d_{ijk}^2 + \sum_{j=1}^{N} \sum_{i=1}^{C} \beta_i u_{ij}^m \left(\sum_{k=1}^{K} \omega_{ik} y_{kj} - t_3 \right)^2 + \sum_{i=1}^{C} \eta_i \sum_{j=1}^{N} (1 - u_{ij})^m
$$

$$
+ \mu \left[\sum_{(X_t, X_k \in NL)} \sum_{i=1}^{C} u_{ij}^m u_{kj}^m + \sum_{(X_t, X_k \in SL)} \sum_{i=1}^{C} \sum_{p=1, p \neq i}^{C} u_{ij}^m u_{kj}^m \right]
$$

(1)

subject to $\sum_{i=1}^{C} u_{ij} = 1 \forall j, u_{ij} \in [0, 1] \forall i, j,$

$\sum_{k=1}^{K} v_{ik} = 1 \forall i, v_{ik} \in [0, 1], \sum_{k=1}^{K} \omega_{ik} = 1 \forall i.$

In (1), u_{ji} represents the possibilistic membership of X_j in cluster i [6]. The $C \times N$ matrix, $U = [u_{ij}]$ is named a possibilistic partition if it satisfies:

$$\begin{cases} u_{ij} \in [0,1], \forall j \\ 0 < \sum_{i=1}^{C} u_{ij} < N, \forall i, j \end{cases} \quad (2)$$

On the other hand, the $C \times d$ matrix of feature subset weight, $V = [v_{ik}]$ satisfies

$$\begin{cases} v_{ik} \in [0,1], \forall i, k \\ \sum_{k=1}^{K} v_{ij} = 1, \forall i \end{cases} \quad (3)$$

The first term in (1) corresponds to the objective function of the SCAD algorithm [7]. It aims to categorize the N instances into C clusters centered in c_i such that each sample x_j is assigned to all clusters with fuzzy membership degrees. Also, it is intended to simultaneously optimize the feature relevance weights with respect to each cluster. SCAD term is minimized when a partition of C compact clusters with minimum sum of intra-cluster distances is discovered. The second term in (1) intends to learn cluster-dependent aggregation weights of the K algorithm outputs. ω_{ik} is the aggregation weight assigned to classifier k within cluster i. This term is minimized when the aggregated partial output values match the desired output. The third term in (1) yields the generation of the possibilistic memberships u_{ji} which represent the degrees of typicality of each data point within every cluster, and reduce the effect of outliers on the learning process. In (1), $m \in [1, \infty)$ is called the fuzzier, and η_i are positive constants that control the importance of the third term with respect to the first/second one. This term is minimized when u_{ij} are close to 1, thus, avoiding the trivial solution of the first term (where $u_{ij} = 0$). Note that $\sum_{i=1}^{C} u_{ij}$ is not constrained to be 1. In fact, instances that are not representative of any cluster will have $\sum_{i=1}^{C} u_{ij}$ close to zero and will be considered as noise. This constraint relaxation overcomes the disadvantage of the constrained fuzzy membership approach which is the high sensitivity to noise and outliers. The parameter η_i is related to the resolution parameter in the potential function and the deterministic annealing approaches. A point X_j will have little influence on the estimates of the model parameters of a cluster if $\sum_{k=1}^{K} v_{ik}^2 \left(d_{ijk}^s\right)^2$ is large when compared with η_i. On the other hand, the "fuzzier" m determines the rate of decay of the membership value. When $m = 1$, the memberships are crisp. When $m \to \infty$, the membership function does not decay to zero at all. In this possibilistic approach, increasing values of m represents increased possibility of all points in the data set completely belonging to a given cluster. The last term in (1) represents the cost of violating the pairwise *SL*, and *NL* constraints. These penalty terms are weighted by the membership values of the instances that violate the constraints. In other words, typical instances of the cluster which have high memberships yield larger penalty term. The value of μ controls the importance of the supervision information compared to the other terms.

The performance of this algorithm relies on the value of β. Overrating it results in the domination of the multi-algorithm fusion criteria which yields non-compact clusters. Also, underestimating β decreases the impact of the proposed method and increases the effect on the distances in the feature space. When appropriate β is chosen, the algorithm yields compact and homogeneous clusters and optimal aggregation weights for each algorithm within each cluster. Minimizing J with respect to U yields the following necessary condition to update u_{ij}:

$$u_{ij} = \frac{1}{1 - \left(\frac{D_{ij}^2}{\eta_i}\right)^{\frac{1}{m-1}}} \tag{4}$$

where

$$D_{ij} = \sum_{k=1}^{K} v_{ik}^q d_{ijk}^2 + \beta_i \sum_{k=1}^{K} v_{ik}^q \left(\sum_{l=1}^{K} \omega_{il} y_{lj} - t_j\right)^2 + \mu \left[\sum_{(X_t, X_k \in NL)} u_{kj}^m + \sum_{(X_t, X_k \in SL)} \sum_{p=1, p \neq i}^{C} u_{kp}^m \right] \tag{5}$$

D_{ij} represents the total cost when we consider instance X_j in cluster i. As it can be seen, this cost depends on the distance between point X_j and the cluster's centroid c_i, the cost of violating the pairwise *SL*, and *NL* constraints (weighted by μ), and the deviation of the combined algorithms' decision from the desired output (weighted by β). More specifically, instances to be assigned to the same cluster: (*i*) are close to each other in the feature space, and (*ii*) their confidence values could be combined linearly with the same coefficients to match the desired output. Minimizing J with respect to the feature weights

$$v_{ik} = \sum_{t=1}^{K} \left[(D_{ik}^2 / D_{il}^2)^{\frac{1}{q-1}} \right] \tag{6}$$

where $D_{il} = \sum_{j=1}^{N} u_{ij}^m d_{ijl}^2$. Minimization of J with respect to the prototype parameters, and the aggregation weights yields

$$c_{ik} = \frac{\sum_{j=1}^{N} u_{ij}^m X_{ik}}{\sum_{j=1}^{N} u_{ij}^m} \tag{7}$$

where

$$w_{ik} = \frac{\sum_{j=1}^{N} u_{ij}^m y_{kj} \left(t_j - \sum_{\substack{l=1 \\ l \neq k}}^{K} \omega_{il} y_{lj} \right) - \zeta_i}{\sum_{j=1}^{N} u_{ij}^m y_{kj}^2} \tag{8}$$

where ζ_i is a multiplier that assures the constraint (2) is satisfied, and is defined as

$$\zeta_i = \frac{\sum_{k=1}^{K} \left(\sum_{j=1}^{N} u_{ij}^m y_{lj} \left(t_j - \sum_{k=1}^{K} \omega_{ik} y_{kj} \right) \right) \left(\sum_{j=1}^{N} u_{ij}^m y_{lj}^2 \right)^{-1}}{\sum_{l=1}^{K} \left(\sum_{j=1}^{N} u_{ij}^m y_{lj}^2 \right)^{-1}} \tag{9}$$

The obtained iterative algorithm starts with an initial partition and alternates between the update equations of u_{ij}; v_{ik}; w_{ik} and c_{ik} as shown in Fig. 1.

Inputs: *X: The data instances.*
Y: The confidences obtained using the different classifiers.
NL: The set of ShouldNot-Link constraints.
SL: The set of Should-Link constraints.
T: The labels of the data instances.
C: The number of clusters.
m: The fuzzyfier.
q: The exponent of the feature weights.
T: The labels of the data instances.
β: The weight assigned to the second term of the objective function (1).
η: The weight assigned to the third term of the objective function (1).
Outputs: *U: The possibilistic membership matrix of the data instances.*
c_i: The Clusters centers.
V : The feature weights.
W: The aggregation weights.
Begin
Initialize the centers;
Initialize the possibilistic partition matrix U;
Initialize the relevance weights;
Repeat
Compute d_{ijk}^2, for $1 \leq i \leq C$ and $1 \leq j \leq N$ and $1 \leq k \leq K$;
Update the relevance weights v_{ik} using equation (6);
Compute D_{ij}^2
Update the partition matrix U using equation (4);
Update the aggregation weights matrix W and the feature
weights matrix and V matrix using equations (8) and (6), respectively;
Update the centers using equation (7);
Until (centers stabilize)
End

Fig. 1. The proposed semi-supervised possibilistic clustering.

The time complexity of one iteration of this first component is $O(N \times d \times K \times C)$, where N is the number of data points, C is the number of clusters, d is the dimensionality of the feature space, and K is the number of feature subsets. The computational complexity of one iteration of other typical clustering algorithms (e.g. FCM [4], PCM [5]) is $O(N \times d \times C)$. Since we use small number of feature subsets ($K = 3$), one iteration of our algorithm has a comparable time complexity to other similar algorithms. However, we should note that since we optimize for more parameters, it may require a larger number of iterations to converge.

After training the algorithm described above, the proposed local fusion approach adopts the steps below in order to generate the final decision for test samples:

1. Run the different classifiers on the test sample within the corresponding feature subset space, and obtain the decision values, $Y^j = \{y_{kj}|k = 1, \ldots .k\}$.
2. The unlabeled test sample inherits the class label of the nearest training sample.
3. Assign the membership degrees u_{ij} to test sample j in each cluster i using Eq. (4).
4. Aggregate the output of the different classifiers within each cluster using

$$\hat{y}_{ij} \sum_{k=1}^{K} w_{ik} y_{kj}.$$

5. The final decision confidence is estimated using $\hat{y} = \sum_{i=1}^{C} u_{ij} \hat{y}_{ij}$.

The flowchart in Fig. 1 describes the proposed method.

3   Experiments

We illustrate the performance of the proposed algorithm using synthetic datasets. For these datasets, we compare our approach to individual classifiers.

In this experiment, we illustrate the need for semi-supervised possibilistic local fusion. We use our approach to classify the synthetic 2-dimensional dataset in Fig. 2 (Left). Let each sample be processed by two single algorithms (K-Nearest Neighbors (K-NN) with $K = 3$). Each algorithm, k, considers one feature X_k; and assigns one

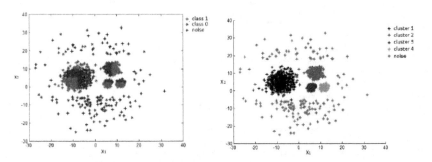

Fig. 2. Synthetic 2-dimensional dataset. Class 0 samples are shown as blue dots and class 1 samples are shown as red dots (Left). Clustering results of the synthetic data using the method in [3]. Magenta points correspond to the identified noise samples (threshold = 0.1) (Right) (Color figure online).

output value y_k. As shown in Fig. 2 (Left), samples from Class 0 are represented using blue dots and samples from Class 1 are displayed in red. Black samples represent noise samples. The dataset consists of four clusters. Each of them is a set of instances from the two classes. In Fig. 2, we show the clustering result of this dataset using possibilistic clustering and feature weighting algorithm [8]. As it can be seen, points assigned low memberships (< 0.1) with respect to all clusters (i.e. noise points) are shown in magenta.

Figure 3 shows the classification results obtained using individual learners. As one can notice, both learners fail to optimally categorize the data, and their accuracies are 69 % and 81 %, for learner 1 and learner 2, respectively. The accuracy of each learner depends on its region of feature space. More specifically, Fig. 3(a) illustrates how learner 1 classifies correctly most of the instances in the top right ellipsoidal cluster. However, it achieves 48 % accuracy on the three spherical clusters. Also, learner 1 performs better for the top right ellipsoidal cluster as shown in Fig. 3(b). This example proves the need for local fusion approach combine strengths of the classifiers in different regions of the feature space. In order to construct the set pairwise constraints, we randomly select samples that are at the boundary of each cluster. We consider 7 % of the total number of instances as *SL* and *NL* sets. Pairs of instances belonging to the

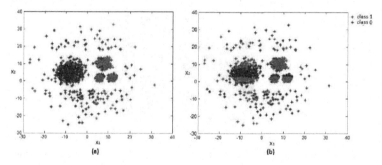

Fig. 3. Classification result of (a) the first algorithm (based on feature x_1). (b) the second algorithm (based on feature x_2).

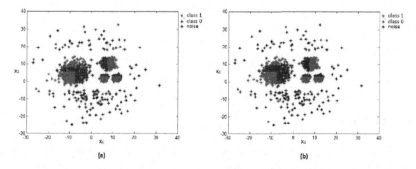

Fig. 4. Local possibilistic fusion results (threshold = 0.1) using (a) method in [6] and (b) the proposed semi-supervised approach with 7 % pairwise constraints

same cluster (based the ground truth) form the *SL* set. Similarly, pairs that belong to different clusters form the *NL* set. The results obtained using the unsupervised local fusion approach (with a threshold = 0.1) in [6] and the proposed approach are shown in Fig. 4. As it can be seen in Fig. 4(b), the supervision information has improved the overall performance compared to the method in [6].

We use the accuracy as performance measure to evaluate the performance of our semi-supervised method. The overall accuracy of the partition is computed as the average of the individual class rates weighted by the class cardinality. To take into account the sensitivity of the algorithm to the initial parameters, we run the algorithm 10 times using different random initializations. Then, we compute the average accuracy values for each supervision rate. As it can be seen in Fig. 5, the accuracy increased at a much lower rate with supervision rate larger than 7 %. Thus, for the rest of the experiments we set the supervision rate used to guide our clustering algorithm to 7 %. We compare the obtained average accuracy, precision, recall, and F-measure values obtained using individual K-NN learners, the method in [6], and the proposed method with the SONAR dataset in Table 1. Our semi-supervised approach outperforms other classifiers on this dataset based on the four performance measures.

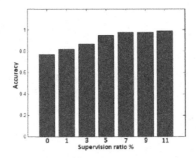

Fig. 5. Accuracy of our method on dataset in Fig. 2 varying supervision rate.

Table 1. Performance comparison of the learners for SOANR dataset.

	Accuracy	Precision	Recall	F-measure
1NN	82.69	76.80	88.03	82.03
2NN	84.16	79.72	88.42	83.84
3NN	85.11	81.42	88.08	84.61
[6]	86.04	86.36	84.31	85.32
Our Approach	90.24	90.90	89.47	90.17

4 Conclusion

In this paper we have proposed a novel approach in ensemble learning. This approach consists in a semi-supervised local fusion algorithm which categorizes the feature space into homogeneous clusters, learns optimal aggregation weights for individual classifiers and optimal fusion parameters for each context in a semi supervised manner. The experiments have shown that the semi-supervised fusion approach yields more accurate classification than the unsupervised version in [6] and the individual classifiers on synthetic and real datasets.

References

1. Frigui, H., Zhang, L., Gader, P.D., Ho, D.: Context-dependent fusion for landmine detection with ground penetrating radar. In: Prooceedings of the SPIE Conference on Detection and Remediation Technologies for Mines and Minelike Targets, FL, USA (2007)
2. Lange, T., Law, M., Jain, A., Buhmann, J.: Learning with constrained and unlabelled data. In: IEEE Computer Society Conference on Computer Vision and Pattern Recognition, 2005. CVPR 2005, vol. 1, pp. 731– 738 (2005)
3. Aridgides, T., Fernandez, M., Dobeck, G.J.: Volterra fusion of processing strings for automated sea mine classification in shallow water. In: Proceedings of the SPIE 5794 (2005)
4. Ji, C., Ma, S.: ombined Weak Classifiers, in Advances in Neural Information Processing Systems. MIT Press, Cambridge (1997)
5. Kuncheva, L.I.: Switching between selection and fusion in combining classifiers: an experiment. IEEE Trans. Syst. Man CYbern.-Part B $32(2)$, 146–156 (2002)
6. Ben Ismail, M.M., Bchir, O.: Insult detection in social network comments using possibilistic based fusion approach. In: Lee, Roger (ed.) CIS 2015. Studies in Computational Intelligence, vol. 566, pp. 15–25. Springer, Switzerland (2015)
7. Frigui, H., Nasraoui, O.: Unsupervised learning of prototypes and attribute weights. Pattern Recogn. J. 37, 567–581 (2004)
8. Ben Ismail, M.M., Bchir, O., Emam, A.Z.: Endoscopy video summarization based on unsupervised learning and feature discrimination. In: IEEE Visual Communications and Image Processing. VCIP 2013, Malaysia (2013)

Mining Unstructured Data via Computational Intelligence

Angel Kuri-Morales[✉]

Instituto Tecnológico Autónomo de México, Río Hondo No. 1,
01000 México, D.F., Mexico
akuri@itam.mx

Abstract. At present very large volumes of information are being regularly produced in the world. Most of this information is unstructured, lacking the properties usually expected from, for instance, relational databases. One of the more interesting issues in computer science is how, if possible, may we achieve data mining on such unstructured data. Intuitively, its analysis has been attempted by devising schemes to identify patterns and trends through means such as statistical pattern learning. The basic problem of this approach is that the user has to decide, a priori, the model of the patterns and, furthermore, the way in which they are to be found in the data. This is true regardless of the kind of data, be it textual, musical, financial or otherwise. In this paper we explore an alternative paradigm in which raw data is categorized by analyzing a large corpus from which a set of categories and the different instances in each category are determined, resulting in a structured database. Then each of the instances is mapped into a numerical value which preserves the underlying patterns. This is done using a genetic algorithm and a set of multi-layer perceptron networks. Every categorical instance is then replaced by the adequate numerical code. The resulting numerical database may be tackled with the usual clustering algorithms. We hypothesize that any unstructured data set may be approached in this fashion. In this work we exemplify with a textual database and apply our method to characterize texts by different authors and present experimental evidence that the resulting databases yield clustering results which permit authorship identification from raw textual data.

Keywords: Data bases · Neural networks · Genetic algorithms · Categorical encoding

1 Introduction

The problem of analyzing large sets of unstructured data sets has grown in importance over the last years. As of April 2014 there was an estimated 958,919,789 sites in the world [1]. Due to corrections to Metcalfe's law [2], which states that the value of a telecommunications network is proportional to $n \ (log_2 \ n)$ of the number of connected users of the system, there is a network world value of $O(28.9e + 09)$. The associated amount of data generated may be inferred from this number and even conservative metrics yield very large estimates. Most of these data are unstructured and recent commercial [3] approaches to the problem attest to the increasing importance assigned to this fact. In the computer science community, data mining of texts [4], music [5] and general information [6, 7] is being approached with growing interest. In the vast majority of the cases,

© Springer International Publishing Switzerland 2015
G. Sidorov and S.N. Galicia-Haro (Eds.): MICAI 2015, Part I, LNAI 9413, pp. 518–529, 2015.
DOI: 10.1007/978-3-319-27060-9_43

information extraction (IE) is highlighted and emphasizes the use of anaphora: the use of an expression the interpretation of which depends upon another expression in context. This approach, although intuitive and natural, suffers from the obvious disadvantage of being case-based. That is, a method developed for, say, texts in English will not be directly applicable to other languages and much less to other kinds of information. For example, even when limiting our range of study to, say, (a) Texts stemming from corporate finance (i.e. mining industry literature for business intelligence), (b) "Horizontal" test mining (i.e. patent analysis) or (c) Life sciences research (i.e. mining biological pathway information) every one of (a), (b) or (c) relies on a case-by-case determination of the anaphoric usage.

The problem at the very heart of this issue is the fact that we must preserve the patterns underlying the information and it had not been treated with success in the past. In [8], however, a method to encode non-numerical data in mixed (numerical and categorical) data bases was shown to be effective in preserving the embedded patterns. In what follows, we denote with G the number of generations of a genetic algorithm (EGA), with n the number of attributes in the database. MLP denotes a multi-layered perceptron network. MD denotes a data base where some of the attributes *may* be numerical and others *are* categorical. ND denotes the data base where all instances of the categories have been replaced by a numerical code. The algorithm developed therein was dubbed CENG and may be succinctly described as follows.

CENG: An algorithm for categorical encoding
1. Specify the mixed database MD.
2. MD is analyzed to determine c (the number of categorical attributes) and t (the number of instances of all categories). The size of the genome (the number of bits needed to encode the solution) is $L=22ct$. EGA (the *Eclectic* Genetic Algorithm [9]) is programmed to *minimize* the fitness function; it randomly generates a set of PS (the number of individuals) strings of size L. This is population P_0. Every one of the PS strings is an individual of EGA.

for $i=1$ to G
  for $j=1$ to PS
      From individual j, ct numerical codes are extracted and ND_{ij} is generated by replacing the categorical instances with their numerical counterparts. Numerical variables are left undisturbed.
      MLP$_{ij}$'s architecture (for EGA's individual j) is determined.
      for $k=1$ to $n-1$
          MLP$_{ij}$ is fed with a data matrix in which the *k-th* attribute of ND is taken as a variable dependent on the remaining $n-1$. MLP$_{ij}$ is trained and the maximum error e_{ijk} (i.e. the one resulting by feeding the already trained MLP$_{ij}$ with all tuples vs. the dependent variable) is calculated.
      endfor
      Fitness(j) = max(e_{ijk})
  Endfor
  If an ending condition is reached the EGA ends. Otherwise the PS individuals of P_i are selected, crossed over and mutated yielding the new P_i.
endfor

CENG delivers the codes for every one of the *ct* instances of the categorical variables and ND: a version of MD in which all categorical instances are replaced by the proper numerical codes.

An example of a Mixed Database and the resulting Numerical Database after CENG is shown in Fig. 1. All numerical values have been mapped into [0,1).

Age	Place	Educa-tion	Race	Sex	Income	Age	Place	Educa-tion	Race	Sex	Income
55	North	9	White	M	2932.49	0.4928	0.0002	0.2000	0.8304	0.1332	0.0226
62	North	7	Asian	F	23453.37	0.5942	0.0002	0.1200	0.0668	0.1283	0.1896
57	South	24	Indian	F	1628.61	0.5217	0.2209	0.8000	0.4084	0.1283	0.0120
56	Center	18	White	M	4069.62	0.5072	0.2691	0.5600	0.8304	0.1332	0.0318
49	South	22	Indian	F	3650.23	0.4058	0.2209	0.7200	0.4084	0.1283	0.0284

Fig. 1. Example of Mixed and Numerical Data after CENG.

The corresponding codes are shown in Fig. 2.

North	0.0002	Indian	0.4084
South	0.2209	Other	0.7472
Center	0.2691	M	0.1332
White	0.8304	F	0.1283
Asian	0.0668		

Fig. 2. Code for categorical instances.

Once having shown that CENG does find the correct codes for categorical attributes in mixed data bases, a corollary is that classic numerical clustering algorithms (such as Fuzzy C-Means [10], Self-Organizing Maps [11] or Entropy Based Clustering [12]) may be used and, furthermore, any text (indeed, any collection of tokenizable data) may be treated as a set of categorical variables provided categories and their corresponding instances are identified.

The rest of the paper is organized as follows. In Sect. 2 we describe the method we applied to tokenize Spanish texts. In Sect. 3 we describe the process of encoding the tokenized data base to obtain the corresponding clusters. In Sect. 4 we present an algorithm developed to identify the correspondence of the clusters in a labeled data base. In Sect. 5 we describe the experiments we performed to test the viability of our method. In Sect. 6 we present our conclusions.

2 Tokenizing Spanish Texts

To tokenize unstructured data we first have to find a representative sample which adequately characterizes the universe of data (*U*). Once having done so we select the number of categories (*c*). The next step is to determine the instances within every category (*t*). The number of tokens (*k*) per tuple determines the form of the structured data base. The final step is to select the text to tokenize and identify the tokens which will populate the structured data base. Notice that these steps are independent of the nature of *U*.

2.1 Tokenizing the Universe of Data

We started by selecting a collection of Spanish texts from different authors: Gabriel García Márquez, Julio Cortázar, Miguel de Cervantes, Jorge Luis Borges, Amado Nervo and Spanish translations of James Joyce and William Shakespeare. 125,882 words were extracted, from which 15,031 distinct ones were identified (i.e. $|U|$ = 15,301). We then made $c = 12$ and $t = 4$. This was achieved by obtaining the frequencies of every one of the 15,301 words and dividing them into 12 equally distributed intervals. That is, every one of the intervals in category i consists of as many words as those needed to account for 1/12 of the total. An index was generated wherein up to 4 equally spaced subintervals were defined. This translates into the fact that there are more words in the initial intervals (more finely split frequencies) whereas those intervals where the more probable words lie consist of less words. An example taken from the actual database is shown in Fig. 3.

word	category	token		word	category	token		word	category	token
ESTIRABAN	1	3		GRITAR	3	15		LOS	11	59
ESTIRANDO	1	3		GUSTARIA	3	15		EN	11	60
ESTIRO	1	3		GENERO	3	15		A	12	61
ESTORBADA	1	3		HABRIAN	3	15		EL	12	62
ESTORBADO	1	3		HERIDO	3	15		QUE	12	63
ESTORNUDAR	1	3		HIPOTESIS	3	15		LA	13	64
ESTRADOS	1	3		HUELLAS	3	15		Y	13	65
ESTRAÑO	1	3		HUIR	3	15		DE	14	66

Fig. 3. An example of categories and instances.

In the third column we find the token number. In the category there are one or more tokens. In category 1, for instance all the words illustrated ("ESTIRABAN",...., "ESTRAÑO") map into token 3 ("T3"). On the other hand, category 12 consists of three tokens and category 14 consists of only one token. Any word in the text may be either matched up with a token (if it is found in the catalog) or is assigned a special "null" token. There is one possible null token for every category. Under this classification, the sentence *"Tomaré el autobús a las dos y llegaré por la tarde"* is represented by the set of tokens <T6> <T62> <T21> <T61> <T54> <T42> <T65> <T4> <T56> <T64> <T34> . However, this simple approach is not the one we took. Rather, we define *<zentence ≡ 12 tokens>*. Our program reads words from a text and would "like" to find one representative for every category. This is attempted by reading up to 26 words or when all the 12 categories are filled-in. The number "26" was calculated so that the average number of unfulfilled categories is approximately 15 %. If, after having read 26 words, a category is still not yet filled-in, a null token is assigned to the empty position of the zentence. If a word is a representative of a category which has already been filled-in, that word is not discarded and a new one is read. A zentence has the structure illustrated in Table 1.

Table 1. Structure of a zentence

Zentence No.	Token No.											
1	1	2	3	4	5	6	7	8	9	10	11	12
2	1	2	3	4	5	6	7	8	9	10	11	12

2.2 Obtaining the Tokenized Data Base

As described, not all zentences include instances of all categories and, therefore, a special token ("nul_i") may appear in the i-th position of the zentence. That is, if no representative of category 1 appears in the zentence, it will be filled-in with the first null; if no representative of category 2 appears it will be filled-in with the second null and so on. In other words, there are up to $(c + 1)t$ symbols present in the database. In the example database there are up to 60 different categorical instances present. This is illustrated in Fig. 4.

T4	T6	T44	T14	T18	T24	T26	T28	T32	T37	T52	T41
T2	T6	T10	T45	T46	T21	T26	T28	T32	T37	T38	T53
T42	T8	T11	T15	T20	T22	T48	T49	T34	T35	T52	T53
T42	T5	T44	T16	T20	T47	T25	T29	T50	T35	T39	T53
T3	T5	T10	T45	T46	T21	T27	T28	T50	T35	T40	T41
T2	T5	T44	T16	T19	T23	T48	T28	T31	T35	T38	T41
T3	T43	T12	T15	T18	T21	T48	T31	T32	T35	T40	T41
T2	T43	T12	T15	T19	T24	T27	T28	T33	T37	T38	T53

Fig. 4. A segment of a tokenized data base.

Once U is determined and categorized any given selected text in Spanish may be mapped into a relational data base formed of zentences. We selected three texts by García Márquez and three by Julio Cortázar and tokenized them accordingly. These texts were then encoded by CENG and finally clustered using Self-Organizing Maps. The resulting clusters were labeled and then tested for similarity. Clusters whose tuples are similarly labeled indicate the same author; different authors otherwise.

3 Coding and Clustering the Tokenized Data Base

Once the tokenized data base has been obtained we proceed to encode the attributes, which correspond to the tokens determined as above. These tokenized database is one in which all attributes are categorical. The idea is to find a set of codes (one for each different instance of all categories) such that the structures present in the non-numerical data set are preserved when every instance of every category is replaced by its numerical counterpart. CENG is an algorithm based on the premise that patterns are preserved if all attributes are adequately expressed as a function of all others and that this is true for all attributes simultaneously. Let us assume that we have a hypothetical *perfect* set of pattern preserving codes. Assume, also, that there are n attributes and p tuples. Given such *perfect* set it would be, in principle, possible to express attribute i as a function of the remaining $n - 1$ with high accuracy since this *perfect* code set will lend itself to a close approximation. Therefore, the first problem to solve, in this approach, is to find $f_1 = f$ $(x_2...,x_n)$: a multivariate function with no predefined model for f_1; that is to say, without restricting the form of the approximant. In this regard Cybenko [13] showed that a 3-layered perceptron network (MLP) is able to approximate arbitrarily closely a function from a known data set. This theorem is not constructive and one has to design the MLP adequately. The issues involved in its design are discussed and solved in [14]. To complete the argument regarding the preservation of patterns we must find the whole collection $f_2, ..., f_n$ where $f_i = f(x_1, ..., x_{i-1}, x_{i+1}, ..., x_n)$ such that the approximation error should be the smallest for all attributes given the same fixed codes. This multi-objective optimization problem [since minimizing the approximation error for f_i may be in conflict with minimizing the corresponding error for f_j $(i \neq j)$] is the second problem to solve. On the other hand, it is clear that we do not know the values of what we have called the *perfect* code. These issues are solved in CENG by using EGA and MLPs.

In every generation PS individuals are delivered to a MLP for evaluation. Every individual consists of a set of possible codes which are to be assigned to every instance in the database. An individual for the database illustrated in Fig. 5a is shown in Fig. 5b. Figure 5c illustrates the database resulting from replacing the instances of MD with the codes of Fig. 5b. The numbers illustrated in Fig. 5b are actually encoded in binary with 22 bits each. Numerical variables are mapped into [0,1) so that all numbers lie in the same range.

Every (binary string) individual of EGA is transformed to a decimal number and its codes are inserted into MD, which now becomes a candidate numerical data base. A MLP (whose architecture is determined as per [14]) is trained (for 1000 epochs with backpropagation [15]) using the first attribute as the output and the remaining $n - 1$ as inputs to the MLP. The associated absolute error is calculated and temporarily stored. This process is repeated $n - 1$ more times using every attribute as the output of a MLP and the remaining $n - 1$ as its inputs. The largest of the stored errors is returned to EGA as the fitness of the individual. EGA runs for 500 generations thus minimizing the maximum absolute error. This strategy guarantees that the resulting set of codes corresponds to the best global behavior. That is, the final set of codes encompasses the best combinations of the f_i's minimizing the approximation error and the multi-objective optimization is solved within the practical limits of the EGA. Additionally it delivers a practical approximation of the *perfect* set: the one preserving the patterns embedded in the data base.

Since both initial values of the weights during the training phase of the MLPs and the initial population of EGA are random any two runs of CENG, in general, will result in different sets of codes, say S1 and S2. This fact allows us to verify that, as postulated, patterns will be preserved. This is done by applying a clustering algorithm which

Age	Place of Birth	Years of Study	Race	Sex	Salary
55	North	9	White	M	2,932.49
62	North	7	Asian	F	23,453.37
57	South	24	Indian	F	1,628.61
56	Center	18	White	M	4,069.62
49	South	22	Indian	F	3,650.23

Fig. 5a. A mixed database (MD)

North	Center	South	White	Asian	Indian	Other	M	F
0.0002	0.2691	0.2209	0.8304	0.0668	0.4084	0.7472	0.1332	0.1283

Fig. 5b. Instances of MD and possible codes

Age	Place of Birth	Years of Study	Race	Sex	Salary
0.4928	0.0002	0.2000	0.8304	0.1332	0.0226
0.5942	0.0002	0.1200	0.0668	0.1283	0.1896
0.5217	0.2209	0.8000	0.4084	0.1283	0.0120
0.5072	0.2691	0.5600	0.8304	0.1332	0.0318
0.4058	0.2209	0.7200	0.4084	0.1283	0.0284
0.0870	0.0002	0.8400	0.0668	0.1332	0.2306

Fig. 5c. Numerical database (ND) with codes from Fig. 2b

yields an assignment of every tuple to one of m clusters. Under the assumption of pattern preservation, clustering with S1 and S2 should yield analogous clusters. This is, indeed, the fact, as was shown in [8].

4   Identification of Cluster Matching in Labeled Databases

The correct identification of analogous clusters is compulsory if, as intended, we are to determine whether two texts correspond (or not) to the same author. Texts T1A and T2A both authored by A should correspond to similar clusters whereas texts T1A and T1B (authored, respectively, by A and B) should correspond to different clusters. To test the purported cluster similarity poses the technical problem we describe in what follows.

4.1   The Problem of Cluster Matching

Assume that tables T1 and T2 consisting of attributes V1,...,VC have been classified into 4 clusters and labeled as illustrated in Figs. 6a and 6b. This labeling convention is

V1	V2	V3	V4	V5	V6	V7	V8	V9	VA	VB	VC	LABEL SET 1			
												C11	C12	C13	C14
0.513	.41	.39	.37	.00	.67	.83	.03	.83	.57	.83	0.007	1	0	0	1
0.513	.41	.39	.81	.51	.19	.27	.08	.36	.35	.83	0.288	0	1	0	0
0.513	.41	.11	.81	.51	.11	.56	.09	.83	.07	.63	0.028	0	1	0	0
0.513	.16	.83	.20	.00	.11	.27	.03	.36	.57	.63	0.288	0	0	0	1
0.513	.41	.39	.20	.51	.19	.56	.03	.36	.57	.63	0.606	0	1	0	0
0.160	.64	.11	.20	.51	.11	.56	.08	.36	.35	.63	0.028	0	0	0	1
0.160	.41	.16	.20	.87	.11	.27	.09	.01	.03	.83	0.028	1	0	0	0
0.284	.32	.11	.20	.08	.19	.27	.41	.35	.35	.39	0.288	0	0	0	1
0.160	.41	.11	.81	.00	.11	.56	.09	.95	.57	.36	0.288	1	0	0	0
0.513	.12	.16	.20	.51	.11	.56	.03	.95	.57	.83	0.007	0	0	0	1
0.160	.41	.39	.81	.51	.11	.56	.08	.01	.07	.36	0.007	0	1	0	0
0.513	.41	.11	.81	.51	.11	.27	.09	.95	.57	.16	0.288	0	1	0	0

Fig. 6a. A segment of labeled Numerical Data Base T1.

V1	V2	V3	V4	V5	V6	V7	V8	V9	VA	VB	VC	LABEL SET 2			
												C21	C22	C23	C24
0.053	.32	.06	.02	.04	.27	.53	.05	.08	.63	.75	0.852	1	0	0	1
0.053	.32	.06	.02	.47	.27	.48	.05	.08	.23	.20	0.852	0	0	1	0
0.717	.32	.02	.56	.04	.27	.48	.05	.31	.31	.58	0.295	0	0	1	0
0.017	.32	.06	.02	.47	.65	.53	.13	.08	.32	.01	0.260	1	0	0	0
0.053	.32	.02	.02	.47	.26	.48	.33	.08	.23	.75	0.295	0	0	1	0
0.717	.03	.06	.56	.04	.27	.48	.05	.36	.63	.01	0.295	1	0	0	0
0.017	.20	.06	.56	.04	.26	.48	.13	.03	.23	.01	0.852	0	0	0	1
0.017	.32	.06	.03	.01	.65	.48	.08	.31	.23	.23	0.852	1	0	0	0
0.053	.20	.06	.56	.01	.65	.48	.08	.36	.63	.58	0.295	0	0	0	1
0.053	.20	.06	.56	.12	.26	.48	.05	.36	.28	.01	0.852	1	0	0	0
0.053	.32	.02	.02	.01	.65	.48	.00	.31	.23	.20	0.852	0	0	1	0
0.017	.32	.06	.03	.47	.65	.53	.33	.08	.23	.75	0.260	0	0	1	0

Fig. 6b. A segment of labeled Numerical Data Base T2.

convenient since one may easily count the number of matches between two clusters. However, clustering algorithms do not necessarily yield the same order of the label columns. For example, in Fig. 7 we have compared column C11 to C21, on the one hand and C11 to C24 on the other. The first choice yields a count of 6 matches leading us to the conclusion that sets C11 and C21 do not match and that, therefore, T1 and T2 do not share the same clusters.

The second choice, however, yields the full 12 matches. Therefore, in this instance one must conclude that column C11 (from set 1) actually corresponds to column C24 (from set 2). Accordingly, we should also conclude that T1 and T2 correspond to the same set for cluster 1. The correct pairing has to be achieved in similar fashion for all clusters.

If there are m clusters and p tuples there are m^p possible combinations of valid labeling sets. We need to investigate which of these does actually correspond to the proper matching of the m clusters in T1 with those of T2. Only then we may compare

C11	C21	Same		C11	C24	Same
1	1	1		1	1	1
0	0	1		0	0	1
0	0	1		0	0	1
0	1	0		0	0	1
0	0	1		0	0	1
0	1	0		0	0	1
1	0	0		1	1	1
0	1	0		0	0	1
1	0	0		1	1	1
0	1	0		0	0	1
0	0	1		0	0	1
0	0	1		0	0	1

Fig. 7. Similarity for different choices of cluster columns

T1 and T2 and determine their similarity. To achieve this identification we designed the following algorithm.

4.2   An Algorithm to Optimize Cluster Matching

1. Create a matching table "MT" of dimensions $m \times m$.
   Make $MT(i,j) \leftarrow 0$ for all i, j.
2. For $i \leftarrow 1$ to m
     For $j \leftarrow 1$ to m
       If column i = column j
         $MT(i,j) \leftarrow MT(i,j) + 1$
       endif
     endfor
   endfor
$MT(i,j)$ will contain the number of matches between cluster i of table T1 and cluster j of table T2.
3. Create a table "Scores" of dimension Q $(Q >> 0)$.
4. For $i \leftarrow 1$ to Q
     4.1. Set a random valid sequence S_i of m possible matching sequences between the clusters of T1 and those of T2.
     4.2. Find the number of matches M_i between T1 and T2 from table MT as per S_i.
     4.3. Make Scores(i) $\leftarrow M_i$.
   endfor
5. $I \leftarrow$ index of max(Scores(i)) for all i.
6. Select S_I. This is the matching set which maximizes the number of coincidences between the clusters of T1 and T2.   □

The core of the algorithm lies in step 4.1 where the valid matching sequences are determined. This algorithm will find the sequence which maximizes the number of matches between the clusters of T1 and T2 with high probability provided Q is large enough. In our experiments we made $Q = 1000$. Given the large number of possible pairings between the clusters of T1 and T2 the algorithm is a practical way to select which cluster of T1 should be paired with which cluster of T2.

5   Experimental Authorship Identification

At this point we are in a position which allows us to test the initial hypothesis of authorship identification. As already stated, we selected 3 texts from Gabriel García Márquez (GM) and 3 from Julio Cortázar (JC). These were, consecutively, tokenized, CENG-encoded, clustered with SOMs and labeled. Previous analysis led us to the conclusion that there were 4 clusters, as may be seen from the graph in Fig. 8.

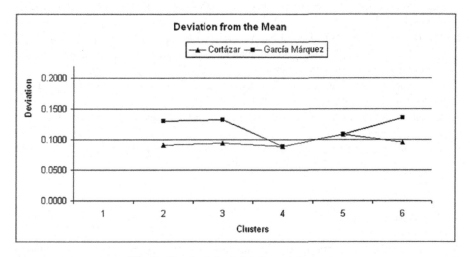

Fig. 8. Standard deviation for training errors

In this graph we display the results of having trained texts from GM and JC for up to 6 clusters with SOMs. The maximum errors relative to the mean were smallest for 4 clusters and the calculated standard deviation with a 0.05 *p-value* [16] was, likewise, smallest for the same number.

The texts we selected were of roughly the same size: $\approx$ 16,000 words. They were then tokenized and CENG-encoded. The resulting data bases were clustered and labeled. Next the cluster matching was performed and adjusted when needed. We then proceeded to obtain a matrix of coincidences for the 15 possible combinations of the 6 texts. These are shown in Table 2. GM_i denotes the *i-th* text by García Márquez; likewise JC_i denotes the texts by Cortázar.

Table 2. Comparison of clusters obtained

	Text 1	Text 2	Cluster matches		Text 1	Text 2	Cluster matches
1	JC1	JC2	98.23 %	9	GM2	JC1	57.14 %
2	JC2	JC3	86.43 %	10	GM3	JC2	57.14 %
3	JC1	JC3	82.50 %	11	GM1	JC2	54.29 %
4	GM1	GM2	78.54 %	12	GM2	JC3	54.29 %
5	GM1	GM3	74.69 %	13	GM3	JC1	54.29 %
6	GM3	JC3	68.60 %	14	GM1	JC1	51.52 %
7	GM2	GM3	66.77 %	15	GM2	JC2	48.57 %
8	GM1	JC3	65.71%				

The texts pairings were ordered according to the percentage of matches we obtained. We observed the following behavior:

- All matching text matches were higher when the authors were the same, with the exception of item 6, where the texts by GM vs JC had higher matches than expected.
- The correct assessment of authorship matches for the first 5 couples remains very close or above 75 % Therefore, a matching percentage of 75 % appears to be sufficient to ascertain similar authorship.
- There appears to be no possible definitive conclusions of the purported authorship in the borderline percentages for items 6-8.
- Matching percentages below 60 % seem to imply negative authorship for the analyzed couples.
- The identification percentage falls smoothly so that there is not a clear cut threshold dividing correctly assessed authorship from the alternative.

6   Conclusions

We have described a method to identify the authorship of selected Spanish texts which is not based on linguistic considerations. Rather, it relies on the identification and preservation of the patterns embedded in the texts by the intelligent encoding of the data. This method is computationally intensive, requiring the training of a large set of candidate codes and, therefore, CPU consuming. Execution time was improved using parallel computation from which genetic algorithms benefit considerably. On the other hand, there are several parameters which were heuristically determined and have to be further explored. For instance, the size of the zentences is arbitrary. Likewise, the fact of having defined the number of categories and the corresponding instances as they were is arbitrary and we expect that a more elaborate selection of these (after systematic experimental tests) may improve the algorithm significantly. Furthermore, the selected texts and their lengths may affect the efficiency of the algorithm one way or the other. Finally, the results, which seem to be promising, are only valid, in general, if we assume that the method will behave similarly if the restricted number of authors we selected were to be expanded. Even if it is not reasonable to assume that the reported results should be much different for a different selection of authors it could be that such is the case. Much experimental work remains to be done.

At any rate this is a novel and possibly promising alternative. Particularly in view of the fact, that as pointed out in the introduction, it may be applied to any kind of unstructured data. We expect to report on the application of our method to more general and non-textual data in the near future.

References

1. http://news.netcraft.com/archives/2014/04/02/april-2014-web-server-survey.html. Accessed 18 June 2015
2. Odlyzko, A., Tilly, B.: A refutation of Metcalfe's Law and a better estimate for the value of networks and network interconnections. Manuscript, 2 March 2005
3. http://www-03.ibm.com/press/us/en/pressrelease/46205.wss. Accessed 18 June 2015
4. Tan, A.H.: Text mining: The state of the art and the challenges. In: Proceedings of the PAKDD 1999 Workshop on Knowledge Disocovery from Advanced Databases, vol. 8, p. 65, April 1999
5. Pachet, F., Westermann, G., Laigre, D.: Musical data mining for electronic music distribution. In: First International Conference on Web Delivering of Music, 2001, Proceedings, pp. 101–106. IEEE, November 2001
6. Lei-da Chen, T.S., Frolick, M.N.: Data mining methods, applications, and tools (2000)
7. Feldman, R., Sanger, J.: The Text Mining Handbook: Advanced Approaches in Analyzing Unstructured Data. Cambridge University Press, Cambridge (2007)
8. Kuri-Morales, A.: categorical encoding with neural networks and genetic algorithms. In: Proceedings of AICT 2015 (Applications of Computer and Computer Theory), Salerno, Italy, pp. 167–175. WSEAS, June 2015
9. Kuri-Morales, A., Aldana-Bobadilla, E.: The best genetic algorithm I. In: Castro, F., Gelbukh, A., González, M. (eds.) MICAI 2013, Part II. LNCS, vol. 8266, pp. 1–15. Springer, Heidelberg (2013)
10. Bezdek, J.C., Ehrlich, R., Full, W.: FCM: the fuzzy c-means clustering algorithm. Comput. Geosci. **10**(2), 191–203 (1984)
11. Ritter, H., Martinetz, T., Schulten, K.: Neural Computation and Self-Organizing Maps. An introduction (1992)
12. Aldana-Bobadilla, E., Kuri-Morales, A.: A clustering method based on the maximum entropy principle. Entropy **17**(1), 151–180 (2015)
13. Cybenko, G.: Approximation by superpositions of a sigmoidal function. Math. Control Signals Systems **2**(4), 303–314 (1989)
14. Kuri-Morales, A.F.: The best neural network architecture. In: Gelbukh, A., Espinoza, F.C., Galicia-Haro, S.N. (eds.) MICAI 2014, Part II. LNCS, vol. 8857, pp. 72–84. Springer, Heidelberg (2014)
15. Hecht-Nielsen, R.: Theory of the backpropagation neural network. In International Joint Conference on Neural Networks, 1989, IJCNN, pp. 593–605. IEEE, June 1989
16. Westfall, P.H., Young, S.S.: Resampling-Based Multiple Testing: Examples and Methods for P-Value Adjustment, vol. 279. Wiley, New York (1993)

EFIM: A Highly Efficient Algorithm
for High-Utility Itemset Mining

Souleymane Zida[1], Philippe Fournier-Viger[1]([✉]), Jerry Chun-Wei Lin[2],
Cheng-Wei Wu[3], and Vincent S. Tseng[3]

[1] Department of Computer Science, University of Moncton, Moncton, Canada
{esz2233,philippe.fournier-viger}@umoncton.ca
[2] School of Computer Science and Technology, Harbin Institute of Technology
Shenzhen Graduate School, Shenzhen, China
jerrylin@ieee.org
[3] Department of Computer Science, National Chiao Tung University,
Hsinchu, Taiwan
silvemoonfox@gmail.com, vtseng@cs.nctu.edu.tw

Abstract. High-utility itemset mining (HUIM) is an important data
mining task with wide applications. In this paper, we propose a novel
algorithm named EFIM (EFficient high-utility Itemset Mining), which
introduces several new ideas to more efficiently discovers high-utility
itemsets both in terms of execution time and memory. EFIM relies on
two upper-bounds named *sub-tree utility* and *local utility* to more effectively prune the search space. It also introduces a novel array-based utility counting technique named *Fast Utility Counting* to calculate these
upper-bounds in linear time and space. Moreover, to reduce the cost of
database scans, EFIM proposes efficient database projection and transaction merging techniques. An extensive experimental study on various datasets shows that EFIM is in general two to three orders of
magnitude faster and consumes up to eight times less memory than
the state-of-art algorithms d²HUP, HUI-Miner, HUP-Miner, FHM and
UP-Growth+.

Keywords: High-utility mining · Itemset mining · Pattern mining

1 Introduction

Frequent Itemset Mining (FIM) [1] is a popular data mining task that is essential
to a wide range of applications. Given a transaction database, FIM consists of
discovering frequent itemsets. i.e. groups of items (itemsets) appearing frequently
in transactions [1,14]. However, an important limitation of FIM is that it assumes
that each item cannot appear more than once in each transaction and that all
items have the same importance (weight, unit profit or value). To address these
issues, the problem of *High-Utility Itemset Mining* (HUIM) has been defined
[2,6–9,11,12]. As opposed to FIM [1,14], HUIM considers the case where items
can appear more than once in each transaction and where each item has a

© Springer International Publishing Switzerland 2015
G. Sidorov and S.N. Galicia-Haro (Eds.): MICAI 2015, Part I, LNAI 9413, pp. 530–546, 2015.
DOI: 10.1007/978-3-319-27060-9_44

weight (e.g. unit profit). Therefore, it can be used to discover itemsets having a high-utility (e.g. high profit), that is *High-Utility Itemsets*. HUIM has a wide range of applications [2,7,12]. The problem of HUIM is more difficult than the problem of FIM because the utility of an itemset is neither monotonic or anti-monotonic (a HUI may have a superset or subset with lower, equal or higher utility) [2,7,12]. Thus techniques to prune the search space developed in FIM based on the anti-monotonicity of the support cannot be directly applied to HUIM.

Several algorithms have been proposed for HUIM. A popular approach to HUIM is to discover high-utility itemsets in two phases. This approach is adopted by algorithms such as PB [6], Two-Phase [9], BAHUI [11], UP-Growth and UP-Growth+ [12]. However, the two-phase model suffers from the problem of generating a huge amount of candidates and repeatedly scanning the database. Recently, to avoid the problem of candidate generation, the HUI-Miner [7] and d^2HUP [8] algorithms were proposed to mine high-utility itemsets directly using a single phase. Then, improved versions of HUI-Miner named HUP-Miner [8] and FHM [2] were proposed, and are to our knowledge the current best algorithms for HUIM. However, despite all these research efforts, the task of high-utility itemset mining remains very computationally expensive.

In this paper, we address this need for more efficient HUIM algorithms by proposing a one-phase algorithm named EFIM (EFficient high-utility Itemset Mining), which introduces several novel ideas to greatly decrease the time and memory required for HUIM. First, we propose two new techniques to reduce the cost of database scans. EFIM performs database projection and merges transactions that are identical in each projected database using a linear time and space implementation. Both operations reduce the size of the database as larger itemsets are explored. Second, we propose two new upper-bounds on the utility of itemsets named *sub-tree utility* and *local utility* to more effectively prune the search space. Third, we introduce a novel array-based utility counting technique named *Fast Utility Counting* (FAC) to calculate these upper-bounds in linear time and space.

We conducted an extensive experimental study to compare the performance of EFIM with the state-of-the-art algorithms d^2HUP, HUI-Miner, HUP-Miner, FHM and UP-Growth+ on various datasets. Results show that EFIM is in general two to three orders of magnitude faster than these algorithms, consumes up to eight times less memory.

The rest of this paper is organized as follows. Sections 2, 3, 4, 5 and 6 respectively presents the problem of HUIM, the related work, the EFIM algorithm, the experimental evaluation and the conclusion.

2   Problem Statement

The problem of high-utility itemset mining is defined as follows. Let I be a finite set of items (symbols). An itemset X is a finite set of items such that $X \subseteq I$. A *transaction database* is a multiset of transactions $D = \{T_1, T_2, ..., T_n\}$ such

Table 1. A transaction database

TID	Transaction
T_1	$(a, 1)(c, 1)(d, 1)$
T_2	$(a, 2)(c, 6)(e, 2)(g, 5)$
T_3	$(a, 1)(b, 2)(c, 1)(d, 6)(e, 1)(f, 5)$
T_4	$(b, 4)(c, 3)(d, 3)(e, 1)$
T_5	$(b, 2)(c, 2)(e, 1)(g, 2)$

Table 2. External utility values

Item	a	b	c	d	e	f	g
Profit	5	2	1	2	3	1	1

that for each transaction T_c, $T_c \subseteq I$ and T_c has a unique identifier c called its TID (Transaction ID). Each item $i \in I$ is associated with a positive number $p(i)$, called its *external utility* (e.g. unit profit). Every item i appearing in a transaction T_c has a positive number $q(i, T_c)$, called its *internal utility* (e.g. purchase quantity). For example, consider the database in Table 1, which will be used as the running example. It contains five transactions ($T_1, T_2..., T_5$). Transaction T_2 indicates that items a, c, e and g appear in this transaction with an internal utility of respectively 2, 6, 2 and 5. Table 2 indicates that the external utility of these items are respectively 5, 1, 3 and 1.

Definition 1 (Utility of an item/itemset). The *utility of an item i in a transaction T_c* is denoted as $u(i, T_c)$ and defined as $p(i) \times q(i, T_c)$ if $i \in T_c$. The *utility of an itemset X in a transaction T_c* is denoted as $u(X, T_c)$ and defined as $u(X, T_c) = \sum_{i \in X} u(i, T_c)$ if $X \subseteq T_c$. The *utility of an itemset X* is denoted as $u(X)$ and defined as $u(X) = \sum_{T_c \in g(X)} u(X, T_c)$, where $g(X)$ is the set of transactions containing X.

For example, the utility of item a in T_2 is $u(a, T_2) = 5 \times 2 = 10$. The utility of the itemset $\{a, c\}$ in T_2 is $u(\{a, c\}, T_2) = u(a, T_2) + u(c, T_2) = 5 \times 2 + 1 \times 6 = 16$. Furthermore, the utility of the itemset $\{a, c\}$ is $u(\{a, c\}) = u(\{a, c\}, T_1) + u(\{a, c\}, T_2) + u(\{a, c\}, T_3) = u(a, T_1) + u(c, T_1) + u(a, T_2) + u(c, T_2) + u(a, T_3) + u(c, T_3) = 5 + 1 + 10 + 6 + 5 + 1 = 28$.

Definition 2 (Problem definition). An itemset X is a *high-utility itemset* if $u(X) \geq minutil$. Otherwise, X is a *low-utility itemset*. The *problem of high-utility itemset mining* is to discover all high-utility itemsets.

For example, if $minutil = 30$, the high-utility itemsets in the database of the running example are $\{b, d\}$, $\{a, c, e\}$, $\{b, c, d\}$, $\{b, c, e\}$, $\{b, d, e\}$, $\{b, c, d, e\}$, $\{a, b, c, d, e, f\}$ with respectively a utility of 30, 31, 34, 31, 36, 40 and 30.

3   Related Work

HUIM is harder than FIM since the utility measure is not monotonic or anti-monotonic [9,12], i.e. the utility of an itemset may be lower, equal or higher than the utility of its subsets. Thus, strategies used in FIM to prune the search space based on the anti-monotonicity of the frequency cannot be applied to the utility measure to discover high-utility itemsets. Several HUIM algorithms circumvent this problem by overestimating the utility of itemsets using the *Transaction-Weighted Utilization* (TWU) measure [6,9,11,12], which is anti-monotonic, and defined as follows.

Definition 3 (Transaction weighted utilization (TWU)). The *transaction utility* of a transaction T_c is defined as $TU(T_c) = \sum_{x \in T_c} u(x, T_c)$. The TWU of an itemset X is defined as $TWU(X) = \sum_{T_c \in g(X)} TU(T_c)$.

Example 1. The TU of transactions T_1, T_2, T_3, T_4 and T_5 for our running example are respectively 8, 27, 30, 20 and 11. $TWU(a) = TU(T_1) + TU(T_2) + TU(T_3) = 8 + 27 + 30 = 65$.

For any itemset X, it can be shown that $TWU(X) \geq u(Y) \forall Y \supseteq X$ (the TWU of X is an upper-bound on the utility of X and its supersets) [9]. The following properties of the TWU is used to prune the search space.

Property 1 (Pruning search space using TWU). For any itemset X, if $TWU(X) < minutil$, then X is a low-utility itemset as well as all its supersets [9].

Algorithms such as PB [6], Two-Phase [9], BAHUI [11], UP-Growth and UP-Growth+ [12] utilize Property 1 to prune the search space. They operate in two phases. In the first phase, they identify candidate high-utility itemsets by calculating their TWUs. In the second phase, they scan the database to calculate the exact utility of all candidates to filter low-utility itemsets. UP-Growth is one of the fastest two-phase algorithm. Recent two-phase algorithms such as PB and BAHUI only provide a small speed improvement.

Recently, algorithms that mine high-utility itemsets using a single phase were proposed to avoid the problem of candidate generation. The d²HUP and HUI-Miner algorithms were reported to be respectively up to 10 and 100 times faster than UP-Growth [7,8]. Then, improved versions of HUI-Miner named HUP-Miner [8] and FHM [2] were proposed to reduce the number of join operations performed by HUI-Miner, and are to our knowledge the current best algorithm for HUIM. In HUI-Miner, HUP-Miner and FHM, each itemset is associated with a structure named *utility-list* [2,7]. Utility-lists allow calculating the utility of an itemset by making join operations with utility-lists of smaller itemsets. Utility-lists are defined as follows.

Definition 4 (Remaining utility). Let $\succ$ be a total order on items from I, and X be an itemset. The *remaining utility* of X in a transaction T_c is defined as $re(X, T_c) = \sum_{i \in T_c \wedge i \succ x \forall x \in X} u(i, T_c)$.

Definition 5 (Utility-list). The *utility-list* of an itemset X in a database D is a set of tuples such that there is a tuple $(c, iutil, rutil)$ for each transaction T_c containing X. The $iutil$ and $rutil$ elements of a tuple respectively are the utility of X in T_c ($u(X, T_c)$) and the remaining utility of X in T_c ($re(X, T_c)$).

For example, assume the lexicographical order (i.e. $e \succ d \succ c \succ b \succ a$). The utility-list of $\{a, e\}$ is $\{(T_2, 16, 5), (T_3, 8, 5)\}$.

To discover high-utility itemsets, HUI-Miner, HUP-Miner and FHM perform a database scan to create utility-lists of patterns containing single items. Then, larger patterns are obtained by joining utility-lists of smaller patterns (see [7,8] for details). Pruning the search space is done using the following properties.

Definition 6 (Remaining utility upper-bound). Let X be an itemset. Let the *extensions* of X be the itemsets that can be obtained by appending an item i to X such that $i \succ x$, $\forall x \in X$. The *remaining utility upper-bound* of X is defined as $reu(X) = u(X) + re(X)$, and can be computed by summing the $iutil$ and $rutil$ values in the utility-list of X.

Property 2 (Pruning search space using utility-lists). If $reu(X) < minutil$, then X is a low-utility itemset as well as all its extensions [7].

One-phase algorithms [2,7,8,10] are faster and generally more memory efficient than two phase algorithms. However, mining HUIs remains very computationally expensive. For example, HUI-Miner, HUP-Miner, and FHM still suffer from a high space and time complexity. The size of each utility-list is in the worst case $O(n)$, where n is the number of transactions (when a utility-list contains an entry for each transaction). The complexity of building a utility-list is also very high [2]. In general, it requires to join three utility-lists of smaller itemsets, which thus requires $O(n^3)$ time in the worst case.

4   The EFIM Algorithm

We next present our proposal, the EFIM algorithm. It is a one-phase algorithm, which introduces several novel ideas to reduce the time and memory required for HUIM. Subsection 4.1 briefly reviews definitions related to the depth-first search of itemsets. Subsections 4.2 and 4.3 respectively explain how EFIM reduces the cost of database scans using an efficient implementation of database projection and transaction merging. Subsection 4.4 presents two new upper-bounds used by EFIM to prune the search space. Subsection 4.5 presents a new array-based utility counting technique named *Fast Utility Counting* to efficiently calculate these upper-bounds in linear time and space. Finally, Subsect. 4.6 gives the pseudocode of EFIM.

4.1   The Search Space

Let $\succ$ be any total order on items from I. According to this order, the search space of all itemsets 2^I can be represented as a *set-enumeration tree*. For example, the set-enumeration tree of $I = \{a, b, c, d\}$ for the lexicographical order is

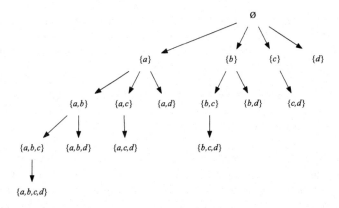

Fig. 1. Set-enumeration tree for $I = \{a, b, c, d\}$

shown in Fig. 1. The EFIM algorithm explores this search space using a depth-first search starting from the root (the empty set). During this depth-first search, for any itemset α, EFIM recursively appends one item at a time to α according to the $\succ$ order, to generate larger itemsets. In our implementation, the $\succ$ order is defined as the order of increasing TWU because it generally reduces the search space for HUIM [2,7,12]. However, we henceforth assume that $\succ$ is the lexicographical order, for the sake of simplicity. We next introduce definitions related to the depth-first search exploration of itemsets.

Definition 7 (Items that can extend an itemset). Let be an itemset α. Let $E(\alpha)$ denote the set of all items that can be used to extend α according to the depth-first search, that is $E(\alpha) = \{z | z \in I \wedge z \succ x, \forall x \in \alpha\}$.

Definition 8 (Extension of an itemset). Let be an itemset α. An itemset Z is an *extension* of α (appears in a sub-tree of α in the set-enumeration tree) if $Z = \alpha \cup W$ for an itemset $W \in 2^{E(\alpha)}$ such that $W \neq \emptyset$. Furthermore, an itemset Z is a *single-item extension* of α (is a child of α in the set-enumeration tree) if $Z = \alpha \cup \{z\}$ for an item $z \in E(\alpha)$.

For example, consider the database of our running example and $\alpha = \{d\}$. The set $E(\alpha)$ is $\{e, f, g\}$. Single-item extensions of α are $\{d, e\}$, $\{d, f\}$ and $\{d, g\}$. Other extensions of α are $\{d, e, f\}$, $\{d, f, g\}$ and $\{d, e, f, g\}$.

4.2   Reducing the Cost of Database Scans Using Projections

As we will explain, EFIM performs database scans to calculate the utility of itemsets and upper-bounds on their utility. To reduce the cost of database scans, it is desirable to reduce the database size. An observation is that when an itemset α is considered during the depth-first search, all items $x \notin E(\alpha)$ can be ignored when scanning the database to calculate the utility of itemsets in the sub-tree of α, or upper-bounds on their utility. A database without these items is called a *projected database*.

Definition 9 (Projected database). The *projection of a transaction T using an itemset* α is denoted as α-T and defined as α-$T = \{i | i \in T \wedge i \in E(\alpha)\}$. The *projection of a database D using an itemset* α is denoted as α-D and defined as the multiset α-$D = \{\alpha$-$T | T \in D \wedge \alpha$-$T \neq \emptyset\}$.

For example, consider database D of the running example and $\alpha = \{b\}$. The projected database α-D contains three transactions: α-$T_3 = \{c, d, e, f\}$, α-$T_4 = \{c, d, e\}$ and α-$T_5 = \{c, e, g\}$.

Database projections generally greatly reduce the cost of database scans since transactions become smaller as larger itemsets are explored. However, an important issue is how to implement database projection efficiently. A naive and inefficient approach is to make physical copies of transactions for each projection. An efficient approach used in EFIM is to sort each transaction in the original database according to the $\succ$ total order beforehand. Then, a projection is performed as a *pseudo-projection*, that is each projected transaction is represented by an offset pointer on the corresponding original transaction. The complexity of calculating the projection α-D of a database -D is linear in time and space with respect to the number of transactions. The proposed database projection technique generalizes the concept of database projection from pattern mining [14] for the case of transactions with internal/external utility values. Note that FP-growth based HUIM algorithms [6,12] and hyper-link based HUIM algorithms [8] also perform projections but differently than the proposed EFIM algorithm.

4.3   Reducing the Cost of Database Scans by Transaction Merging

To further reduce the cost of database scans, EFIM also introduce an efficient transaction merging technique. It is based on the observation that transaction databases often contain identical transactions. The technique consists of identifying these transactions and to replace them with single transactions. In this context, a transaction T_a is said to be *identical to* a transaction T_b if it contains the same items as T_b (i.e. $T_a = T_b$) (but not necessarily the same internal utility values).

Definition 10 (Transaction merging). *Transaction merging* consists of replacing a set of identical transactions $Tr_1, Tr_2, ...Tr_m$ in a database D by a single new transaction $T_M = Tr_1 = Tr_2 = ... = Tr_m$ where the quantity of each item $i \in T_M$ is defined as $q(i, T_M) = \sum_{k=1...m} q(i, Tr_k)$.

But to achieve higher database reduction, we also merge transactions in projected databases. This generally achieves a much higher reduction because projected transactions are smaller than original transactions, and thus are more likely to be identical.

Definition 11 (Projected transaction merging). *Projected transaction merging* consists of replacing a set of identical transactions $Tr_1, Tr_2, ...Tr_m$ in a database α-D by a single new transaction $T_M = Tr_1 = Tr_2 = ... = Tr_m$ where the quantity of each item $i \in T_M$ is defined as $q(i, T_M) = \sum_{k=1...m} q(i, Tr_k)$.

For example, consider database D of our running example and $\alpha = \{c\}$. The projected database α-D contains transactions α-$T_1 = \{d\}$, α-$T_2 = \{e, g\}$, α-$T_3 = \{d, e, f\}$, α-$T_4 = \{d, e\}$ and α-$T_5 = \{e, g\}$. Transactions α-T_2 and α-T_5 can be replaced by a new transaction $T_M = \{e, g\}$ where $q(e, T_M) = 3$ and $q(g, T_M) = 7$.

Transaction merging is obviously desirable. However, a key problem is to implement it efficiently. The naive approach to identify identical transactions is to compare all transactions with each other. But this is inefficient ($O(n^2)$, where n is the number of transactions). To find identical transactions in $O(n)$ time, we propose the following approach. We initially sort the original database according to a new total order $\succ_T$ on transactions. Sorting is achieved in $O(n\ log(n))$ time, and is performed only once.

Definition 12 (Total order on transactions). The $\succ_T$ order is defined as the lexicographical order when the transactions are read backwards. Formally, let be two transactions $T_a = \{i_1, i_2, ...i_m\}$ and $T_b = \{j_1, j_2, ...j_k\}$. The total order $\succ_T$ is defined by four cases. The first case is that $T_b \succ T_a$ if both transactions are identical and T_b is greater than the TID of T_a. The second case is that $T_b \succ_T T_a$ if $k > m$ and $i_{m-x} = j_{k-x}$ for any integer x such that $0 \leq x < m$. The third case is that $T_b \succ_T T_a$ if there exists an integer x such that $0 \leq x < \min(m, k)$, where $j_{k-x} \succ i_{m-x}$ and $i_{m-y} = j_{k-y}$ for all integer y such that $x < y < \min(m, k)$. The fourth case is that otherwise $T_a \succ_T T_b$.

For example, let be transactions $T_x = \{b, c\}$, $T_y = \{a, b, c\}$ and $T_z = \{a, b, e\}$. We have that $T_z \succ_T T_y \succ_T T_x$.

A database sorted according to the $\succ_T$ order provides the following property (proof omitted due to space limitation).

Property 3 (Order of identical transactions in a $\succ_T$ sorted database). Let be a $\succ_T$ sorted database D and an itemset α. Identical transactions appear consecutively in the projected database α-D.

Using the above property, all identical transactions in a (projected) database can be identified by only comparing each transaction with the next transaction in the database. Thus, using this scheme, transaction merging can be done very efficiently by scanning a (projected) database only once (linear time). It is interesting to note that transaction merging as proposed in EFIM cannot be implemented efficiently in utility-list based algorithms (e.g. FHM and HUP-Miner) and hyperlink-based algorithms (e.g. d²HUP) due to their database representations.

4.4   Pruning Search Space Using Sub-tree Utility and Local Utility

To propose an efficient HUIM algorithm, a key problem is to design an effective pruning mechanism. For this purpose, we introduce in EFIM two new upper-bounds on the utility of itemsets named *sub-tree utility* and *local utility*. The key difference with previous upper-bounds is that they are defined w.r.t the sub-tree of an itemset α in the search-enumeration tree.

Definition 13 (Sub-tree utility). Let be an itemset α and an item z that can extend α according to the depth-first search ($z \in E(\alpha)$). The *Sub-tree Utility* of z w.r.t. α is $su(\alpha, z) = \sum_{T \in g(\alpha \cup \{z\})} [u(\alpha, T) + u(z, T) + \sum_{i \in T \wedge i \in E(\alpha \cup \{z\})} u(i, T)]$.

Example 2. Consider the running example and $\alpha = \{a\}$. We have that $su(\alpha, c) = (5 + 1 + 2) + (10 + 6 + 11) + (5 + 1 + 20) = 61$, $su(\alpha, d) = 25$ and $su(\alpha, e) = 34$.

The following theorem of the sub-tree utility is proposed in EFIM to prune the search space (proof ommited due to space limitation).

Property 4 (Overestimation using the sub-tree utility). Let be an itemset α and an item $z \in E(\alpha)$. The relationship $su(\alpha, z) \geq u(\alpha \cup \{z\})$ holds. And more generally, $su(\alpha, z) \geq u(Z)$ holds for any extension Z of $\alpha \cup \{z\}$.

Theorem 1 (Pruning a sub-tree using the sub-tree utility). *Let be an itemset α and an item $z \in E(\alpha)$. If $su(\alpha, z) < minutil$, then the single item extension $\alpha \cup \{z\}$ and its extensions are low-utility. In other words, the sub-tree of $\alpha \cup \{z\}$ in the set-enumeration tree can be pruned.*

Thus, using Theorem 1, we can prune some sub-trees of an itemset α, which reduces the number of sub-trees to be explored. To further reduce the search space, we also identify items that should not be explored in any sub-trees.

Definition 14 (Local utility). Let be an itemset α and an item $z \in E(\alpha)$. The *Local Utility* of z w.r.t. α is $lu(\alpha, z) = \sum_{T \in g(\alpha \cup \{z\})} [u(\alpha, T) + re(\alpha, T)]$.

Example 3. Consider the running example and $\alpha = \{a\}$. We have that $lu(\alpha, c) = (8 + 27 + 30) = 65$, $lu(\alpha, d) = 30$ and $lu(\alpha, e) = 57$.

Property 5 (Overestimation using the local utility). Let be an itemset α and an item $z \in E(\alpha)$. Let Z be an extension of α such that $z \in Z$. The relationship $lu(\alpha, z) \geq u(Z)$ holds.

Theorem 2 (Pruning an item from all sub-trees using the local utility). *Let be an itemset α and an item $z \in E(\alpha)$. If $lu(\alpha, z) < minutil$, then all extensions of α containing z are low-utility. In other words, item z can be ignored when exploring all sub-trees of α.*

The relationship between the proposed upper-bounds and the main ones used in previous work is the following.

Property 6 (Relationships between upper-bounds). Let be an itemset $Y = \alpha \cup \{z\}$. The relationship $TWU(Y) \geq lu(\alpha, z) \geq reu(Y) = su(\alpha, z)$ holds.

Given, the above relationship, it can be seen that the proposed local utility upper-bound is a tighter upper-bound on the utility of Y and its extensions compared to the TWU, which is commonly used in two-phase HUIM algorithms. Thus the local utility can be more effective for pruning the search space. Besides, one can ask what is the difference between the proposed su upper-bound and the *reu* upper-bound of HUI-Miner and FHM since they are mathematically equivalent. The major difference is that su is calculated when the depth-first search is at itemset α in the search tree rather than at the child itemset Y. Thus, if $su(\alpha, z) < minutil$, EFIM prunes the whole sub-tree of z including node Y rather than only pruning the descendant nodes of Y. Thus, using su instead of *reu* is more effective for pruning the search space. In the rest of the paper, for a given itemset α, we respectively refer to items having a sub-tree utility and local-utility no less than *minutil* as *primary* and *secondary* items.

Definition 15 (Primary and secondary items). Let be an itemset α. The *primary items of* α is the set of items defined as $Primary(\alpha) = \{z | z \in E(\alpha) \land su(\alpha, z) \geq minutil\}$. The *secondary items of* α is the set of items defined as $Secondary(\alpha) = \{z | z \in E(\alpha) \land lu(\alpha, z) \geq minutil\}$. Because $lu(\alpha, z) \geq su(\alpha, z)$, $Primary(\alpha) \subseteq Secondary(\alpha)$.

For example, consider the running example and $\alpha = \{a\}$. $Primary(\alpha) = \{c, e\}$. $Secondary(\alpha) = \{c, d, e\}$.

4.5 Calculating Upper-Bounds Efficiently Using Fast Utility Counting

In the previous subsection, we introduced two new upper-bounds on the utility of itemsets to prune the search space. We now present a novel efficient array-based approach to compute these upper-bounds in linear time and space that we call Fast Utility Counting (FUC). It relies on a novel array structure called utility-bin.

Definition 16 (Utility-Bin). Let be the set of items I appearing in a database D. A *utility-bin array* U for database D is an array of length $|I|$, having an entry denoted as $U[z]$ for each item $z \in I$. Each entry is called a *utility-bin* and is used to store a utility value (an integer in our implementation, initialized to 0).

A utility-bin array can be used to efficiently calculate the following upper-bounds in $O(n)$ time (recall that n is the number of transactions), as follows.

Calculating the TWU of all Items. A utility-bin array U is initialized. Then, for each transaction T of the database, the utility-bin $U[z]$ for each item $z \in T$ is updated as $U[z] = U[z] + TU(T)$. At the end of the database scan, for each item $k \in I$, the utility-bin $U[k]$ contains $TWU(k)$.

Calculating the Sub-tree Utility w.r.t. an Itemset α. A utility-bin array U is initialized. Then, for each transaction T of the database, the utility-bin $U[z]$ for each item $z \in T \cap E(\alpha)$ is updated as $U[z] = U[z] + u(\alpha, T) + u(z, T) + \sum_{i \in T \land i \succ z} u(i, T)$. Thereafter, we have $U[k] = su(\alpha, k) \ \forall k \in I$.

Calculating the Local Utility w.r.t. an Itemset α. A utility-bin array U is initialized. Then, for each transaction T of the database, the utility-bin $U[z]$

for each item $z \in T \cap E(\alpha)$ is updated as $U[z] = U[z] + u(\alpha, T) + re(\alpha, T)$. Thereafter, we have $U[k] = lu(\alpha, k) \; \forall k \in I$.

Thus, by the above approach, the three upper-bounds can be calculated for all items that can extend an itemset α with only one (projected) database scan. Furthermore, it can be observed that utility-bins are a very compact data structure ($O(|I|)$ size). To utilize utility-bins more efficiently, we propose three optimizations. First, all items in the database are renamed as consecutive integers. Then, in a utility-bin array U, the utility-bin $U[i]$ for an item i is stored in the i-th position of the array. This allows to access the utility-bin of an item in $O(1)$ time. Second, it is possible to reuse the same utility-bin array multiple times by reinitializing it with zero values before each use. This avoids creating multiple arrays and thus reduces memory usage. In our implementation, only three utility-bin arrays are created, to respectively calculate the TWU, sub-tree utility and local utility. Third, when reinitializing a utility-bin array to calculate the sub-tree utility or the local utility of single-item extensions of an itemset α, only utility-bins corresponding to items in $E(\alpha)$ are reset to 0, for faster reinitialization of the utility-bin array.

4.6. The Proposed Algorithm

In this subsection, we present the EFIM algorithm, which combines all the ideas presented in the previous section. The main procedure (Algorithm 1) takes as input a transaction database and the *minutil* threshold. The algorithm initially considers that the current itemset α is the empty set. The algorithm then scans the database once to calculate the local utility of each item w.r.t. α, using a utility-bin array. Note that in the case where $\alpha = \emptyset$, the local utility of an item is its TWU. Then, the local utility of each item is compared with *minutil* to obtain the secondary items w.r.t to α, that is items that should be considered in extensions of α. Then, these items are sorted by ascending order of TWU and that order is thereafter used as the $\succ$ order (as suggested in [2,7]). The database is then scanned once to remove all items that are not secondary items w.r.t to α since they cannot be part of any high-utility itemsets by Theorem 2. If a transaction becomes empty, it is removed from the database. Then, the database is scanned again to sort transactions by the $\succ_T$ order to allow $O(n)$ transaction merging, thereafter. Then, the algorithm scans the database again to calculate the sub-tree utility of each secondary item w.r.t. α, using a utility-bin array. Thereafter, the algorithm calls the recursive procedure *Search* to perform the depth first search starting from α.

The *Search* procedure (Algorithm 2) takes as parameters the current itemset to be extended α, the α projected database, the primary and secondary items w.r.t α and the *minutil* threshold. The procedure performs a loop to consider each single-item extension of α of the form $\beta = \alpha \cup \{i\}$, where i is a primary item w.r.t α (since only these single-item extensions of α should be explored according to Theorem 1). For each such extension β, a database scan is performed to calculate the utility of β and at the same time construct the β projected database. Note that transaction merging is performed whilst the β projected

---

Algorithm 1. The EFIM algorithm

---

input : D: a transaction database, $minutil$: a user-specified threshold
output: the set of high-utility itemsets

1 $\alpha = \emptyset$;
2 Calculate $lu(\alpha, i)$ for all items $i \in I$ by scanning D, using a utility-bin array;
3 $Secondary(\alpha) = \{i | i \in I \wedge lu(\alpha, i) \geq minutil\}$;
4 Let $\succ$ be the total order of TWU ascending values on $Secondary(\alpha)$;
5 Scan D to remove each item $i \notin Secondary(\alpha)$ from the transactions, and delete empty transactions;
6 Sort transactions in D according to $\succ_T$;
7 Calculate the sub-tree utility $su(\alpha, i)$ of each item $i \in Secondary(\alpha)$ by scanning D, using a utility-bin array;
8 $Primary(\alpha) = \{i | i \in Secondary(\alpha) \wedge su(\alpha, i) \geq minutil\}$;
9 **Search** $(\alpha, D, Primary(\alpha), Secondary(\alpha), minutil)$;

---

database is constructed. If the utility of β is no less than $minutil$, β is output as a high-utility itemset. Then, the database is scanned again to calculate the sub-tree and local utility w.r.t β of each item z that could extend β (the secondary items w.r.t to α), using two utility-bin arrays. This allows determining the primary and secondary items of β. Then, the *Search* procedure is recursively called with β to continue the depth-first search by extending β. Based on properties and theorems presented in previous sections, it can be seen that when EFIM terminates, all and only the high-utility itemsets have been output.

Complexity. A rough analysis of the complexity is as follows. To process each primary itemset α encountered during the depth-first search, EFIM performs database projection, transaction merging and upper-bound calculation in $O(n)$ time. In terms of space, utility-bin arrays are created once and require $O(|I|)$ space. The database projection performed for each primary itemset α requires at most $O(n)$ space. In practice, this is small considering that projected databases become smaller as larger itemsets are explored, and are implemented using offset pointers.

5   Experimental Results

We performed experiments to evaluate the performance of the proposed EFIM algorithm. Experiments were carried out on a computer with a fourth generation 64 bit core i7 processor running Windows 8.1 and 16 GB of RAM. We compared the performance of EFIM with the state-of-the-art algorithms UP-Growth+, HUP-Miner, d^{2}HUP, HUI-Miner and FHM.

Algorithms were implemented in Java and memory measurements were done using the Java API. Experiments were performed using a set of standard datasets used in the HUIM literature for evaluating HUIM algorithms, namely (*Accident, BMS, Chess, Connect, Foodmart* and *Mushroom*). Table 3 summarizes their characteristics. *Foodmart* contains real external/internal utility values. For other

Algorithm 2. The *Search* procedure

> **input** : α: an itemset, α-D: the α projected database, $Primary(\alpha)$: the primary items of α, $Secondary(\alpha)$: the secondary items of α, the *minutil* threshold
>
> **output**: the set of high-utility itemsets that are extensions of α

1 **foreach** *item* $i \in Primary(\alpha)$ **do**
2      $\beta = \alpha \cup \{i\}$;
3   Scan α-D to calculate $u(\beta)$ and create β-D; // uses transaction merging
4   **if** $u(\beta) \geq minutil$ **then** output β;
5   Calculate $su(\beta, z)$ and $lu(\beta, z)$ for all item $z \in Secondary(\alpha)$ by scanning β-D once, using two utility-bin arrays;
6      $Primary(\beta) = \{z \in Secondary(\alpha) | su(\beta, z) \geq minutil\}$;
7      $Secondary(\beta) = \{z \in Secondary(\alpha) | lu(\beta, z) \geq minutil\}$;
8   Search $(\beta, \beta$-$D, Primary(\beta), Secondary(\beta), minutil)$;
9 **end**

Table 3. Dataset characteristics

Dataset	# Transactions	# Distinct items	Avg. trans. length
Accident	340,183	468	33.8
BMS	59,601	497	4.8
Chess	3,196	75	37.0
Connect	67,557	129	43.0
Foodmart	4,141	1,559	4.4
Mushroom	8,124	119	23.0

datasets, external/internal utility values have been respectively generated in the $[1,000]$ and $[1,5]$ intervals using a log-normal distribution, as done in previous state-of-the-art HUIM studies [2,7,12]. The datasets and the source code of the compared algorithms can be downloaded as part of the SPMF data mining library http://goo.gl/rIKIub [3].

Influence of the *minutil* Threshold on Execution Time. We first compare execution times of the various algorithms. We ran the algorithms on each dataset while decreasing the *minutil* threshold until algorithms were too slow, ran out of memory or a clear winner was observed. Execution times are shown in Fig. 2. Note that for UP-Growth+, no result is shown for the connect dataset and that some results are missing for the chess dataset because UP-Growth+ exceeded the 16 GB memory limit. It can be observed that EFIM clearly outperforms UP-Growth+, HUP-Miner, d²HUP, HUI-Miner and FHM on all datasets. EFIM is in general about two to three orders of magnitude faster than these algorithms. For *Accident, BMS, Chess, Connect, Foodmart* and *Mushroom*, EFIM is respectively up to 15,334, 2, 33,028, –, 17 and 3,855 times faster than UP-Growth+, 154,

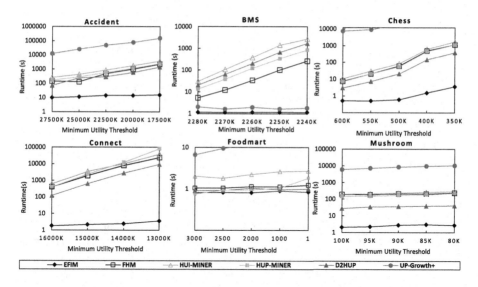

Fig. 2. Execution times on different datasets

741, 323, 22,636, 2 and 85 times faster than HUP-Miner, 89, 1,490, 109, 2,587, 1 and 15 times faster than d^2HUP, 236, 2,370, 482, 10,586, 3 and 110 times faster than HUI-Miner and 145, 227, 321, 6,606, 1 and 90 times faster than FHM. An important reason why EFIM performs so well is that the proposed upper-bounds allows EFIM to prune a larger part of the search space compared to other algorithms (as will be shown). The second reason is that the proposed transaction merging technique often greatly reduces the cost of database scans. It was observed that EFIM on *Chess*, *Connect* and *Mushroom*, EFIM is up to 116, 3,790 and 55 and times faster than a version of EFIM without transaction merging. For other datasets, transaction merging reduces execution times but by a lesser amount (EFIM is up to 90, 2 and 2 times than a version of EFIM without transaction merging on *Accident*, *BMS* and *Foodmart*). The third reason is that the calculation of upper-bounds is done in linear time using utility-bins. It is also interesting to note that transaction merging cannot be implemented efficiently in utility-list based algorithms such as HUP-Miner, HUI-Miner and FHM, due to their vertical database representation, and also for hyperlink-based algorithms such as the d^2HUP algorithm.

Influence of the *minutil* Threshold on Memory Usage. In terms of memory usage, EFIM also clearly outperforms other algorithms as shown in Table 4. For *Accident*, *BMS*, *Chess*, *Connect*, *Foodmart* and *Mushroom*, EFIM uses 1.8, 4.4, 14.9, 27.0, 1.3 and 6.5 times less memory than the second fastest algorithm (d^2HUP). Moreover, EFIM uses 1.6, 9.2, 4.6, 8.1, 3.2 and 3.1 times less memory than the third fastest algorithm (FHM). It is also interesting that EFIM utilizes less than 100 MB on four out of the six datasets, and never more than 1 GB, while other algorithms often exceed 1 GB.

Table 4. Comparison of maximum memory usage (MB)

Dataset	HUI-MINER	FHM	EFIM	UP-Growth+	HUP-Miner	d^2HUP
Accident	1,656	1,480	**895**	765	1,787	1,691
BMS	210	590	**64**	64	758	282
Chess	405	305	**65**	–	406	970
Connect	2,565	3,141	**385**	–	1,204	1,734
Foodmart	808	211	**64**	819	68	84
Mushroom	194	224	**71**	1,507	196	468

Table 5. Comparison of visited node count

Dataset	HUI-MINER	FHM	EFIM	UP-Growth+	HUP-Miner	d^2HUP
Accident	131,300	128,135	**51,883**	3,234,611	113,608	119,427
BMS	2,205,782,168	212,800,883	**323**	91,195	205,556,936	220,323,377
Chess	6,311,753	6,271,900	**2,875,166**	–	6,099,484	5,967,414
Connect	3,444,785	3,420,253	**1,366,893**	–	3,385,134	3,051,789
Foodmart	55,172,950	1,880,740	**233,231**	233,231	1,258,820	233,231
Mushroom	3,329,191	3,089,819	**2,453,683**	13,779,114	3,054,253	2,919,842

A reason why EFIM is so memory efficient is that it use a simple database representation, which does not requires to maintain much information in memory (only pointers for pseudo-projections). Other algorithms relies on complex structures such as tree-structures (e.g. UPGrowth+) and list-structures (e.g. HUP-Miner, HUI-Miner and FHM), which requires additional memory. Moreover, projected databases generated by EFIM are often very small due to transaction merging. Another reason is that the number of projected databases created by EFIM is small, because EFIM visits less nodes of the search-enumeration tree (as we will show later). EFIM is also more efficient than two-phase algorithms such as UPGrowth+ since it is a one-phase algorithm. Lastly, another important characteristic of EFIM in terms of memory efficiency is that it reuses some of its data structures. For example, FAC only requires to create three arrays that are reused to calculate the upper-bounds of each itemset considered during the depth-first search.

Comparison of the Number of Visited Nodes. We also performed an experiment to compare the ability at pruning the search space of EFIM to other algorithm. Table 5 shows the number of nodes of the search-enumeration tree (itemsets) visited by EFIM, UP-Growth+, HUP-Miner, d^2HUP, HUI-Miner and FHM for the lowest *minutil* values on the same datasets. It can be observed that EFIM is much more effective at pruning the search space than the other algorithms, thanks to its proposed sub-tree utility and local utility upper-bounds.

6   Conclusion

We have presented a novel algorithm for high-utility itemset mining named EFIM. It relies on two new upper-bounds named *sub-tree utility* and *local utility*. It also introduces a novel array-based utility counting approach named *Fast Utility Counting* to calculate these upper-bounds in linear time and space. Moreover, to reduce the cost of database scans, EFIM introduces techniques for database projection and transaction merging, also performed in linear time and space. An extensive experimental study on various datasets shows that EFIM is in general two to three orders of magnitude faster and consumes up to eight times less memory than the state-of-art algorithms UP-Growth+, HUP-Miner, d^{2}HUP, HUI-Miner and FHM. The source code of all algorithms and datasets used in the experiments can be downloaded as part of the SPMF data mining library http://goo.gl/rIKIub [3]. For future work, we will extend EFIM for popular variations of the HUIM problem such as mining closed+ high-utility itemset [13], high-utility sequential rules [15], generators of high-utility itemsets [5], and on-shelf high-utility itemsets [4].

Acknowledgement. This work is financed by a National Science and Engineering Research Council (NSERC) of Canada research grant.

References

1. Agrawal, R., Srikant, R.: Fast algorithms for mining association rules in large databases. In: Proceedings of the International Conference on Very Large Databases, pp. 487–499 (1994)
2. Fournier-Viger, P., Wu, C.-W., Zida, S., Tseng, V.S.: FHM: faster high-utility itemset mining using estimated utility co-occurrence pruning. In: Andreasen, T., Christiansen, H., Cubero, J.-C., Raś, Z.W. (eds.) ISMIS 2014. LNCS, vol. 8502, pp. 83–92. Springer, Heidelberg (2014)
3. Fournier-Viger, P., Gomariz, A., Gueniche, T., Soltani, A., Wu, C.-W., Tseng, V.S.: SPMF: a java open-source pattern mining library. J. Mach. Learn. Res. **15**, 3389–3393 (2014)
4. Fournier-Viger, P., Zida, S.: Foshu: faster on-shelf high utility itemset mining with or without negative unit profit. In: Proc. 30th ACM Symposium on Applied Computing, pp. 857–864 (2015)
5. Fournier-Viger, P., Wu, C.-W., Tseng, V.S.: Novel concise representations of high utility itemsets using generator patterns. In: Luo, X., Yu, J.X., Li, Z. (eds.) ADMA 2014. LNCS, vol. 8933, pp. 30–43. Springer, Heidelberg (2014)
6. Lan, G.C., Hong, T.P., Tseng, V.S.: An efficient projection-based indexing approach for mining high utility itemsets. Knowl. Inform. Syst. **38**(1), 85–107 (2014)
7. Liu, M., Qu, J.: Mining high utility itemsets without candidate generation. In: Proceedings of 22nd ACM International Conference on Information on Knowledge and Management, pp. 55–64 (2012)
8. Krishnamoorthy, S.: Pruning strategies for mining high utility itemsets. Expert Syst. Appl. **42**(5), 2371–2381 (2015)

9. Liu, Y., Liao, W., Choudhary, A.K.: A two-phase algorithm for fast discovery of high utility itemsets. In: Ho, T.-B., Cheung, D., Liu, H. (eds.) PAKDD 2005. LNCS (LNAI), vol. 3518, pp. 689–695. Springer, Heidelberg (2005)
10. Liu, J., Wang, K., Fung, B.: Direct discovery of high utility itemsets without candidate generation. In: Proceedings of the 12th IEEE International Conference on Data Mining (ICDM), pp. 984–989 (2012)
11. Song, W., Liu, Y., Li, J.: BAHUI: fast and memory efficient mining of high utility itemsets based on bitmap. Int. J. Data Warehous. Min. **10**(1), 1–15 (2014)
12. Tseng, V.S., Shie, B.-E., Wu, C.-W., Yu, P.S.: Efficient algorithms for mining high utility itemsets from transactional databases. IEEE Trans. Knowl. Data Eng. **25**(8), 1772–1786 (2013)
13. Tseng, V., Wu, C., Fournier-Viger, P., Yu, P.: Efficient algorithms for mining the concise and lossless representation of closed+ high utility itemsets. IEEE Trans. Knowl. Data Eng. **27**(3), 726–739 (2015)
14. Uno, T., Kiyomi, M., Arimura, H.: LCM ver. 2: efficient mining algorithms for frequent/closed/maximal itemsets. In: Proceedings of the ICDM 2004 Workshop on Frequent Itemset Mining Implementations. CEUR (2004)
15. Zida, S., Fournier-Viger, P., Wu, C.-W., Lin, J.C.-W., Tseng, V.S.: Efficient mining of high-utility sequential rules. In: Perner, P. (ed.) MLDM 2015. LNCS, vol. 9166, pp. 157–171. Springer, Heidelberg (2015)

Improving Label Accuracy by Filtering Low-Quality Workers in Crowdsourcing

Bryce Nicholson[1]([✉]), Victor S. Sheng[1], Jing Zhang[2],
Zhiheng Wang[3], and Xuefeng Xian[4]

[1] Computer Science Department, University of Central Arkansas, Conway, USA
{bnicholson1,ssheng}@uca.edu
[2] School of Computer Science and Engineering,
Nanjing University of Science and Technology, Nanjing, China
jingzhang.cs@gmail.com
[3] IT Department, China Executive Leadership Academy Pudong, Shanghai, China
zhwang@celap.org.cn
[4] College of Computer Engineering, Suzhou Vocational University, Suzhou, China
xianxuefeng@jssvc.edu.cn

Abstract. Filtering low-quality workers from data sets labeled via crowdsourcing is often necessary due to the presence of low quality workers, who either lack knowledge on corresponding subjects and thus contribute many incorrect labels to the data set, or intentionally label quickly and imprecisely in order to produce more labels in a short time period. We present two new filtering algorithms to remove low-quality workers, called Cluster Filtering (CF) and Dynamic Classification Filtering (DCF). Both methods can use any number of characteristics of workers as attributes for learning. CF separates workers using k-means clustering with 2 centroids, separating the workers into a high-quality cluster and a low-quality cluster. DCF uses a classifier of any kind to perform learning. It builds a model from a set of workers from other crowdsourced data sets and classifies the workers in the data set to filter. In theory, DCF can be trained to remove any proportion of the lowest-quality workers. We compare the performance of DCF with two other filtering algorithms, one by Raykar and Yu (RY), and one by Ipeirotis et al. (IPW). Our results show that CF, the second-best filter, performs modestly but effectively, and that DCF, the best filter, performs much better than RY and IPW on average and on the majority of crowdsourced data sets.

1 Introduction

Crowdsourcing is "an online, distributed problem-solving and production model that has emerged in recent years" [2]. It allows simple tasks to be outsourced to online workers at a very cheap price. Any cognitive task that has value and that an ordinary person is capable of can be crowdsourced. Just a few tasks to which crowdsourcing has been applied with success include the production of quality photographs and videos [7], rating the quality of images [10], gathering

© Springer International Publishing Switzerland 2015
G. Sidorov and S.N. Galicia-Haro (Eds.): MICAI 2015, Part I, LNAI 9413, pp. 547–559, 2015.
DOI: 10.1007/978-3-319-27060-9_45

geographic information for creating maps to aid disaster relief [14], and translating text [13].

Crowdsourcing is proof that ordinary people are capable of extraordinary things. Alonso and Mizzaro [1] experimented on Amazon Mechanical Turk, a popular crowdsourcing platform, having workers assess the relevance of a set of documents regarding a specific topic. The authors compared the workers' answers with that of experts and concluded that in some cases the workers were capable of being "more precise than the original experts".

However, not all workers can contribute such good work. One study of American and Indian workers showed that 75 % of Indian workers had an accuracy of less than 50 %, and only one worker had an accuracy of more than 60 % while performing 250 or more tasks [4]. Downs et al. [5] stated that some workers do not perform their tasks with the appropriate rigor. That is, they might just answer with random, meaningless clicks. The authors suggested that factors contributing to this behavior include easy cash, anonymity, and lack of accountability. These workers, who consciously output bad responses, are referred to as spammers in this paper. Workers may have low quality for other reasons as well, including carelessness and lack of knowledge on corresponding subjects. Spammers tend to perform the worst simply because they expend no effort in their annotations. Their responses are therefore worthless at best, and detrimental at worst.

These findings imply a need for detecting and removing low-quality workers, so that requesters will see an improvement in the overall quality of their results. The goal of our research, then, is to discover a method to find the low-quality workers and to filter them out. Given the versatility of crowdsourcing, it is unlikely that one single method can detect low-quality workers for any type of task—we must narrow our focus. In this paper, we focus on the crowdsourcing scenario in which a worker is presented with a number of tasks and is asked to label them. The task could be a text document, a picture, or any other digital object. The worker is asked to classify the object of the task by annotating it with one label. That is, we consider only the single-label scenario.

Our research drove us to analyze characteristics of workers, and how they might provide clues as to their quality. The characteristics we define measure how evenly distributed the workers' labels are among the possible class values, how different the workers' labels are from the average, what proportion of the data set the workers labeled, and how accurate the worker is estimated to be using an EM learning algorithm. We find that these characteristics can often be good predictors of the workers' quality. We define the workers' quality as the accuracy of their labels, defined as the proportion of their labels that match the true label for the corresponding task.

Next, we take a machine learning approach to discover which workers are of low quality based on their known characteristics. We develop two algorithms: one uses unsupervised learning, and the other uses supervised learning. Our first algorithm, which we call Cluster Filtering (CF), performs k-means clustering, treating each worker as a data point, and the characteristics of the worker are the attributes of each point. CF separates the workers into two groups, which conceptually signify the group of high-quality workers and the group of low-quality workers. CF filters the group belonging to the low-quality worker cluster. Our second algorithm, called Dynamic Classification Filtering (DCF), requires a crowdsourced set of auxiliary data, so that the characteristics of workers from other sets can help DCF learn a model to detect low-quality workers. The characteristics for these workers are treated as attributes, and a training set is formed in which the workers are instances. Then, DCF requires the workers of the data set in which the true labels are unknown in the form of a testing set. This testing set contains workers as instances with the same attributes (based on their characteristics) as in the training set. DCF then builds a model repeatedly on the training set, adjusting the proportion of workers who are classified as being of low quality until some predefinded proportion of the labels belong to one of the workers whom the classifier believes is of low-quality. Note that this predefined proportion is not a parameter we focus on finding an optimal value for. Instead, we use the value 50 % for simplicity. Finally, those labels that belong to a worker who was classified as being of low quality are filtered. Because any number of worker characteristics and any type of classifier can be used with DCF, the algorithm has a lot of versatility.

Finally, we compare the effectiveness of CF and DCF with that of Raykar and Yu (2011) and Ipeirotis et al. (2010). Overall, we achieve superior label quality improvement over their methods.

2 Related Work

One indirect method of dealing with low-quality workers is to retrieve multiple labels for each task, and to use a consensus method to infer one integrated label for each task [11]. The authors show that higher-quality results can be achieved by this method. Worker filtering would not be effective without this method, because if each task has only one label, removing a worker will leave several tasks without a label.

Venetis and Garcia-Molina [12] perform some experiments in improving data quality by removing low-quality workers. Specifically, they compare two metrics for detecting low-quality workers: gold standard performance and plurality answer agreement. Gold standard performance uses a gold set, which is a set of tasks whose true labels are already known, and calculates the proportion of these tasks each worker labels correctly. Gold standard tasks should appear no different from normal tasks so that spammers cannot pay special attention in answering them correctly. Plurality answer agreement calculates the proportion of tasks on which each worker agreed with the most commonly chosen label. Using this metric, workers who disagree with the majority are assumed to be of low quality, roughly speaking. The authors conclude that although the worker's gold standard performance has a higher correlation with the worker's accuracy on average than plurality agreement does, the cost of generating gold standard tasks outweighs the accuracy benefit. They determined that filtering by plurality agreement has a lower cost/benefit ratio, making it more efficient than using gold standard sets. In another concluding remark, they stated that although they were able to improve the data accuracy after removing labels from low-quality workers, the improvements were minimal.

Raykar and Yu [9] proposed the idea of a "spammer score," a quantitative, scalar measurement of how much a given worker resembles a spammer in his or her work. Below is their spammer score calculation formula:

$$S^j = \frac{1}{K(K-1)} \sum_{c<c'} \sum_k (a^j_{ck} - a^j_{c'k})^2$$

where S^j is the spammer score of worker j, K is the number of possible values a label can take (i.e., the number of classes), c and c' are two distinct label values, and a^j_{ck} is the probability that worker j assigns label k to a task given that the ground truth label is c. The calculation is normalized such that the most spam-like workers receive a score of 0, and the least spam-like workers receive a score of 1. In their paper, Raykar and Yu maintained the notion that a spammer is a worker whose labels are completely random. While a worker who labels completely randomly represents one kind of spammer, there are other types, such as a worker who chooses one label and assigns that label to every task he or she labels. Regardless, we use their method of calculating the spammer score (to later filter workers) and compare it to our method of filtering low-quality workers. We refer to their method as RY in the remainder of this paper.

Ipeirotis, Provost, and Wang [8] took the approach of identifying bias within a worker's labeling habits, and eliminating the bias by converting all labels to "soft" labels. Specifically, their approach converts labels as follows.

$$\langle \pi^j_{1c} Pr\{C = 1\}, \cdots, \pi^j_{Lc} Pr\{C = L\} \rangle$$

given that worker j assigned label c and $\pi^j_{c'c}$ is the probability that worker j assigns label c to a task whose ground truth label is c'. These soft labels must be normalized such that the components sum to 1. In effect, this process creates a weighted label resulting from the removal of detected bias of a worker. They then define the cost of a soft label as the following:

$$Cost(\mathbf{p}) = \sum_{m=1}^{L} \sum_{n=1}^{L} p_m p_n \theta_{mn}$$

where the soft label $\mathbf{p}$ has the form $< p_1, p_2, \cdots, p_L >$. θ_{mn} is the cost of assigning label n to a task with ground truth label m, which is defined to be 0 if $m = n$ and 1 otherwise. Finally, they define the total cost of a worker j as the following:

$$Cost(j) = \sum_c \left[Cost(\mathbf{soft}^j(c)) \times Pr\{AC = c\} \right]$$

where c is the value of each label, $\mathbf{soft}^j(c)$ is worker j's label c converted to a soft label, and $Pr\{AC = c\}$ is the prior probability that worker j labels a task as c. As a threshold for determining which workers are good quality and which are low quality (perhaps spammers), the authors suggest using the total cost of a worker who always uses the label with the highest prior probability (i.e., the majority class, or the mode). In our experiments, we calculate the total cost of the workers using this method, filter workers based on the suggested threshold, and compare it to our method. Throughout the rest of this paper, we refer to their method as IPW.

3   Characteristics of Workers

In our research, we analyze several characteristics of workers from nine crowd-sourced data sets, shown in Table 1. Table 1 shows the number of workers, the total number of tasks, and the distribution of true class values for each data set. We will analyze four different characteristics of workers from these data sets and discuss what the characteristics imply about the quality of the labels the workers provide.

Table 1. Summary of crowdsourced data sets

Data Set	#Workers	#Classes	Distribution
Adult2	269	4	187:61:36:49
FEJ2013	48	3	19:531:26
Anger	38	2	96:4
Duck	53	2	100:140
Disgust	38	2	96:4
Fear	38	2	91:9
Joy	38	2	87:13
Sadness	38	2	92:8
Surprise	38	4	91:9

3.1   Evenness

The evenness of a worker is a measure we devise to quantify how equally distributed a worker's labels are among the possible classes. Suppose $\mathbf{v}$ is a vector where v_c contains the proportion of tasks labeled c by worker j, and l, the length of $\mathbf{v}$, is the number of classes. Then the evenness is calculated by

$$Evenness(j) = \frac{l}{C(l,2)} \sum_{c=1}^{l} \sum_{c'=c+1}^{l} (1 - |v_c - v'_c|)(min(v_c, v'_c))$$

The constant $\frac{l}{C(l,2)}$ represents the number of classes divided by the number of pairs of classes (l choose 2, denoted as $C(l,2)$). The evenness calculation sums over each pair. Based on how large or small the difference between the distributions of the two elements of each pair, the total will be inversely small or large. The evenness is therefore 1 if and only if all of the proportions are equal. Also, a proportion of 1 for one class value and 0 for all others results in an evenness value of 0. Any other distribution of classes results in an intermediate evenness value. Evenness can also be applied to individual workers. A worker supplies labels, and each label corresponds to a class value. Therefore, the distribution of class values of a worker's labels has an evenness value as well.

Note that in our experiments, we do not use the raw evenness measure. We instead compute the average evenness over all workers in the data set, then find the difference of each worker's evenness from the average, or $|Evenness(j) - avgEvenness|$ and use that as the evenness metric.

3.2   Log Distance

The log distance of a worker is used to measure how far away the worker is from the rest of the workers in terms of label similarity. If the worker's labels agree with most or all of the other workers' labels, then the log distance will be small. Likewise, if the worker's labels are drastically different from that of most workers, then the log distance will be large. The log distance formula is given by:

$$ld(j) = -\frac{1}{n} \sum_{i=1}^{n} ln(p(t_i))$$

where j is the worker in question, n is the total number of tasks labeled by j, t_i is task i, and $p(t_i)$ is the proportion of labels that are the same as j's (including j's own label).

Intuitively, workers who are of low quality have a high probability of contributing minority labels in most cases. That is, workers whose labels are different from the others are likely to be of low quality. Indeed, using random guessing techniques instead of human reason is likely to lead to anomalous results. Also, non-spammers who have poor judgment regarding a task will tend to differ in their annotations from those who apply good judgment when labeling. Therefore, spammers and other low-quality workers should tend to have high log distance measures.

3.3   Proportion

The proportion characteristic for a worker is used to analyze the number of labels the worker has contributed. We calculate it by dividing the number of labels the worker has given by the total number of labels contributed by all workers in the data set.

3.4   EM Accuracy

Dawid and Skene [3] used an Expectation Maximization (EM) technique to infer the true labels of tasks after several workers have labeled them. From this estimation of the true labels, it becomes possible to estimate the accuracy of workers.

The more reliable the true label estimation, the more reliable the worker accuracy estimate is.

We define EM accuracy as the estimated accuracy of a worker after using Dawid and Skene's consensus method to estimate the true labels.

3.5 Correlation Summary

Table 2 shows the correlation coefficients of each characteristic with accuracy of all workers for all the data sets in our experiments. The correlations for all data sets are calculated, using Pearson's R value, by the following formula:

$$\frac{cov(char, acc)}{\sigma_{char}\sigma_{acc}}$$

where $cov(char, acc)$ is the covariance between all workers' values for the given characteristic and all workers' accuracy values, σ_{char} is the standard deviation of all workers' values for the given characteristic, and σ_{acc} is the standard deviation of all workers' accuracy values. The most clear relationship here is the negative correlation between log distance (LD) and accuracy. In every case, log distance is negatively correlated with accuracy. This means that as a worker's labels become more dissimilar with the other workers' labels, his accuracy tends to decrease. Difference from average evenness (DAE) is also usually somewhat strongly associated with accuracy, but the direction of the correlation is not uniform. On heavily biased data sets such as the emotion sets (e.g. *Anger, Disgust,* and *Fear*), there is a relatively strong negative correlation between evenness and accuracy. Proportion is correlated with accuracy to the weakest degree. This is due in part to the fact that most workers contributed a relatively small number of labels, and the accuracy of those workers tends to vary a lot. Even so, it still shows some indication of being able to predict a worker's accuracy, because the correlation is almost always positive. Finally, EM accuracy is usually positively correlated with accuracy to a considerable degree. Again, the reliability of this metric is dependent on how well the true labels were predicted in the first place. These four characteristics together contain a lot of information that can be used to determine whether the worker is low quality or not.

4 Detecting and Filtering Low-Quality Workers

To detect low-quality workers, we have two different methods: one supervised, and one unsupervised. With both, we use the characteristics we describe in the previous sections, but the methods are general enough so that any characteristic of workers could be used for learning and predicting worker quality.

4.1 Cluster Filtering

Our first low-quality worker filtering method consists of constructing a data set of workers, where the workers' characteristics represent attributes. We perform

Table 2. Correlation coefficient of all four characteristics vs. accuracy.

Data Set	DAE	LD	Prop.	EM Acc.
Adult2	$-.0303$	$-.4673$	$.0450$	$.3828$
FEJ2013	$.0760$	$-.1261$	$.0220$	$-.0548$
Anger	$-.4433$	$-.7912$	$.1274$	$.2786$
Duck	$.1831$	$-.2329$	$.1280$	$-.1970$
Disgust	$-.3415$	$-.7206$	$.0084$	$.0950$
Fear	$-.0852$	$-.4528$	$.0338$	$.3845$
Joy	$-.5331$	$-.5625$	$-.0586$	$.1006$
Sadness	$-.5454$	$-.6021$	$-.0898$	$.3558$
Surprise	$-.5435$	$-.8405$	$.1551$	$.7766$

k-means clustering on the data set, with 2 centroids. This separates all workers into two groups of points in $\mathbb{R}^n$ where n is the number of attributes all workers have. Conceptually, one group corresponds to the workers who have a set of characteristics generally held by high-quality workers, and one group corresponds to the set of workers whose attributes generally correspond to those held by low-quality workers. We then predict the cluster that corresponds to the low-quality workers by computing the average EM accuracy for each cluster, and picking the cluster that has the lower average EM accuracy. Finally, we filter all workers who belong to that cluster.

4.2 Dynamic Classification Filtering

Our second low-quality worker filtering method, called Dynamic Classification Filtering (DCF), uses a supervised learning approach. We construct a testing data set of workers who labeled the data set we requested labels for, where the attribute values are three of the values of the characteristics we discussed earlier: difference from average evenness, log distance, and proportion. We use EM accuracy to estimate the true labels of the tasks. Then, we train a classifier on a training data set of workers who have the same attribute types. That is, we use other crowdsourced data sets, calculate the same characteristic values for all of the workers, and form a training set from the workers in the crowdsourced data sets. Therefore, the algorithm relies upon other crowdsourcing data. Note that we do not use the true labels for the tasks in the training set. We use the EM-estimated labels instead because they are inexpensive to obtain, whereas true labels are not always known and may be very expensive to obtain. Thus, our method can be more widely applied using EM-estimated labels in the training set.

DCF removes a fixed proportion, say p, of all labels in a data set. That is, we identify some number of workers as low quality such that the total number of labels they contribute is arbitrarily close to p. The proportion we choose in our experiments is 50 %, but our method can operate using any proportion. The process of our method (DCF) is depicted in Fig. 5. First, we sort the workers in the training set according to their EM accuracy. Then, we label the lower half (i.e., the workers who fall below the median in EM accuracy) as being of low quality. We train a classifier on these workers, and classify the workers in the testing set. We count the number of labels contributed by the workers in the testing set who are classified as being of low quality. If it is approximately equal (we use a tolerance of ± 5 % in our experiments) to the desired amount (50 % in our case), then we filter those workers from the data set. In other words, we throw away their labels. If the number of labels contributed by the workers in the testing set who are classified as being of low quality is less than the desired amount, we only label the lowest quarter of workers in the training set as low quality this time. Likewise, if the number of labels is greater than the desired amount, we label the lowest three quarters of workers as low quality. As DCF continues to search for the perfect threshold, it uses the same binary-search process to select the cutoff point regarding which workers to label as being of low quality.

Dynamic Classification Filtering represents a novel use of classifiers. True to its name, DCF *dynamically* selects class values for instances in the training set, in order to achieve a desired result for the classifier it uses. This differs from traditional classification, which is to build one model and to classify members of the testing set without any expectations as to the classifier's behavior except its precision. Our dynamic use of classifiers is necessitated by the unclear boundary between high-quality and low-quality workers; our method, which coerces the classifier into classifying a fixed number of workers as being of low quality, can be modified to fit the expected proportion of labels that are contributed by low-quality workers. By finding this boundary, the classifier can achieve the best accuracy regarding the particular data set.

DCF's use of crowdsourced data sets for building a classifier gives it an advantage over the other filtering methods. Given enough data, DCF is easily able to learn patterns regarding workers' characteristics and their resulting accuracy, which is crucial to determining which workers are of low quality. Underlying behaviors of low-quality workers that other techniques might not detect can be detected by DCF, using knowledge from workers in other crowdsourced data sets.

Although we discuss four specific characteristics of workers in this paper, any number of characteristics of workers can be used with DCF. The resulting effectiveness of the algorithm depends highly upon how correlated with worker quality the characteristics are. In fact, in our experiments, we also use the two quantities on which the filtering algorithms RY and IPW rest upon: spammer score and worker cost, respectively, to train our classifier.

5   Experiments

Our results consist of a comparison for each dataset between the consensus accuracy using Dawid and Skene's method (DS) before filtering the workers, and consensus accuracy using DS again after filtering workers. We compare our spam-filtering method DCF with that of Raykar and Yu (RY) and Ipeirotis et al. (IPW).

5.1   Experimental Setup

Raykar and Yu discuss in their paper a possible threshold for filtering spammers. A worker's threshold spammer score is the score he would obtain if he were to label all tasks as belonging to the majority class. We calculate that score and compare it to the worker's actual score. If the worker's actual spammer score is less than or equal to the threshold score, he is filtered (using the RY method), i.e., his labels are not considered in consensus. Ipeirotis et al. also mention the same threshold as being a good baseline for filtering spammers. To apply it to their method, we calculate the total cost of each worker given the labels he provided, and the total cost each worker would have if he had labeled all tasks as belonging to the majority class. If the worker's cost is greater than or equal to the cost he would have if he had labeled all tasks as the majority class, he is filtered (using the IPW method).

In our Cluster Filtering implementation, we use the characteristics of proportion, difference from average evenness, log distance, EM accuracy, spammer score, and worker cost as our attributes. We perform clustering using the k-means algorithm, with 2 centroids.

For our DCF method, we allow a 5 % tolerance from exactly half of the testing data set workers being labeled as being of low quality. We allow the binary-search process to continue for 10 iterations, saving the proportion of labels belonging to workers classified as being of low quality each time. If the algorithm cannot find a case in which 45-55 % of labels belong to workers classified as low quality, we select the training set that yielded the value closest to 50 %, then filter using the classifier's model built from that training set. We use a holdout scheme in our experiments, treating each of our data sets as the test set once, and combining the remaining data sets into the training set. As our attributes, we use the characteristics of proportion, difference from average evenness, log distance, spammer score, and worker cost. We do not use EM accuracy as an attribute, because we use that characteristic to determine which workers in the training set to label as being of low quality, and that would give the classifier unwanted bias.

The consensus method used is Dawid and Skene's label integration algorithm [3]. The clustering algorithm we used is Weka's SimpleKMeans algorithm [6]. For our classifier, we use Weka's IBk algorithm [6], with k set at 7.

5.2   Experimental Results

The results are shown in Table 3. Our DCF method performs best overall, achieving the best label quality improvement on four of the nine data sets. DCF's and CF's greatest improvements are made on the emotion data sets. One reasons for this is that the workers on the emotion data sets are most predictably correlated with the characteristics we chose for learning. Another reason DCF is able to perform so well on the emotion data sets is because there are six emotion data sets, and a large proportion of the training set is composed of workers from these data sets, which helps the classifier learn a better model for the workers

Table 3. Accuracy increase after filtering low-quality workers using three filtering techniques

Data Set	DS	DCF	CF	RY	IPW
Adult2	.736	.745	.742	**.748**	.742
FEJ2013	.877	.885	.885	.877	.877
Anger	.820	**.860**	.820	.830	.820
Duck	.608	.604	.588	.608	.608
Disgust	.840	.820	.830	**.860**	.840
Fear	.870	**.900**	.880	.890	.870
Joy	.830	**.870**	.850	.830	.830
Sadness	.850	.850	**.880**	.850	.850
Surprise	.880	**.900**	.890	.860	.880
Average	.812	**.826**	.818	.817	.813

of the emotion testing set. The label quality of the data sets *Disgust* and *Duck* is slightly reduced by DCF.

Although RY performs best on two data sets (*Adult2* and *Disgust*), and CF only performs best on one (*Sadness*), CF performs slightly better on average. It is the second best low-quality worker filtering algorithm.

Raykar and Yu's method is third best overall. It performs best on the emotional data sets also. On four out of the nine data sets, it cannot improve data set label quality at all. This is likely because it does not filter any workers on these data sets, a sign that the threshold is inappropriate for those data sets. On one data set, it harms label quality.

Ipeirotis et al.'s method performs worst overall. It can only improve accuracy on the data sets that are improved by Raykar and Yu's method (except *Surprise*), indicating a similarity in the two methods. This similarity likely lies in the method of calculating the threshold for filtering. At least on these data sets, a more aggressive threshold is needed to make significant accuracy improvement possible.

In summary, our supervised method of detecting and filtering low-quality workers, DCF, has proven to be very successful. It performs better than all other methods on four of the nine data sets. On three of the data sets, our method was able to achieve great gains in accuracy (3 % or more). CF typically improves label quality modestly, outperforming the other three methods on only one data set, but performing second best on average. The other two filtering methods we considered, Raykar and Yu's method and Ipeirotis et al.'s method, usually fail to increase label quality significantly. In Ipeirotis et al.'s defense, they use a technique to generate soft labels with which to perform consensus that we did not analyze in this paper, because it went beyond our focus. The issue with both Raykar and Yu's and Ipeirotis et al.'s methods is their technique of calculating the threshold with which to filter workers, a topic discussed very briefly in both their papers but a topic definitely worth exploring in more detail.

6   Conclusions

The advent of crowdsourcing has greatly increased labeling productivity. However, with increased efficiency comes increased risk due to spammers and other low-quality workers. To greatly benefit overall label quality of data, we seek to detect and filter spammers and other low-quality workers from data sets so that their labels are thrown away.

Before we developed our worker filtering methods, we analyzed four characteristics of workers who label crowdsourced data sets: label evenness, log distance, proportion of labels contributed, and EM accuracy. We showed that these characteristics are generally correlated with worker accuracy. Therefore, we use these characteristics to predict whether a worker is of low quality.

We composed two methods to filter low-quality workers: Cluster Filtering (CF) and Dynamic Classification Filtering (DCF). CF separates the workers into two groups based on their characteristics. The algorithm chooses the cluster of workers that is approximately more similar to low-quality workers, and filters all workers in that cluster. DCF uses a classifier in a unique manner, repeatedly building a model from a training set of workers until it classifies an appropriate number of workers as low quality. DCF is very powerful, because it learns a model from workers in other crowdsourced data sets, which provides a diverse set of data to build a classifier.

We compared overall label quality improvement (determined by performing Dawid and Skene's consensus method without and with filtering) with Raykar and Yu's method (RY) and Ipeirotis et al.'s method (IPW). Our results showed that DCF performs the best out of all four methods on average, making it a viable algorithm for filtering low-quality workers. CF is the second best. It performs better than the other three methods on only one data set, whereas DCF outperforms the other three methods on four data sets. RY is the third best, improving overall label quality on only about half of all data sets. Finally, IPW performs the worst, barely imroving overall label quality from DS at all.

References

1. Alonso, O., Mizzaro, S.: Can we get rid of trec assessors? using mechanical turk for relevance assessment. In: Proceedings of the SIGIR 2009 Workshop on the Future of IR Evaluation, vol. 15, p. 16 (2009)
2. Brabham, D.C.: Crowdsourcing as a model for problem solving an introduction and cases. Convergence: Int. J. Res. New Media Technol. **14**(1), 75–90 (2008)
3. Dawid, A.P., Skene, A.M.: Maximum likelihood estimation of observer error-rates using the em algorithm. Appl. Stat. **28**, 20–28 (1979)
4. Difallah, D.E., Demartini, G., Cudre-Mauroux, P.: Mechanical cheat: spamming schemes and adversarial techniques on crowdsourcing platforms. In: CrowdSearch, pp. 26–30 (2012)
5. Downs, J.S., Holbrook, M.B., Sheng, S., Cranor, L.F.: Are your participants gaming the system?: screening mechanical turk workers. In: Proceedings of the SIGCHI Conference on Human Factors in Computing Systems, pp. 2399–2402. ACM (2010)

6. Hall, M., Frank, E., Holmes, G., Pfahringer, B., Reutemann, P., Witten, I.H.: The weka data mining software: an update. ACM SIGKDD Explor. Newsl. **11**(1), 10–18 (2009)
7. Howe, J.: The rise of crowdsourcing. Wired Mag. **14**(6), 1–4 (2006)
8. Ipeirotis, P.G., Provost, F., Wang, J.: Quality management on amazon mechanical turk. In: Proceedings of the ACM SIGKDD workshop on human computation, pp. 64–67. ACM (2010)
9. Raykar, V.C., Yu, S.: Ranking annotators for crowdsourced labeling tasks. In: Advances in neural information processing systems, pp. 1809–1817 (2011)
10. Ribeiro, F., Florencio, D., Nascimento, V.: Crowdsourcing subjective image quality evaluation. In: 2011 18th IEEE International Conference on Image Processing (ICIP), pp. 3097–3100. IEEE (2011)
11. Sheng, V.S., Provost, F., Ipeirotis, P.G.: Get another label? improving data quality and data mining using multiple, noisy labelers. In: Proceedings of the 14th ACM SIGKDD International Conference on Knowledge Discovery and Data Mining, pp. 614–622. ACM (2008)
12. Venetis, P., Garcia-Molina, H.: Quality control for comparison microtasks. In: Proceedings of the First International Workshop on Crowdsourcing and Data Mining, pp. 15–21. ACM (2012)
13. Zaidan, O.F., Callison-Burch, C.: Crowdsourcing translation: professional quality from non-professionals. In: Proceedings of the 49th Annual Meeting of the Association for Computational Linguistics: Human Language Technologies, vol. 1, pp. 1220–1229. Association for Computational Linguistics (2011)
14. Zook, M., Graham, M., Shelton, T., Gorman, S.: Volunteered geographic information and crowdsourcing disaster relief: a case study of the haitian earthquake. World Med. Health Policy **2**(2), 7–33 (2010)

An Embedded Application System for Data Collection of Atmospheric Pollutants with a Classification Approach

Eduardo Solórzano-Alor[1]([✉]), Amadeo José Argüelles-Cruz[2],
María Isabel Cajero-Lázaro[3], and Miguel Sánchez-Meraz[4]

[1] Centro de Innovación y Desarrollo Tecnológico en Cómputo, CIDETEC,
Instituto Politécnico Nacional, IPN, México City, México
eduardosolorzano22@hotmail.com
[2] Centro de Investigación en Computación, CIC, Instituto Politécnico Nacional, IPN,
México City, México
jamadeo@cic.ipn.mx
[3] Unidad Profesional Interdisciplinaria de Ingeniería y Ciencias Sociales y
Administrativas, UPIICSA, México City, México
mcajero10900@alumno.ipn.mx
[4] Escuela Superior de Ingeniería Mecánica y Eléctrica, ESIME,
Instituto Politécnico Nacional, IPN, México City, México
mmeraz@ipn.mx

Abstract. This paper shows the application of an embedded system
with a wireless sensor network to collect atmospheric pollutants data
obtained from sensors placed into micro-climates; such dataset provides
the information required to test classification algorithms, that helps to
develop applications to improve air quality in specific areas.

Keywords: Embedded system · Waspmote · Classifier algorithms ·
Atmospheric pollutants · Micro-climates

1 Introduction

Throughout the history, man has created devices that help to track the action
course, as time goes by, of several phenomena, some of those devices that include a
group of computing resources, peripherals, and sensors received the name of embedded systems. According to the task required, some of those embedded systems has
been incorporated to consumer electronics such as cell phones, calculators, audio
players [3], major household appliances, smart thermostats, video surveillance,
lighting systems, among others [18,26]. It is important to mention that an embedded system is less expensive than a computer equipment, and have specific characteristics which distinguishes it of a general-purpose computer [20]. An embedded system can be used for several tasks, the goal is turn easy users work in all of
them, as in the case of monitoring air pollutants. To perform this tasks, sensors and
new technologies are combined to monitor and quantify pollutants under demand

© Springer International Publishing Switzerland 2015
G. Sidorov and S.N. Galicia-Haro (Eds.): MICAI 2015, Part I, LNAI 9413, pp. 560–571, 2015.
DOI: 10.1007/978-3-319-27060-9_46

[2, 21]. Human activities have dealing with enhance the quality of life around the world, however in recent years pollution has increased and is an important factor that affect the health of most vulnerable society groups, so public policies should be applied to decrease their effects, supporting their actions by means of environmental alerts, problems identification to fight them and apply security protocols for contingency [14]. All these effects are present in a more specific level such a micro-climate, that is, a climate variation in small area. Some examples of micro-climates are housing, industrial areas, shopping areas, schools, research centers, and green areas in citis [1, 19]. Those micro-climates are susceptible of being analyzed using a wireless sensor network and an embedded system. This paper presents a case of study where data, obtained and processed inside a research building facility, is taken as an example of school's micro-climate.

2 Development Platform

The use of data acquisition equipment is common to data measurement and registration processes. There are several examples where such technologies are used for environmental purposes, not only to characterize certain situations, as climate fluctuations, but also to have data that can be process to help us understand some phenomena, to support decision making. Examples of these applications include: portable and wireless sensors system to monitor volatile organic compounds [24], geo-sensors network for air pollutants, which sends automatic alarm messages depending on the type of pollutant detected in the field [12], wireless embedded microprocessors network, composed of multiple sensors, which monitors and transmits atmospheric environmental parameters to a control center [9], the use of ZigBee networks to cover a larger urban area [7], and others. It is important to have specific environmental information of our living place, that can be used to apply statistical analysis, classification and prediction methods that help to identify instantly the health risks that pollutants levels produced.

2.1 Waspmote

Waspmote was the platform defined in this work for data acquisition, due to their characteristics. It is a module-based hardware and an open source technology,

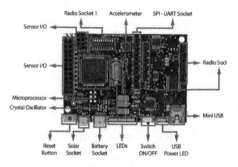

Fig. 1. Waspmote top view (Libelium's courtesy).

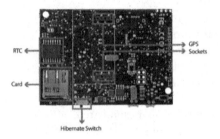

Fig. 2. Waspmote bottom view (Libelium's courtesy).

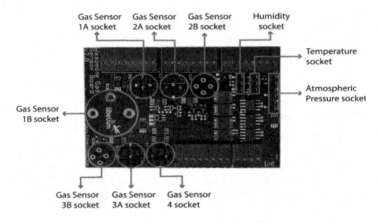

Fig. 3. Gas sensor board V2.0 (Libelium's courtesy).

which has been developed in order to be the spearhead for smart cities, Figs. 1 and 2. Waspmote has different parameters and characteristics similar to other well known platform called Arduino [17]. Many authors compare this boards with commercial platforms mentioned before. The main difference between Arduino and Waspmote is that the former has been developed to create small-scale projects, and it is consider accessible for developers, while the latter was developed for durability and deployment in real scenarios, such as a smart cities. Waspmote present terminals that are use to connect several boards for different

Table 1. Features Waspmote platform [27]

Features	Waspmote
Microcontroller	ATmega 1281
SRAM	8 KB
Storage	Micro-SD
Dimensions	$73.5 \times 51 \times 13$ mm
Clock	RTC(32 KHz)
Consumption	ON: 15 mA

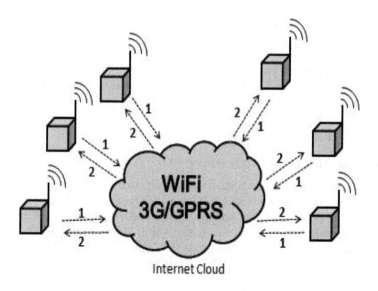

Fig. 4. Waspmote 3G/Cloud.

applications: security, industrial control, environment, mining, and others. This work used a gas sensor board v 2.0, Fig. 3.

Table 1 shows main characteristics of the used platform.

When two or more sensors are connected through Waspmote, it is possible to communicate the measurements through a wireless sensor network, capturing data over a specific geographic area, and as seen in Fig. 4. It is possible to transmit such data by using the 3G protocol to the cloud, and all this under the coordination of a gateway called Meshlium. There are different communication protocols for the target platform: ZigBee, Wi-Fi, and 3G protocols. In the case of this work ZigBee protocol was used.

The main characteristics of platform communication protocols used are presented (Table 2):

Table 2. Comparative of characteristics of communication protocols in Waspmote [27]

Features protocols	ZigBee	WI-FI	3G
Protocols	ZigBee-PRO	802.11b/g - 2.4 GHz	3G
TX Power	50 mW	0 dBm–12 dBm	GSM 850 MHz/900 MHz 2 W
Security	AES128	WEP, WPA, WPA2	-
Topologies	Star, Tree, etc	AP and Adhoc	-

To collect data, the gas sensor board used a ZigBee protocol, so it is possible to detect atmospheric pollutants levels. Data collected has several uses:

- To compare pollutants levels with the recommended ones according to the norm provided by local environmental authorities.
- From the previous point, be aware of an environmental emergency, or if there is specific conditions that must be critical to human health.
- To take actions according to the environmental situation, aimed to human health and improving life's quality.

3   Algorithms Classifiers

3.1   Machine Learning Algorithms

This section shows a brief description of each algorithms used during the experimental phase. It must be mentioned that a Java Data Mining Software platform called WEKA 3 (Waikato Environment for Knowledge Analysis) [29] is the software tool that supports tests. It has collection of state-of-art machine learning algorithms implemented, but we only test the following nine algorithms for comparison purposes.

3.2   Bagging

Bagging predictors is a method that generates multiple versions of a predictor and uses these to obtain an associated predictor. When it is predicting a numerical outcome, the multiple versions of a predictor are averaged by contrast when it is predicting a class, each predictor takes a plurality voting scheme. The multiple versions are formed by making bootstrap replicates of the learning set and using these as new learning sets [4].

3.3   BayesNet

Bayesian networks are a different form to represent a conditional probability distribution through directed acyclic graphs (DAGs). In graphical model, each node represents a random variable and there are two kinds of nodes: parent and child node. Arrow between them shows its relationship [6], calculated in terms of conditional probability of these two variables.

3.4   Dagging

Ting and Witten [23], proposed this meta-classifier, that creates a number of disjoint, stratified folds out of the data and feeds each amount of data to a copy of the supplied base classifier. The majority votes made predictions, since all the generated base classifiers are put into the Vote meta-classifier.

3.5   Decision Stump

It is an operator that can take any type of data and is used for generating one-level decision trees. The resulting tree can be used for classifying unseen examples. The leaf nodes of a decision tree contain the class name whereas a non-leaf node is a decision node. The decision node is an attribute test with each branch (to another decision tree) being a possible value of the attribute [13].

3.6   IBK

It is a kind of K-NN algorithm (supervised learning algorithm), where user separates his dataset in a specified number of clusters (K) [10]. Training phase of the classifier stores the features and the class label of the training sets. New objects are classified based on the voting criteria [15].

3.7   Logistic

This algorithm builds and uses a multinomial logistic regression model with a ridge estimator. Le Cessie and van Houwelingen [5] showed how ridge estimators improve the estimate parameters in a logistic regression and decrease error of further predictions.

3.8   Multilayer Perceptron

It is a finite directed acyclic graph and the most use type of Neural Networks, because is a general-purpose model, with a huge number of applications, able to modeling complex functions. Has robustness and can adapt its weights and/or topology in response to environmental changes [8].

3.9   Naive Bayes

Algorithm NaiveBayes assumes that predictive attributes are conditional, independent of the given class, and it proposes that no hidden or latent attributes that influence the prediction process [11]. Numeric estimator precision values are chosen based on analysis of training data.

3.10   Simple Logistic

LogitBoost with simple regression functions as base learners is used for fitting the logistic models. The optimal number of LogitBoost iterations to perform is cross-validated, which leads to automatic attribute selection. For more information, see [16, 22].

4   Dataset and Wireless Sensor Network

The topology used for data collection is describe below, where three boards Waspmote are used with their respective sensor board gas V 2.0 distributed in the research center, specifically in a computer lab (micro-climate), covering most of it, these platforms collect data in a 6 min interval each of them because embedded system needs 120 s to take measurements, and are sent through the Zigbee protocol to the aforementioned Gateway (Meshlium), which contains a database where the frames, obtained by the sensors are stored as shown in Fig. 5.

The gas sensor board v 2.0. has the capacity to contain multiple gas sensors, which are not by themselves calibrated for detection thereof, the calibration

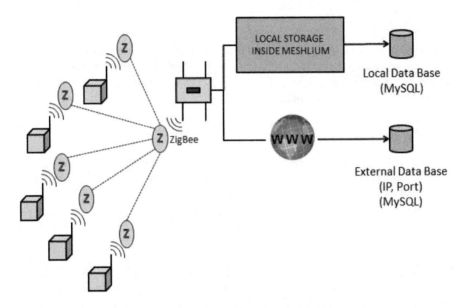

Fig. 5. Topology of the entire nodes used for the application.

of each sensor is performed in programming of the platform and according to manufacturer specifications, assigning resistance and gain [28].

Dataset has 830 instances, 5 numerical attributes, and 3 categorical classes (Fig. 6). Data obtained could be used as a time series, however they were classified

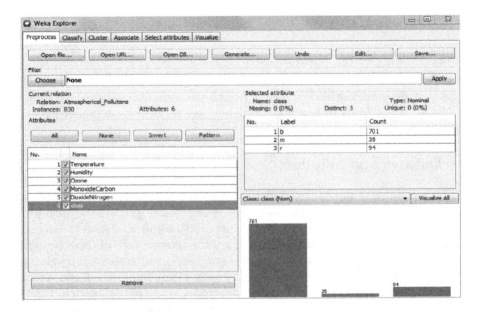

Fig. 6. Dataset shown in WEKA interface

and assigned to three different class labels (bad, regular and good) taking three Mexican Standards as a reference (NOM-020-SSA1-2014, NOM-021-SSA1-1993 and NOM-023-SSA1-1993) that need a 75 % of the concentrations data in an hour, for some of the most important atmospheric pollutants: O_3, CO and NO_2. Each dataset register has the average information of 8 h of the air pollutants concentration measurement, to comply with air quality regulations mentioned before, to establish previous labels.

Samples of atmospheric pollutants and weather factors (WF) (temperature and humidity), were taken inside the building of a research and education center. Data obtained were organized in 8 h periods in order to have a good contrast with Mexican Environmental Regulations for permissible concentrations levels.

This is an example of a frame obtained from Waspmote:

```
<=>#TIME:7-6-8+31#TCA:24.97#HUMA:46.8#O3:0.275#CO:0.512#NO2:1.413#
```

Pollutants monthly average registrations are presented in Tables 3 and 4 shows weather factors average found.

Table 3. Atmospheric pollutants monthly average concentration registered during 10 months (ppm) and NO_2 (ppb)

Month	O_3	CO	NO_2
February	0.02184	0.512	1.413
March	0.03681	0.459	1.393
April	0.02915	0.415	1.355
May	0.02656	0.343	1.329
June	0.01986	0.330	1.231'
July	0.02103	0.327	1.139
August	0.01953	0.332	1.028
September	0.01493	0.324	1.216
October	0.01265	0.336	1.298
November	0.01789	0.342	1.355

5   Experimental Phase

The experimental phase was conducted with nine previous algorithms, all of them are different methods of classification and other datasets obtained from the UCI: Machine Learning Repository [25]; these algorithms are implemented in JAVA (WEKA), that test the efficiency of each one of them. In order to explore results, test was evaluated with the validation method: k-fold cross validation.

Table 4. Monthly average of weather factors found during 10 months

Month	°C	RH %
February	24.5739	28.6540
March	25.9254	27.7649
April	25.3562	37.2448
May	25.5793	39.2659
June	25.5154	47.1457
July	24.9795	45.1539
August	26.1798	40.7152
September	25.8456	44.2424
October	25.3956	45.2533
November	24.4285	39.3901

Table 5. Efficiency of classifier algorithms with k-fold cross validation (k = 10)

Algorithm	Atmospheric Pollutants*	Breast-cancer	Iris-Plant	Parkinson
Bagging	99.63	96.63	93.28	87.69
BayesNet	97.46	97.21	94.63	80
Dagging	84.09	96.77	87.24	85.12
DecisionStump	92.16	91.65	66.44	83.07
IBK (K = 1)	93.37	95.75	95.30	96.41
IBK (K = 3)	93.25	96.92	95.97	93.33
IBK (K = 5)	93.49	97.21	95.30	93.33
Logistic	90.72	96.63	97.98	86.66
MultilayerPerceptron	97.59	96.33	96.64	91.28
NaiveBayes	94.21	96.19	94.63	69.23
SimpleLogistic	90.72	96.63	95.97	84.61

Table 5 shows the efficiency results of the algorithms executed under WEKA environment with the dataset proposed* and other UCI datasets.

6   Results, Analysis and Conclusions

Data inconsistencies coming from the measurements were checked and cleaned using the mean of data, in order to have good results in the experimental phase. As it is shown in Fig. 7, classification algorithms applied over the dataset (Atmospheric Pollutants*) results in a good performance, where Bagging, Multilayer Perceptron and BayesNet algorithms had the best performance with the dataset proposed.

The algorithms used in the dataset, provides good performance in comparison with other datasets used for other applications and validated many times, this results in a dataset that represents reliability and also guarantees reliable data, and can be used in conjunction with algorithms for classification analysis.

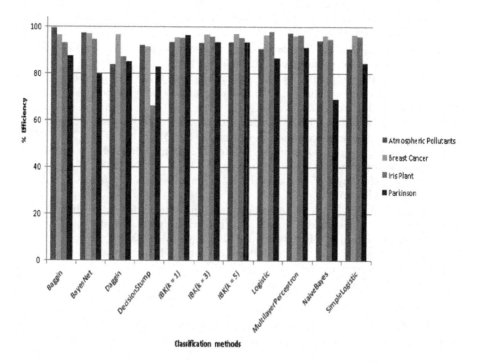

Fig. 7. Efficiency of classifier algorithms with k-fold cross validation (k = 10)

Dataset obtained by the aforementioned embedded system, provides good performance when classification algorithms are implemented regardless validation method applied, therefore this system could be used in cooperation with Mexico City Atmospheric Monitoring System (SIMAT: Sistema de Monitoreo Atmosférico) for micro-climates in small areas areas. This open up a range of different applications for the proposed dataset, that can be collected with Waspmote from the atmospheric pollutants in different environments, implementing predictive algorithms for time series, or establish levels of pollutant classes supported by national environmental standards.

Acknowledgments. The authors of the present paper would like to thank the following institutions for their support to develop this work: Consejo Nacional de Ciencia y Tecnología (CONACyT), SNI, Instituto Politécnico Nacional (COFAA, SIP, CIDETEC, CIC, AND ESIME).

References

1. Microclimate (1993). http://www.gardening.cornell.edu/weather/microcli.pdf. Accessed 16 May 2015
2. Amigoni, F., Brandolini, A., Caglioti, V., Di Lecce, V., Guerriero, A., Lazzaroni, M., Lombardi, F., Ottoboni, R., Pasero, E., Piuri, V., Scotti, O., Somenzi, D.: Agencies for perception in environmental monitoring. IEEE Trans. Instrum. Meas. **55**(4), 1038–1050 (2006)
3. Bertolotti, I.C., Hu, T.: Modular design of an open-source, networked embedded system. Comput. Stan. Interfaces **37**, 41–52 (2015)
4. Breiman, L.: Baggin predictors. Mach. Learning **24**(2), 123–140 (1996)
5. Le Cessie, S., van Houwelingen, J.C.: Ridge estimators in logistic regression. Appl. Stat. **41**(1), 191–201 (1992)
6. Christofides, N.: Graph Theory: An Algorithmic Approach. Computer Science and Applied Mathematics. Academic Press, London (1975)
7. Chung, W.-Y., Sung-Ju, O.: Remote monitoring system with wireless sensors module for room environment. Sens. Actuators, B **113**(1), 64–70 (2006)
8. Cortez, P.: Multilayer Perceptron. http://www3.dsi.uminho.pt/pcortez/mg.pdf. Accessed 16 May 2015
9. Gao, M., Zhang, F., Tian, J.: Environmental monitoring system with wireless mesh network based on embedded system. In Fifth IEEE International Symposium on Embedded Computing, SEC 2008, pp. 174–179, October 2008
10. Jiawei, H., Micheline, K.: Data Mining-Concepts and Techniques. Elsevier Publishers, San Francisco (2008)
11. John, G., Langley, P.: Estimating continuous distributions in bayesian classifiers. In: Proceedings of the Eleventh Conference on Uncertainty in Artificial Intelligence, pp. 338–345. Morgan Kaufmann (1995)
12. Jung, Y.J., Lee, Y.K., Lee, D.G., Ryu, K.H., Nittel, S.: Air pollution monitoring system based on geosensor network. In: IEEE International Geoscience and Remote Sensing Symposium, IGARSS 2008, vol. 3, pp. III - 1370–III - 1373, July 2008
13. Iba, W., Langley, P.: Induction of one-level decision trees. In: Sleeman, D., Edwards, P. (eds.) Machine Learning: Proceedings of the Ninth International Workshop, pp. 233–240. Morgan Kaufmann, San Mateo (1992)
14. Kelly, F.J., Fuller, G.W., Walton, H.A., Fussell, J.C.: Monitoring air pollution: use of early warning systems for public health. Respirology **17**(1), 7–19 (2012)
15. Förster, K., et al.: Incremental kNN classifier exploiting correct-error teacher for activity recognition. In: Proceedings of the 9th International Conference on Machine Learning and Applications (ICMLA), pp. 445–450 (2010)
16. Landwehr, N., Hall, M., Frank, M.: Logistic Model Trees. Mach. Learn. **59**(1), 161–205 (2005). Springer
17. University of Pau: Communication performance of low-resource sensor motes for data-intensive applications (1993). http://cpham.perso.univ-pau.fr/Paper/WD13.pdf. Accessed 16 May 2015
18. Pandharipande, A., Caicedo, D.: Daylight integrated illumination control of led systems based on enhanced presence sensing. Energ. Build. **43**(4), 944–950 (2011)
19. Salata, F., et al.: How high albedo and traditional buildings' materials and vegetation affect the quality of urban microclimate. A case study. Energy Build. **99**, 32–49 (2015). Elsevier

20. Shafik, R.A., et al.: Design considerations for reliable embedded systems. In: Swingler, J. (ed.) Reliability Characterisation of Electrical and Electronic Systems, pp. 169–194. Woodhead Publishing Series in Electronic and Optical Materials, London (2014)

21. Sukwon, C., Nakyoung, K., Hojung, C., Rhan, H.: Micro sensor node for air pollutant monitoring: hardware and software issues. Sensors **9**(10), 7970–7987 (2009). 14248220

22. Sumner, M., Frank, E., Hall, M.: Speeding up logistic model tree induction. In: Jorge, A.M., Torgo, L., Brazdil, P.B., Camacho, R., Gama, J. (eds.) PKDD 2005. LNCS (LNAI), vol. 3721, pp. 675–683. Springer, Heidelberg (2005)

23. Ting, K.M., Witten, I.H.: Stacking bagged and dagged models. In: Proceedings of 14th International Conference on Machine Learning, pp. 367–375. Morgan Kaufmann (1997)

24. Tsow, F., Forzani, E., Rai, A., Wang, R., Tsui, R., Mastroianni, S., Knobbe, C., Gandolfi, A.J., Tao, N.J.: A wearable and wireless sensor system for real-time monitoring of toxic environmental volatile organic compounds. IEEE Sensors J. **9**(12), 1734–1740 (2009)

25. UCI: Machine learning repository (2007). http://archive.ics.uci.edu/ml/. Accessed on 16 May 2015

26. Venetianer, P.L., Deng, H.: Performance evaluation of an intelligent video surveillance system - a case study. Comput. Vis. Image Understand. **114**(11), 1292–1302 (2010). Special Issue on Embedded Vision

27. Libelium: Waspmote-Datasheet, Libelium Comunicaciones Distribuidas S.L., Document version V5.5 - 10/2015 (2015)

28. Waspmote: Waspmote documentation (1999). http://www.libelium.com/development/waspmote/documentation/gases-board-technical-guide/. Accessed on 16 May 2015

29. Witten, I.H., Frank, E., Hall, M.A.: Data Mining: Practical Machine Learning Tools and Techniques, 3rd edn. The Morgan Kaufmann Series in Data Management Systems, San Francisco (2011)

Author Index

Printed in the United States
By Bookmasters